AIDS and STIs

A GLOBAL PERSPECTIVE

Sixth Edition

Edited by

DONNA A. CHAMPEAU, Ph.D.

KAREN ELLIOTT, Ph.D.

Taken from:

AIDS Update 2003: An Annual Overview of Acquired Immune Deficiency Syndrome
by Gerald J. Stine

Choices: Sex in the Age of STDs, Second Edition
by Jeffrey S. Nevid and Fern Gotfried

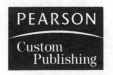
PEARSON

Custom
Publishing

Cover images: Cuzco, Java Market, Nigeria, Morocco

Excerpts taken from:

AIDS Update 2003: An Annual Overview of Acquired Immune Deficiency Syndrome
by Gerald J. Stine
Copyright © 2002 by Benjamin Cummings
A Pearson Education Company
San Francisco, California 94111

Choices: Sex in the Age of STDs, Second Edition
by Jeffrey S. Nevid and Fern Gotfried
Copyright © 1998 by Allyn and Bacon
A Pearson Education Company
Boston, Massachusetts 02116

Printed in the United States of America

10 9 8 7 6 5 4 3

ISBN 0-536-49758-3

2007280072

JK/SB

Please visit our web site at *www.pearsoncustom.com*

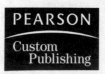
PEARSON CUSTOM PUBLISHING
501 Boylston Street, Suite 900, Boston, MA 02116
A Pearson Education Company

Copyright Acknowledgments

"HIV as an STD," by Sten H. Vermund, Sibylle Kristensen, and Madhav P. Bhatta, reprinted from *The Emergence of AIDS: The Impact on Immunology, Microbiology, and Public Health*, edited by Kenneth H. Mayer, MD and H.F. Pizer (2000), by permission of the American Public Health Association.

"Global Prevalence and Incidence of Selected Curable Sexually Transmitted Infections: Overview and Estimates," by the World Health Organization: Department of Communicable Disease Surveillance and Response (2001).

"Ensuring Access to HPV Vaccines Through Integrated Services: A Reproductive Health Perspective," by Amy E. Pollack, Miranda Balkin, Lindsay Edouard, Felicity Cutts, and Nathalie Broutet, reprinted from *Bulletin of The World Health Organization* 85, no.1 (January 2007), World Health Organization.

"Syndemics, Sex and the City: Understanding Sexually Transmitted Diseases in Social and Cultural Context," by Merrill C. Singer, Pamela I. Erickson, Louise Badiane, Rosemary Diaz, Dugeidy Ortiz, Traci Abraham, Anna Marie Nicolaysen, reprinted from *Social Science and Medicine* 63 (2006), Elsevier Science, Ltd.

"Understanding the Immune System: How It Works," reprinted from *NIH Publication*, no. 03-5423, National Institute of Allergy and Infectious Disease.

"The Disease and Its Epidemiology," by Tony Barnett and Alan Whiteside, reprinted from *AIDS in the Twenty-First Century: Disease and Globalization* (2002), by permission of Palgrave Publishers.

"Transmission of HIV," by Darrell Ward, reprinted from *The AmFAR AIDS Handbook* (1999), W.W. Norton & Company.

"Comprehensive HIV Prevention," reprinted from *2006 Report on the Global AIDS Epidemic* (2006), United Nations Publications.

"New Approaches to HIV Prevention: Global HIV Prevention Working Group," reprinted from *Gatesfoundation.org*, August 2006, Bill & Melinda Gates Foundation.

"Unfinished Business—Expanding HIV Testing in Developing Countries," by Kevin M. De Cock, Rebecca Bunnell, and Jonathan Mermin, reprinted from *New England Journal of Medicine* 345, no. 5 (February 2, 2006), Massachusetts Medical Society.

"The Search for Effective HIV Vaccines," by Howard Markel, reprinted from *New England Journal of Medicine* 353 (August 25, 2005), Massachusetts Medical Society.

"Treatment of HIV Disease," by Darrell Ward, reprinted from *The Am FAR AIDS Handbook* (1999), W.W. Norton & Company.

"Women, Inequality, and the Burden of HIV," by Bisola O. Ojikutu, Valerie E. Stone, reprinted from *New England Journal of Medicine* 352, no. 7 (February 17, 2005), Massachusetts Medical Society.

"Understanding and Addressing AIDS-Related Stigma: From Anthropological Theory to Clinical Practice in Haiti," by Arachu Castro and Paul Farmer, reprinted from *American Journal of Public Health* 95, no. 1 (January 2005).

"I Have an Evil Child at My House: Stigma and HIV/AIDS Management in a South African Community," by Catherine Campbell, Carol Ann Foulis, Sbongile Maimane, and Zweni Sibiya, reprinted from *American Journal of Public Health* 95, no. 5 (May 2005).

"Culture, Poverty, and HIV Transmission: The Case of Rural Haiti," by Paul Farmer, reprinted from *Infections and Inequalities: The Modern Plagues* (2001), by permission of the University of California Press.

Contents

Introduction

Putting Infectious Disease in Perspective

Donna A. Champeau

Throughout time sickness and death have been two factors of life that we all must face. These are realities that nobody can escape and in most cases we go about life as if it will never happen to us. Then one day it hits. We get sick, we have an accident, we lose a loved one to disease. In most cases, we talk about it, seek support, and grieve appropriately. Society has given us a set of rules and social norms in which to deal with these tragedies of life but not all sicknesses are created equally. Some diseases are different. Sexually Transmitted infections have always been and still remain the most stigmatized grouping of infectious diseases throughout the world. When someone gets sick, is debilitated, or even dies of one of many sexually transmitted infections, the rules don't apply. There is isolation, denial, and even shame attached to the receptacle of these diseases. So why is this the case? Should we not treat all illnesses the same? What is it that we fear so much about these diseases that could warrant isolation, harassment and even death to the afflicted individual?

Today we are still faced with the challenge of addressing these questions through research, education, and policy. We still have stigma, isolation, harassment, and yes, even the threat of bodily harm to those who acquire these diseases. The challenge to stop the spread of these infections is a huge and is only being complicated by new diseases as well as old ones that have reinvented themselves.

The "super bugs" of today have become more virulent and deadly than similar pathogens of the past. There are new drug resistant strains of gonorrhea and in the early 1980's, before many of you were born, a new disease emerged that was also sexually transmitted, it was HIV/AIDS. That was over 25 years ago and we are still searching for a way to stop the spread of the disease. Never before has there ever been a disease that has challenged us medically and socially as does HIV/AIDS.

In this text we approach the sexually transmitted infections from a Public Health Perspective. The readings in this text have been selected based on a Public Health Philosophy. That philosophy states that we must assure safe conditions for people to be healthy in society. Public Health operates from three core functions.

- Assessing and monitoring the health of communities and populations at risk to identify health problem and priorities.
- Formulating public policies, in collaboration with community and government leaders, designed to solve identified local, national and international problems and priorities.
- Assuring that all populations have access to appropriate and cost-effective care, including health promotion and disease prevention services, and evaluation of effectiveness of these.

In this text we will challenge you to think critically about the issues that are central to the prevention and treatment of these diseases while keeping in mind the public health philosophy.

When discussing HIV/AIDS and STIs, it is important to remember that while we can work with individuals to educate them about risk, reduce apathy, and motivate them toward risk reduction behaviors, the true impact of prevention/intervention activities will not be recognized through myopic or individual-centered approaches. While medicine and research will continually try to unlock the answers to treatment and reduce risks of infection, public health will focus on the environmental supports for health. Globally, these approaches to stop the spread of these diseases are different and sometimes complex.

The task to reduce the spread of STIs around the world is formidable. These diseases touch every corner of the earth and the global pandemic is increasing. New challenges emerge every day creating tremendous barriers. This text is designed to expose you to information surrounding STIs. It is also designed to increase your cultural sensitivity and recognition about the spread of diseases that know no borders, have no special considerations for men or women, no racial barriers, no special affinity for persons of various sexual orientations, and no apparent "end" in sight. To reduce the threat from these diseases, we must increase our understanding, remove biases, myths, and misperceptions, think globally, consider individual, community, and system responsibility for change, and use sound public health principles in our efforts.

In 25 years there have been countless numbers of articles and books written on the topic of STIs. We have attempted to collect what we believe to be an assortment of readings that will give you a global perspective on these diseases. We have also included in the text at the end of each section additional readings and questions to guide you in the understanding of the material in each section.

In **Part One**, **Chapter One**, *Historical Perspective,* we take you through the history of sexually transmitted infections. The readings will examine where we have been and where we are today with respect to sexually transmitted infections. Hopefully, these readings will give you a good understanding of the past and provide you with a sense of what may come in the future with respect to these infections. The discussions in **Chapter Two**, *Ethical Principles,* will pave a way for your understanding of the ethics of Public Health in which all aspects of Public Health practice must abide by. Then in **Chapter Three**, *Case Studies with Ethical Implications,* we provide examples of historical practices that were questionable and indeed unethical yet were carried out in a time before the protection of human subjects existed. Hopefully, you will be able to connect the relevance of the information in these readings with the issues in today's

Public Health research and practice. In **Part Two, Chapters Four, Five, and Six**, we separate the sexually transmitted infections by the pathogen that causes each one. In these chapters the readings will examine the etiology, prevention and treatment of the diseases. In **Chapter Seven**, the reading will give you a clear picture of the global nature of selected STIs and in **Chapter Eight**, *Social Implications of STIs* the readings will focus on how our social norms sometimes clash with the contextual realities of individuals and their risk taking behaviors. In **Part Three**, we wanted to focus primarily on HIV/AIDS. Although it is among the list of sexually transmitted infections, it has morphed over the last 25 years to become one of the most complex and puzzling challenges for scientists all over the world. **Chapters Nine** through **Thirteen** will provide an overview of the pathology, transmission, testing, treatment and prevention. Finally, in the last **Part Four**, we provide you with a small representative sample of some of the issues and topics that are of global importance in the battle to address the ill effects of HIV/AIDS and its progression. This section will hopefully get you to ponder many issues such as social conditions, stigma, poverty, child headed households, and more. These issues have been central to the HIV/AIDS epidemic over the years.

Obviously, in a book like this, it is impossible to cover every issue we would have liked to address; therefore, in each chapter we have suggested further readings to take you deeper into the topics that are discussed. I encourage you to read these and find others of your own choosing to broaden your understanding of the diseases and the social, political, ethical, and medical issues that they present.

PART ONE

Historical and Ethical Considerations

Chapter

1

Historical Perspective

The HIV–AIDS Pandemic at 25—The Global Response

Michael H. Merson, M.D.

On June 5, 1981, when the Centers for Disease Control reported five cases of *Pneumocystis carinii* pneumonia in young homosexual men in Los Angeles, few suspected it heralded a pandemic of AIDS. In 1983, a retrovirus (later named the human immunodeficiency virus, or HIV) was isolated from a patient with AIDS. In the 25 years since the first report, more than 65 million persons have been infected with HIV, and more than 25 million have died of AIDS. Worldwide, more than 40 percent of new infections among adults are in young people 15 to 24 years of age.

Ninety-five percent of these infections and deaths have occurred in developing countries. Sub-Saharan Africa is home to almost 64 percent of the estimated 38.6 million persons living with HIV infection (see Figure 1-1). In this region, women represent 60 percent of those infected and 77 percent of newly infected persons 15 to 24 years of age.

AIDS is now the leading cause of premature death among people 15 to 59 years of age. In the hardest-hit countries, the foundations of society, governance, and national security are eroding, stretching safety nets to the breaking point, with social and economic repercussions that will span generations.

This crisis demanded a unique and truly global response to meld the resources, political power, and technical capacity of wealthy countries with the needs and capacities of developing countries. Such a response would have required policymakers to address taboos concerning sexual behavior, drug use, power relations between the sexes, poverty, and death. Instead, AIDS often engendered stigma, discrimination, and denial, because of its association with marginalized groups, sexual transmission, and lethality. The result was two decades of a slow, insufficient, inconsistent, and often inappropriate response.

In 1987, six years into the pandemic, the World Health Organization (WHO) established the Global Program on AIDS. This program, of which I was executive director from 1990 to 1995, raised awareness about the pandemic; formulated evidence-based policies; provided technical and financial support to countries; initiated relevant social, behavioral, and biomedical

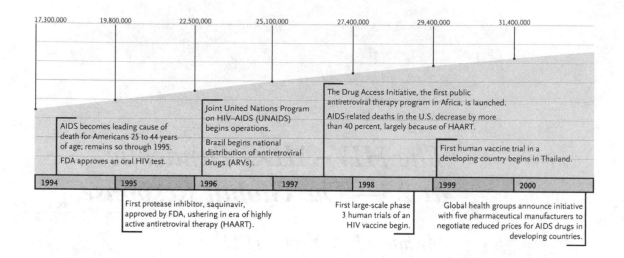

research; promoted participation by nongovernmental organizations; and championed the rights of those living with HIV. Among other efforts, the program provided assistance to two countries—Uganda and Thailand—that successfully reversed their epidemics.

Despite its achievements, the Global Program on AIDS was unable to muster the necessary political will in donor and affected countries, and its effectiveness was compromised by rivalries with other United Nations (U.N.) organizations, concern about the senior leadership of the WHO, and an increasing preference of wealthy governments for bilateral aid programs. So in 1996, the program was replaced by the Joint United Nations Programme on HIV/AIDS (UNAIDS), initially cosponsored by 6 U.N. agencies (now 10), with a mandate to lead an expanded, better-coordinated, multisectoral global response. UNAIDS found this task difficult. Its resources were limited, and resolving strategic conflicts among U.N. partners proved nearly impossible. Moreover, wealthy countries became disenchanted with the U.N. system and, as their own AIDS-related mortality declined, disengaged from the global response to the pandemic.

Then, around the turn of the millennium, four key developments inspired a new receptivity to the advocacy of UNAIDS. First, the World Bank became more active in AIDS-related lending, increasing its commitments from $500 million in 1998 to $2.7 billion today, much of it for sub-Saharan Africa. Second, in 2000, the XIII International AIDS Conference, in Durban, South Africa, raised global public consciousness about Africa's upward-spiraling AIDS-related mortality and the need for accessible, affordable antiretroviral drugs. Around the same time, Brazil reported that its use of antiretroviral drugs had dramatically reduced AIDS-related mortality and hospitalizations, providing hope for other developing countries. Emboldened nongovernmental organizations then agitated for the purchase of lower-cost, generic antiretroviral drugs and price reductions for brandname products, while the Doha Declaration concerning the Agreement on the Trade-Related Aspects of Intellectual Property Rights and Public Health permitted broader access to antiretroviral drugs.

Third, politically powerful religious groups, particularly in the United States, that had long been reluctant to support condom distribution and other sex-related prevention programs

Estimated number of adults and children living with HIV globally

| 33,300,000 | 34,800,000 | 36,200,000 | 37,300,000 | 38,600,000 | | |

40,000,000

35,000,000

30,000,000

President George W. Bush announces
the President's Emergency Plan for
AIDS Relief (PEPFAR).

Indian manufacturer Ranbaxy gains FDA
approval to produce generic antiretroviral
for PEPFAR.

25,000,000

20,000,000

The Global Fund to Fight AIDS,
Tuberculosis, and Malaria
begins operations.

"3 by 5" Initiative announced by World
Health Organization, to bring
treatment to 3 million people by 2005.

1.3 million people in low- and middle-
income countries have access to ARVs.

15,000,000

HIV infection is leading cause
of death worldwide among
persons 15 to 59 years of age.

10,000,000

5,000,000

| 2001 | 2002 | 2003 | 2004 | 2005 | 2006 | 2007 |

The World Trade Organization announces
Doha Agreement, allowing developing
countries to buy or manufacture generic
HIV–AIDS medications.

June 5 marks a quarter-century
since first AIDS case reported.

Expanded timeline available with the full text of this article at www.nejm.org. Adapted with permission from the Henry J. Kaiser Family Foundation (whose complete Global HIV/AIDS Timeline is available at www.kff.org/hivaids/timeline) and from UNAIDS.

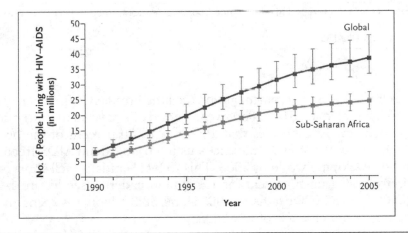

FIGURE 1-1 Number of People Living with HIV or AIDS, Globally and in Sub-Saharan Africa.
The I bars indicate the ranges around the estimates. The wider the range, the greater the uncertainty surrounding the estimate. Data are from UNAIDS.

embraced the need for global treatment, largely in order to reduce the numbers of children being orphaned by AIDS. And fourth, the spread of HIV into Russia, China, and India prompted concern that AIDS could destabilize global political and economic systems beyond sub-Saharan Africa, threatening global security.

These developments generated a long-needed enhanced response. Shortly after the Organization of African Unity declared the AIDS situation in Africa a state of emergency, U.N. Secretary-General Kofi Annan convened a U.N. Special Session on HIV/AIDS in June 2001. There, political leaders from 180 governments adopted a declaration of commitment that set program targets for affected countries and funding levels for donor governments. Soon thereafter, the multilateral Global Fund to Fight AIDS, Tuberculosis and Malaria was established to provide money rapidly for country-owned initiatives. As of March 2006, the fund had committed $5.2 billion to 131 countries, 57 percent of it for AIDS programs.

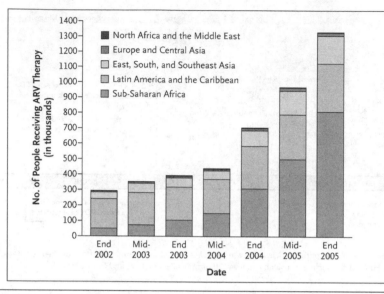

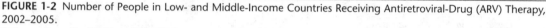

FIGURE 1-2 Number of People in Low- and Middle-Income Countries Receiving Antiretroviral-Drug (ARV) Therapy, 2002–2005.
Data are from the WHO and UNAIDS.

In January 2003, the U.S. government announced the President's Emergency Plan for AIDS Relief, through which it pledged $15 billion over a period of five years to prevention, treatment, and care, with a focus on 15 countries that are home to 80 percent of the people requiring treatment. Later that year, the WHO announced its intent to extend AIDS treatment to 3 million persons in the developing world by 2005. This "3 by 5" initiative fell short of its target but resulted in antiretroviral-drug treatment for 1.3 million patients (see Figure 1-2), preventing an estimated 250,000 to 350,000 deaths. In 2005 alone, $8.3 billion was spent on AIDS—about 30 times as much as at the creation of UNAIDS.

Despite recent gains in treatment, only about one in five people in low- and middle-income countries who need antiretroviral drugs are receiving them. A renewed emphasis on the prevention of HIV infection is critical. There is good evidence that available behavioral prevention strategies are effective, yet key prevention services currently reach less than 10 percent of persons at risk. Expanding these strategies worldwide would avert more than half the HIV infections projected to occur by 2015 and save $24 billion in treatment costs. Prevention programs must engage civil society and be evidence-based (not moralistic), locally planned, and linked to efforts to reduce stigma and elevate the status of women. Treatment programs, by increasing demand for HIV testing, can enhance prevention, provided that they minimize the high-risk sexual behavior that can result from the availability of antiretroviral drugs.

There is also a need for research on new approaches to prevention. Adult male circumcision, preexposure antiretroviral prophylaxis against sexual transmission in high-risk populations, acyclovir treatment for herpes simplex virus type 2, and microbicidal agents all hold promise. Although a preventive vaccine has been elusive, there is optimism that one will be developed within a decade.

Better international coordination remains imperative. Donors must align their assistance with and support robust, nationally led strategies, policies, and plans. UNAIDS should continue to enhance its coordination, technical support, monitoring, and leadership.

A quarter century into the pandemic, the global response stands at a crossroads. More new infections and deaths occurred in 2005 than ever before. A year ago, the Group of 8 (G8) countries and the U.N. World Summit embraced the goal of implementing "a package for HIV prevention, treatment and care, with the aim of as close as possible to universal access to treatment . . . by 2010." Such a package will require more resources—an estimated $18.1 billion in 2007 and $22.1 billion in 2008. As AIDS becomes a chronic disease, this funding must be used in part to strengthen fragile health care systems. The progress of the past five years provides a solid foundation on which to build the comprehensive and sustainable response vital to ultimate control of this pandemic. Without this response, many millions more will die of AIDS or be catastrophically affected by its consequences.

▶ An Interview with Dr. Merson Is Available at www.nejm.org.

Dr. Merson is a professor at the Yale School of Public Health, New Haven, Conn., and director of Yale's Center for Interdisciplinary Research on AIDS.

1. Pneumocycstis pneumonia—Los Angeles. MMWR Morb Mortal Wkly Rep 1981; 30:250–2.

2. 2006 Report on the global AIDS epidemic. Geneva: UNAIDS, 2006. (Accessed May 18, 2006, at http://www.unaids.org/en/.)

3. Declaration of Commitment on HIV/AIDS. "Global crisis—global action." New York: United Nations, 2001. (Accessed May 18, 2006, at http://www.un.org/ga/aids/coverage/FinalDeclarationHIVAIDS.html.)

4. Stover J, Bertozzi S, Gutierrez JP, et al. The global impact of scaling up HIV/AIDS prevention programs in low- and middle-income countries. Science 2006;311:1474–6.

5. The Gleneagles communiqué on Africa. Climate change, energy, and sustainable development. G8 Gleneagles Summit, 2005. (Accessed May 18, 2006 at http://www.fco.gov.uk/Files/kfile/PostG8_Gleneagles_Communique,0.pdf.)

Pioneers in AIDS Care—Reflections on the Epidemic's Early Years

Ronald Bayer, Ph.D., and Gerald M. Oppenheimer, Ph.D., M.P.H.

In 1995, Constance Wofsy, who had been a leader in San Francisco's response to AIDS in the 1980s, recalled the way she and other physicians had been drawn to the nascent epidemic. "How gripped we were," she said, "How separate we were from everyone who wasn't part of the thing. There were the involved and uninvolved, and they just didn't understand one another."

In July, a tape recording of these recollections, made a year before Wofsy's death, was heard by 17 doctors who had come together in New York to commemorate the 25th anniversary of the first reported AIDS cases. The participants were among 76 first-generation AIDS doctors whom we had interviewed in the 1990s for an oral history documenting the U.S. epidemic. At the day-long July meeting, they looked back on their work, shared memories of the darkest years, recalled the exhilaration of the first prospects for effective AIDS treatment, and ruminated about who would step in to care for future patients.

The group vividly recalled pervasive institutional and professional resistance to caring for patients with AIDS during the early 1980s. How could they explain why they had decided to take on this burden—a decision that had shaped their lives in unanticipated ways? At the time, most were young and beginning their careers, unencumbered by established commitments. But there was more to it than that. For gay and lesbian doctors, the suffering in their community provided sufficient motivation. For others, the AIDS crisis tapped into long-held views about the social mission of medicine and the need to care for the marginalized and despised. Wafaa El-Sadr, who developed the AIDS program at Harlem Hospital, said the epidemic had opened new worlds to her by demonstrating the importance of engaging in a genuine way with patients and drawing on their strengths.

Many felt compelled by geography: being in New York, Los Angeles, San Francisco, or Miami made the epidemic hard to ignore. Pediatrician James Oleske remembers feeling that in the impoverished community of Newark, New Jersey, he had no alternative but to care for babies and children with AIDS.

One thread that ran through the varied explanations was a deep sense of duty—of the doctor's moral responsibility. In 1981, Molly Cooke, a San Francisco physician, was pregnant with her first child. Given how little was known about the risk of transmission, she was understandably fearful of taking on patients with AIDS. Yet she remembered saying to her husband, Paul Volberding, an oncologist who would help to shape San Francisco General Hospital's response to AIDS, "If not us, who? What's the justification for saying someone else should do this?"

Whatever induced these physicians to make the initial commitment, perhaps a more difficult question is what sustained their engagement in patient care and advocacy in an era when medicine was all but impotent against AIDS. Some, like Donna Mildvan, an infectious-disease specialist in New York, felt a strong need to "bear witness; we were seeing stuff that nobody else in the world was seeing." Through clinical treatment and careful observation, she believed, "We were going to solve this, and that was the commitment that kept me alive and kicking." Volberding, for his part, felt the pull of treating a disease that constantly challenged his competence: "The thrill of this was the care of these patients; they needed us so much. We couldn't cure or treat HIV effectively, but we managed a lot of problems."

Some credited the compelling characteristics of their patients with keeping them in the field. Pediatrician Hermann Mendez, who worked in Brooklyn, recalled, "You respected the people you were working with; you loved them, and you hated what was happening, and it was that love that kept you there and keeps me there." Like Mendez, Gerald Friedland, who worked with drug users in the Bronx, remembered the emotional draw: "The kind of suffering that people endured and the courage that most of our patients actually had [were] extraordinary and inspired me."

> I was in Newark, New Jersey. I was committed to working in an underserved area. I love children. All I remember was that there was one sick child after another coming in. It wasn't a conscious decision that I wanted to work with AIDS or not work with AIDS. It was there, and you had to do it. You didn't have a choice.
>
> —James Oleske, New Jersey Medical School, University of Medicine and Dentistry of New Jersey, Newark

These physicians also found their commitment strengthened by the camaraderie that developed among them, fueled by mutual need and professional succor. Most recalled forming friendships within the AIDS-care community because the "uninvolved" didn't understand what they were doing or why they were doing it.

> HIV touched something inside each of us that's more than the profession that we chose. It might be that keen interest in people's lives and wanting to talk to people and understand why they are what they are, and how they relate to their world, where they live, what they do. Maybe it was their stories. [In the early years] I was afraid that AIDS was just going to take over the world and what's going to happen? What brought solace to our lives was talking to the patients and that optimism of how they struggled and how they dealt with this, and how we helped them deal with it. I think in a way that kept our fear in check.
>
> —Wafaa El-Sadr, Mailman School of Public Health, Columbia University, and Harlem Hospital, New York

Their inability to change the course of the disease forced doctors to seek other ways to meet patients' needs. Today, more than a decade after the introduction of antiretroviral therapy transformed the landscape of AIDS treatment, the memories these pioneers retain are vivid. Howard Grossman, who had a Manhattan-based private practice for gay men, recalled, "We got thrown back to an earlier time of medicine"—to an era when the doctor was more magician than scientist. Simple acts such as holding patients' hands and listening to their stories were critical. Those who cared for poor patients, including drug users and their families, say the demands they confronted went far beyond the clinical interventions they had been trained to provide. Gwendolyn Scott, a pediatric infectious-disease specialist from Miami, remarked that she became a sort of social worker for affected families: "They were living in cars, they didn't have food, they didn't have roofs over their heads. I couldn't give them medical care when they didn't have a place to live and food to put in their mouths."

Of course, it was the tide of death during the epidemic's early years that left the most haunting memories. Although he had tried "to take pain and put it back in its own compartment," Volberding said, "there were horrible, horrible moments" during those years. Just as they strove to offer clinical care in the absence of effective medicine, many sought, in Friedland's words, "to arrange for a good death." Mendez was brought to tears as he recalled a young girl in Brooklyn who had died in the hospital just 1 hour after a brief reunion with her imprisoned mother: "We learned the lesson the hard way, how to allow them to die at home in their room with their siblings, with everybody understanding what is going on. From then on, we didn't and couldn't allow anybody to die in the hospital." El-Sadr recalled with anguish the surviving children of her patients and wondered what had happened to them. "Where are they now?" she asked. "Are they being taken care of? Are they healthy? Are they in jail?"

> A patient of mine was admitted, blind and demented, because his AZT had worn off. I think that was the most depressing, horrifying experience of my whole career—having gone on that roller coaster, having been so excited, it was as if the whole bottom was just ripped out from under me, and there was nothing in sight that was really going to alter this.
>
> —Donna Mildvan, Beth Israel Medical Center, New York

Commitments were tested in the late 1980s and early 1990s, not only by the emotional demands of a disease that mocked medicine's therapeutic aspirations but also by the dashed hopes for progress in attacking the underlying cause of AIDS. It was hard to forget the exhilaration many had felt when zidovudine (earlier known as azidothymidine, or AZT), the first antiretroviral drug, seemed to be effective. Alexandra Levine, an oncologist from Los Angeles, remembered a patient who had called because he had survived to celebrate his birthday. But it was also hard to forget the despair of learning that AZT's benefits were limited. Mildvan said she found the experience personally painful and "professionally humbling."

With the development of effective antiretroviral therapy in the mid-1990s, many saw AIDS as having been normalized, rendered just another chronic disease. The crisis that had drawn these doctors and sustained their sense of mission had passed. For a few pioneers, this sense of mission retains something of its original excitement. Mildvan, for example, said, "This has never been a boring disease; it keeps evolving into new questions." Others, however, see the epidemic against which they struggled as fundamentally changed. AIDS care, observed Donna Futterman, a New York–based specialist in adolescent medicine, is now "about managing extremely technical combinations of doses"—a far cry from the multidisciplinary demands that once seemed to mean that "to know HIV was to know society." Friedland registered the irony: "It's clear that something has been lost. Honestly, at this point I miss it, even though I never thought I would, with all the death and dying." Nothing underscored this ironic sense of nostalgia more dramatically than the startling announcement by Donald Abrams, a prominent gay physician and researcher in San Francisco, that he would be leaving HIV medicine imminently because it no longer spoke to his "need to be a healer."

> HIV care doesn't grab me and doesn't move me and doesn't excite me or challenge me the way it used to. So I, in fact, will be seeing my last HIV clinic on August 8, and I will no longer be doing HIV research or care. I'm happy for the patients, fortunately, that you can see them and say, "I'll see you in 4 months. Here's your lab slip. Here's your prescription refill." But for me, that doesn't speak to my need to be a healer, and it doesn't excite me the way it did at the very beginning, when there was so much uncertainty.

> —Donald Abrams, San Francisco General Hospital,
> University of California, San Francisco

Many of these pioneers feel that something has gone awry, and they despair about the next generation. "I'm not finding a lot of medical students and residents who want to do what I do," said Oleske. "They actually say, 'This isn't for me.' I don't know how we're going to change that, but I worry very much." The sense of urgency that drew Oleske and his generation to the care of patients with AIDS in its early years no longer defines the world encountered by young doctors.

Some veterans of the U.S. epidemic have found their idealism revitalized by a commitment to the global epidemic. El-Sadr, for example, who has thrown herself into the struggle against AIDS in southern Africa, is "driven to make it happen there for all those people like we really did here. There are so many more similarities between Harlem and Maputo than there are between Harlem and San Francisco."

For others, the shifting of attention to the global epidemic implies that the challenge at home is no longer compelling. Oleske confronted that position directly, reminding his colleagues that AIDS remains embedded in America's poorest communities. "I'm not here to celebrate that HIV is over," he concluded. "In Newark, New Jersey, AIDS is alive and well."

▶ An Interview with Drs. El Sadr and Oleske Can Be Heard at www.nejm.org.

Dr. Bayer is a professor at the Center for the History and Ethics of Public Health, Department of Sociomedical Sciences, Mailman School of Public Health, Columbia University, New York. Dr. Oppenheimer is a professor in the Department of Health and Nutrition Sciences at Brooklyn College and the Graduate Center, City University of New York, and an associate professor of clinical public health in the Department of Sociomedical Sciences at the Mailman School of Public Health, Columbia University, New York.

1. Bayer R, Oppenheimer GM. AIDS doctors: voices from the epidemic. Oxford, England: Oxford University Press, 2000.

AIDS in Historical Perspective: Four Lessons from the History of Sexually Transmitted Diseases

Allan M. Brandt

It has become abundantly clear in the first six years of the AIDS (acquired immunodeficiency syndrome) epidemic that there will be no simple answer to this health crisis. The obstacles to establishing effective public health policies are considerable. AIDS is a new disease with a unique set of public health problems. The medical, social, and political aspects of the disease present American society and the world community with an awesome task.

The United States has relatively little recent experience dealing with health crises. Since the introduction of antibiotics during World War II, health priorities shifted to chronic, systemic diseases. We had come to believe that the problem of infectious, epidemic disease had passed—a topic of concern only to the developing world and historians.

In this respect, it is not surprising that in these first years of the epidemic there has been a desire to look for historical models as a means of dealing with the AIDS epidemic. Many have pointed to past and contemporary public health approaches to sexually transmitted diseases (STDs) as important precedents for the fight against AIDS. And indeed, there are significant similarities between AIDS and other sexually transmitted infections which go beyond the mere fact of sexual transmission. Syphilis, for example, also may have severe pathological effects. In the first half of the twentieth century, it was both greatly feared and highly stigmatized. In light of these analogues, the social history of efforts to control syphilis and other STDs may serve to inform our assessments of the current epidemic.

But history holds no simple truths. AIDS is not syphilis; our responses to the current epidemic will be shaped by contemporary science, politics, and culture. Yet the history of disease does offer an important set of perspectives on current proposals and strategies. Moreover, history points to the range of variables that will need to be addressed if we are to create effective and just policies.

In these early years of the AIDS epidemic, there has been a tendency to use analogy as a means of devising policy. It makes sense to draw upon past policies and institutional arrangements to address the problems posed by the current crisis. But we need to be sophisticated in drawing analogues; to recognize not only how AIDS is like past epidemics, but the precise ways in which it is different. This article draws four "lessons" from the social history of sexually transmitted disease in the United States and assesses their relevance for the current epidemic.

▶ Lesson #1—Fear of Disease Will Powerfully Influence Medical Approaches and Public Health Policy

The last years of the nineteenth century and the first of the twentieth witnessed considerable fear of sexually transmitted infection, not unlike that which we are experiencing today. A series of important discoveries about the pathology of syphilis and gonorrhea had revealed a range of alarming pathological consequences from debility, insanity, and paralysis, to sterility and blindness. In this age of antibiotics, it is easy to forget the fear and dread that syphilis invoked in the past. Among the reasons that syphilis was so greatly feared was the assumption that it could be casually transmitted. Doctors at the turn of the twentieth century catalogued the various models of transmission: pens, pencils, toothbrushes, towels and bedding, and medical procedures were all identified as potential means of communication. As one woman explained in an anonymous essay in 1912:

> At first it was unbelievable. I knew of the disease only through newspaper advertisements [for patent medicines]. I had understood that it was the result of sin and that it originated and was contracted only in the underworld of the city. I felt sure that my friend was mistaken in diagnosis when he exclaimed, "Another tragedy of the public drinking cup!" I eagerly met his remark with the assurance that I did not use public drinking cups, that I had used my own cup for years. He led me to review my summer. After recalling a number of times when my thirst had forced me to go to the public fountain, I came at last to realize that what he had told me was true.

The doctor, of course, had diagnosed syphilis. One indication of how seriously these casual modes of transmission were taken is the fact that the US Navy removed doorknobs from its battleships during World War I, claiming that they had become a source of infection for many of its sailors. We now know, of course, that syphilis cannot be contracted in these ways. This poses a difficult historical problem: Why did physicians believe that they could be?

Theories of casual transmission reflect deep cultural fears about disease and sexuality in the early twentieth century. In these approaches to venereal disease, concerns about hygiene, contamination, and contagion were expressed, anxieties that reflected a great deal about the contemporary society and culture. Venereal disease was viewed as a threat to the entire late Victorian social and sexual system, which placed great value on discipline, restraint, and homogeneity. The sexual code of that era held that sex would receive social sanction only in marriage. But the concerns about venereal disease and casual transmission also reflected a pervasive fear of the urban masses, the growth of the cities, and the changing nature of familial relationships.

Today, persistent fears about casual transmission of AIDS reflect a somewhat different, yet no less significant, social configuration. First, AIDS is strongly associated with behaviors which have been traditionally considered deviant. This is true for both homosexuality and intravenous drug use. After a generation of growing social tolerance for homosexuality, the epidemic has generated new fears and heightened old hostilities. Just as syphilis created a disease-oriented xenophobia in the early twentieth century, AIDS has today generated a new homophobia. AIDS has recast anxiety about contamination in a new light. Among certain social critics, AIDS is seen as "proof" of a certain moral order.

Second, fears are fanned because we live in an era in which the authority of scientific expertise has eroded. This may well be an aspect of a broader decline in the legitimacy of social institutions, but it is clearly seen in the areas of science and medicine. Despite significant evidence that HIV (human immunodeficiency virus) is not casually transmitted, medical and public health experts have been unable to provide the categorical reassurances that the public would like. But without such guarantees, public fear has remained high. In part, this reflects a misunderstanding of the nature of science and its inherent uncertainty. While physicians and public health officials have experience tolerating such uncertainty, the public requires better education in order to effectively evaluate risks.

Third, as a culture, we Americans are relatively unsophisticated in our assessments of relative risk. How are we to evaluate the risks of AIDS? How shall social policy be constructed around what are small or unknown risks? The ostracism of HIV-infected children from their schools in certain locales, the refusal of some physicians to treat AIDS patients, job and housing discrimination against those infected (and those suspected of being infected) all reveal the pervasive fears surrounding the epidemic. Clearly, then, one public health goal must be to address these fears. Addressing such fears means understanding their etiology. They originate in the particular social meaning of AIDS—its "social construction." We will not be able to effectively mitigate these concerns until we understand their deeper meaning. The response to AIDS will be fundamentally shaped by these fears; therefore, we need to develop techniques to assist individuals to distinguish irrational fears of AIDS from realistic and legitimate concerns. In this respect, many have focused on the need for more education.

▶ Lesson #2—Education Will Not Control the AIDS Epidemic

Early in the twentieth century, physicians, public health officials, and social reformers concerned about the problem of syphilis and gonorrhea called for a major educational campaign. They cogently argued that the tide of infection could not be stemmed until the public had adequate knowledge about these diseases, their mode of transmission, and the means of prevention. They called for an end to "the conspiracy of silence"—the Victorian code of sexual ethics—that considered all discussion of sexuality and disease in respectable society inappropriate. Physicians had contributed to this state of affairs by hiding diagnoses from their patients and families, and upholding what came to be known as the "medical secret." One physician described the nature of the conventions surrounding sexually transmitted diseases:

> Medical men are walking with eyes wide open along the edge of despair so treacherous and so pitiless that the wonder can only be that they have failed to warn the world away. Not a signboard! Not a caution spoken above a whisper! All mystery and seclusion. . . . As a result of this studied propriety, a world more full of venereal infection than any other pestilence.

Prince Morrow, the leader of the social hygiene movement, the antivenereal disease campaign, concluded, "Social sentiment holds that it is a greater violation of the properties of life publicly to mention venereal disease than privately to contract it."

During this period, the press remained reticent on the subject of sexually transmitted infections, refusing to print accounts of their effects. Reporters employed euphemisms such as "rare blood disorder," when forced to include a reference to a venereal infection. Nevertheless, magazines and newspapers did accept advertisements for venereal nostrums and quacks. In 1912, the US Post Office confiscated copies of birth control advocate Margaret Sanger's *What Every Girl Should Know,* because it considered the references to syphilis and gonorrhea "obscene" under the provisions of the Comstock law.

Enlightened physicians vigorously called for an end to this hypocrisy. "We are dealing with the solution of a problem," explained Dr. Egbert Grandin, "where ignorance is *not* bliss but is misfortune, and where, therefore, it is folly not to be wise." Social reformers viewed education and publicity as a panacea; forthright education would end the problem of sexually transmitted infection. If parents failed to perform their social responsibilities and inform their children, then the schools should include sex education. By 1919, the US Public Health Service endorsed sex education in the schools, noting, "As in many instances the school must take up the burden neglected by others." By 1922, almost half of all secondary schools offered some instruction in sex hygiene.

Educational programs devised by the social hygienists emphasized fear of infection. Prince Morrow, for example, called fear "the protective genius of the human body." Another physician explained, "The sexual instinct is imperative and will only listen to fear." Margaret Cleaves, a leading social hygienist, argued, "There should be taught such disgust and dread of these conditions that naught would induce the seeking of a polluted source for the sake of gratifying a controllable desire."

In this sense, educational efforts may have actually contributed to the pervasive fears of infection, to the stigma associated with the diseases, and to the discrimination against its victims. Indeed, educational materials produced throughout the first decades of the twentieth century emphasized the inherent dangers of all sexual activity, especially disease and unwanted pregnancy. In this respect, such educational programs, rather than being termed sex education were actually antisex education. Pamphlets and films repeatedly emphasized the "loathsome" and disfiguring aspects of sexually transmitted disease; the most drastic pathological consequences (insanity, paralysis, blindness, and death); as well as the disastrous impact on personal relations.

This orientation toward sex education reached its apogee during World War I, when American soldiers were told, "A German bullet is cleaner than a whore." Despite their threatening quality, these educational programs did not have the desired effect of reducing the rates of infection. And indeed, sexual mores in the twentieth century have responded to a number of social and cultural forces more powerful than the fear of disease.

There are, nonetheless, some precedents for successful educational campaigns. During World War II, the military initiated a massive educational campaign against sexually transmitted disease. But unlike prior efforts, it reminded soldiers that disease could be prevented through the use of condoms, which were widely distributed. The military program recognized that sexual behaviors could be modified, but that calls for outright abstinence were likely to fail. Given the need for an efficient and healthy army, officials maintained a pragmatic posture that separated morals from the essential task of prevention. As one medical officer explained, "It is difficult to make the sex act unpopular."

Today, calls for better education are frequently offered as the best hope for controlling the AIDS epidemic. But this will only be true if some resolution is reached concerning the specific content and nature of such educational efforts. The limited effectiveness of education which merely encourages fear is well-documented. Moreover, AIDS education requires a forthright confrontation of aspects of human sexuality that are typically avoided. To be effective, AIDS education must be explicit, focused, and appropriately targeted to a range of at-risk social groups. As the history of sexually transmitted diseases makes clear, we need to study the nature of behavior and disease. If education is to have a positive impact, we need to be far more sophisticated, creative, and bold in devising and implementing programs.

Education is not a panacea for the AIDS epidemic, just as education did not solve the problem of other sexually transmitted diseases earlier in the twentieth century. It is one critical aspect of a fully-articulated program. As this historical vignette makes clear, we need to be far more explicit about what we mean when we say "education." Certainly education about AIDS is an important element of any public health approach to the crisis, but we need to substantively evaluate a range of educational programs and their impact on behavior for populations with a variety of needs.

Because the impact of education is unclear and the dangers of the epidemic are perceived as great (see lesson #1), there has been considerable interest in compulsory public health measures as a primary means of controlling AIDS.

▶ Lesson #3—Compulsory Public Health Measures Will Not Control the Epidemic

Given the considerable fear that the epidemic has generated and its obvious dangers, demands have been voiced for the implementation of compulsory public health interventions. The history of efforts to control syphilis during the twentieth century indicates the limits of compulsory measures which range from required premarital testing to quarantine of infected individuals.

Next to programs for compulsory vaccination, compulsory programs for premarital syphilis serologies are probably the most widely known of all compulsory public health measures in the twentieth century United States. The development of effective laboratory diagnostic measures stands as a signal contribution in the history of the control of sexually transmitted diseases. With the development of the Wassermann test in 1906, there was a generally reliable way of detecting the presence of syphilis. The achievement of such a test offered a new series of public health potentials. No longer would diagnosis depend on strictly clinical criteria. Diagnosis among the asymptomatic was now possible, as was the ability to test the effectiveness of treatments. The availability of the test led to the development of programs for compulsory testing.

Significantly, calls for compulsory screening for syphilis predated the Wassermann exam. Beginning in the last years of the nineteenth century, several states began to mandate premarital medical examinations to assure that sexually transmitted infections were not communicated in marriage. But without a definitive test, such examinations were of limited use. With a laboratory test, however, calls were voiced for requiring premarital blood tests. In 1935, Connecticut became the first state to mandate premarital serologies of all prospective brides and grooms. The rationale for premarital screening was clear. If every individual about to be married were tested, and, if found to be infected, treated, the transmission of infection to marital partners and offspring would be halted. The legislation was vigorously supported by the public health establishment, organized women's groups, magazines, and the news media. Many clinicians, however, argued against the legislation, suggesting that diagnosis should not rely exclusively on laboratory findings which were, in some instances, incorrect. N.A. Nelson of the Massachusetts Department of Public Health explained, "Today, it is becoming the fashion to support, by law, the too common notion that the laboratory is infallible." Despite such objections, by the end of the World War II, virtually all the states had enacted provisions mandating premarital serologies.

Legislation is currently pending in 35 state legislatures that would require premarital HIV serologies. The rationale for such programs is often the historical precedent of syphilis screening. The logic seems intuitively correct: We screen for syphilis. AIDS is a far more serious disease; we should therefore screen for AIDS. In this respect it is worth reviewing the effectiveness of premarital syphilis screening as well as those factors that distinguish syphilis from AIDS.

Mandatory premarital serologies never proved to be a particularly effective mechanism for finding new cases of syphilis. First, physicians and public health officials recognized that there was a significant rate of false positive tests which occurred because of technical inadequacies of the tests themselves or as a result of biological phenomena (such as other infections). As the concepts of sensitivity (the test's performance among those with the disease) and specificity (the test's performance among those free of infections) came to be more fully understood in the 1930s, the oversensitivity of tests like the Wassermann was revealed. As many as 25 per cent of individuals determined to be infected with syphilis by the Wassermann test were actually free of infection; nevertheless, these individuals often underwent toxic treatment with arsenical drugs, assuming the tests were correct. Beyond this, individuals with false positive tests often suffered the social repercussions of being infected: deep stigma and disrupted relationships. As many physicians pointed out, a positive serology did not always mean that an individual could transmit the disease. Because the tests tended to be mandated for a population at relatively low risk of infection, their accuracy was further compromised. Some individuals reportedly avoided the test altogether. Many of the difficulties associated with the high numbers of false positives were alleviated as new, more specific tests were developed in the 1940s and 1950s, but the central problem remained. Premarital syphilis serologies failed to identify a significant percentage of the infected population. In 1978, for example, premarital screening accounted for only 1.27 per cent of all national tests found to be positive for syphilis. The costs of these programs were estimated at $80 million annually. Another study in California projected the costs per case found through premarital screening to be $240,000. Moreover, premarital screening for syphilis continued to find a significant number of false positives. As these studies indicated, the benefits of screening programs are dependent on the prevalence of the disease in the population being screened. In this respect, it seems unlikely that premarital screening effectively served the function of preventing infections within marriage that its advocates assumed it would. These data led a number of states to repeal mandatory premarital serologies in the early 1980s.

Compulsory premarital syphilis serologies thus offer a dubious precedent for required HIV screening. The point, of course, is *not* that the test is inaccurate. ELISA (enzyme-linked immunosorbent assay) testing coupled with the Western Blot *can be* quite reliable, but only when applied to populations which are likely to have been' infected. Screening of low-prevalence populations, like premarital couples, is unlikely to have any significant impact on the course of the epidemic. Not only will such programs find relatively few new cases; they will also reveal large numbers of false positives. A recent study concluded that a national mandatory premarital screening program would find approximately 1,200 new cases of HIV infection, one-tenth of 1 per cent of those currently infected. But it would also incorrectly identify as many as 380 individuals—actually free of infection—as infected, even with supplementary Western blot tests. Such a program would also falsely reassure as many as 120 individuals with false negative results. Moreover, the inability to treat and render non-infectious those individuals who are found to be infected severely limits the potential benefits of such mandatory measures. With syphilis serologies, the rationale of the program was to treat infected individuals.

This, of course, is *not* to argue that testing has no role in an effective AIDS public health campaign. During the late 1930s, a massive voluntary testing campaign heightened consciousness of syphilis in Chicago, bringing thousands of new cases into treatment. AIDS testing, conducted voluntarily and confidentially, targeted to individuals who have specific risk factors for infection, may have significant public health benefits. Compulsory screening, however, could merely discourage infected individuals from being tested. This makes clear the need to enact legislation guaranteeing the confidentiality of those who volunteer to be tested and prohibiting discrimination against HIV-infected individuals.

As a mandatory measure, premarital screening is a relatively modest proposal. During the course of the twentieth century, more radical and intrusive compulsory measures to control STDs, such as quarantine, have also been attempted. These, too, have failed. During World War I, as hysteria about the impact of STDs rose, Congress passed legislation to support the quarantine of prostitutes suspected of spreading disease. The Act held that anyone suspected of harboring a venereal infection could be detained and incarcerated until determined to be non-infectious. During the course of the War, more than 20,000 women were held in camps because they were suspected of being "spreaders" of venereal disease.

The program had no apparent impact on rates of infection, which actually climbed substantially during the War. In sexually transmitted infections, the reservoir of infection is relatively high, modes of transmission are specific, and infected individuals may be healthy. In the case of AIDS, where there is no medical intervention to render individuals non-infectious, quarantine is totally impractical because it would require life-long incarceration of the infected.

Compulsory measures often generate critics because such policies may infringe on basic civil liberties. From an ethical and legal viewpoint, the first question that must be asked about any potential policy intervention is: Is it likely to work? Only if there is clear evidence to suggest the program would be effective does it make sense to evaluate the civil liberties implications. Then it is possible to evaluate the constitutional question: Is the public health benefit to be derived worthy of the possible costs in civil liberties? Is the proposed compulsory program the least restrictive of the range of potential measures available to achieve the public good?

In this respect, it is worth noting that compulsory measures may actually be counterproductive. First, they require substantial resources that could be more effectively allocated. Second, they have often had the effect of driving the very individuals that the program hopes to reach farther away from public health institutions. Ineffective draconian measures would serve only to augment the AIDS crisis. Nevertheless, despite the fact that such programs offer no benefits, they may have substantial political and cultural appeal (see lesson #1).

Because compulsory measures are controversial and unlikely to control the epidemic, there is considerable hope that we will soon have a "magic bullet"—a biomedical "fix" to free us of the hazards of AIDS.

▶ Lesson #4—The Development of Effective Treatments and Vaccines Will Not Immediately or Easily End the AIDS Epidemic

As the history of efforts to control other sexually transmitted diseases makes clear, effective treatment has not always led to control. In 1909, German Nobel laureate Paul Ehrlich discovered Salvarsan (arsphenamine), an arsenic compound which killed the spirochete, the organism which causes syphilis. Salvarsan was the first effective chemotherapeutic agent for a specific disease. Ehrlich called Salvarsan a "magic bullet," a drug which would seek out and destroy its mark. He claimed that modern medicine would seek the discovery of a series of such drugs to eliminate the micro-organisms which cause disease. Although Salvarsan was an effective treatment, it was toxic and difficult to administer. Patients required a painful regimen of injections, sometimes for as long as two years.

Unlike the arsphenamines, penicillin was truly a wonder drug. In early 1943, Dr. John S. Mahoney of the US Public Health Service found that penicillin was effective in treating rabbits infected with syphilis. After repeating his experiments with human subjects, his findings were announced and the massive production of penicillin began.

With a single shot, the scourge of syphilis could be avoided. Incidence fell from a high of 72 cases per 100,000 in 1943 to about 4 per 100,000 in 1956. In 1949, Mahoney wrote, "as a result of antibiotic therapy, gonorrhea has almost passed from the scene as an important clinical and public entity. An article in the *American Journal of Syphilis* in 1951 asked, "Are Venereal Diseases Disappearing?" Although the article concluded that it was too soon to know, by 1955 the *Journal* itself had disappeared. *The Journal of Social Hygiene,* for half a century the leading publication on social dimensions of the problem, also ceased publication. As rates reached all time lows, it appeared that venereal diseases would join the ranks of other infectious diseases that had come under the control of modern medicine.

Although there is no question that the nature and meaning of syphilis and gonorrhea underwent a fundamental change with the introduction of antibiotic therapy, the decline of venereal diseases proved short-lived. Rates of infection began to climb in the early 1960s. By the late 1950s much of the machinery, especially procedures for public education, case-finding, tracing and diagnosis had been severely reduced.

In 1987, the Centers for Disease Control (CDC) reported an increase in cases of primary and secondary syphilis. The estimated annual rate per 100,000 population rose from 10.9 to 13.3 cases, the largest increases in 10 years. These figures are particularly striking in that they come in the midst of the AIDS epidemic which many have assumed has led to a substantial decline in sexual encounters. Moreover, after an eight-year decline, rates of congenital syphilis have also reportedly risen since 1983. The CDC concluded that individuals with a history of sexually transmitted infection are at increased risk for infection with the AIDS virus.

Despite the effectiveness of penicillin as a cure for syphilis, the disease has persisted. The issue, therefore, is not merely the development of effective treatments but the *process* by which they are deployed; the means by which they move from laboratory to full allocation to those affected. Effective treatments without adequate education, counseling, and funding may not reach those who most need them. Even "magic bullets" need to be effectively delivered. Obviously effective treatments should be a priority in a multifaceted approach to AIDS and will ultimately be an important component in its control; but even a magic bullet will not quickly or completely solve the problem.

No doubt, new and more effective treatments for AIDS will be developed in the years ahead, but their deployment will raise a series of complex issues ranging from human subject research to actual allocation. And while effective treatments may help to control further infection, as they do for syphilis and gonorrhea, treatments which prolong the life of AIDS patients may have little or no impact on the rates of transmission of the virus, which occurs principally among individuals who have no symptoms of disease.

This suggests certain fundamental flaws in the biomedical model of disease. Diseases are complex bio-ecological problems that may be mitigated only by addressing a range of scientific, social, and political considerations. No single intervention—even an effective vaccine—will adequately address the complexities of the AIDS epidemic.

▶ Conclusions

As these historical lessons make clear, in the context of fear surrounding the epidemic (lesson #1), the principal proposals for eradicating AIDS (lessons #2–4) are unlikely to be effective, at least in the immediate future. These lessons should not imply, however, that nothing will work; they make evident that no single avenue is likely to lead to success. Moreover, they suggest that in considering any intervention we will require sophisticated research to understand its potential impact on the epidemic. While education, testing, and biomedical research all offer some hope, in each instance we will need to fully consider their particular effectiveness as measures to control disease.

Simple answers based upon historical precedents are unlikely to alleviate the AIDS crisis. History does, however, point to a range of variables which influence disease, and those factors which require attention if it is to be effectively addressed. Any successful approach to the epidemic will require a full recognition of the important social, cultural, and biological aspects of AIDS. A public health priority will be to lead in the process of discerning those programs likely to have a beneficial impact from those with considerable political and cultural appeal, but unlikely to positively affect the course of the epidemic. Only in this way we will be able to devise effective and humane public policies.

▶ References

1. Cutler JC, Arnold RC: Venereal disease control by health departments in the past: Lessons for the present. *Am J Public Health* 1988; 78:372–376.
2. Bulkey LD: *Syphilis of the Innocent.* New York: Bailey and Fairchild, 1894.
3. Anon: What one woman has had to bear. *Forum* 1912; 68:451–454.
4. Brandt AM: *No Magic Bullet: A Social History of Venereal Disease in the United States Since 1880.* New York: Oxford University Press, 1985, Rev. Ed. 1987.
5. Eisenberg KE: The genesis of fear: AIDS and public's response to science. Law, *Med Health Care* 1986; 14:243–249.
6. Becker MH, Joseph JG: AIDS behavioral change to reduce risk: A review. *Am J Public Health* 1988; 78:394–410.
7. Yankauer A: AIDS and Public Health. (editorial) *Am J Public Health* 1988; 78:364–366.

8. Willson RN: The relationship of the medical profession to the social evil. *JAMA* 1906; 47:32.

9. Morrow PA: Publicity as a factor in venereal prophylaxis. *JAMA* 1906; 47:1246.

10. Grandin E: Should the Great Body of the General Public Be Enlightened? *Charities and Commons,* February 24, 1906.

11. US Public Health Service: *The Problem of Sex Education in the Schools.* Washington, DC, 1919; p. 9.

12. Cleaves M: *Transactions of the American Society for Social and Moral Prophylaxis* 1910; 3:31.

13. Pappas JP: The venereal problem in the US Army. *Milit Surg,* August 1943; 93:182.

14. Nelson NA: Marriage and the laboratory. *Am J Syphilis:* 1939; 23:289.

15. Kolmer JA: The problem of falsely doubtful and positive reactions in the serology of syphilis. *Am J Public Health* 1944; 34:510–526.

16. Felman Y: Repeal of mandated premarital tests for syphilis: A survey of state health officers. *Am J Public Health* 1981; 71:155–159.

17. Haskell RJ: A cost benefit analysis of California's mandatory premarital screening program for syphilis. *West J Med* 1984; 141:538–541.

18. Cleary PD, Barry MJ, Mayer KH, Brandt AM, Gostin L, Fineberg HV: Compulsory premarital screening for the human immunodeficiency virus. *JAMA* 1987; 258:1757–1762.

19. Gostin L. Curran W: *The Limits of Compulsion in Controlling AIDS.* Hastings Center Report 1986; 16(suppl):24–29.

20. Marquardt M: Paul Ehrich. New York: Henry Schuman, 1951.

21. Dowling H: *Fighting Infection.* Cambridge: Harvard University Press, 1977.

22. Brown WJ, Donohue JF, Axnick NW, Blount JH, Jones OG, Ewen NJ: *Syphilis and Other Venereal Diseases.* Cambridge: Harvard University Press (APHA), 1970.

23. Mahoney JF: The effect of antibiotics on the concepts and practices of public health. *In:* Galdston I (ed): *The Impact of Antibiotics on Medicine and Society.* New York: 1958; 98–120.

24. USPHS, Centers for Disease Control: *MMWR* 1987; 36:393.

The AIDS Memorial Quilt

Elizabeth Fee, Ph.D.

The AIDS Memorial Quilt was conceived in November 1985 by San Francisco, Calif, gay activist Cleve Jones. Jones had helped organize the annual march honoring Mayor George Moscone and gay San Francisco Supervisor Harvey Milk, who were assassinated in 1978. When planning the march, Jones learned that more than 1000 San Franciscans had died of AIDS, and he asked the marchers to write on their placards the names of friends, partners, and family members who had died of the disease. After the march, the marchers taped their placards onto the walls of the San Francisco Federal Building. The wall of names looked like a patchwork quilt.

Jones and his fellow activists gathered in a San Francisco storefront to plan a more permanent memorial to those who had died of AIDS and to publicize the devastating impact of the disease. They created the NAMES Project AIDS Memorial Quilt. Generous donors supplied sewing machines and materials, and volunteers over the years have created more than 46 000 individual 3- by 6-foot memorial panels, most of them honoring one particular person who died of AIDS. Some 35 countries, from Argentina to Japan to Uganda, have contributed panels.

The quilt was displayed for the first time on the National Mall in Washington, DC, on October 11, 1987, during the National March on Washington for Lesbian and Gay Rights. In 1988, the quilt went on a national tour during which it was displayed in 20 cities. This tour raised $500 000 for AIDS service organizations. The quilt would return to Washington in 1988, 1989, 1992, and 1996. Each time it returned, the quilt had grown larger. Every panel is different, and the panels feature a multitude of materials: feather boas, lace, leather, love letters, cowboy boots, buttons and bows, paintings, photographs, fishnet, and fur are but a few of the materials used and objects attached. Each display of the quilt features celebrities, politicians, and family members, friends, and lovers reading aloud the names of the people for whom the quilt panels were made. The largest community art project in the world, the AIDS Memorial Quilt was nominated for the Nobel Peace Prize in 1989. In the last 20 years, the quilt has been viewed by more than 15 million people and has raised more than $3 million for AIDS service organizations.

The AIDS Memorial Quilt is an overwhelming sight, both a joyful remembrance and a reminder of the tragedy of lives lost. It is a beautiful broad expanse of color and feeling, each panel made with love for the person being honored and celebrated. The quilt is a powerful statement; its image serves as a memorial to all the people and their loved ones whose lives have been transformed by this epidemic over the past 25 years.

► About the Authors

Requests for reprints should be sent to Elizabeth Fee, PhD, History of Medicine Division, National Library of Medicine, National Institutes of Health, 8600 Rockville Pike, Bethesda, MD 20894 (e-mail: feee@mail.nih.gov).
doi: 10.2105/AJPH.2006.088575

► References

1. The AIDS Memorial Quilt: The Names Project Foundation. Available at: http://www .aidsquilt.org. Accessed February 14, 2006.

The Just Rewards of Unbridled Lust: Syphilis in Early Modern Europe

Peter Allen

Shortly after Christopher Columbus and his sailors returned from their voyage to the New World, a horrifying new disease began to make its way around the Old. The "pox," as it was often called, erupted with dramatic severity. According to Ulrich von Hutten (1488–1523), a German knight, revolutionary, and author who wrote a popular book about his own trials with syphilis and the treatments he underwent, the first European sufferers were covered with acorn-sized boils that emitted a foul, dark green pus. The secretion was so vile, von Hutten affirmed, that even the burning pains of the boils troubled the sick less than the horror at the sight of their own bodies. Yet this was only the beginning. People's flesh and skin filled with water; their bladders developed sores; their stomachs were eaten away. Girolamo Fracastoro, a professor at the University of Padua, described the onward march of symptoms: syphilis pustules developed into ulcers that dissolved the skin, muscle, bone, palate, and tonsils—even lips, noses, eyes, and genital organs. Rubbery tumors, filled with a white, sticky mucus, grew to the size of rolls of bread. Violent pains tormented the afflicted, who were exhausted but could not sleep, and suffered starvation without feeling hunger. Many of them died

The public was appalled by this scourge. Physicians too, von Hutten reported, were so revolted that they would not even touch their patients. As in the earlier Middle Ages, divines quickly announced that the extraordinary sins of the age were responsible for the new plague; others blamed the stars, miasmas, and various other causes. Barrels of medical ink were spilled on the question of where the disease had come from. Treatments, preventions, and cures were sought. The idea of infection began to be taken far more seriously than it ever had before. Hospitals transformed themselves in response to the new plague—sometimes for the better, often for the worse, as when, in fear, they cast their ulcerated patients out into the streets. Most of all, people continued to follow their old ways: in the face of this new threat, they castigated and persecuted the sick. As infection spread, so did fear; and where fear went, blame followed close behind.

Perhaps more than any other disease before or since, syphilis in early modern Europe provoked the kind of widespread moral panic that AIDS revived when it struck America in the 1980s. Syphilitics were condemned from pulpits and from chairs in university medical schools. John Calvin (1509–1564) announced that "God has raised up new diseases against debauchery"; medical authorities willingly agreed. The greatest English surgeon of the sixteenth century, William Clowes (1540–1604) who counted Queen Elizabeth among his patients, announced to his colleagues and patients that syphilis was "loathsome and odious, yea troublesome and dangerous, a notable testimony of the just wrath of God." A century later, a French physician, M. Flamand, summed up this point of view concisely by announcing that venereal diseases were "the just rewards of unbridled lust." Disease commonly invited theological speculation, but in the case of syphilis people felt that little speculation was necessary. Just as fornication opened the door to pox, so the pox opened the door to chastisement and blame.

Motivated by these fears, panicky towns and hospitals barred their gates against syphilitics. Within two years of the first reported cases, cities from Geneva to Aberdeen evicted the pox-ridden. Often, city fathers blamed their prostitutes for the disease, and some threatened to brand their cheeks with hot iron if they did not desist from the vices. Sexual morality was becoming stricter, and prostitutes were usually condemned far more savagely than the men who used their services.

What was more extraordinary, however, was that hospitals refused to admit syphilis patients. Hospitals in early modern Europe were charitable institutions, designed to provide care and shelter to the sick poor. The most famous of them, the Paris Hôtel-Dieu prided itself, with one single exception, on the breadth of its generosity. This hospital boasted that it "receives, feeds, and tends all poor sufferers, wherever they come from and whatever ailment they may have, even plague victims—though not if they have the pox." The Hôtel-Dieu expelled its syphilitic patients in 1496, and, after relenting briefly, expelled them again in 1508. Two years after that, another Parisian hospital shunted its pox victims off to the stables, to sleep with the animals. Many cities threw the poxy poor into leper houses that for years and years had housed only ghostly memories; Toulouse kept its infected prostitutes in a ward that was little more than a high-security prison. Two infamous hospitals in Paris, Bicêtre and the Salpétrière, had patients "piled upon one another," in the words of historian Michel Mollat, "like a cargo of Negroes in an African slave ship." And another, the Petites Maisons, which warehoused syphilitics and the mentally ill from the 1550s until the 1800s, became known as the "pox-victims' Bastille."

Fear of contact was one reason for this behavior. Even more than this, however, the sick—like lepers—were often reviled because people believed that they had brought their torments upon themselves. Some pundits, early on, announced that blasphemy was the vice that had called down this new torment from heaven, but most often syphilis was attributed to the sin of lust. This was certainly a logical assumption: soldiers and prostitutes, traditionally associated with sexual license and moral disorder, were among the first victims, and the connection became even closer when people noticed that the disease's first sores often turned up on the genital organs. The loathsome symptoms were taken as signs that the sick housed debauched and sinful souls. The reasoning stood behind many of the cruelties that individuals, doctors, hospitals, priests, ministers, and even entire town and cities inflicted on people with the pox, as the stories in this chapter will show.

▶ The Source of This Distemper

Horror was the first emotion the pox provoked among the general public, but what the medical community first felt was confusion. Was this an old disease, and, if so, which one? If it was new, what did that say about the state of medical knowledge? And in any case, how could physicians make sense of it?

Medical research in the twentieth century mostly takes place in the lab; in the Renaissance, though, researchers went first and foremost to the library to see what the ancients had said. The problem, however, was that is was not clear that in this case the ancients had anything useful to offer. Nothing the Greek and Arabic authorities had described seemed very similar to the cases turning up in increasing numbers on the physicians' rounds and in the streets, and so it was hard to affirm that the old remedies would do any good.

If the pox was a new disease, how had it arisen? Some cast the blame on supernatural powers—the planets, the stars, God, or even witches. Galenists claimed that the pox came from corrupted air, or even, like lovesickness, from an excess of black bile. Some said the disease was God's punishment for sin; others attributed it to the recent and risky voyages to the New World.

The theories that tied the disease to the Americas were the most innovative, since they focused on the new idea that diseases could travel from one person to another. (They may also have been the most accurate: many scientists today believe that the New World was the source of the syphilis bacterium, or of a new strain or cofactor that triggered the epidemic of the 1490s.) In a quirky 1672 screed entitled *Great Venus Unmasked*, the English writer Gideon Harvey looked backward to argue that it was Columbus's Neapolitan sailors who had acquired this "new pretty toy." With it, he reasoned, they had infected the prostitutes of their native city, which was under siege by the French in 1494–1495: when provisions in Naples ran out, wrote Harvey, the whores crept over to the besiegers' camp, and offered their services to the French soldiers. If the Neapolitan prostitutes were hungry for food, Harvey explained, the French soldiers were "almost starved for want of women's flesh, which they found so well seasoned, and daubed with mustard, that in a few weeks it took 'em all by the nose."

Other exotic theories abounded. One Leonardo Fioravanti (1518–1588) claimed that the French soldiers became sick because they had devoured the rotten carcasses of their enemies. Some said the malady had been bred when a French leper had sex with a Neapolitan whore. Others said soldiers became sick from drinking Greek wine adulterated with lepers' blood; still others blamed the "entailed manginess" of the French, who—has Harvey reminded his English readers—"are slovens in their linen." One anonymous author even suggested that syphilis was spontaneously generated by promiscuous sex.

This wild proliferation of theories showed that nobody really knew where the pox had come from; it also showed that people were deeply troubled by it, and thought that something had gone gravely amiss in the world to provoke such a strange and awful evil. Their confusion and anxiety were also revealed by the names that people gave the new arrival. The name most commonly used today, syphilis, came from an Italian poem, written in 1530, which traced the disease to a punishment inflicted by Jupiter on a fictional character named Syphilus, an impious shepherd. More commonly, however, the pox was called after whichever country people wanted to blame for the disease. To the French, it was the *mal de Naples*, the sickness from Naples; to many others, it was the *morbus gallicus*, the French disease. But also accused were the Americans, the Mexicans, the Spanish, the Germans, the Poles, and the Portuguese.

Everyone, observed the astute author of *A New Method of Curing the French-Pox* (1690), "to excuse himself, is forward to ascribe to his neighbors the source and original of this distemper."

Regardless of its geographic origin, people quickly began to notice that the pox traveled from one person to another. They sometimes blamed transmission on common and morally innocuous practices—drinking from a common cup, kissing friends in church, following a syphilitic comrade on the latrine. But from 1495 on, the route of transmission people talked about most was sex. Von Hutten noticed that men in their sexually active years were much more susceptible to the French disease than boys or the elderly; soldiers and prostitutes remained highly suspect. As early as 1504, infection became grounds for breaking off engagements, and even saying that someone was infected was enough to provoke a lawsuit. Syphilis was well on its way to becoming a "venereal" disease, and a public mark of shame.

▶ A Moral Revolution

It seems likely that these developments were related to a dramatic change of moral climate that was sweeping over Europe. Though it is impossible to know all the details of this picture, particularly five hundred years after the fact, an educated guess would suggest that this major new public health problem contributed to people's increasingly negative attitudes toward sex, a shift in views that revolutionized people's lives. For heterosexual men, at least, the 1400s had been an era of comparatively free sexuality. In part, this was because people married late: men often waited to wive until their fathers had died and had and left property and businesses to them. As a result, many men remained unmarried long after they reached sexual maturity, and a male-dominated social structure left these single men free to find ways to satisfy their urges.

Historical records show that young men had a number of common sexual outlets. One was masturbation, which young men (though not young women) could practice without attracting much condemnation. Another was rape. Young men—groups of adolescents, especially—frequently assaulted poor girls who had no male protection, and the perpetrators generally suffered far less than their victims for the consequences of their actions. For example, in the little city of Dijon, which in the fifteenth century contained fewer than three thousand households, at least twenty rapes were reported every year. Who knows how many more actually occurred? More commonly still, men used prostitutes, whether these were elegant courtesans, whores they met in the brothels or—even further down the social ladder—poor women who made a seedy living servicing male customers at the baths. Men scarcely needed to be married to have sex.

Women were not necessarily sexually monogamous either, though when they were promiscuous it was often less out of choice than from obligation, whether through rape or the force of circumstances. In theory, girls remained virgins until they were married, passing directly from their fathers' control to their husbands'; in practice, however, many did not manage to remain on this straight and narrow path. Rape was one common ambush, especially for poor girls, and this often led them even further afield, to prostitution. The same was true of girls who had lost their place in society by being orphaned, wives who fled husbands who abused them, and women who were discharged, penniless, from public hospitals. The oldest profession extended its lucrative embrace to the homeless, the victimized, and the poor.

Prostitution was not a very respectable way for women to earn a living in the fifteenth century, but it was not exceptionally shameful, and it paid well. In half an hour, a prostitute could make as much money as a woman laboring in a vineyard could earn in half a day. The financial rewards were so tempting, in fact, that in lean times even married women sometimes joined this labor force.

In addition, prostitution was tolerated, and often even actively promoted, by town and church leaders, who felt that society would collapse if unmarried men did not have this squalid but essential outlet for their sexual desires. This view had a prestigious heritage, having been articulated by none other than St. Augustine. Before his conversion to Christianity, Augustine had accumulated substantial experience in the pleasures of the flesh, as witnessed by his famous prayer, "Lord, give me chastity and continence—but not just yet." Even in his maturer years, the saint felt that men's nature was such that whores were an unfortunate social necessity. "What is more sordid, more worthless, more full of shame and disgrace than prostitutes, pimps, and other plagues of this kind?" Augustine rhetorically inquired, disapproval dripping from his episcopal pen. "If, however," he went on to warn, "you remove prostitutes from human society, you will overturn everything with lust." Prostitution, Augustine argued, was like a city sewer system— disgusting, but essential to maintaining cleanliness and order in every other area.

Late medieval town leaders even argued that prostitution was a public good—perhaps because it was a way to appease the sexual urges of the working men the upper classes had driven out of the marriage market. Cities owned and operated brothels. Bishops and abbots owned bathhouses, and supported themselves on their profits; the fact that these establishments made getting dirty as much fun as getting clean was not considered a problem. Many clergymen, in fact, were among the baths' and brothels' clientele: at certain times and in certain places, in fact, one customer in five was a cleric.

In the early 1500s, however, chillier moral winds began to blow. The public, which in the past had tolerated brothels as a fact of life, began to consider them shameful. Prostitutes were denounced and arrested; the Bishop of Winchester's London bordellos were shut down. French cities closed their brothels; Geneva expelled its whores. The freeze affected more than just prostitutes; increasingly, women in general were blamed as a corrupting influence on men. And in 1539, only five years after its creation, Michelangelo's *Last Judgment* was declared obscene; the offending parts were painted over. Old-fashioned sexual license was as out of place in this new era as painted and gilded statues of the Virgin Mary and the saints would have been in an austerely undecorated Protestant church.

Part of this change was the result of religious developments. Protestants made much of the sins of the flesh: lust so afflicted humankind, preached Martin Luther (1483–1546), that God had been obliged to create matrimony as "a hospital for incurables." Calvin saw sexual vices everywhere: the young, he preached, were tormented by "boiling affections," while fornicators were pigs who soiled the very blood of Christ by mixing it with "the stinking mire." Even in the holy city of Geneva—even in his own church council—Calvin believed he was surrounded by "fornicators, wife-beaters, idolaters, and heretics."

Did syphilis contribute to these changes? Obviously, not all can be attributed to the new disease: the rise of Protestantism was a far larger and more influential matter than any bacterium. But a new, virulent, sexually transmitted infection can only have reinforced people's increasing fears and anxieties about sex.

Neither preachers nor physicians had the slightest hesitation about announcing that syphilis—and syphilitics—were wicked. Both Catholics and Protestants endorsed this view and proclaimed it from their pulpits. One of the most popular Catholic preachers of the day, a Franciscan monk named Michel Menot, focused on the "Naples pox" in a sermon delivered during the penitential Lenten season of 1508. The sins of the flesh, proclaimed Brother Michel, made the body leprous, stinking, and infirm; the pox simply worked God's will. "Lust short-ens the days of mankind," he concluded, Q.E.D. The Catholic queen of Navarre, Marguérite d'Angoulême (1492–1549), agreed. Fornication led to infection, she wrote in her poetic con-fession, *The Mirror of a Sinful Soul* (1531), a book Elizabeth I of England (1533–1603) found so moving and persuasive that she translated it into English herself.

Protestants also enthusiastically linked sickness with immorality: Calvin warned Geneva that the new and strange diseases showed clearly that "God is more angry than ever" with the sins of humankind. A century later, in England, Edward Lawrence (1623–1695) phrased the same sentiment in even more inflammatory language. Through the filthy sin of whoredom, he fulminated, "men and women sacrifice their health, estates, names, bodies, and souls to their stinking lusts, carrying a filthy and guilty soul in a rotten body whilst they live, and shutting themselves out of heaven and into hell when they die." The torments of the body merely showed the public the inner degradation of the soul.

▶ The Morality of Medicine

Some physicians took a more tolerant stance than these vitriolic preachers. Others, however, were even more censorious than the men of the cloth, and warned that pox victims were so sinful that they did not even deserve medical treatment. Syphilis revived the old questions that lovesickness had raised centuries before: should the doctor do what was best for his patients' bodies, or should he attend to their souls? If they tried to care for both, would there be con-flicts? And when the patient's life was at stake, which side would win?

Like attitudes throughout society, doctors' views on syphilis grew more severe as time went on. Few physicians ever felt that syphilis was a morally neutral issue, but some of the earliest writers were at least willing to separate their spiritual concerns from their medical prac-tice. For example, Johannes Widman (professor at the University of Tübingen, ca. 1460–ca. 1500), wrote around 1500 that "a doctor, as a doctor, does not cure much" by arguing about whether a disease is caused by human sin or by the wheeling of the constellations in the heav-ens. If doctors simply removed the bodily causes of disease, he asserted, their patients would recover far more quickly than if the doctor tried to redeem his patient's virtue first.

Widman's willingness to cure pox was seconded by Gaspare Torrella (1440–1524), a Span-ish physician who was also a bishop. Ever a self-promoter, Torrella reassured his readers that, "with the help of all-powerful God and his mother, the most glorious Virgin Mary, the pox can be cured if the doctor is clever and follows all the instructions I provide." Torrella's close ties with the Borgia family—not a notoriously clean-living bunch—may have taught him tol-erance, or at least expedience: within a single two-month period, the doctor-bishop treated for syphilis not only the cardinal of Valencia, who happened to be Pope Alexander VI's illegit-imate son, but also seventeen other Borgias and members of the papal court. Presumably, Torrella understood that it did not pay to preach at the pope's family. A physician from Geneva, Jacobus Catenus de Lacumarino, also argued (around 1504) that he had an obligation to treat syphilitics, regardless of how they had become infected. For these men, religious morality did not necessarily determine how they carried out their professional responsibilities.

Other doctors, however, feared the hand of God they saw in this disease. The famous anatomist Gabriel Fallopius (1523–1562), who had succeeded to Vesalius's chair at the Uni-versity of Padua, announced that God had sent the "French scab" expressly to teach people to beware his wrath and abandon venereal lust. Juan Almenar (another of Pope Alexander VI's doctors, fl. ca. 1500), believed that vices and diseases came in pairs, like the animals on Noah's ark. Thus pride was matched with fever, sloth with gout, and lust with leprosy and its modern reincarnation, the pox. These views—a throwback to ancient ideas of disease that are still echoed by the self-help preacher-healers of today—made offering a cure a moral dilemma: what if doing so endangered the patient's soul—not to mention that of the doctor, who fostered sin by curing the afflictions it caused?

Sin also haunted those Englishmen who wrote on syphilis. English doctors feared that if they provided medical care to those "wicked and sinful creatures" who brought this disease down upon themselves, the abetting physicians would be standing directly in the way of God's will. William Clowes, for example, had no interest in encouraging "rogues and idle persons, men and women," to wallow in the muck and continue to live the beastly lives that had made them sick. He published his remedies, he explained, only for the honest and good. His contemporary William Bullein (d. 1576), an English physician and botanist, read his lesson from the same text. No one who had gotten sick with the "filthy, rotten burning of harlots," Bullein argued, had any right to seek a cure: such people should not even expect to find one in his book. He provided his remedies only for the blameless, the ignorant, and the unfortunate—those who had contracted the pox through no fault of their own. The rest would have to suffer. These views were fully backed by the greatest scientific laureates of the day, such as the French surgeon Ambroise Paré (ca. 1510–1590) and the Flemish chemist and physicist Jan Baptista van Helmont (1577–1644). They too were convinced that syphilis was God's way of punishing the deadly and all-too-human affliction of lust.

▶ Innocent Victims

The fact that babies and faithful wives could contract syphilis made it impossible to condemn every single person who came down with the disease. But babies had little in common, surely, with prostitutes and adulterers, so medical authorities divided syphilitics into two groups, and treated them accordingly: the "guilty," who had earned the pox by their sinful behavior, and the "innocent," who had done nothing to deserve it. Along with drugs, these physicians also dispensed moral advice that would provide a model for social views of venereal disease in the centuries to come.

Medical writers' remarks on syphilis were a real window into their views of human nature. Some tolerance, for example, was shown by the English doctor "L. S.," author of a book called *Prophylaktikon* (1673). He reminded his fellow doctors to show patience to men who had been led by passion to commit foolish acts. The debauched husband and his lusts were detestable, of course; still, L.S. could find it in his heart to hate such a man's sins while yet loving the sinner. But the prostitutes who led these men to their destruction—theirs was a different story: the milk of this physician's kindness curdled in his breast when he thought of these pocky and infectious whores. If he had his wish, Dr. S. wrote, prostitutes would do themselves a favor and die of the pox, or do a courtesy to humankind and hang themselves. And if fortune was not so cooperative—well, Dr. S. had a remedy of his own to suggest: why not transport all the infected prostitutes away from England to the royal plantations in the New World? There they could engage in productive work, while the balmy climate improved their health. There was an added bonus, as well: the example of these sinful whores, ripped from the breast of Mother England, would terrorize lustful women and, perhaps, "fright them into better manners." Men could be cured, but wicked women must be sent far away.

The good and the wicked received their own due justice from a French medical moralist, too. In her *Collection of Easy and Domestic Remedies* (1678), Marie de Maupeou Fouquet (1590–1681) made it clear that venereal diseases were different from others. In most of her book's entries, Mme. Fouquet would simply list a disease's symptoms, and then offer a few home remedies that would cure the ill without straining a middle-class pocketbook. Venereal diseases, however, provoked a fierce and furious sermon. These ills, she explained, were not simply a health problem, but rather the natural and just consequences of the most fatal of sins, the sin that "sent more souls tumbling headlong into hell than all others combined." The proper way to treat the venereally afflicted, she declared, was not to comfort them with mild remedies, but instead to increase their torments by meting out the rigorous penances they deserved. Mme. Fouquet's flinty sense of justice, however, was melted by the warmth of divine mercy (on which, perhaps, she had learned to rely as she suffered through the long, public, and scandalous embezzlement trial of her son, Louis XIV's discredited minister of finances). Charity toward the innocent victims of syphilis led Mme. Fouquet to offer remedies for the pox, even though the guilty would unfairly benefit as a result of her kindness.

▶ Worse Than the Disease

Treatments for the pox were often more excruciating than the disease's symptoms. According to their place in society, early modern Europeans received varying types of medical care, but all were problematic. The rich were seen by physicians, whose treatments ranged from the useless to the deadly; the middle class could consult self-help books, or hire barber-surgeons to torture them with knives, drills, and white-hot cautery irons. The poor had to deal with charity hospitals. If admitted to these institutions, they were housed and fed, but they also shared beds and germs with all the other diseased patients in their ward, and often received little medical help; if they were refused admission, they suffered and died in the streets. It was hard to say which was worse—to languish untreated, as syphilis ate its way through one's organs, or to be tortured by poisonous and savage remedies administered by physicians and surgeons who often believed that their job was to punish their patients for their sins. To have syphilis in early modern Europe was a torment and a tragedy for rich and poor alike.

Doctors did not use harsh remedies at first, perhaps because the disease had not yet earned real opprobrium, or perhaps because these early cures derived from the Galenic model, which, whatever its limitations, at least employed fairly gentle methods. Physicians who viewed the disease as a humoral imbalance recommended baths, chicken broth, bloodletting, syrups, the milk of a woman who had given birth to a daughter, and even that old standby used for curing lovesickness, sexual intercourse. (This last piece of medical foolishness, fortunately, did not garner many endorsements.) Others warned of the dangers of promiscuous sex, particularly with prostitutes; some even proposed safer sex techniques for preventing the pox, such as washing the genitals, before or after intercourse, in hot vinegar or white wine. It probably took physicians awhile to realize that these mild remedies, while doing no harm, did little good either. Syphilis was new, after all, and nobody knew at first that the disease passed through primary, secondary, and tertiary stages, each with distinct symptoms and with quiescent periods in between. Eventually, though, physicians did realize that they were doing their patients no particular service with remedies of this sort.

Gradually doctors came to understand that, once aquired, syphilis tended to persist, and gradually its severe symptoms and venereal taint attracted much more aggressive medical treatment. Some doctors, for example, injected drugs directly into male patients' infected urethras. A character in the writings of the Dutch humanist scholar Desiderius Erasmus (1469–1536) spoke in favor of binding female syphilitics in chastity belts, and of deporting, castrating, and even burning pox-ridden men alive. Surgeons treated racking syphilis headaches by trepanation, the ancient practice of boring holes into the skull. Oozing ulcers in skin and bone were cauterized with fearsome, white-hot irons. Milk remedies quickly gave way to these treatments, which at least showed that doctors were doing something their patients could *feel*.

▶ These Bitter Pains and Evils

Bleeding, bathing, cautery, and herbs were used now and then, but most often, physicians fought syphilis with two important drugs: mercury, and the wood of the Central American guaiac, or *lignum vitae,* tree. Ulrich von Hutten was well acquainted with these, having suffered though the appalling mercury vapor treatment eleven times in nine years. As he explained the process in his book, patients were shut in a "stew," a small steam room, for twenty or thirty days at a time. Seated or lying down, they were spread from head to foot with a mercury-based ointment, swathed in blankets, and left until the sweat poured down; often they fainted from the heat. Disgusting secretions issued from their mouths and noses; sores filled their throats and tongues, their cheeks and lips, and the rooves of their mouths. Their jaws swelled; often their teeth fell out. Everything stank.

Many patients, von Hutten observed, decided they would rather die than undergo this torture. Others went through it, and died as a result. Von Hutten knew of one anointer, for example, who killed three men in a single day by overheating the stew. His patients suffered silently, believing that, the hotter the room, the sooner they would be cured; but though their patience lasted, their hearts gave way under the strain. Others strangled when their throats swelled so much from mercury poisoning that they could not breathe. And others still died of kidney failure when their urination was blocked too long. "Very few there were," von Hutten lamented, "that got their health, if they passed through these jeopardies, these bitter pains and evils."

Stranger methods for applying mercury were dreamed up, too. It could be taken internally, for example: one eighteenth-century recipe called for mixing the liquid metal with hot chocolate, though the author cautioned against this exotic beverage because he felt that the *chocolate* was too dangerous for those afflicted with the French disease. One entrepreneurial medic marketed underpants coated inside with a mercury ointment. All these remedies were based on the theory that, once inside the body, quicksilver atoms spread through it, eliminating the "pocky miasmas" through sweat and the copious salivation that the heavy metal provoked.

These doctors were not wrong about the virtues of mercury, which Arab physicians had used for centuries to treat diseases of the skin: mercury kills the syphilis bacterium *in vitro*, and it may also help the body's immune system to attack the microorganism. The problem, however, is that mercury is a deadly poison, particularly in vapor form or when combined with other substances. (Mercuric chloride, for example, commonly prescribed as "corrosive sublimate" in early modern medical handbooks, is fatal in doses as small as a single gram.) Von Hutten correctly noted such symptoms of mercury poisoning as excessive salivation, loosening of the teeth, pain and numbness in the extremities, uremia, and renal damage; other toxic effects include vomiting, dizziness, convulsions, tremors, liver damage, anorexia, severe diarrhea, and mental deterioration. This remedy may have helped cure skin problems, but it also hastened syphilitics to their death.

Doctors warned of these dangers as early as the 1490s. Bishop Torrella, for example, noted that mercury had killed numerous syphilis patients he knew of, including a cardinal and two members of the Borgia family. Others cautioned against excessive and internal use. But despite the suffering it caused—if not because of it—many physicians enthusiastically endorsed mercury in all of its forms, and patients continued to seek out and undergo these treatments, at the cost of their financial resources, their remaining health, and, often, their lives.

In 1517 a much-heralded new treatment for syphilis arrived in Europe, championed by many as less deadly and more effective than mercury. Von Hutten was one of these champions: his book about his experiences of syphilis was an enthusiastic testimonial for the new wonder drug, which he also endorsed as a remedy for gallstones, palsy, leprosy, dropsy, epilepsy, and gout. If we ought to give thanks upward to God for all the good and evil in this life, urged von Hutten, how much more grateful we must be for the mercy God as shown in granting us this happy remedy!

Many echoed these sentiments, reasoning that a New World medicine must be sovereign against what was perceived as a New World disease. Guaiac wood and bark were imported into Europe at staggering prices by a monopoly controlled by the House of Fugger, a mining and banking family who were the Rockefellers of their day. The syphilitic rich imbibed guaiac cocktails as often as they could, and the city of Strasbourg even provided these decoctions free of charge to all of its citizens who were afflicted with the pox.

There were, however, two drawbacks to guaiac. One was that, in actuality, it had no effect against syphilis; about all it did was to induce sweating. (The cynical and eccentric physician-alchemist Paracelsus [1493–1541] suggested—cynically but perhaps accurately—that the only people who benefited from the use of guaiac were the Fuggers.) The other problem was that the regimen under which this new drug was administered was almost as harsh as the awful mercury cure. Patients were once again installed in small heated rooms; they were placed on a rigid diet, or even kept from eating anything at all. Purged with powerful laxatives, they drank large doses of the decoction and sweated profusely for thirty or forty days in a row. Von Hutten cautioned that wine and women were to be strictly avoided during this time, lest such moral impurities anger the generous God who had provided this cure. The punitive nature of the remedy was shown even more strongly by a strange book written in 1527 by Dr. Jacques de Béthencourt, *The New Lent of Penance*. This treatise featured an argument between guaiac and mercury over which one of them cured syphilis more effectively—and which had the dubious merit of making patients suffer more in the process. Syphilitic bodies had to be purified of the disease, but they also needed to be taught a lesson; the harsher that lesson, medics obviously believed, the better.

▶ Strict Charity

For better or worse, not everyone had access to these treatments. The drugs were dreadfully expensive, and a doctor's visit could cost even more. In seventeenth-century England, for example, a single appearance by a physician might cost twenty times the daily income of a poor family of seven. Who could give up enough bread to pay such fees? The middle classes relied on healers with less formal training—surgeons, midwives, herbalists, and so on—and on the increasingly popular medium of the medical self-help book, which retailed to a popular audience the drugs and the judgmental attitudes that physicians could deliver personally to the wealthy. But it was the poor who received the largest dose of spiritual direction when they went to seek health care. This was true, most of all, in French hospitals, of which the most important by far was the Paris Hôtel-Dieu, the hospital that barred syphilis patients from its gates in 1496. On the face of things, it was shocking that the Hôtel-Dieu refused to admit these men and women, since the institution was far more tolerant than almost any other of its time. In subtler ways, however, the Hôtel-Dieu's treatment of syphilis patients simply revealed the pervasive and underlying flaws and weaknesses of the era's medical care for the poor.

Did this religious orientation affect the treatment of patients suffering from the physical and moral scourge of syphilis? It seems likely. Why else would hospitals admit plague victims, swollen, vomiting, and quick to die, yet turn away from those afflicted with the pox? It was not a question of the patient's adherence to the one true faith: the Hôtel-Dieu took in not only Christians, but even Moslems and Jews, and kept an assortment of clergymen on staff to tend to their spiritual needs. The pox, however, was evidence of a kind of sin the hospital feared even more than heresy or death.

True, there were complicating factors. Hospitals generally tried to avoid taking in patients with chronic or incurable diseases. Then as now, hospitals preferred those who would recover quickly, and who would not be a long-term drain on their resources. Moreover, syphilis arrived at a particularly inconvenient time. French hospitals had been badly hurt by the long financial depression caused by the Hundred Years' War (1337–1453), and, starting in the 1490s, the Paris Hôtel-Dieu was racked by accounting scandals and ferocious staff disputes; one unpopular new purser was greeted, on his first day of work, with insults, daggers, and an axe. The ecclesiastical mismanagement and corruption were so appalling, in fact, that over the first decades of the 1500s, public officials took these hospitals over and barred churchmen from holding any administrative posts. The last thing these chaotic institutions needed was a new onslaught of patients afflicted with a virulent, contagious, and disgusting venereal disease.

Most of all, however, syphilis patients were turned away because their disease was a moral problem so severe that it barred even charity itself. Part of this rejection was caused by revulsion; part was caused by the fact that charity was becoming a much more selective enterprise than it had been. Starting in the 1500s, those who gave imposed increasingly high moral standards on those who received, and poor syphilitics were obvious targets for the judgmental upper class. In the Middle Ages, giving away money had been seen as a virtuous end in itself, and monasteries and the rich willingly distributed largesse. But this system, though based in generosity, was often ineffectual: it had no mechanisms to ensure that money went where it was most needed. As the Middle Ages gave way to the Renaissance, and close-knit feudal society yielded to capitalist economies, rich and poor led increasingly separate lives. Inflation increased, and so did begging—and crime. Charity was viewed, more and more, as a way to control social problems linked with the poor.

The Protestant Reformation played its part in these changing attitudes. Luther constantly reminded those with means that they had to care for those without, but he also stressed the moral responsibilities of the poor. Writing on welfare reform in 1520, he reminded the public of St. Paul's dictum "Whoever will not work shall not eat." Cities had to care for the unfortunate, said Luther, but they also had the right to determine who was truly deserving and who was not. The poor who passed muster were given food and services; the rest (foreigners, malingerers, the idle) were driven away, ridiculed, punished, or even locked up. Women who were considered to be "in danger of becoming lost" were carted off to institutions for "correction," sometimes at the instigation of their husbands. Seventeenth-century English laws ordered that vagabonds be whipped and paraded through town with the letter "V" fastened to their breast, a model for Hawthorne's adulterous Hester Prynne and her scarlet "A." A 1635 English legal handbook distinguished those who were "poor by impotency and defect" (the blind, the lame, the aged, the diseased) and the "poor by casualty" (the victims of accidents, etc.) from "the thriftless poor"—the slothful, the dissolute, vagabonds, and drunks. Judgment and care were appointed accordingly. Those who were sick and poor might merit charity, or they might merit punishment, depending on whether they were viewed as being innocent or at fault. Poverty was no longer an unfortunate state that merited help from the lucky; instead, as one historian of the period explains, it had become "a moral condition to be evaluated and judged."

Who was easier to judge than the pox-ridden? Already suspect, the poor were seen as idlers, wastrels, or worse; those with syphilis bore the signs of their vices on their suppurating bodies. It was better for all concerned simply to exclude them from care. Many people felt that there was no good reason to shelter and feed these dangerous and wicked sinners, and, often enough, institutions and municipalities acted according to these beliefs.

▶ Doctors, Patients, and Expectations

How did the treatment of syphilis square with the social and medical expectations of the time? How did it relate to the diseases that had gone before, and what kind of model did it provide for those to come?

These are not easy questions to answer. Even at the beginning of the twenty-first century, the study of "outcomes evaluation" is still a new and uncertain part of health care management; for times long past, standards and results are even more difficult to evaluate. Still, we have enough information to gain insights into what people expected medicine to accomplish in these centuries, and to evaluate whether syphilis was handled appropriately for the standards of the day.

Compared to today, people in Renaissance Europe expected relatively little of medicine. They saw health and illness, explains medical historian Katharine Park, not as polar opposites, but as variable points along a continuum. Moving patients from one point on this scale to another at which they felt more comfortable was probably seen as successful treatment by patient and practitioner alike. Probably few people expected to live lives free of pain and suffering; if physicians, surgeons, and herbalists could free them from their more acute and pressing problems, patients probably felt they had been treated properly.

Still, many were discontented with those who provided health care—particularly with physicians, who were often seen as arrogant and grasping. When epidemics struck, people looked to medical men for protection, but they were usually disappointed in the results. Even in 1370, for example, plague prompted the Italian humanist Francis Petrarch (1304–1374) to send the following accusation to a professor of medicine: "Doctors promote themselves shamelessly, making exorbitant claims about their competence. Yet when faced with an emergency like plague, they can only inveigle the trustful out of their money and watch them die." Three centuries later, Thomas Sydenham (1624–1689), the "English Hippocrates," admitted that many poor people were alive precisely because they could not afford to pay for medical treatment. As time went on, hopes rose higher, but this often led to greater disappointments. One eighteenth-century French doctor wrote that he could handle the expectations of the general public. He complained, however, that "what is annoying about the upper classes if that, when they come to be sick, they absolutely want their doctors to cure them."

Treatments for syphilis provoked similar reactions, as von Hutten's bitter recriminations about mercury plainly showed. The punitive harshness of syphilis treatments, combined with the expense and the judgmental attitudes with which medical authorities commonly administered them, speaks ill of the times, as does the expulsion of the pox-ridden from hospitals, cities, and towns. Physicians and surgeons multiplied the torments of the sick; quacks exploited them for easy cash. Doctors and divines alike reminded the sufferers and their neighbors that the pox was a sign of wickedness. Von Hutten died, penniless and syphilitic, at the age of thirty-five, sheltered by the Swiss reformer Hyldrich Zwingli but rejected by Erasmus, his former friend. Summing up his experiences with the clergy, von Hutten bitterly remarked, "The divines did interpretate this to be the wrath of God, and to be his punishment for our evil living. And so did openly preach, as though they, admitted into that high council of God, had there learned, that men never lived worse." The physical burdens of syphilis were thus made even heavier by social, medical, and moral torment. To a modern viewer, certainly, it seems that the social response to syphilis—like the response to leprosy—revealed not only a failure of health care, but also a failure of the most basic Christian virtue of all, the virtue of charity. Moralizing, for many, took precedence over the fundamental commands to feed the hungry, clothe the naked, and heal the sick.

Europe was not alone in this regard. Islamic nations judged syphilis as harshly as Christian ones did, just as the faraway societies of East Asia and India had viewed leprosy as divine punishment. The fact that European prejudice against syphilitics was not unique, however, did not make it right—nor did it make it any easier for the rejected to bear.

There were some bright spots in the gloom. Some physicians were moved to compassion for their syphilitic patients. Even the misogynistic Dr. L. S., for example, argued that "the more loathsome the disease, the more commiseration is required, and the physician is obliged to a more tender care." Some cities *were* charitable. Strasbourg opened a special hospital for its syphilitics; Lyon and Frankfurt, soon after the epidemic hit, cut taxes for the sick. The new disease may also have helped to advance medical knowledge and health care, as physicians thought more carefully about infectious diseases, and cities and hospitals developed specialized clinics, rather than treat all the sick poor together in the same infectious wards.

All too often, however, syphilis provoked responses reminiscent of the most brutal and unfeeling reactions to leprosy and plague. Charity and compassion were often overpowered by prejudice and fear. The limits of medical knowledge and old histories of anger and terror at disease proved almost irresistible, and syphilis created even more panic by mixing terror about physical illness with Christian culture's ancient and profound anxieties about sex. The unfortunate Europeans who suffered from syphilis experienced the worst of disease, medicine, and religious condemnation all at once—a deadly mixture, and a dangerous model for the centuries ahead.

Chapter 2

Ethical Principles

Ethics and Public Health: Forging a Strong Relationship

Daniel Callahan, Ph.D., and Bruce Jennings, M.D.

Ethics and Public Health

The field of bioethics arose in the late 1960s in response to the emerging ethical dilemmas of that era. The field for many years focused in general on the dilemmas generated by high-technology medicine rather than on issues of population health and the ethical problems of public health programs and regulations. The time has come to more fully integrate the ethical problems of public health into the field of public health and, at the same time, into the field of bioethics. Public health raises a number of moral problems that extend beyond the earlier boundaries of bioethics and require their own form of ethical analysis.

When the field of bioethics emerged in the late 1960s and early 1970s, it represented a significant broadening of medical ethics. It moved the subject beyond the doctor-patient relationship and medical professionalism into the new territory of, among other things, organ transplants, genetics, reproductive biology, and resource allocation. But little attention was paid by bioethics in its early years to the distinctive ethical problems inherent in public health. That is perhaps not surprising. Bioethics received its initial stimulus from the abuses of human subjects research, the emergence of the patients' rights movement and the drama of high-technology medicine. That focus on technology has continued, as has a lack of thoroughgoing engagement with issues of social and economic inequality, which have been staples of attention in public health since the 19th century.

In early bioethics, the good of the individual, and particularly his or her autonomy, was the dominant theme, not population health. The bioethics movement, moreover, shadowed the rapid expansion of the biomedical research enterprise, first in the search for cures through better biological understanding and technological innovation and then in the ensuing struggle over issues of equitable access as the cost of health care steadily rose. Meanwhile, the field of public health—though sporadically brought to public attention by the polio epidemics of the 1950s, by the smoking and lung cancer reports, and by the AIDS pandemic—was moved to the shadows to some extent by the drama of advances in biomedicine.

But the times are changing, as they should, and some fresh winds are blowing. The last decade or so has produced a much needed resurgence of public visibility for public health. There are at least 2 reasons for this. One is the unwelcome reminder that infectious disease has not, in fact, been conquered. The second is the recognition that the health of populations is a function more of good public health measures and socioeconomic conditions than of biomedical advances, even though it is true that public health needs biomedicine to do its work fully, especially through disease screening programs and the biomedical techniques they require. This has long been commonplace within the public health community, but it has been a neglected truth by most outside the field.

As the concern of health policymakers turns toward health outcomes, cost-effectiveness, and preventive measures throughout the life cycle (primary, secondary, and tertiary prevention), the field of public health is gaining increased public and legislative attention. Research!America, a leading advocacy group long focused on biomedical research advocacy, is now working with a strong coalition to promote health and disease prevention research, and many private foundations are giving such research a more conspicuous position on their agendas.

Of course, the prominence of public health has not displaced that of biomedicine, which, during this same period, has had the Human Genome Project, among other things, to sustain it. Nonetheless, public health is once more a force to be reckoned with, and it is increasingly apparent that public health must contribute to the definition of the ends as well as the means of health policy. It is hard to overestimate the chastening effect that HIV/AIDS, multiple-drug–resistant tuberculosis, Lyme disease, and other serious infectious diseases have had on this development. Nor should we forget how much research in the field of public health has, since the 1960s, taught us about the looming challenges of health care in an aging society: chronic illness, high-risk health-related behavior, injuries, and the interaction between health and the environment.

As the field of public health becomes more prominent, so will the ethical issues associated with it.[1] As more teaching and research are done on ethics in public health, it is important to begin a focused conversation within the field and between the field and others. What are the basic ethical issues of public health? What ethical orientations are most helpful in the clarification and resolution of these issues? How are ethical principles and concepts incorporated into decision making in public health agencies and programs? How adequately are the ethical dimensions of public health policy identified and debated? What are the chances for a fruitful collaboration between public health and bioethics, and what factors would be conducive to its success?

For its part, bioethics has become restless for change, and it is particularly looking for a value orientation that may bring it into closer proximity with public health. There has always been an undercurrent of resistance to the individualistic, autonomy-driven mainstream orientation within bioethics, and that orientation has held sway. And why not? In keeping with the cultural trends of the 1970s and 1980s, it has often brought together the political left and the market-oriented right in a celebration of choice and freedom. But the obvious need for universal health care, the persistence of racial and ethnic disparities in health status, and the importance of background social and economic factors have caught the eye of many.[2] A shift of direction in the field of bioethics was called for, and it has already begun. By the mid-1990s, increased interest in population health had emerged, the ethical dilemmas faced by public health programs were attracting attention, and courses on ethics and public health had begun to appear with greater frequency in the curriculum of schools of public health.

Although interest in public health and ethics has been present in the field for many years—one thinks of the long-standing concern among epidemiologists—those in the field of public health seem to welcome the growing interest among their colleagues in bioethics. There is a small but growing cadre of ethicists writing and teaching within the field of public health itself. In the 1980s, the American Public Health Association established a special primary interest group on bioethics, the Forum on Bioethics (now called the Forum on Ethics), that certainly facilitated the discussions and networking of public health ethics scholars.

The importance of ethics was recognized again in 1997, when the Centers for Disease Control and Prevention (CDC) established an ethics subcommittee of the Director's Advisory Committee. Ethical guidelines have been developed by the American College of Epidemiology and the American Statistical Association. Most recently, a work group of the Public Health Leadership Society established a group to develop a code of ethics for the field, and the Association of Schools of Public Health (ASPH) initiated a curriculum development project designed to advance the teaching of ethics in public health.

The interest in ethics and public health is clearly there, and the question now is how to bring it to maturity so that it can make the most helpful contributions. The benefits can and should run in 2 directions, toward illuminating some important problems in public health and enriching and expanding bioethics. Still, it is fair to say that there are some significant obstacles to such a dialogue. We have already alluded to one such obstacle, namely, the difference between the individualistic orientation of bioethics and the population and societal focus of public health. This is not so much an intrinsic difference between the 2 fields as it is a difference between the perspectives of the public health and policy world, on the one hand, and the world of clinical medicine (in which bioethics has principally operated), on the other.

More difficult will be the tension produced by the predominant orientation in favor of civil liberties and individual autonomy that one finds in bioethics, as opposed to the utilitarian, paternalistic, and communitarian orientations that have marked the field of public health throughout its history.[3] The ethical and policy issues concerning, for example, HIV and multidrug-resistant tuberculosis already have thrust public health ethics into the thick of this clash of values. And, if the issue of paternalism (limiting the freedom of the individual for the sake of his or her own greater good or best interests) were not enough, the cognate clash between individualistic civil liberties and a communitarian orientation (limiting the freedom of the individual for the sake of the common good or public interest) will also provoke lively discussion.

Neither of these conflicts are intractable, however. Beginning with the civil libertarian concerns of the AIDS epidemic in the 1980s, a rights-based orientation has made a strong mark, occasioning some important struggles about the relationship between individual and society and seeking better ways to balance community health needs and individual rights. Moreover, the international human rights framework, which has been given serious consideration in public health by Jonathan Mann, Lawrence Gostin, Sophia Gruskin, and others, is one potential path of synthesis among these conflicting ethical perspectives, and other frameworks described later in this commentary, such as the analytic and critical ethical frameworks, may be able to come to the same resolution as well.[4]

▶ The Scope of Public Health Ethics

Just as public health is broad in its scope, the range of ethical issues in the field is uncommonly wide, encompassing ethics in public health as well as the ethics of public health. If ethics is understood to be a search for those values, virtues, and principles necessary for people to live together in peace, mutual respect, and justice, then there are few issues in public health that do not admit of an ethical perspective. To begin to map the scope of this broad terrain, 4 general categories of such issues should be noted: health promotion and disease prevention, risk reduction, epidemiological and other forms of public health research, and structural and socioeconomic disparities in health status.

Health Promotion and Disease Prevention

Programs designed to promote health and prevent disease and injury raise questions about the responsibility of individuals to live healthy lives; about the government's role in creating an environment in which individuals are able to exercise their health related responsibility; about the role of government in coercing or influencing health-related behavior or in developing educational programs; about the use of incentives, economic or otherwise, to promote good health; and about the relative importance for society of pursuing good health, particularly in a culture that prizes autonomy and does not always look fondly on government intervention.[5]

Risk Reduction

Risks to the health of the public are many, and many methods are used to reduce or eliminate them.[6] Almost all can pose one or more ethical problems. The concept of risk itself is seemingly impossible to define in value-neutral terms and is inherently controversial. Even more ethically charged is the question of what level or degree of risk is socially acceptable to individuals and communities. Who should decide about that and how should exposure to risk be distributed across the affected population?[7] Researchers in epidemiology are often reluctant to draw broad general conclusions from their data, but pressure from policymakers on public health professionals is often intense to provide a definitive recommendation or answer.

A significant debate in public health ethics is whether and to what extent the so-called "precautionary principle" should be followed. In essence, this principle places the burden of proof on those who would initiate risk to demonstrate that the benefits will outweigh the dangers and that the risk is rationally worth taking. There is, however, often an inconsistency in that those who propose the removal of risk find that the burden is on them to prove that their cause is worth spending money on.

Routine public health practice entails a number of interventions and policies designed to prevent harm to individuals and to lower health risks within the population. These include various forms of screening and testing of different age groups, many of which are legally mandatory and paternalistic or are administered in a way that does not follow the requirements of informed consent. Epidemiologic practice, especially when mandated by state laws, may not always follow appropriate ethical protocols on the rights of human subjects, and the collection of health information may sometimes put the public health practitioner in a position of possessing information that certain individuals (e.g., employers, insurance providers) might have an interest in knowing. The responsibilities of the public health researcher regarding individual notification and protection of personal privacy and confidentiality are not yet clearly set out as a matter of consensus within the profession. The experience with HIV/AIDS in the past 2 decades has shown how problematic it can be when public health officials seek to employ fairly standard practices such as contact tracing and partner notification to curb the spread of sexually transmitted diseases.[8,9]

Epidemiological and Other Public Health Research

Research with human subjects has been a central ethical problem for biomedicine for at least 100 years, but particularly since World War II. Yet, is the biomedical model—focused on individual informed consent and tightly regulated research with those at risk of exploitation—an appropriate model for public health, one that may either pose no medical or other risks to individuals or make consent impractical to gain in research encompassing large communities? And should the research standards used in the United States be exactly the same for research in other countries, particularly developing countries?

Structural and Socioeconomic Disparities

It has been known for many years that socioeconomic disparities have a major impact on health status. Equitable access to decent health care and reductions in health status disparities have been long-sought goals in American society but have not always been dealt with in the context of socioeconomic disparities. What is the appropriate role for the public health community in seeking greater justice in health care, and how should it balance its fact-finding and educational role with its historically strong advocacy mission?

To some, for example, it is surprising and disturbing that more attention has not been paid by the public health community and in the ethics literature to ethical issues of occupational health and safety and to the ethical problems that arise when considering the health implications of environmental policy. These are 2 major areas in which the following of lines of inquiry on ethical and social value issues is likely to expose the need for far more attention to empirical research than public health specialists have yet provided. Finally, to what extent, if any, should the field adopt a politically partisan posture, taking a public stand on important policy issues and legislative initiatives?

▶ Types of Ethical Analysis

While the preceding classification of broad issues by no means exhausts the possible categories of topics, it is sufficient to make evident that no single method of ethical analysis can be used for all of them (or even for the great variety of subtopics involved with any of the particular issues). In our pluralistic society, numerous ethical perspectives coexist on matters of such widespread interest and importance as public health. Ethical analysis can be usefully divided into a number of different types, depending on the point of view and needs from which it originates. One or more of them might be appropriate for any specific ethical problem.

Professional Ethics

The study of professional ethics tends to seek out the values and standards that have been developed by the practitioners and leaders of a given profession over a long period of time and to identify those values that seem most salient and inherent in the profession itself. Applied to public health, this perspective entails identifying the central mission of the profession (e.g., protection and promotion of the health of all members of society) and building up a body of ethical principles and standards that would protect the trust and legitimacy the profession should maintain.

Applied Ethics

Another approach to public health ethics comes from the field that has emerged in recent years as applied or practical ethics. Bioethics is one area among others within this domain of ethics. The applied ethics perspective differs from the professional ethics perspective principally in that it adopts a point of view from outside the history and values of the profession. From this more general moral and social point of view, applied ethics seeks to devise general principles that can then be applied to real-world examples of professional conduct or decision making. These principles and their application are designed to give professionals guidance and to provide those individuals affected by professional behavior, as well as the general public, with standards to use in assessing the professions. Thus, in applied ethics, there is a tendency to reason abstractly and to draw from general ethical theories rather than from the folkways and knowledge base of the professions. The emphasis tends to be on professional conduct rather than on the virtues of professional character.

Advocacy Ethics

If there is a characteristic ethical orientation within the field of public health today, it is probably less theoretical or academic than either professional ethics or applied ethics. While on occasion it can pose difficulties for civil servants, the ethical persuasion most lively in the field is a stance of advocacy for those social goals and reforms that public health professionals believe will enhance general health and well-being, especially among those least well off in society. Such advocacy is in keeping with the natural priorities of those who devote their careers to public health. It has a strong orientation toward equality and social justice. Much of the research and expertise in public health throughout its history has shown how social deprivation, inequality, poverty, and powerlessness are directly linked to poor health and the burden of disease. In recent years, a growing international movement in support of human rights has exerted an important influence on public health as well.

Critical Ethics

Finally, we would distinguish yet another possible perspective on ethics that could be directed toward the distinctive issues and problems of public health. For want of a better term, we label it "critical ethics." In many ways, it attempts to combine the strengths of the other perspectives mentioned. Like professional ethics, it is historically informed and practically oriented toward the specific real-world and real-time problems of public health, but, like applied ethics, it brings larger social values and historical trends to bear in its understanding of the current situation of public health and the moral problems faced. These problems are not only the result of the behavior of certain disease organisms or particular individuals. They are also the result of institutional arrangements and prevailing structures of cultural attitudes and social power.

The perspective of critical ethics has much in common with the egalitarian and human rights–oriented discourse of advocacy ethics in public health. One possible advantage of critical ethics is its call for discussions of ethics and public health policy to be genuinely public or civic endeavors: not the advocacy of a well-intentioned elite on behalf of needy clients, but a search for forums and programs of meaningful participation, open deliberation, and civic problem solving and capacity building. Some of the best examples of public health practice, from this point of view, grow out of efforts to champion communities as places of mutual support, respect, and self-esteem, thereby reinforcing health-promoting behaviors among their individual members.

We submit that a rich discourse on ethics and public health cannot be advanced without relating it to the background values of the general society, and the particular communities, in which it will be carried out. Our Canadian neighbors in public health have much more consciously attempted to relate public health and the sociopolitical values of that country's society.[10] It is one thing to say that public health rests on a communitarian foundation and quite another to determine how best to relate that foundation to our individualist culture, particularly in that members of this culture have been historically hostile toward government. The conflict, long endemic in our society, between the right of individuals to be left alone and the needs of the larger public does not make it easy to develop population-based health strategies that must, on occasion, ignore the special needs of individuals.

▶ An Ethical Code?

The work of the Public Health Leadership Society in initiating a process to establish a code of ethics for public health is important. Where does a code of ethics fit into a broader confrontation with ethical issues? Most professions have a code, and of course many professionals in public health belong to one or another of such professions. Considering this, is there any need for an additional code for public health? There are at least 3 reasons to have a code. One of them is to respond to scandals in a field, aiming to ensure better future conduct. Some business and governmental codes of ethics had that aim as their origin. Another is to help establish the moral credibility of a field and its professional status and to provide principles to deal with common dilemmas. Such was the 19th-century origin of the code of ethics of the American Medical Association. Still another purpose is to provide a profession with a moral compass and to set forth its ideals. Some professional codes, such as that of the American Bar Association, include a large number of concrete rules to deal with almost every kind of ethical problem.

This is not the place to discuss ethics codes in detail, but some general considerations are worth noting. Public health has rarely been attacked for a lack of professionalism or for scandals, and the field is unlikely to be attracted to a code similar to that of the American Bar Association. The greatest challenge in writing a code is to specify clearly the ideals of the field and then to specify some general guidelines that will be illuminating for the wide array of problems practitioners can encounter. Historically, many if not most professional codes have been written because of structural changes in a profession that have generated new ethical problems and made it necessary to shore up public confidence in the profession's integrity.

We believe that the integrity of the profession of public health is sound, but the changing situation of public health practice may be a good reason to more precisely specify the ethical obligations that those in the field take on when they become practitioners. Code developments and revisions, it might be noted, have often been most successful when they are accompanied by lengthy and strenuous debate engaging the entire professional community and not simply those with a special interest in ethics.

▶ Science and Public Ethics

Public health ethics and public health science are often connected. A good example is the ethics of public health decision making. Public health professionals recommend preventive interventions that presumably will—on balance—benefit the public's health. Existing scientific evidence and, especially, its interpretation play important roles in these decisions.

What makes the ethics of decision making so difficult is the presence of scientific complexity and scientific uncertainty. The evidence used in making claims about disease causation and about the efficacy of preventive interventions typically arises from several sources: biological (laboratory) science, epidemiological and clinical sciences, and the social and behavioral sciences. Furthermore, the methods used to summarize evidence are more qualitative than quantitative. Making valid and reliable claims under those circumstances is difficult.[11] Public health decisions carry with them varying levels of empirical uncertainty. The extent to which the public's health ultimately benefits or does not benefit in the face of such uncertainty is not well established.

There are other ethical concerns that emerge from public health's strong connection to science. Research ethics provides many examples, such as scientific misconduct.[12] The choice of research topics is another. The values that determine where and how public health research dollars are spent have important ethical implications.

▶ Law and Ethics

Public health is one of the few professions that has, in many matters, legal power—in particular, the police power of the state—behind it. It can, through use of the law, coerce citizens into behaving in some approved, healthy way: for example, by forcing immunization on their children, by restricting their right to smoke in public places, or by quarantining them to stop the spread of infectious disease. Public health also has the distinction, along with a few others—such as city management, public administration, and law enforcement—of being a profession in which many practitioners are government employees and officials. It thus has an obligation both toward government, which controls it, and toward the public that it serves.

Because of its public and governmental roles, public health has ethical problems unlike those of most other professions. The relationship between ethics and law is a long and tangled one, but it is safe to say that most public health laws and regulations have behind them an explicitly moral purpose: that of promoting and protecting the lives of citizens. Because the police power of the state is involved, however, a number of moral conflicts are generated. The tension between individual health and rights, on the one hand, and government obligations and population health, on the other, is an obvious instance of this kind of conflict The economic and social impact on communities of public health measures, requiring some form of cost-benefit analysis, is another.

Health is an important human need, and good health is highly valued. But health is not the only need or good health the only value. Laws must always find ways of balancing various goods, and the centrality of laws for the work of public health brings uncommon visibility to its actions and an uncommon need for public accountability.

▶ Politics and Public Health

As public arguments over fluoridation or HIV disease amply demonstrate, public health measures can quickly become politicized. Political controversy is often treated as some kind of disaster for calm reflection and measured rationality. This is sometimes in fact the case, but given the governmental role of public health and its use of coercion for many purposes, politics is unavoidable and necessary. It is unavoidable because there is no way to stop the public from turning to legislatures or the courts to express their values and needs; nor should there be. Politics is a necessary component of public health, moreover, precisely in order to achieve public health policies and practices consistent with American traditions and values. Politics is the messy arena in which ultimate questions of the public good are worked out. Ethics, Aristotle wrote 2500 years ago, is a branch of politics—a shrewd insight—and it is surely true in this country that the most important moral struggles almost always end in the public arena.

Yet, there can be responsible and irresponsible politics. Public health can best serve the cause of responsible politics, even when it has a self-interested stake in the outcome, when it makes available good data, when it is sensitive to community sentiments, and when it makes clear by all of its actions that it is not (as the stereotype would have it) just one more self-serving, distant government bureaucracy. Public health receives its money from the public, gains its legal powers from the public, and must be judged by the effectiveness of its service to the public. As long as this is kept clearly in mind, public health can survive the imposition of politics on its work and can, in fact, flourish.

▶ Curriculum Development

One crucial question toward which the preceding discussion points is how to promote a greater awareness and a more sustained, sophisticated discussion of ethical issues among public health practitioners and researchers themselves, as well as among the broader public. In any professional field, ethical sensitivity and discernment exist, to the extent that they exist, only if they begin early in the educational and socialization processes of the field and only if ethics is a discipline that is taken seriously both by the academic wing of the profession in its writing and teaching and by the practice wing of the profession in its conduct. In these respects, we reluctantly observe, the field of public health has an important opportunity for advancement. Ethics education has a university-based ("preservice") component and a workplace-based or continuing education ("in-service") component. Both are essential, and the in-service setting is particularly crucial in public health because so many practitioners receive their academic training in cognate fields.

The Teaching of Public Health Ethics

An obvious and crucial step to take is to promote the teaching of ethics in all schools of public health in the United States. In the past decade, a handful of public health programs have integrated some ethics education into their course offerings, but not to the extent of their close neighbors, medical and nursing schools. Much more needs to be done if there is going to be serious study and discussion of the myriad ethical issues arising in public health comparable to the impressive body of work achieved by medical ethics and bioethics.

In the first place, the teaching of ethics in public health is still quite limited. In a 1999 study, 24 schools of public health were surveyed to assess their formal ethics instruction. Only 8 schools required course work in ethics, and only 1 school required it of all students. Fourteen more schools offered an elective course. Many schools had occasional ethics lectures and symposia.[14] This means that a significant percentage of each graduating class at the master's level has not been exposed to a systematic and sustained analysis of ethical issues in the field, led by a faculty member with sufficient training in ethics.

Moreover, a review of syllabi collected through an ASPH-conducted project revealed that most of the courses listed in the curricula of schools of public health are in fact primarily courses in medical ethics. While it is beneficial for members of the public health community to be aware of bioethical issues, it is even more important to isolate those practice and policy issues that are distinctive to public health or that set up a balance between the interests of health care consumers and the public health objectives of the society as a whole. In a number of cases, the teaching of ethics in public health is not strictly speaking, public health ethics but rather some generic offering of bioethics with one or two public health topics salted in. Such courses will introduce students of public health to the rudiments of ethical reasoning but will do little to advance ethical solutions to dilemmas that arise in public health practice. Of course, there are prominent exceptions to this general observation, but their example has not been widely followed.

Why has more not been done? The fact is that the teaching of ethics in any professional school is controversial, intellectually difficult, institutionally challenging, and expensive. (The same is true for ethics education in in-service settings.) Nonetheless, there are good reasons why ethics in public health can and should be taught.

The teaching of ethics is controversial primarily because the dominant ethos of most professions is empiricist, quantitative, and oriented toward precise, definitive solutions to discrete problems. This often does not comport well with the intellectual characteristics of ethical analysis, which focus on the multifaceted nature of problems—the difficulty in finding definitive solutions to problems that take complex forms as analogies, narratives, or dilemmas—and on the qualitative and interpretative character of moral judgment in contrast to the quantitative knowledge that carries legitimacy in most professional fields. In public health there is an opening for the teaching of ethics in part because it has been so well accepted in medicine, which still exerts a powerful influence in the field of public health, and in part because public health is itself a multidisciplinary field. Although there are certainly strongly quantitative elements present in public health, there is also a substantial influence from history, law, and the social sciences, areas in which qualitative reasoning akin to ethics is well regarded.

Beyond these academic considerations, however, support for the teaching of ethics in many fields has come from students themselves, on the one side, and from practitioners, on the other. Students want to engage the value and social issues of their chosen profession and not merely its most technical aspects. For their part, practitioners well recognize the inevitability of the ethical quandaries in the world beyond graduate preparation. They need and expect young professionals to emerge from their training with more than technical information and intelligence. They want precisely the kinds of reasoning ability and capacity for judgment that ethics education, properly conducted, provides. There is no reason why the combined forces of student interest and the practice needs of the profession should not succeed in prompting the addition of ethics to the public health curriculum as well.

The teaching of ethics in schools of public health will be intellectually challenging for many of the reasons we have reviewed here. The field is not well unified and does not have a clear consciousness of itself as a profession. The conceptual and intellectual framework necessary to develop a public health ethics is not yet in place. In consequence, the academic qualifications appropriate for faculty in public health ethics and a solid body of written work for students to study are lacking. Rarely will existing faculty in schools of public health step forward to teach a course in ethics. Qualified people will have to be brought in from the outside or recruited from other faculties within the university. Those who have been teaching bioethics in medical school or at the undergraduate level will find that a substantially new and different course should be created for public health students.

Institutionally, any change in an already crowded and overtaxed curriculum is difficult. Qualified faculty must be put in place, and that costs money. Ethics faculty may not be able to bring in the kinds of research grants that scholars in other disciplines can generate. Moreover, if space is to be made for ethics, some other work may have to give way. The advance of biomedical science is unrelenting; arguably, subjects such as genetics need much more attention in the public health curriculum than they have had before. The same could be said for economics or health services research.

If a case is to be made for giving time to ethics in a crowded scientific curriculum, it must be made on the basis of a conception of the profession that is richer than the mastery of technical knowledge and skills. It also must be made on the basis of a conception of the qualities and abilities that a public health professional should possess if he or she is to be truly educated toward public service: sound judgment, ability to recognize and analyze ethical issues, tolerance for ambiguity, and capacity for a moral imagination with which seemingly isolated issues or events can be placed in a broader context of human experience and value. These are educational goals worthy of an attempt to overcome whatever institutional or financial challenges curriculum innovation in public health may require.

Continuing Ethics Education

Another step that can be taken to encourage better discussion of and sensitivity toward ethical issues in public health is to promote, insofar as is practical, continuing education materials and programs for public health practitioners in the field. Because the profession is so dispersed in its work—from employment in private managed care organizations and clinics to international nongovernmental organizations and federal, state, and local agencies—it is difficult to know where to begin with this in-service ethics education effort. Perhaps state departments of health would be as good a place as any to start. And university graduate schools of public health should do more to reach out to the practice community and support the development of in-service ethics programs.

▶ Recommendations

To promote the discussion and advancement of ethics in public health, we offer the following recommendations.

1. Leaders in public health should support the development of conferences and symposia on the theme of ethics and public health. Creating these forums will encourage both scholars and practitioners to turn their attention to original research and writing, will help to sharpen the issues, and will attract the attention of scholars in other fields such as bioethics, history, sociology, and political science, encouraging them to undertake new work on topics relating to public health and public health ethics. The US Public Health Service, the surgeon general, and the CDC could take the lead in this effort. Such symposia could be sponsored and supported by federal and state agencies, schools of public health, the leading public health professional journals, and major foundations that have an abiding interest in the field of public health as a scientific and professional resource for the country.

2. The editors of leading public health and bioethics journals should give high priority to accepting and soliciting rigorous work in public health ethics for publication. This type of recognition will lead to the acceptance of work in public health ethics as valid scholarship within the field, and it will produce the reading materials that courses in public health ethics can use.

3. Efforts should be undertaken to compile a set of case materials for ethics discussion and teaching. These materials, in fact, have pedagogical uses that are not limited to ethics. They could be akin to the case studies developed by the Harvard Business School, and they should explore in detail the complexity of public health practice and the ethical issues that are embedded within it.

4. The specific topic of ethical issues in public health research should be a focus. This topic certainly deserves fresh attention, and it should be part of the current agenda for the various governmental and private bodies that oversee the human subjects research area. There is a tremendous resurgence of interest in research ethics in biomedicine across the board today, and epidemiological and public health research should be firmly included on that agenda as well.

5. The accreditation process for schools of public health should involve an increase in ethics instruction requirements. It may be premature to mandate that all students take required course work in ethics, but all schools of public health should give priority to ethics in their curriculum development planning. Ethics-related learning objectives could at least be incorporated into existing courses in the curriculum. This indirect approach should give way to more systematic instruction once the field has had time to develop the necessary faculty expertise and literature in ethics.

6. As a profession, public health should develop continuing education requirements and make ethics prominent among them. This type of initiative could start at the governmental level: anyone employed as a public health officer or professional should attend periodic programs designed to educate practitioners on ethical issues they face.

7. Public health agency managers and supervisors at the federal, state, and local levels should be encouraged to provide the time and resources necessary for periodic in-service ethics sessions. There is value in having in-service programs conducted at workplaces so that discussions can involve multidisciplinary and multilevel coworkers. With the right support and leadership, such sessions can create an atmosphere of trust and candor so that problems can be addressed and solutions sought. Those involved with similar programs in other professions have discovered that such sessions not only serve to provide education about ethics but also can improve working relations and morale.

8. Scholars in the field of ethics should educate themselves about public health and develop a more sophisticated understanding of how ethical issues in public health might best be approached. Throughout, all activities should run a strong and imaginative effort to better specify the nature and range of ethical issues and how they might best be analyzed. The field of public health ethics has great promise. Careful thought, blended with experience, will be necessary to fulfill that promise. Academics, practitioners, and ethicists within the field and those outside it should cooperate in this important endeavor.[15]

Contributors

D. Callahan and B. Jennings both led the writing of this commentary.

Acknowledgement

We wish to acknowledge the generous support of the Robert Wood Johnson Foundation.

References

1. Beauchamp TE, Steinbock B, eds. *New Ethics for the Public's Health.* New York, NY: Oxford University Press Inc; 1999.
2. Faden R. "Bioethics and public health in the 1980s: resource allocation and AIDS." *Annu Rev Public Health* 1991;12:335–360.
3. Leichter H. *Free to Be Foolish.* Princeton, NJ: Princeton University Press; 1992.
4. Mann J, Gruskin S, Grodin MA, eds. *Health and Human Rights: A Reader.* New York, NY: Routledge; 1999.
5. Faden R. "Ethical issues in government sponsored public health campaigns." *Health Educ Q.* 1987;14:27–37.
6. Leviton L, Needleman CE, Shapiro MA. *Confronting Public Health Risks: A Decision Makers Guide.* Thousand Oaks, Calif: Sage Publications; 1998.
7. Stem PC, Fineberg HV, eds. *Understanding Risk: Informing Decisions in a Democratic Society.* Washington, DC: Academic Press; 1996.
8. Fox DM. "From TB to AIDS: value conflicts in reporting disease." *Hastings Center Rep.* 1986;11:11–16.
9. Bayer R, Toomey KE. "HIV prevention and the two faces of partner notification." *Am Public Health.* 1995;85: 1569–1576.
10. Robertson A. "Health promotion and the common good: reflection on the politics of need." In: Callahan D, ed. *Promoting Health Behavior.—How Much Freedom? Whose Responsibility?* Washington DC: Georgetown University Press; 2001;76–94.
11. Weed DL. "Epistemology and virtue ethics." *Int J Epidemiol.* 1998;27:343–349.
12. Weed DL. "Epistemology and ethics in epidemiology." In: Coughlin SS, Beauchamp TL, eds. *Ethics and Epidemiology.* New York, NY: Oxford University Press Inc; 1998:79–94.
13. Gostin LO. *Public Health Law: Power, Duty, Restraint.* Berkeley, Calif: University of California Press/Milbank Memorial Fund; 2000.
14. Coughlin SS, Katz VVH, Mattison DR. "Ethics instruction at schools of public health in the United States." *Am J Public Health.* 2000;90:768–770.
15. Coughlin SS. "Model curricula in public health ethics." *Am J Prev Med.* 1996;12:247–251. Daniel Callahan, PhD, and Bruce Jennings, MD.

About the Authors

The authors are with The Hastings Center, Garrison, NY. They are writing for members of the Hastings Center Project on Ethics and Public Health: Ronald Bayer, Columbia University School of Public Health; Allan Brandt, Harvard Medical School; Daniel Callahan, The Hastings Center; Ruth R. Faden, Johns Hopkins University; Lawrence O. Gostin, Georgetown University Law School and Johns Hopkins University; Bruce Jennings, The Hastings Center; Jeffrey Kahn, University of Minnesota; Jan Malcolm, Minnesota State Department of Health; Donald R. Mattison, March of Dimes; Thomas L. Milne, National Association of County and City Health Officials; Phillip Nieburg, Centers for Disease Control and Prevention; Margaret Pappaianau, Centers for Disease Control and Prevention: Ann Robertson, University of Toronto; Dixie E. Snider, Centers for Disease Control and Prevention; Bonnie Steinbock, State University of New York at Albany; and Douglas L. Weed, National Cancer Institute.

Requests for reprints should be sent to Daniel Callahan, The Hastings Center, 21 Malcolm Gordon Road, Garrison, NY 10524-5555 (e-mail: Callahand@thehastingscenter.org). This commentary was accepted October 4, 2001.

Principles of the Ethical Practice of Public Health

▶ Preamble

This code of ethics states key principles of the ethical practice of public health. An accompanying statement lists the key values and beliefs inherent to a public health perspective upon which the Ethical Principles are based. Public health is understood within these principles as what we, as a society, do collectively to assure the conditions for people to be healthy. We affirm the World Health Organization's understanding of health as a state of complete physical, mental, and social well-being, and not merely the absence of disease or infirmity.[1]

The Code is neither a new nor an exhaustive system of health ethics. Rather, it highlights the ethical principles that follow from the distinctive characteristics of public health. A key belief worth highlighting, and which underlies several of the Ethical Principles, is the interdependence of people. This interdependence is the essence of community. Public health not only seeks to assure the health of whole communities but also recognizes that the health of individuals is tied to their life in the community.

The Code is intended principally for public and other institutions in the United States that have an explicit public health mission. Institutions and individuals that are outside of traditional public health, but recognize the effects of their work on the health of the community, may also find the Code relevant and useful.

▶ Values and Beliefs Underlying the Code

The following values and beliefs are key assumptions inherent to a public health perspective. They underlie the 12 Principles of the Ethical Practice of Public Health.

Health

1. *Humans have a right to the resources necessary for health.* The Public Health Code of Ethics affirms Article 25 of the Universal Declaration of Human Rights, which states in part

Principles of the Ethical Practice of Public Health, Version 2.2. © 2002 Public Health Leadership Society

"Everyone has the right to a standard of living adequate for the health and well-being of himself and his family . . ."

Community

2. *Humans are inherently social and interdependent.* Humans look to each other for companionship in friendships, families, and community; and rely upon one another for safety and survival. Positive relationships among individuals and positive collaborations among institutions are signs of a healthy community. The rightful concern for the physical individuality of humans and one's right to make decisions for oneself must be balanced against the fact that each person's actions affect other people.

3. *The effectiveness of institutions depends heavily on the public's trust.* Factors that contribute to trust in an institution include the following actions on the part of the institution: communication; truth telling; transparency (i.e., not concealing information); accountability; reliability; and reciprocity. One critical form of reciprocity and communication is listening to as well as speaking with the community.

4. *Collaboration is a key element to public health.* The public health infrastructure of a society is composed of a wide variety of agencies and professional disciplines. To be effective, they must work together well. Moreover, new collaborations will be needed to rise to new public health challenges.

5. *People and their physical environment are interdependent.* People depend upon the resources of their natural and constructed environments for life itself. A damaged or unbalanced natural environment, and a constructed environment of poor design or in poor condition, will have an adverse effect on the health of people. Conversely, people can have a profound effect on their natural environment through consumption of resources and generation of waste.

6. *Each person in a community should have an opportunity to contribute to public discourse.* Contributions to discourse may occur through a direct or a representative system of government. In the process of developing and evaluating policy, it is important to discern whether all who would like to contribute to the discussion have an opportunity to do so, even though expressing a concern does not mean that it will necessarily be addressed in the final policy.

7. *Identifying and promoting the fundamental requirements for health in a community are of primary concern to public health.* The way in which a society is structured is reflected in the health of a community. The primary concern of public health is with these underlying structural aspects. While some important public health programs are curative in nature, the field as a whole must never lose sight of underlying causes and prevention. Because fundamental social structures affect many aspects of health, addressing the fundamental causes rather than more proximal causes is more truly preventive.

Bases for Action

8. *Knowledge is important and powerful.* We are to seek to improve our understanding of health and the means of protecting it through research and the accumulation of knowledge. Once obtained, there is a moral obligation in some instances to share what is known. For example, active and informed participation in policy-making processes

requires access to relevant information. In other instances, such as information provided in confidence, there is an obligation to protect information.

9. *Science is the basis for much of our public health knowledge.* The scientific method provides a relatively objective means of identifying the factors necessary for health in a population, and for evaluating policies and programs to protect and promote health. The full range of scientific tools, including both quantitative and qualitative methods, and collaboration among the sciences is needed.

10. *People are responsible to act on the basis of what they know.* Knowledge is not morally neutral and often demands action. Moreover, information is not to be gathered for idle interest. Public health should seek to translate available information into timely action. Often, the action required is research to fill in the gaps of what we don't know.

11. *Action is not based on information alone.* In many instances, action is required in the absence of all the information one would like. In other instances, policies are demanded by the fundamental value and dignity of each human being, even if implementing them is not calculated to be optimally efficient or cost-beneficial. In both of these situations, values inform the application of information or the action in the absence of information.

PRINCIPLES OF THE ETHICAL PRACTICE OF PUBLIC HEALTH

1. Public health should address principally the fundamental causes of disease and requirements for health, aiming to prevent adverse health outcomes.
2. Public health should achieve community health in a way that respects the rights of individuals in the community.
3. Public health policies, programs, and priorities should be developed and evaluated through processes that ensure an opportunity for input from community members.
4. Public health should advocate and work for the empowerment of disenfranchised community members, aiming to ensure that the basic resources and conditions necessary for health are accessible to all.
5. Public health should seek the information needed to implement effective policies and programs that protect and promote health.
6. Public health institutions should provide communities with the information they have that is needed for decisions on policies or programs and should obtain the community's consent for their implementation.
7. Public health institutions should act in a timely manner on the information they have within the resources and the mandate given to them by the public.
8. Public health programs and policies should incorporate a variety of approaches that anticipate and respect diverse values, beliefs, and cultures in the community.
9. Public health programs and policies should be implemented in a manner that most enhances the physical and social environment.
10. Public health institutions should protect the confidentiality of information that can bring harm to an individual or community if made public. Exceptions must be justified on the basis of the high likelihood of significant harm to the individual or others.
11. Public health institutions should ensure the professional competence of their employees.
12. Public health institutions and their employees should engage in collaborations and affiliations in ways that build the public's trust and the institution's effectiveness.

▶ Rationale for a Public Health Code of Ethics

The mandate to assure and protect the health of the public is an inherently moral one. It carries with it an obligation to care for the well being of others and it implies the possession of an element of power in order to carry out the mandate. The need to exercise power to ensure health and at the same time to avoid the potential abuses of power are at the crux of public health ethics.

Until recently, the ethical nature of public health has been implicitly assumed rather than explicitly stated. Increasingly, however, society is demanding explicit attention to ethics. This demand arises from: technological advances that create new possibilities, and with them, new ethical dilemmas; new challenges to health such as the advent of human immunodeficiency virus; abuses of power, such as the Tuskegee study of syphilis; and an increasingly pluralistic society in which we can no longer simply adopt the values from a single culture or religion, but we must work out our common values in the midst of diversity.

Historically, medical institutions have been more explicit about the ethical elements of their practice than have public health institutions. The concerns of public health are not fully consonant with those of medicine, however, thus we cannot simply translate the principles of medical ethics to public health. For example, in contrast to medicine, public health is concerned more with populations than with individuals, and more with prevention than with cure. Thus, the purview of public health includes those who are not presently ill, and for whom the risks and benefits of medical care are not immediately relevant.

What Does a Code of Ethics Accomplish?

A code of ethics for public health clarifies the distinctive elements of public health and the ethical principles that follow from or respond to those distinct aspects. It makes clear to populations and communities the ideals of the public health institutions that serve them. A code of ethics thus serves as a goal to guide public health institutions and practitioners and as a standard to which they can be held accountable.

Codes of ethics are typically relatively brief; they are not designed to provide a means of untangling convoluted ethical issues. That process requires deliberation and debate over the multitude of factors relevant to a particular issue. Nor does a code typically provide a means of resolving a particular dispute. It does, however, provide those in a dispute over a public health concern with a list of issues and principles that should be considered in the dispute.

A Living Document

Many public health professionals, most of them associated with the Public Health Leadership Society (PHLS), came together to initiate the process of writing the Code. Represented on the PHLS Public Health Code of Ethics Committee are public health professionals from local and state public health, public health academia, the Centers for Disease Control and Prevention (CDC), and the American Public Health Association (APHA). They were formally encouraged in this effort during a town hall meeting attended by representatives from a wide variety of public health organizations at the 2000 APHA annual meeting. A draft code was reviewed and critiqued in May 2001 by 25 public health professionals and ethicists in a CDC-funded meeting held in Kansas City. A revised version of the Code was presented for discussion at another town hall meeting at the 2001 APHA annual meeting. Prior to the meeting, the Code was published on the APHA Website and an e-mail address was provided for reactions and feedback. The present code reflects the input and discussion from all of these forums. It is now being presented to various organizations for adoption or endorsement. Even so, there are ongoing opportunities to provide feedback (see page 10 for details), and an updating of the Code is anticipated. Tools for teaching about the Code and ensuring its practical utility are currently in the making.

▶ Notes on the Individual Ethical Principles

1. This Principle gives priority not only to prevention of disease or promotion of health, but also at the most fundamental levels. Yet the principle acknowledges that public health will also concern itself with some immediate causes and some curative roles. For example, the treatment of curable infections is important to the prevention of transmission of infection to others. The term "public health" is used here and elsewhere in the Code to represent the entire field of public health, including but not limited to government institutions and schools of public health.

2. This Principle identifies the common need in public health to weigh the concerns of both the individual and the community. There is no ethical principle that can provide a solution to this perennial tension in public health. We can highlight, however, that the interest of the community is part of the equation, and for public health it is the starting place in the equation; it is the primary interest of public health. Still, there remains the need to pay attention to the rights of individuals when exercising the police powers of public health.

3. A process for input can be direct or representative. In either case, it involves processes that work to establish a consensus. While democratic processes can be cumbersome, once a policy is established, public health institutions have the mandate to respond quickly to urgent situations. Input from the community should not end once a policy or program is implemented. There remains a need for the community to evaluate whether the institution is implementing the program as planned and whether it is having the intended effect. The ability for the public to provide this input and sense that it is being heard is critical in the development and maintenance of public trust in the institution.

4. This Principle speaks to two issues: ensuring that all in a community have a voice; and underscoring that public health has a particular interest in those members of a community that are underserved or marginalized. While a society cannot provide resources for health at a level enjoyed by the wealthy, it can ensure a decent minimum standard of resources. The Code cannot prescribe action when it comes to ensuring the health of those who are marginalized because of illegal behaviors. It can only underscore the principle of ensuring the resources necessary for health to all. Each institution must decide for itself what risks it will take to achieve that.

5. This Principle is a mandate to seek information to inform actions. The importance of information to evaluate programs is also implied.

6. This Principle is linked to the third one about democratic processes. Such processes depend upon an informed community. The information obtained by public health institutions is to be considered public property and made available to the public. This statement is also the community-level corollary of the individual-level ethical principle of informed consent. Particularly when a program has not been duly developed

with evaluation, the community should be informed of the potential risks and bene-fits, and implementation of the program should be premised on the consent of the community (though this principle does not specify how that consent should be obtained).

7. Public health is active rather than passive, and information is not to be gathered for idle interest. Yet the ability to act is conditioned by available resources and opportu-nities, and by competing needs. Moreover, the ability to respond to urgent situations depends on having established a mandate to do so through the democratic processes of Ethical Principle number three.

8. Public health programs should have built into them a flexibility that anticipates diver-sity in those needs and perspectives having a significant impact on the effectiveness of the program. Types of diversity, such as culture and gender, were intentionally not mentioned. Any list would be arbitrary and inadequate.

CORRESPONDENCE OF THE 12 ETHICAL PRINCIPLES WITH THE 10 ESSENTIAL PUBLIC HEALTH SERVICES

Essential Public Health Services[2] | *Ethical Principle*

1. Monitor the health status to identify community health problems — (5) collect information; (7) act on information
2. Diagnose and investigate health problems and health hazards in the community — (5) collect information
3. Inform, educate, and empower people about health issues — (4) advocacy and empowerment; (6) provide information
4. Mobilize community partnerships to identify and solve health problems — (12) collaboration
5. Develop policies and plans that support individual and community health efforts — (1) protect and promote health; address fundamental causes of health risks; (3) processes for community input; (5) collect information
6. Enforce laws and regulations that protect health and ensure safety — (2) achieve community health with respect for individual rights; (3) feedback from the community; (7) act upon information
7. Link people to needed personal health services and assure the provision of health care when otherwise unavailable — (4) advocate for and empower; basic resources available to all; (8) incorporate diversity
8. Assure a competent public health and personal health care workforce — (11) professional competence
9. Evaluate effectiveness, accessibility, and quality of personal and population-based health services — (3) community feedback; (5) collect information
10. Research for new insights and innovative solutions to health problems — (5) collect information

No corresponding essential public health service — (9) enhance physical and social environments; (10) protect confidentiality

9. This Principle stems from the assumptions of interdependence among people, and between people and their physical environment. It is like the ethical principle from medicine, "do no harm," but it is worded in a positive way.
10. This statement begs the question of which information needs to be protected and what the criteria are for making the information public. The aims of this statement are modest: to state explicitly the responsibility inherent to the "possession" of information. It is the complement to Ethical Principles 6 and 7, about acting on and sharing information.
11. The criteria for professional competence would have to be specified by individual professions, such as epidemiology and health education.
12. This statement underscores the collaborative nature of public health while also stating in a positive way the need to avoid any conflicts of interest that would undermine the trust of the public or the effectiveness of a program.

▶ Contact for Further Information and Feedback

Visit **www.phls.org** for:

- Ways to provide feedback to inform ongoing development of the 12 Ethical Principles
- Information on aligning your organization's public health practice with the 12 Ethical Principles
- Permission to reprint the 12 Ethical Principles and supporting documentation
- Requests for further information about public health ethics or the Public Health Leadership Society
- Public Health Leadership Society contact information

▶ Acknowledgements

The development and dissemination of the Principles of the Ethical Practice of Public Health is funded by a cooperative agreement between the Centers for Disease Control and Prevention and the Public Health Leadership Society (PHLS). The Center for Health Leadership & Practice, Public Health Institute is acknowledged for its role in the initial development of the Principles. PHLS also acknowledges the work of the members of the original PHLS Ethics Work Group (responsible for drafting the Code) and the current members of the PHLS standing Committee on Public Health Ethics. Specifically, PHLS acknowledges the following contributors: Elizabeth Bancroft (Centers for Disease Control and Prevention, Los Angeles County), Terry Brandenburg (West Allis Health Department), Kitty Hsu Dana (American Public Health Association), Jack Dillenberg (Arizona School of Health Sciences), Joxel Garcia (Connecticut Department of Health), Kathleen Gensheimer (Maine Department of Health), V. James Guillory (University of Health Sciences, Kansas City, MO), George Hardy (Association of State and Territorial Health Officers), Joseph Kimbrell (Louisiana Public Health Institute and National Network of Public Health Institutes), Teresa Long (Columbus, OH, Department of Health), Alan Melnick (Oregon Health and Science University, School of Medicine), Susan Myers (University of Pittsburgh), Ann Peterson (Virginia Department of Health), Michael Sage (Centers for Disease Control and Prevention), Margaret Schmelzer (Wisconsin Department of Health and Family Services), Liz Schwarte (Center for Health Leadership & Practice, Public Health Institute), James Thomas (University of North Carolina), Kathy Vincent (Alabama Health Department), and Carol Woltring (Center for Health Leadership and Practice, Public Health Institute).

▶ Notes

1. From *The Future of Public Health*, Institute of Medicine, 1988.
2. Developed by the Essential Public Health Services Work Group of the Public Health Functions Steering Committee, 1994.

Chapter 3

Case Studies with Ethical Implications

Controversies Surrounding Laud Humphreys' Tearoom Trade: An Unsettling Example of Politics and Power in Methodological Critiques

Michael Lenza, University of Missouri-Columbia

Laud Humphreys' *Tea Room Trade: Impersonal Sex In Public Places* (1970) is commonly presented in many sociological methods texts as an example of covert and deceptive research methods that endangered subjects without their consent. The following excerpt is reasonably representative of how this work tends to be presented:

> "In Laud Humphreys' tearoom trade study (a study of male homosexual encounters in public restrooms), about 100 men were observed engaging in sexual acts as Humphreys pretended to be a "watchqueen" (a voyeur and lookout). Subjects were followed to their cars, and their license numbers were secretly recorded. Names and addresses were obtained from police registers when Humphreys posed as a market researcher. A year later, in disguise, Humphreys used a deceptive story about a health survey to interview the subjects in their homes. Humphreys was careful to keep names in safety deposit boxes, and identifiers with subject names were burned. He significantly advanced knowledge of homosexuals who frequent "tearooms" and overturned previous false beliefs about them. There has been controversy over the study: The subjects never consented; deception was used; and the names could have been used to blackmail subjects, to end marriages, or to initiate criminal prosecutions" (Neuman 1997: 447).

Regarding these issues surrounding research on human subjects, this paper will argue that this dominant view of Humphreys' tearoom trade study, focusing primarily upon respect for autonomy (informed consent), misinforms the reader as much as it informs of the underlying moral and ethical foundations for research with human subjects. Three moral and ethical principles provide the foundations for most medical, scientific, and social research methodologies: beneficence, justice, and respect for autonomy (informed consent) (Faden and Beauchamp 1986: 5). I will first review each of these three ethical foundations for sociological research, then, I will examine Humphreys' Tearoom Trade study through the vantage point of each and the historical facts surrounding the controversies.

Humphreys' study in casual public sex, when historically situated and examined through each of the three ethical and moral pillars, will provide a more balanced framework from which to view his work. In addition, this more balanced view may promote better understanding of how ethical and methodological dilemmas arise when the underlying principles for human research come into conflict with each other.

▶ The Pillar of Beneficence

Beneficence carries within it perhaps the most basic ethical and moral consideration before a social researcher. It requires the researcher avoid harming the subject. *Beneficence* also carries with it a stipulation that research activities decidedly benefit others:

> "The principle of beneficence includes the following four elements, all linked through the common theme of promoting the welfare of others: (1) one ought not to inflict evil or harm; (2) one ought to prevent evil or harm; (3) one ought to remove evil or harm; (4) one ought to do or promote good. (Faden and Beauchamp 1986: 10)

These four elements are not so much a hierarchical ordering of considerations as an interconnected pattern of considerations that should be weighed and present in all stages of research. A small potential for harm can be acceptable if it serves to prevent, remove, or correct a larger harm or evil likely to be experienced by the subjects. There is an unavoidable element of paternalism in *beneficence* that can, and often does, create conflicts with respect for autonomy.

The Pillar of Respect for Autonomy

Rooted in our principle of respect for autonomy, *informed consent* is believed to protect a subject's right to make autonomous decisions so as not to infringe upon self-determination (Faden and Beauchamp 1986: 8–9, 27–28). Although research involving human subjects is as old as medicine itself, institutional concerns and formal requirements for *informed consent* for human subjects is a relatively recent development that grew out of accounts of misconduct uncovered at the Nuremberg trials of Nazi physician's experiments with human subjects.

It is interesting to note that it was actually Germany, in 1931, who were the first modern nation to enact strict regulations on the use of human subjects in medical research. These regulations specifically required researchers obtain the willing consent "in a clear and undebatable manner" before human subjects could be used (Sass 1983; Faden and Beauchamp 1986: 154). This fact is omitted in historical revisionist reviews of *informed consent* that present the Nuremberg Code of 1947 as the first major code addressing this issue (Belmont Report 1979).

It is important to recognize that horrific human experimentations, conducted by the Nazis, were carried out in the presence of strict legal doctrine prohibiting such crimes. History should inform and temper researchers' beliefs that bureaucratic structures function independent of the social and political events surrounding them. As history indicates, Internal Review Boards and Professional Codes of Ethics, though helpful, cannot serve to replace the ethics of individual researchers.

The Pillar of Justice

The concept of *justice,* as addressed in the literature on human subjects, is problematic for sociologists. It is approached principally from an economic and rational choice model for distributive justice. For example, the Belmont Report (1979) discusses Justice in Section B, Part 3:

> "**Justice.**—Who ought to receive the benefits of research and bear its burdens? This is a question of justice, in the sense of "fairness in distribution" or "what is deserved." An injustice occurs when some benefit to which a person is entitled is denied without good reason or when some burden is imposed unduly" (Belmont Report 1979).

The subsequent discussion following the above quote is relevant to medical, biological, and social scientific research projects that are developing new products or procedures, but has limited value in guiding social research. The American Sociological Association (ASA) code of Ethics does not have an explicit section on justice or beneficence, though it does address informed consent at considerable length (ASA 2003).

In a search of the JSTOR database of 24 sociological journals, for articles with the keyword *justice,* 135 articles were returned representing all major paradigms in sociology. The bulk of publications prove to be concerned with social justice. However, *justice,* as defined above is not a primary concern of sociology's acknowledged governing professional body. It is therefore both curious and disheartening to see an explicit emphasis on *informed consent* within the ASA Code of Ethics, which fulfills federal funding requirements, while discussion of justice and beneficence, arguably the heart and soul of the sociological endeavor, is conspicuously absent. Although there are numerous differences and debates about what social justice entails, too numerous for this writing, it is possible to recognize what should be a modest point of agreement: social justice entails an understanding of what is or was, combined with a view to what could be, for human benefit.

An Examination of Humphreys' Tearoom Trade Through the Three Ethical Pillars of Social Science Research

An examination of Humphreys' study through all three of the moral pillars underlying social research will establish that his research did not violate any premise of either beneficence or the sociological interest in social justice. His methods in interviewing subjects within their homes under the guise of conducting a health care survey did violate respect for autonomy. However, it is necessary to recognize that there were no federal or professional guidelines requiring informed consent in human research at that time.

Research that conducted a review of studies published in the *Journal of Personality and Social Psychology* in 1971 established that deception was used in 47% of the articles published that year (Menges 1973). Exemplary work in sociology commonly utilized deception. Goffman (1961) posed as an athletic director in his fieldwork for *Asylums.* Gusfield (1955) in *Symbolic Crusade,* informed the Woman's Christian Temperance Union (WCTU) he was a disinterested investigator of social movements (Gusfield 1955: 29; Mitchell 1993: 3). There was nothing exceptional in Laud Humphreys' use of deception in his fieldwork. It fell well within the accepted methodologies of that time period. Further, a more recent in-depth review of secrecy and fieldwork (Mitchell 1993), firmly establishes that secrecy remains to this day an essential element of most research involving human subjects. A belief that informed consent fully informs human subjects and in practice protects their right to autonomy is more a methodological myth than fact:

The following five elements have been identified as the concepts analytical components:

1. Disclosure
2. Comprehension
3. Voluntariness
4. Competence
5. Consent (Faden and Beauchamp 1986: 274)

Research indicates that what *informed consent* really means to subjects is closer to a release, "by letting the doctor do whatever is necessary, best, or whatever he sees fit" (Faden and Beauchamp 1986: 277). While the actual practice of gaining informed consent from patients tended to boil down to merely a ritual of "obtaining a signature on a consent form" (Zussman 1997: 178; Faden and Beauchamp 1986: 277; Mitchell 1993). *Informed consent* implies that subjects understand and agree to every facet of an experiment. This is clearly not true.

The underlying focus and function of *informed consent* is based in its legalistic importance as a signed contract establishing proof of voluntary cooperation protecting the researcher and the sponsoring institution from liability, aligning sociological research with the current funding requirements (Mitchell 1993: 35, 28).

Despite a recent institutional focus upon informed consent as the principle means to protect subjects, beneficence remains the most achievable and strongest moral principle protecting human subjects in social research: (1) one ought not to inflict harm; (2) one ought to prevent harm; (3) one ought to remove harm; (4) one ought to do or promote good.

The issue of inflicting harm on his subjects revolves around Humphreys' commitment and ability to protect their identity. Humphreys kept the list of his subjects' identities in a locked box, at a secret location, 1000 miles away from where his research was conducted. He destroyed the list when a possibility arose that there could be outside interests in the list. He took the identity of his subjects with him to the grave (Reiss 1978: 175; Mitchell 1993: 53). The facts clearly show Humphreys was absolutely committed to the protection of his subjects and did not allow harm to befall them through his actions. Regardless of one's position on the issues surrounding his methodology, one has to admit he admirably upheld that tenant, "one ought not to harm," (Faden and Beauchamp 1986: 10) and successfully protected his subjects' identities.

It was the publicity and homophobic hysteria surrounding Humphreys' dissertation work at Washington University that created a dangerous situation for the subjects. One should ask whether Alvin Gouldner's revelations to Nicholas von Hoffman and the resulting public scandal created a greater potential for harm to subjects than actions by Humphreys (see Goodwin et al. 1991). Metaphorically, if one were to become aware of possible fire hazards and lack of exits in a given building, it would be highly inappropriate to then run through the building screaming "Fire," and thereby actually creating a more immediately dangerous situation. Gouldner's actions in communicating his opinion of Humphreys's study outside of department to Von Hoffman, away from structures of confidentiality for subjects, intentionally created a public scandal where no protections for subjects existed. This could have brought serious harm to Humphreys' participants, as newspapers are exempt from libel if reporting is absent malice. In reality, the publicity generated by Gouldner and Von Hoffman posed a greater danger to participants than Humphreys' observations and follow-up interviews ever did.

Warwick (1982) notes the importance of recognizing the difference between "harms that are *intrinsic* to the research process and those that are *extrinsic* to that process" (Warwick 1982: 121) and even directly quotes Humphreys on the extrinsic publicity intentionally brought by others:

> "In the wake of front-page publicity, *fostered by members of the administration and faculty* at Washington University soon after the completion of the research, I am surprised that no such investigation followed" (emphasis my own; Warwick 1982: 108; Humphreys 1975: 229).

Despite this recognition of these extrinsic forces in play, Warwick, who engages in unfettered exposition of imagined harms, does not address or discuss the evidence of actual harms that resulted from these intentional extrinsic acts by others. In fact, the only substantive evidence we have of any harm befalling Humphreys' subjects are the anxious phone calls he received from several subjects after the extrinsic sensationalizing this study in the public sphere (Glazer 1972; Humphreys 1975: 215).

Should there not be some reasonable constraints upon critics? Is it proper for professionals to publicly accuse other researchers of possible crimes or harms to subjects with no more substantive proof than their mere imaginations or fanciful what if stories that never occurred? If a professional knowingly presents fabricated claims within the public sphere should they then not be responsible for:

1. The anxiety, fears, and harms to subjects that result from the contrived accusations.
2. The harms they create for the accused researcher's reputation and future.
3. The harm and fears brought to the field of study that arises from these unsubstantiated claims.

Intentionally placing someone in a false light in the public eye is unethical (Pickard 1982: 261). Many ethical critics of sociological research would be well served to turn their imaginative critical musings upon themselves.

If there is a lesson to be learned from this it would be that our first and foremost ethical requirement as practitioners should be the protection of subjects, which would include proper procedures for the bringing about and settling of ethical and methodological disputes. This would be accomplished in a manner that insures the confidentiality and protection of subjects, apart from media attention and personal conflicts.

There is another dilemma in the discussions and presentations of Humphreys' study. Should a possible harm that did not occur take precedence over what actually did occur?

> "The subjects never consented; deception was used; and the names could have been used to blackmail subjects, to end marriages, or to initiate criminal prosecutions" (Neuman 1997: 447).

This presentation, as do most methodological reviews of Humphreys' tearoom trade study, fits what Best (1990) calls "the atrocity tale" which is then tied to a particular policy position (Best 1990: 132–137; Toulmin et al. 1979: 43–56; Mitchell 1993: 27). This presentation clearly ties a violation of informed consent to the atrocity tales of destroyed marriages, blackmail, and criminal prosecutions. Neuman fails to acknowledge that if *informed consent* forms were used in Humphreys' project, it would have constituted a grave danger to the subjects as those records could be subject to subpoena (Bond 1978: 146; Mitchell 1993: 34). It is not that atrocity tales are not useful. They can inform us of all the many things that could possibly go wrong when conducting sociological research. However, critics can themselves make substantive and ethical errors if they present their arguments in a manner that intentionally substitutes their imaginative musings for the actual substantive reality.

On the way to the office yesterday, one could have become distracted, run over, horribly mangled and killed a neighbor's child, destroyed a family, and caused a terrible grief. An interesting element of "what ifs" is that such statements are very difficult to defend against. By the mere telling of the tale one creates and assigns guilt for events that never occurred. Therein lies the power of the "what if" scenario. *The burden of proof shifts from the teller of the tale to the accused.* These types of arguments, substantively based upon nonevents can be inherently unfair, particularly, as in Humphreys' case, when the facts speak to the care and consideration that was undeniably taken to insure that damage to subjects would not occur.

These what if stories surrounding Humphreys' work also provide us with a view to politics and power within our profession. Humphreys had little status or power as a PhD candidate completing his dissertation relative to the status and power of established professionals such as Alvin Gouldner and Nicholas von Hoffman. This difference in power and status allowed his critics to merely imaginatively create what if tales, void of any substantive proofs, to forever cast the specter of ethical impropriety around this work. There is no exoneration from what if. Even when established as untrue the specter of the horror remains. It haunted Humphreys throughout his life (Humphreys 1975: 223–232; Nardi 1995). These fabricated "what if" tales did in reality create more harm to subjects, damage to Laud Humphreys' reputation, and did more to undermine public faith in sociological research than any act by Humphreys in conducting the research itself.

More importantly, from the vantage point of beneficence as well as from a concern with social justice, Humphreys' tearoom study made significant positive contributions to the population he studied. His thorough fieldwork exploded the myth that the populations of men engaging in these casual sexual encounters were criminals, transients, or predatory pedophiles that communities needed to hunt down and criminally prosecute. His study firmly established that this casual sexual behavior was limited to consenting adults that transpired in a manner that made it highly unlikely that youths or disinterested parties would be approached or harassed. Furthermore, he established that this population principally consisted of individuals of good standing within the community, many of which were married, employed, and former members of the armed forces. Humphreys' work seriously questioned the received view that homosexual contact should be subjected to the retributive harms of imprisonment and ultimately created doubt in the dichotomous categories of gender that closely paralleled sexual behavior (Humphreys 1975: 64, and chapters 6 and 7). His conceptualization of the *breastplate of righteousness* was a significant contribution to our understanding that expressed religious and political views sometimes serve as purposeful acts of misdirection. Few studies in sociology have accomplished as much in a single work. Laud Humphreys' *Tearoom Trade* (1970) did not violate the deeper ethical and social concerns of sociology, expressed in the concepts of *beneficence* and *justice,* and it is necessary to recognize both its historical and continuing importance in understanding human sexuality.

► Acknowledgements

I would like to extend special thanks to David Keys, Steven Schacht, and John Galliher for their support and editorial suggestions in preparing this article for publication.

► Biographical Information

I received my undergraduate degree in sociology at Southwest Missouri State University and completed my Masters Degree at the University of Missouri, Columbia where I am presently completing two independent doctorates. In Sociology I am completing a historical, political and statistical analysis of the death penalty in Missouri. Preliminary findings from this work was awarded first prize in 2003 for graduate student research in the Social Sciences at the University of Missouri. For my Rural Sociology dissertation I am completing an inter-generational study of Ozark Folk music, collective memory, and community structures. I anticipate completing both doctorates in 2004.

► References

American Sociological Association Code of Ethics. 2003. *http://www.asanet.org/members/ecostand2.html*.

Belmont Report. 1979. *http://ohrp.osophs.dhhs.gov/humansubjects/guidance/belmont.htm*.

Best, J. 1990. *Threatened Children: Rhetoric and Concern about Child Victims.* Chicago: University of Chicago Press.

Bond, K. 1978. "Confidentiality and the Protection of Human Subjects in Social Science Research: A Report on Recent Developments." *American Sociologist* 13: 14–152.

Faden, Ruth R. and Beauchamp, Tom L. 1986. *A History and Theory of Informed Consent.* New York: Oxford University Press.

Glazer, Myron. 1975. "Impersonal Sex." In Humphreys, L. *Tearoom Trade: Impersonal Sex in Public Places.* pp. 213–222. Chicago: Aldine Publishing Company.

Goffman, Erving. 1961. *Asylums: Essays on the Social Situation of Mental Patients and Other Inmates.* Garden City, N.Y.: Anchor Books.

Goodwin, Glen A., Horowitz, Irving Louis, and Nardi, Peter, M. 1991. "Laud Humphreys: A Pioneer in the Practice of Social Science." *Sociological Inquiry* 61: 139–147.

Gusfield, J. 1955. "Fieldwork Reciprocities in Studying a Social Movement." *Human Organization* 14: 29–33.

Humphreys, Laud. 1970. *Tearoom Trade: Impersonal Sex in Public Places.* Chicago: Aldine Publishing Company.

———. 1975. *Tearoom Trade: Impersonal Sex in Public Places.* Chicago: Aldine Publishing Company.

Menges, Robert J. 1973. "Openness and Honesty Versus Coercion and Deception in Psychological Research." *American Psychologist* 28: 1030–34.

Mitchell, Richard G. 1993. *Secrecy and Fieldwork.* Newbury Park: Sage Publications.

Nardi, Peter, M. 1995. "The Breastplate of Righteousness: Twenty-Five Years After Laud Humphreys' Tearoom Trade Impersonal Sex in Public Places." *Journal of Homosexuality* 30: pp. 1–10.

Neuman, W. Lawrence. 1997. *Social Research Methods: Qualitative and Quantitative Approaches.* 3rd ed. Boston: Allyn and Bacon.

Pickard, Terry. 1982. "Invasions of Privacy in Social Science Research." In Beauchamp, Tom L., R. Faden, R. Wallace, and L. Walters (eds.) *Ethical Issues in Social Science Research.* pp. 257–273. Baltimore: Johns Hopkins University Press.

Reiss, A. J. 1978. "Conditions and Consequences of Consent in Human Subject Research," In K. Wulff (Ed.) *Regulation of Scientific Inquiry.* pp. 161–184. Boulder: Westview Press.

Sass, Hans Martin. 1983. "Reichsrundschreiben 1931: Pre Nuremberg German Regulations Concerning New Therapy and Human Experimentation." *Journal of Medicine and Philosophy* 8: pp. 99–111.

Toulmin, S., Rieke, R., and Janik, A. 1979. *An Introduction to Reasoning.* New York: Macmillan.

Warwick, Donald P. 1982. "Types of Harm in Social Research." In Beauchamp, Tom L., R. Faden, R. Wallace, and L. Walters (eds.) *Ethical Issues in Social Science Research.* pp. 101–124. Baltimore: Johns Hopkins University Press.

Zussman, Robert. 1997. "Sociological Perspectives on Medical Ethics and Decision Making." *Annual Review of Sociology* 23: pp. 171–189.

Public Health Then and Now
The Tuskegee Syphilis Study, 1932 to 1972: Implications for HIV Education and AIDS Risk Education Programs in the Black Community

*Stephen B. Thomas, Ph.D., and
Sandra Crouse Quinn, M.Ed.*

Abstract

The Tuskegee study of untreated syphilis in the Negro male is the longest nontherapeutic experiment on human beings in medical history. The strategies used to recruit and retain participants were quite similar to those being advocated for HIV/AIDS prevention programs today. Almost 60 years after the study began, there remains a trail of distrust and suspicion that hampers HIV education efforts in Black communities.

The AIDS epidemic has exposed the Tuskegee study as a historical marker for the legitimate discontent of Blacks with the public health system. The belief that AIDS is a form of genocide is rooted in a social context in which Black Americans, faced with persistent inequality, believe in conspiracy theories about Whites against Blacks. These theories range from the belief that the government promotes drug abuse in Black communities to the belief that HIV is a manmade weapon of racial warfare.

An open and honest discussion of the Tuskegee Syphilis Study can facilitate the process of rebuilding trust between the Black community and public health authorities. This dialogue can contribute to the development of HIV education programs that are scientifically sound, culturally sensitive, and ethnically acceptable. *(Am J Public Health* 1991;81:1498–1504)

► Background

AIDS Among Black Americans

Since acquired immunodeficiency syndrome (AIDS) was first recognized and reported in 1981, more than 179,000 persons with AIDS have been reported to the Centers for Disease Control (CDC). Of these, more than 63% have died. Infection with the human immunodeficiency virus (HIV) has emerged as a leading cause of death among men and women under 45 years of age and children 1 to 5 years of age.[1]

By May 1991, there were 179,136 cases of AIDS reported in the United States. Of the reported cases, 97,329 (54%) were White and 51,190 (29%) were Black. Thus, although Whites still constitute a majority of the AIDS cases, Blacks are contracting AIDS in numbers far greater than their relative percentage in the population (Blacks constitute 12% of the US population). In addition, 52% of all children (under age 13 at time of diagnosis) and 52% of all women with AIDS are Black.[1] The best data available demonstrate that in the United States, HIV infection is spreading more rapidly among Blacks than among other population groups..

Because of the disproportionate impact of AIDS among Blacks, special emphasis must be placed on reaching this population with effective HIV education and AIDS risk reduction programs. To plan and evaluate these programs effectively, it is crucial to have an understanding of the behavioral risk factors and AIDS knowledge deficiencies in the Black community.

Public health professionals must recognize that the history of slavery and racism in the United States has contributed to the present social environment, in which those Blacks, whose behavior places them at greater risk for HIV infection, are also among the most disadvantaged members of our society. As we enter the new millennium, the promises of opportunity and equality envisioned by the civil rights movement have failed to be realized for the vast majority of American Blacks. Blacks' consequent anger and despair in the face of persistent inequality have contributed to the development of conspiracy theories about Whites (the government) against Blacks. These conspiracy theories range from the belief that the government promotes drug abase in Black communities to the belief that HIV is a manmade weapon of racial warfare.

For example, The Nation of Islam has disseminated literature that describes AIDS as a form of genocide, an attempt by White society to eliminate the Negro race.[2] The mainstream Black media have also contributed to the discussion. "Tony Brown's Journal," a popular Public Broadcast System television show, aired a series of programs debating the issue of AIDS as a form of genocide. The Los Angeles Sentinel, the largest Black newspaper on the West Coast, ran a series of stories beginning March 9, 1989, suggesting that Blacks had been intentionally infected with HIV. *Essence* also ran a story titled "AIDS: Is It Genocide?"[3] In that article, Barbara J. Justice, MD, a New York City physician, asserted that "there is a possibility that the virus was produced to limit the number of African people and people of color in the world who are no longer needed" (p. 78). James Small, PhD, a Black studies instructor at City College of New York, was quoted as saying:

> Our whole relationship to Whites has been that of their practicing genocidal conspiratorial behavior on us from the whole slave encounter up to the Tuskegee Study. People make it sound nice by saying the Tuskegee "Study." But do you know how many thousands and thousands of our people died of syphilis because of that?[3]

The history of the Tuskegee Syphilis Study, with its failure to educate the participants and treat them adequately, helped to lay the foundation for Blacks' pervasive sense of distrust of public health authorities today. Fears about genocide have been reported by public health professionals and community-based-organization staff who work in Black communities. During his 1990 testimony before the National Commission on AIDS, Mark Smith, MD, from the School of Medicine at Johns Hopkins University in Baltimore, described the African American community as "already alienated from the health care system and the government and . . . somewhat cynical about the motives of those who arrive in their communities to help them" (p.19).[4] Smith said that the Tuskegee Syphilis Study "provides validation for common suspicions about the ethical even-handedness in the medical research establishment and in the federal government, in particular, when it comes to Black people" (p. 20).[4]

Harlon Dalton, associate professor of law at Yale University and member of the National Commission on AIDS, eloquently describes the social basis for genocidal theories in his much quoted essay, "AIDS in Blackface."[5] Dalton believes that the Tuskegee Syphilis Study is a reflection of society's historical disregard for the lives of Black people. He accepts the commonly repeated distortion that "the government purposefully exposed Black men to syphilis so as to study the natural course of the disease."[5]

The continuing legacy of the Tuskegee Syphilis Study has contributed to Blacks' belief that genocide is possible and that public health authorities cannot be trusted. These fears and attitudes must be assessed in order to develop AIDS education programs for the Black community. For example, the Southern Christian Leadership Conference (SCLC), a leading civil rights organization founded by Dr. Martin Luther King, Jr, received funding from the CDC to provide HIV education through a national program titled RACE (Reducing AIDS through Community Education). In 1990, the SCLC conducted a survey to determine HIV education needs among 1056 Black church members in five cities (Atlanta, Ga; Charlotte, NC; Detroit, Mich; Kansas City, Mo; and Tuscaloosa, Ala). While 35% of the respondents believed that AIDS is a form of genocide, another 30% were unsure. Additionally, 44% believed that the government is not telling the truth about AIDS, while 35% were unsure. Furthermore, 34% believed that AIDS is a manmade virus, while 44% were unsure.[20]

The results of the SCLC survey strongly suggest that Blacks' belief in AIDS as a form of genocide and their mistrust of the government should be cause for serious concern among public health officials. Within this context, the health professionals responsible for HIV education must be made aware of the history of the Tuskegee Syphilis Study and its implications for HIV education and AIDS risk reduction programs in Black communities. Unfortunately, the details of the Tuskegee study are not well known. Therefore, we utilize the work of historian James Jones, who provides the most comprehensive description of the Tuskegee study in his book, *Bad Blood: The Tuskegee Syphilis Experiment—A Tragedy of Race and Medicine.*[6]

Factors Leading to the Tuskegee Syphilis Study

The Julius Rosenwald Fund, a philanthropic organization in Chicago, Ill, was dedicated to the promotion of the health, education, and welfare of Black Americans. In 1928, the fund's director of medical service approached the United States Public Health Service (PHS) in an effort to expand activities to improve the health status of Blacks in the rural South. At that time the PHS had successfully completed a study of the prevalence of syphilis in over 2000 Blacks employed by the Delta Pine and Land Company in Mississippi. Twenty-five percent of the sample had tested positive for syphilis. The PHS collaborated with the Rosenwald Fund to provide treatment to these people. It was the success of this collaboration that led the PHS to submit a proposal to the Rosenwald Fund for expansion of syphilis control demonstration programs into free counties in the rural South. The Rosenwald Fund approved the proposal with the condition that a Black public health nurse be employed on the project.[6,7]

From 1929 to 1931, the Rosenwald Fund sponsored syphilis control demonstration projects in Albemarle County, Virginia; Glynn County, Georgia; Pitt County, North Carolina; Mason County, Alabama; and Tipton County, Tennessee. The primary goal was to demonstrate that rural Blacks could be tested and treated for syphilis. During the testing phase of the study, it was found that in Mason County, Alabama, 35% to 40% of all age groups tested were positive for syphilis.[6,7] Before the treatment phase of the project could begin, two things happened that led to the Tuskegee Syphilis Study.

First, there was much speculation in the scientific literature on racial differences in the natural history of syphilis. Although some theories suggested that syphilis affected the neurological functioning of whites, there was speculation that latent syphilis had an impact on the cardiovascular systems of Blacks. However, Dr. Bruusgaard in Oslo, Norway, conducted a retrospective study of white men with untreated syphilis which found that cardiovascular damage was common and neurological involvement was rare. This finding, published in 1929, was contrary to the prevailing scientific view in the United States.[6]

Second, the start of the Depression in 1929 devastated the Rosenwald Fund's financial resources, which were needed for the treatment component of the demonstration project. Without financial support from the Rosenwald Fund, the PHS simply did not have the resources to develop treatment programs in all five counties. It was thought that the best chance of salvaging anything of value from the project lay in the conduct of a scientific experiment.

Conflict between findings from the Oslo study and the prevailing scientific view in the U.S. on racial differences led Taliaferro Clark, M.D., of the PHS, to propose that a major improvement on previous syphilis research could be obtained by conducting a prospective study of living patients. Consequently, in 1932, Dr. Clark stated that "the Alabama community offered an unparalleled opportunity for the study of the effect of untreated syphilis" (p. 94).[6]

The original study population consisted of 399 Black men with syphilis and 201 controls. The study was intended to last for 6 to 9 months. However, as Jones demonstrates, the drive to satisfy scientific curiosity resulted in a 40-year experiment that followed these men to "end point" (autopsy). Jones eloquently describes the irony of the Tuskegee Syphilis Study:

> [The] study would be an expression of concern for Negro health problems, keeping the PHS involved as a vital force in promoting medical attention to Blacks. The more damaging the disease was shown to be, the more pressure would build on Southern legislators to fund treatment programs. The study would also permit the PHS to maintain the momentum of public health work in Alabama by continuing the close working relationships with state and local health officials, not to mention Black leaders at the Tuskegee Institute (p. 94).[6]

▶ The Tuskegee Syphilis Study

Strategies Used to Recruit and Track Participants

The 40-year continuation of the Tuskegee Syphilis Study can be attributed to extensive collaboration among government agencies, along with an unprecedented community-based approach that demonstrated a degree of cultural sensitivity toward the poor Black target population in Macon County. The strategies used to recruit and retain participants in the study were quite similar to those being advocated for HIV education and AIDS risk reduction programs today. In addition to the PHS, which served as the lead agency, there was an impressive group of cooperating agencies from state and local levels:

- Macon County Medical Society
- Tuskegee Institute
- Alabama State and Macon County Boards of Health
- The Milbank Memorial Fund
- local Black churches and public schools
- local plantation owners

During the early phase of the project, the PHS decided to ask Tuskegee Institute to participate in the study. It was felt that because Tuskegee Institute had a history of service to Blacks in Macon County, its participation would not threaten white physicians in the county. Furthermore, the PHS felt that the use of Black physicians was necessary to facilitate the cooperation of subjects.[6] Tuskegee Institute benefited from this collaboration by receiving funds, training opportunities for interns, and employment for its nurses. Jones describes the complex political maneuvers involved in setting up the study:

> [By persuading the Tuskegee Institute physicians to cooperate], the old syphilis control demonstration team of (PHS) clinicians would be reunited and the study would have the appearance of a revival of syphilis control work. The true purpose of the experiment would be totally obscured, leaving investigators free to trade upon the goodwill and trust that the Rosenwald Fund's syphilis control demonstration had generated among the Black people of the county and their white employers. Dr. Clark was not the least bit embarrassed by the deceit. (p. 100)[6]

The study included culturally sensitive grassroots approaches to ensure the involvement and continued participation of the men. The study employed Eunice Rivers, a Black public health nurse from Macon County, throughout the entire 40 years. As the primary contact person, she provided transportation, organized the men for examinations by the visiting PHS physicians, provided reassurance, and formed trusting relationships with the men and their families.[8]

The PHS was extremely successful in enlisting Black church leaders, elders in the community, and plantation owners to encourage participation. The plantation owners had an economic incentive to maintain the health of their employees. Often they would give permission for medical examinations while workers toiled in the fields.[7] In addition, physical examinations, including the taking of blood samples, were conducted in Black churches and schools. Jones describes the process through which subjects were recruited: "First the health officials won over local leaders. Then, they used schoolhouses and churches as makeshift clinics, with local schoolteachers and ministers serving as 'advance people' who spread the word about where and when the 'government doctors' would be in the area" (p. 69).[6]

In addition, the fact that Whites ruled Blacks in Macon County, coupled with the Black men's extreme poverty and most total lack of access to health care, made the men willing subjects. As Dr. Frost, a Black physician from the Rosenwald Fund, stated, "as a group, they were susceptible to kindness."[6]

Lack of medical care in Macon County meant that many of the study participants had never been treated by a physician. The PHS physicians, believing that their patients would not understand clinical terms, did not even attempt to educate them about syphilis. Participants were not informed that they suffered from a specific, definable disease that was contagious and transmitted through sexual intercourse. Nor were they told that the disease could be transmitted from mother to fetus. The PHS clinicians translated medical terms into local language. Syphilis became "bad blood," a phrase that Black people of the rural South used to describe a variety of ailments.[9] Consequently, when the PHS physicians announced that they had come to test for "bad blood," people turned out in droves. The PHS also used incentives including free physical examinations, food, and transportation.[8] Burial stipends, provided by the Milbank Memorial Fund, were used to gain permission from family members for autopsies to be performed on study participants who reached "end point."[6]

From the historical and social perspective of the rural South in the early 1930s, the PHS strategies represented a high degree of understanding about the cultural milieu in which the study was being conducted. There is no doubt the approach was a sophisticated demonstration of cultural sensitivity coupled with political savvy and an impressive commitment by collaborating agencies. However, the tragedy was that a project originally intended to meet real health needs ended in a mere attempt to salvage scientific data.

▶ How Did It Go on for So Long?

The Tuskegee study of untreated syphilis in the Negro male is the longest nontherapeutic experiment on human beings in medical history.[6] Numerous factors contributed to the continuation of this experiment over a period of 40 years. However, almost from the outset, its scientific merit was questionable.

The Alabama state health officer and the Macon County Board of Health extracted a promise from the PHS that all who were tested and found to be positive for syphilis, including those selected for the study, would receive treatment. It was understood by all, except the subjects, that the treatment given was less than the amount recommended by the PHS to cure syphilis. By the late 1930s some physicians began to raise concerns regarding the scientific merit of a study about untreated syphilis when it was clear that some subjects had received some form of treatment. In 1938, removal of these men from the experiment was briefly considered, but it was decided that in the interest of maintaining esprit de corps among the participants and in order to avoid suspicion, those men who had received minimal treatment would remain in the experimental group.[6]

The ultimate tragedy of the Tuskegee experiment was exemplified by the extraordinary measures taken to ensure that subjects in the experimental group did not receive effective treatment. During World War II, approximately 50 of the syphilitic cases received letters from the local draft board ordering them to take treatment. At the request of the PHS, the draft board agreed to exclude the men in the study from its list of draftees needing treatment.[6] According to Jones,

> [Preventing] the men from receiving treatment had always been a violation of Alabama's public health statutes requiring public reporting and prompt treatment of venereal diseases. . . . Under the auspices of the law health officials conducted the largest state-level testing and treatment program in the history of the nation [but] state and local health officials continued to cooperate with the study (p. 178).[6]

In 1943, the PHS began to administer penicillin to syphilitic patients in selected treatment clinics across the nation. The men of the Tuskegee Syphilis Study were excluded from this treatment for the same reason other drugs had been withheld since the beginning of the study in 1932—treatment would end the study. Once penicillin became the standard of treatment for syphilis in 1951, the PHS insisted that it was all the more urgent for the Tuskegee study to continue because "it made the experiment a never-again-to-be-repeated opportunity (p. 179).[6]

In 1952, in an effort to reach subjects who had moved out of Macon County, the PHS utilized its entire national network of state and local health departments for the first time in its history in order to bring subjects in for examination. Over the next 20 years, state and local health departments cooperated in keeping the men in the study, yet denying treatment.

According to Jones, the ultimate reason why the Tuskegee Syphilis Study went on for 40 years was a minimal sense of personal responsibility and ethical concern among the small group of men within the PHS who controlled the study. This attitude was reflected in a 1976 interview conducted by Jones with Dr. John Heller, Director of Venereal Diseases at the PHS from 1943 to 1948, who stated, "The men's status did not warrant ethical debate. They were subjects, not patients, clinical material, not sick people"(Heller 179).[6]

Jones details the following chronology of events leading to the end of the Tuskegee Syphilis Study:

- November 1966. Peter Buxtun, a venereal disease interviewer and investigator with the PHS in San Francisco, sent a letter to Dr. William Brown, Director of the Division of Venereal Diseases, to express his moral concerns about the experiment. He inquired whether any of the men had been treated properly and whether any had been told the nature of the study.
- November 1968. Buxtun wrote Dr. Brown a second letter, in which he described the current racial unrest prevalent in the nation. Buxtun made the point that "the racial composition of the study group [100% Negro] supported the thinking by Negro militants that Negroes have long been used for medical experiments and teaching cases in the emergency wards of county hospitals . . ." (p. 193).[6] Dr. Brown showed this letter to the Director at the Centers for Disease Control. For the first time, health officials saw the experiment as a public relations problem that could have severe political repercussions.
- February 1969. The CDC convened a blue-ribbon panel to discuss the Tuskegee study. The group reviewed all aspects of the experiment and decided against treating the men. This decision ended debate on the Tuskegee study's future: it would continue until "end point." The committee also recommended that a major thrust be made to upgrade the study scientifically.
- In the final analysis, it was Peter Buxtun who stopped the Tuskegee Syphilis Study by telling his story to a reporter with the Associated Press. On July 25, 1972, the *Washington Star* ran a front-page story about the experiment. It is important to note that the PHS was still conducting the experiment on the day when the story broke.

The story was picked up off the wire service and became front-page news and the subject of editorials in major newspapers across the nation. It did not take long for officials in the Department of Health, Education, and Welfare (HEW) and the PHS to form a chorus of denunciation in concert with the public outcry condemning the study. Little effort was made directly to defend or justify the experiment. For example, Dr. Donald Printz, an official in the Venereal Disease Branch of the CDC, publicly stated that the experiment was "almost like genocide . . . a literal death sentence was passed on some, of those people" (p. 207).[6]

► Implications for HIV/AIDS Risk Reduction Programs in the Black Community

The historic 1972 disclosure of the Tuskegee study in the national press led to congressional subcommittee hearings held in February and March of 1973 by Senator Edward Kennedy. The result was a complete revamping of HEW regulations on protection of human subjects in experimentation. On July 23, 1973 a $1.8 billion class-action law suit was filed in the U.S. District Court for the Middle District of Alabama on behalf of the men in the study. In December 1974, the government agreed to pay $10 million in an out-of-court settlement. Jones provides a detailed description of the law suit consequences.[6]

There has been relatively little discussion of the Tuskegee Experiment within the public health professional literature since the historic 1972 disclosure of the study in the national press. For example, Cutler and Arnold's 1988 article titled "Venereal Disease Control by Health Departments in the Past: Lessons for the Present"[10] failed to make any mention of the Tuskegee study yet called upon readers of this journal to honor Surgeon General Parran who at one point directed the study. Silver described this omission as evidence of the continued inability to confront our racist past. Silver went on to state that . . .

> the behavior of the PHS officers was no more than representative of the sentiments and prejudices of the times. But not to remember is to forget, and to forget is a disservice to those who suffered the indignities. . . . [In] calling upon us to honor [Parran], one of the participants, we should also mention the context in which the meritorious service was earned.[11]

Both Brandt[12] and Fee[13] emphasize the importance of history in the cultural meaning of disease. Therefore, as the pattern of HIV infection shifts and increasing numbers of Blacks are affected, it will be crucial to understand the historical context in which Black Americans will interpret the disease. The failure of public health professionals to comprehensively discuss the Tuskegee experiment contributes to its use as a source of misinformation and helps to maintain a barrier between the Black community and health care service providers. In presentations at public health professional meetings and interactions with Black community-based-organization staff members, the authors have consistently observed how the Tuskegee Study is used to undermine trust and justify AIDS conspiracy theories. Although there is no evidence to support Dalton's assertion that the men were intentionally infected with syphilis[5] this distortion continues to be disseminated through community discussions and the popular media. There is no need to misrepresent the facts of the study to recognize how it contributes to fears of genocide. Given that the conduct of the study demonstrated little regard for the lives of the men who participated, it is no surprise that Blacks today do not readily dismiss assertions that HIV is a manmade virus intentionally allowed to run rampant in their communities.

Now, almost 70 years after the experiment began, the Tuskegee Syphilis Study's legacy is a trail of distrust and suspicion that hampers HIV education efforts to Black communities. During testimony delivered before the National Commission on AIDS in December 1990, Alpha Thomas, a health educator with the Dallas Urban League, stated: "So many African American people that I work with do not trust hospitals or any of the other community health care service providers because of that Tuskegee Experiment. It is like . . . if they did it then they will do it again" (p. 43).[4]

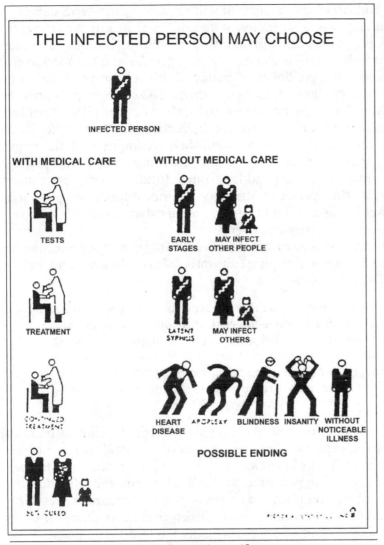

THE INFECTED PERSON MAY CHOOSE

INFECTED PERSON

WITH MEDICAL CARE   WITHOUT MEDICAL CARE

TESTS   EARLY   MAY INFECT
                     STAGES   OTHER PEOPLE

TREATMENT   LATENT   MAY INFECT
                     SYPHILIS   OTHERS

CONTINUED   HEART   APOPLEXY BLINDNESS INSANITY WITHOUT
TREATMENT   DISEASE   NOTICEABLE
                                                    ILLNESS

                     POSSIBLE ENDING

NOT CURED

From Thomas Parran's book, *Shadow on the Land.*[7]

Public health professionals must recognize that Blacks' belief in AIDS as a form of genocide is a legitimate attitudinal barrier rooted in the history of the Tuskegee Syphilis Study. Many public health authorities who work with Black communities are uncomfortable responding to the issue of genocide and the Tuskegee study. The common response is to ignore these issues. This approach may result in a loss of believability and further alienation. One culturally sensitive response would be for public health professionals to discuss the fear of genocide evoked by the AIDS epidemic. They must be willing to listen respectfully to community fears, share the facts of the Tuskegee study when it arises as a justification of those fears, and admit to the limitations of science when they do not have all the answers. This approach may help public health authorities to regain the credibility and the public trust they need to successfully implement HIV risk reduction strategies in the Black community.

The necessary public health science technology and experience exist for the development and implementation of effective community-based HIV education programs that are ethnically acceptable and culturally sensitive. Strategies such as (1) the use of program staff indigenous to the community, (2) the use of incentives, and (3) the delivery of health services within the target community were used to recruit participants in the Tuskegee Syphilis Study. These techniques are being implemented by AIDS risk reduction programs today. The value of these community-based strategies should not be diminished by their association with the Tuskegee study. The impact of HIV infection and AIDS in Black communities is exacerbated by the presence of other sources of poor health status and social inequities. Therefore, AIDS risk reduction programs must be built on solid assessments of community perceptions and needs, and must include ongoing involvement of community members in program planning and evaluation efforts.[14]

Successful HIV education and AIDS risk reduction will require a long-term commitment from and collaboration among federal agencies, state and local health departments, community-based organizations, private industry, philanthropies, and institutions of higher learning. Such collaboration must be based on trust between the agencies and the Black community. Given the legacy of Tuskegee, the credibility of public health service providers from outside the Black community is severely limited. Consequently, CDC's program to provide direct funding to Black community-based organizations (CBOs) to deliver HIV education represents a significant development in the effort to overcome distrust. However, while CBOs may have ready access to a community and may have established credibility with the target population, they often lack the infrastructure necessary for long-term success.[14] Consequently, CBOs will require consistent technical assistance and long-range funding from government and private agencies. To ensure that the specter of Tuskegee will not impede progress, it is crucial that decision-making power be distributed in such a manner that collaborating agencies allow CBOs to maintain control over program integrity.

Distrust of and resistance to involvement with public health programs have a legitimate basis to history; to overcome these feelings will require cultural sensitivity. In testimony before the National Commission on AIDS, Dr. Smith stated:

> [The Black] communities' perspective on medical research has a historical basis which sometimes outweighs the demonstrable integrity and commitment of individual investigators. . . . In light of the historical basis of the suspicion of being guinea pigs, it is particularly ironic to hear the cries for more access to experimental medicines. [This resistance] will only be overcome, frankly, with a more long-range effort to reassure African Americans that they will not be the victims of more Tuskegees.[4] (p. 31)

Public health professionals must support Blacks' increased access to clinical trials so that the AIDS knowledge base can be expanded and the benefits of potential treatments can be realized. The successful inclusion of Blacks in clinical trials will require researchers to conduct their investigations in convenient settings trusted by the Black community. In addition, investigators must recognize that simple compliance with protection of human subjects procedures is not sufficient. The researchers who conducted the Tuskegee study made a conscious decision to withhold information about syphilis from participants. Consequently, Blacks today may not believe that they are being told the whole truth about HIV. To overcome the distrust of community members, researchers must see that they are fully informed about research procedures, costs, and benefits, and that they have representation on research advisory committees. Investigators should conduct their work with an attitude of respect for the humanity of study participants, regardless of the social and cultural gulf that may exist between investigators and subjects. Ultimately, cultural sensitivity can best be manifested through the professional obligation to advocate AIDS policies that provide for the protection of civil rights and access to health care services.[15]

It must be acknowledged that public health research and practice operate in an environment influenced by societal values and political ideology. For example, needle distribution programs for intravenous drug users, along with HIV testing policies and counseling of HIV-infected women, are frequently the subject of political debate. Efforts to develop needle distribution programs have been stymied by political controversy, moral questions, and outraged claims that such programs have a genocidal impact on Black communities. In many communities where drug abuse is epidemic, needle distribution programs are perceived as contributing to the drug problem, particularly when such programs are promulgated in the absence of access to adequate drug treatment services. The image of Black intravenous drug users reaching out for treatment, only to receive clean needles from public health authorities, provides additional fuel for the genocide theory. The emphasis on HIV testing and counseling without adequate access to clinical trials and appropriate therapy for AIDS evokes memories of the deliberate withholding of treatment by the researchers in the Tuskegee study. Public health professionals must ensure that HIV testing and counseling are accompanied by specific informed consent, full discussion of treatment options, and appropriate referrals for primary care and clinical trials.

The reproductive rights of HIV-infected women cannot be separated from societal values, political ideology, moral issues, and concern over access to primary health care. In an effort to prevent perinatal transmission, the CDC and state health departments advocate HIV testing programs and counsel HIV-infected women to avoid pregnancy.[16] However, implementation of these public health policies in the Black community is potentially volatile and disastrous. The promotion of condoms as a means of preventing HIV infection is viewed with suspicion by Blacks. Levine and Dubler state that "many African Americans view any attempt to interfere with or discourage reproduction as part of a plan for genocide" (p. 333).[16] If health care providers demonstrate a lack of sensitivity to these views and continue to advocate HIV testing, contraception, and abortion, the fears of Blacks—who are already alienated from health care providers—will be reinforced.

AIDS in the Black community must be understood within the broader context of other leading causes of preventable death that may result in decreased population growth and decreased lifespan. The failure to close the gap in health status between White and Black Americans can be directly attributed to social inequities and Blacks' lack of access to health care. George Lundberg, editor of the *Journal of the American Medical Association* attributes this lack of access to long-standing, institutionalized racial discrimination.[17] Although the PHS officials who conducted the Tuskegee study were clearly influenced by the racial prejudice of their time, it was their use of institutional power and resources that transformed prejudice into racism. We must guard against prejudicial assumptions about the race, class status, and lifestyle of people at risk for HIV infection. As Allan Brandt states, "the notion that science is a value free discipline must be rejected. The need for greater vigilance in assessing the specific ways in which social values and attitudes affect professional behavior is clearly indicated" (p. 27).[18] A failure to eliminate prejudice aggressively today could lead to repressive AIDS policies, cloaked as traditional public health practices designed to control the epidemic.

As the American public becomes increasingly aware of AIDS as a significant health problem in the Black community, there will be both opportunity and danger. The opportunity is to deal comprehensively rather than haphazardly with the problem as a whole: to see it as a social catastrophe brought on by years of economic deprivation and to meet it as other disasters are met, with adequate resources. The danger is that AIDS will be attributed to some innate weakness of Black people and used to justify further neglect and to rationalize continued deprivation. We must be mindful that the AIDS epidemic has uncovered the harsh reality of diminished economic resources, the limits of medical science, and confusion over how best to attribute responsibility for the prevention of HIV infection. It is within this context that public health must be used as a means for social justice.[19]

The AIDS epidemic has exposed the Tuskegee Syphilis Study as a historical marker for the legitimate discontent of Blacks with the public health system. In the absence of a cure for

AIDS, education remains our best chance to stop the spread of HIV infection. We must discuss the feeling within the Black community that AIDS is a form of genocide, a feeling justified by the history of the Tuskegee study. This dialogue can contribute to a better understanding of how to develop and implement HIV education programs that are scientifically sound, culturally sensitive, and ethnically acceptable.

► Acknowledgments

This study was supported in part by grant 14629 from the Robert Wood Johnson Foundation and a professional service contract from the Southern Christian Leadership Conference. Parts of this work were presented at the American Public Health Association Annual Meeting, New York City, October 1990; the Walter Reed Army Research Institute, Washington. DC, November 1990; and the Association for the Advancement of Health Education Annual Meeting. San Francisco, Calif., April 1991. The authors gratefully acknowledge the assistance of Patricia Mail and Peg Kopf, whose thoughtful criticism contributed significantly to this manuscript.

► References

1. Centers for Disease Control. *HIV/AIDS Surveillance Report.* June 1991. Atlanta, GA.
2. Smith R. Muhammad warns Blacks to beware: social AIDS. *Eclipse: The Black Student News Magazine of the University of Maryland.* November 23, 1988;21:6.
3. Bates K. AIDS: is it genocide? *Essence.* September 1990;21:77–116.
4. National Commission on AIDS. Hearings on HIV Disease in African American Communities. 1990.
5. Dalton H. AIDS in blackface. *Daedalus: J Am Acad Arts and Sci.* 1989 (Summer): 205–228.
6. Jones J. *Bad Blood: The Tuskegee Syphilis Experiment—Tragedy of Race and Medicine.* New York, NY: The Free Press: 1981.
7. Parran T. *Shadow on the Land—Syphilis.* New York, NY: Reynal & Hitchcock: 1937.
8. Rivers E, Schuman S, Olansky S. Twenty years of followup experience in a long-range medical study. *Public Health Rep.* 1953;68:391–395.
9. Johnson C. *Shadow of the Plantation.* Chicago. III: University of Chicago Press: 1934.
10. Cider J. Arnold R. Venereal Disease Control by Health Departments in the Past: Lessons for the Present.

► Editor's Notes

Stephen B. Thomas and Sandra Crouse Quinn are with the Minority Health Research Laboratory, Department of Health Education, University of Maryland.

Requests for reprints should be sent to Stephen B. Thomas. PhD. Department of Health Education. Minority Health Research Laboratory, University of Maryland, College Park, MD 20742.

Elizabeth Fee, PhD. and Robert K. Korstad, PhD. are coeditors of the journal's Public Health Then and Now department. Contributions for this department should be addressed to Dr. Fee as follows: Elizabeth Fee, PhD. The Johns Hopkins University. School of Hygiene and Public Health, 624 North Broadway, Baltimore. MD 21205.

▶ Questions for Discussion Part 1

History, Disease, and the Immune System

- How does HIV/AIDS differ from other epidemics? What is unique about its transmission, treatment, etc.?
- What ethical issues have surfaced as a result of HIV/AIDS?
- What does it mean to use a "Public Health approach" when dealing with issues surrounding HIV/AIDS?
- What factors affect the course of the disease in different individuals and how it affects the immune system? Why do some people who are infected remain healthy for long periods of time, such as Magic Johnson, while others die quickly?
- What can be learned from HIV/AIDS and how people reacted to those infected early on?
- What myths about the virus still exist and how do these myths impede prevention efforts and/or treatment?

▶ Human Subjects Protections—A Brief History

1947	**Nuremberg Code 26** Nazis physicians are tried at Nuremberg, Germany, for research atrocities performed on prisoners of war. This resulted in the Nuremberg Code, the first internationally recognized code of research ethics, issued by the Nazi War Crimes Tribunal.
1955	**The Wichita Jury Study** Researchers audio-taped jurors deliberating on cases, without their permission. Public criticism about the basic problem of deceiving people for research purposes in a setting where privacy and confidentiality were critically important. It is not appropriate to compromise the integrity of important social institutions, even if it's the only way to answer important research questions.
1962	**Kefauver-Harris Bill** The Kefauver-Harris bill is passed to ensure greater drug safety in the United States after thalidomide (a new sleeping pill) is found to have caused birth defects.
1964	**Helsinki Declaration** The 18th World Medical Assembly meets in Helsinki, Finland, and issues recommendations to guide physicians in biomedical research involving human subjects. The guide was known as the Helsinki Declaration.
1966	**The NEJM, Ethics of Clinical Research by Henry Beecher** Described the ethical violations of 22 studies that had been conducted by well-respected researchers and published in prestigious research journals. It was an unprecedented attempt by a respected member of the research community to focus attention on the need to improve ethical standards.
1932–1972	**Tuskegee Syphilis Study, 1932–1972** Public Health Service funded a study to evaluate the natural history of untreated syphilis in human beings. When the study was conceptualized, the basic concept was considered scientifically important and ethically justifiable because there was no known treatment for the disease. The research population included one of the most vulnerable research populations-approximately 300 mostly indigent African-American sharecroppers in Macon County, Alabama. The reality is that the subjects did not know that they were part of a research study designed to understand the natural progression of the disease. Many thought they were receiving beneficial medical care. The subjects were followed, untreated, many years after penicillin was known to cure syphilis. The study was stopped in 1972 after high profile stories in the national media generated public outrage over the blatant exploitation of this vulnerable segment of society. The fact that the federal government directed Tuskegee over such a long period of time has stained the integrity of the American research enterprise . . . it also catalyzed passage of the National Research Act in 1974.

1973	**Congressional Hearings on the Quality of Health Care and Human Experimentation** were held in response to public concern about ethical problems in the way medical and social science research was being conducted. This is a partial list:

Willowbrook Hepatitis Study, 1950s

To understand issues related to the transmission of the hepatitis virus in retarded children who were residents in the Willowbrook state school. The study design involved intentionally infecting health children with hepatitis by feeding them a solution made from the feces of children with active hepatitis.

Jewish Chronic Disease Studies, 1960s

Experiments were performed on chronically ill, mostly demented patients in the Jewish Chronic Disease Hospital. The purpose of the research was to determine how a weakened immune system influenced the spread of cancer. To evaluate this, live cancer cells were injected into the bloodstream of the subjects.

Milgram Studies of Obedience to Authority, 1960s

The purpose of the Milgram studies was to understand why people follow the directions of authority figures even when they are told to do things that are cruel or unethical. Subjects were instructed to deliver, at increasingly higher intensities, shocks to others. After they were "debriefed," subjects complained of extreme psychological distress after understanding the potentially lethal level of shocks administered.

San Antonio Contraceptive Study, 1970s

The purpose of this study was to determine the efficacy of different kinds of contraceptive pills. The clinic served predominantly indigent patients who had no other place to go for contraceptive advice or medication. The randomized design meant some patients received a placebo. As expected, there were a high number of unplanned pregnancies in the placebo group.

Tearoom Trade Study, 1970s

Social scientist, Laud Humphries posed as a "watch queen" outside public restrooms where people gathered to engage in anonymous homosexual behavior. He recorded the license plate numbers and other identifying information, which he used to obtain their names and addresses. He then presented himself at their homes to interview them about their background and family life. Many subjects were living with their family in a situation where it would be devastating to reveal information about homosexual activity. At no time did the subjects understand they were participating in a study about homosexuality. In his published reports, the level of detail was such that the identity of some of the subjects becomes known.

1974	**National Research Act** The National Commission for the Protection of Human Subjects of Biomedical and Behavioral Research is established, and Congress passes the National Research Act. This Act requires that all research involving human participants be regulated.
1979	**Belmont Report** The National Commission for the Protection of Human Subjects of Biomedical and Behavioral Research publishes the Belmont Report: the Ethical Principles and Guidelines for the Protection of Human Subjects of Research.
1993	**Albuquerque Tribunal publicizes Human Radiation Experiments** The Albuquerque Tribunal publicizes 1940s experimentation involving plutonium injections of human research subjects and secret radiation experiments. Indigent patients and mentally retarded children were deceived about the nature of their treatment.
1994	**National Bioethics Advisory Commission Formed** President Clinton creates the National Bioethics Advisory Commission (NBAC).
1995	**Human Radiation Experiments Unethical** The President's Advisory Commission on Human Radiation Experiments concludes that some of the radiation experiments from the 1940s were unethical.
1997	**Apology to Tuskegee Experimental Subjects** President Clinton issues a formal apology to the subjects of the Tuskegee Syphilis Experiments. NBAC continues investigations into genetics, consent, and privacy.
2002	**NBAC Charter Not Renewed** The U.S. Department of Health and Human Services under President Bush appointee Tommy Thompson decides not to renew the charter of the National Bioethics Advisory Commission (NBAC).

▶ **Suggested Readings and Resources for Part 1**

Kim J. Y, & Farmer, P. (2006). AIDS in 2006: Moving Toward One World, One Hope? *The New England Journal of Medicine,* 355:7:645–647.
http://content.nejm.org/cgi/content/full/355/7/645\

AVERT History: March 2007
http://www.avert.org/historyi.htm

CDC Tuskegee
http:www.cdc.gov/nchstp/od/tuskegee/time.htm

CDC Research Implications of Tuskegee Study
http://www.cdc.gov/nchstp/od/tuskegee/after.htm

▶ **Part 1**

Critical Thinking

1. Select one study from the Human Subjects Protection: A Brief History Timeline and look up additional information on the particular study. What are the ethical implications of the study?
2. Do you believe that the participants in the Tuskegee study were treated fairly? Why or why not? Support your conclusions using ethical reasoning.

Questions for Review

1. List and describe the different types of ethical analysis.
2. What was the Tuskegee Syphilis study and why was it considered unethical?
3. What was the Tearoom Trade Study and why was it considered unethical?
4. What are the four lessons from the history of sexually transmitted diseases?
5. What is the importance of ethics in public health?

PART TWO

Pathology of STIs

Chapter
4

Bacterial STIs

What You Should Know About Chlamydia

J. S. Nevid

▶ Did You Know That?

- Chlamydia occurs more commonly than either gonorrhea or syphilis.
- Both men and women can develop chlamydial infections.
- NGU, an infection frequently traced to the chlamydia bacterium, occurs about two or three times as often in men as gonorrhea, although men are more likely to have heard of gonorrhea than NGU.
- If you have gonorrhea, there's a good chance you also have a chlamydial infection.
- The majority of men and women with chlamydial infections experience no symptoms and are generally unaware that they are infected.
- Untreated chlamydia can lead to the development of PID in women, which can result in infertility.

What bacterial STD occurs most often—gonorrhea, syphilis, or chlamydia? Although you may be more familiar with gonorrhea and syphilis, it is chlamydia, in its various forms, that occurs most frequently.[1] The precise prevalences of chlamydial infections are unknown, since physicians are not required to report cases to public health officials. Yet researchers estimate that as many as 4 million cases occur annually in the U.S.[2] Sexually active teenagers and college students constitute two of the highest risk groups for chlamydial infections.[3]

Health Tips

People today stand a greater chance of contracting a chlamydial infection than either gonorrhea or syphilis. Yet fewer people are acquainted with chlamydia than with these other STDs.

► What Is Chlamydia?

Chlamydia is a term used to describe an infection caused by the *Chlamydia trachomatis* bacterium, a unique parasitic organism that survives only within cells.[4] The particular type of infection depends upon the particular organs that are affected by the bacterium. Among the infections caused by *Chlamydia trachomatis* are *nongonococcal urethritis* (NGU) in men and women, *epididymitis* in men (infection of the epididymis), and *cervicitis* (infection of the cervix), *endometritis* (infection of the endometrium, the inner layer of the uterus), and PID (pelvic inflammatory disease) in women.[5]

► Urethral Infections and Chlamydia

Urethritis is a term used to refer to any type of inflammation or infection of the urethra, the canal through which urine is carried from the bladder to the outside world. Nongonococcal urethritis or NGU refers to any type of urethritis not caused by the gonococcal bacterium. (NGU was formerly called nonspecific urethritis or NSU.) While many organisms can cause NGU, *Chlamydia trachomatis* is the most common culprit,[6] accounting for about half of the cases among men.[7] NGU seems to be about two or three times as prevalent among men in the United States as gonorrhea.[8] Men in the 20 to 24 age range are considered most at risk for both gonorrhea and NGU,[9] presumably because of the high level of sexual activity among men in this age range. Teenage men 15 to 19 years of age and men in their late twenties are the two next highest risk groups.[10]

NGU is generally diagnosed only in men. Women with urethritis due to *Chlamydia trachomatis* are generally said to have chlamydia or a chlamydial infection.

Chlamydial infections also frequently occur together with other STDs, most often gonorrhea. As many as 45 percent of cases of gonorrhea involve coexisting chlamydial infections.[11]

► What Are the Symptoms of Chlamydia?

Chlamydial infections may produce symptoms that are similar to those of gonorrhea, but are usually milder. NGU in men may produce a thin, whitish discharge from the penis and some burning or other pain during urination. These symptoms contrast with the yellow-greenish discharge and more intense pain associated with gonorrhea. There may be soreness in the scrotum and feelings of heaviness in the testes. A chlamydial infection can progress to infect the epididymis, causing epididymitis, which is associated in young men with such symptoms as pain, swelling and tenderness of the scrotum, and fever.[12]

Health Tips

The symptoms of chlamydia are similar to those of gonorrhea, but are generally milder.

Women with a chlamydial infection may experience burning sensations when they urinate, irritation in the genitals, and a mild (vaginal) discharge. Women may also encounter pelvic pain and irregular menstrual cycles. The cervix may look swollen and inflamed. Oral sex performed on an infected partner may lead to the development of a throat infection in either gender.

▶ Chlamydia Typically Occurs without Symptoms

Only about *one in three women and men* infected with chlamydia have any noticeable symptoms.[13] For this reason, many refer to chlamydia as the "silent disease." People with asymptomatic chlamydial infections can innocently pass along their infections to other sex partners.

Health Tips

Most people with chlamydial infections, perhaps two in three, have no symptoms. Yet chlamydia can lead to serious consequences, and be passed along to others, whether or not it produces any noticeable symptoms.

▶ How Is Chlamydia Transmitted?

Chlamydial infections are usually transmitted sexually through vaginal or anal intercourse. If a person touches his or her eyes after handling the genitals of an infected partner, chlamydia can also cause an eye infection. Chlamydia can also infect the throat if one has oral-genital sex with an infected partner.[14]

Chlamydial infections frequently have nonsexual origins in underdeveloped countries,[15] where they are often spread by contact with fecal matter or with discharges on the fingers or skin of infected persons, or by insect bites. In industrialized countries like the U.S. and Canada, however, virtually all cases of chlamydial infections in adults are transmitted sexually.[16]

Newborns can acquire potentially serious chlamydial eye infections as they pass through the birth canal of infected mothers during birth. Even newborns delivered by Caesarean section (also called C-section) may be infected if the amniotic sac (the sac holding the fetus) breaks before delivery.[17] Each year, more than 100,000 infants are infected with the bacterium during birth.[18] Of these, about 75,000 develop eye infections (conjunctivitis) and 30,000 develop a form of pneumonia caused by the chlamydial bacterium. Evidence from several studies suggests that between 2 and 26 percent of pregnant women in the United States carry *Chlamydia trachomatis* in their cervix and are thus capable of transmitting the organism to their newborns upon delivery.[19]

▶ What Are the Risks Associated with Untreated Chlamydia?

Because chlamydia is usually asymptomatic, many infected people go untreated. In untreated women, a chlamydial infection, like a gonorrheal infection, can spread to involve the reproductive tract, possibly leading to PID and scarring of the fallopian tubes, which can result in infertility.[20] Researchers estimate that perhaps half of the more than one million cases of PID diagnosed each year are attributable to chlamydial infections.[21] (Untreated gonorrhea is also a principal culprit.) Women with a history of exposure to *Chlamydia trachomatis* also stand twice the chance of incurring an ectopic (tubal) pregnancy, in which the pregnancy develops in a fallopian tube rather than the uterus.[22] Tubal pregnancies must be surgically removed (aborted) to avoid the rupturing of the tube.

Untreated chlamydial infections can also spread internally in men, causing such conditions as epididymitis. Chlamydial infections account for about half of the cases of epididymitis.[23] Swelling, feelings of tenderness, and pain in the scrotum are the principal symptoms. Fever may also be present. Yet only about one or two percent of men with untreated NGU caused by *Chlamydia trachomatis* go on to develop epididymitis.[24] That's no excuse for not seeking treatment, but men do stand a much lesser chance of serious complications from chlamydial infections than do women. Still, evidence concerning the long-term effects of untreated chlamydial infections in men remains inconclusive.

Health Tips

In women, untreated chlamydial infections can lead to PID and result in sterility, as well as increase the risk of tubal pregnancies; in men, the long-term consequences of untreated chlamydial infections remain undetermined.

▶ How Are Chlamydial Infections Diagnosed?

A laboratory test, the Abbott Testpack, permits physicians to verify a diagnosis in women in about 25 or 30 minutes.[25] The test analyzes a cervical smear (like a Pap smear) and identifies about 75 to 80 percent of infected cases, with relatively few *false positives* (incorrect positive findings). In men, a swab is inserted through the penile opening and the extracted fluid is analyzed to detect the presence of *Chlamydia trachomatis*.

▶ How Are Chlamydial Infections Treated?

Antibiotic treatment with a seven-day course of doxycycline, tetracycline, or erythromycin is highly effective in eradicating chlamydial infections.[26] (Penicillin, effective in treating gonorrhea, is ineffective against *Chlamydia trachomatis*.) A person does not acquire immunity to chlamydia as the result of having had the infection or being successfully treated for an infection; hence reinfection is possible following a subsequent exposure to the bacterium.

Treatment of sex partners is considered critical regardless of apparent symptomatology to prevent the infection from being passed back and forth.[27] A woman whose sex partner develops NGU should be examined for a chlamydial infection; at least 30% of these women will test positive for a chlamydial infection even though they (and their partners) may be free of symptoms.[28]

Men whose sex partners develop urethral or cervical infections should be medically evaluated, whether or not they notice any symptoms themselves. With chlamydia, both partners may be unaware that they are infected, and may be oblivious to the damage the infection is causing internally. Because of the risks posed by untreated chlamydial infections, especially to women, and the high rate of asymptomatic infections, many physicians routinely perform diagnostic tests on young women to detect chlamydia during regular check-ups.

Health Tips

If your sexual partner has a chlamydial infection, you should be tested too, whether or not you have any symptoms.

STD FACT SHEET: CHLAMYDIA

What it is	A bacterial STD
What causes it	The bacterium, *Chlamydia trachomatis*
How it is transmitted	Vaginal or anal intercourse or oral-genital contact; touching the eyes after touching the genitals of an infected partner; from infected mother to newborn during childbirth
Signs and symptoms	Women may notice more frequent urination, which may be painful. Lower abdominal pain and pelvic inflammation may occur, as well as a vaginal discharge. Most women, however, are asymptomatic.
	Men may experience symptoms similar to gonorrhea, but generally milder, such as burning or painful urination and a slight penile discharge. Most men, like most women, are symptom free. Either gender may experience a sore throat following oral-genital contact with an infected partner.
How it is diagnosed	In women, analysis of a cervical smear; in men, analysis of an extract of fluid drawn from the penis.
How it is treated	Use of antibiotics, such as doxycycline, tetracycline, or erythromycin.

► Notes

1. USDHHS (1992). *What we have learned from the AIDS community Demonstration Projects.* Atlanta: Center for Disease Control.

2. ABC List. American Social Health Association, 1996.

3. Shafer, M. A., et al. (1993). Evaluation of urine-based screening strategies to detect *Chlamydia trachomatis* among sexually active asymptomatic young men. *Journal of the American Medical Association,* 270, 2065–2070. CDC (1993b). Evaluation of surveillance for *Chlamydia trachomatis* infections in the United States, 1987 to 1991. *Mortality and Morbidity Weekly Report,* 42 (SS-3), 21–27.

4. Yarber, W. L., & Parillo, A. V. (1992). Adolescents and sexually transmitted diseases. *Journal of School Health,* 62, 331–338.

5. Martin, D. H. (1990). Chlamydial infections. *Medical Clinics of North America,* 74, 1367–1387.

6. Martin (1990); Westrom, L. V. (1990). Chlamydia trachomatis-clinical significance and strategies of intervention. *Seminars in Dermatology,* 9, 117–125.

7. Braude, A. I., Davis, C. E., & Fierer, J. (Eds.). (1986). *Infectious diseases and medical microbiology* (2nd ed.) Philadelphia: W. B. Saunders.

8. CDC (1989). Treatment Guidelines for Sexually Transmitted Diseases. *Morbidity and Morality Weekly Report,* 38, No. S–8.

9. CDC (1985). Chlamydia Trachomatis infection. *Morbidity & Mortality Weekly Report,* 34, 53.

10. Bowie, W. R. (1990). Approach to men with urethritis and urologic complications of sexually transmitted diseases. *Medical Clinics of North America, 74*, 1543–1557.

11. Bowie (1990).

12. CDC (1989b).

13. Stamm, W. E., & Holmes, K. K. (1990). *Chlamydia trachomatis* infections of the adult. In K. K. Holmes et al. (Eds.), *Sexually transmitted diseases.* (2nd ed.) (pp. 181–194). New York: McGraw-Hill Information Services Company.

14. American Social Health Association (1996).

15. Handsfield, H. H. (1988). Questions and answers: "Safe sex" guidelines: Mycoplasma and chlamydia infections. *Journal of the American Medical Association, 259*, 2022.

16. Bowie, W. (1984). Epidemiology and therapy of chlamydia trachomatis infections. *Drugs, 27*, 459–468.

17. Schachter, J. (1990). Biology of *Chlamydia trachomatis*. In K. K. Holmes, P. Mardh, P. F. Sparling, & P. J. Wiesner (Eds.). *Sexually transmitted diseases* (2nd Ed.). (pp. 161–180). New York: McGraw-Hill.

18. Reinisch (1990).

19. Graham, J. M., & Blanco, J. D. (1990). Chlamydial infections. *Primary Care: Clinics in Office Practice, 17*, 85–93.

20. Reinisch (1990).

21. CDC. Sexually Transmitted Disease Surveillance 1995, September 1995; Hodgson, R., et al. (1990). Chlamydia trachomatis: The prevalence, trend and importance in initial infertility management. *Australian and New Zealand Journal of Obstetrics and Gynaecology, 30*, 25–254; Garland, S. M., Lees, M. I., & Skurrie, I. J. (1990). Chlamydia trachomatis: Role in tubal infertility. *Australian and New Zealand Journal of Obstetrics and Gynecology, 30*, 83–86.

22. American Social Health Association, 1996.

23. Sherman, K. J., et al. (1990). Sexually transmitted diseases and tubal pregnancy. *Sexually Transmitted Diseases, 17*, 115–121.

24. Crum, C., & Ellner, P. (1985). Chlamydia infections: Making the diagnosis. *Contemporary Obstetrics and Gynecology, 25*, 153–159, 163, 165, 168.

25. Bowie (1990).

26. Reichart, C. A., et al. (1990). Evaluation of Abbott Testpack Chlamydia for detection of chlamydia trachomatis in patients attending sexually transmitted diseases clinics. *Sexually Transmitted Diseases, 17*, 147–151.

27. Centers for Disease Control and Prevention. 1993 Sexually transmitted diseases treatment guidelines. *MMWR*, 1993, 42 (No. RR-14).

28. Martin (1990); CDC (1993a).

29. Stamm & Holmes (1990).

30. CDC (1993a).

What You Should Know About Gonorrhea

J. S. Nevid

▶ Did You Know That?

- If you are 20 to 24 years of age, you are in the age group most at risk of contracting gonorrhea.
- About four of five women who contract gonorrhea experience no symptoms, but are capable of passing the infection along to their sexual partners.
- Gonorrhea can cause internal damage even in the absence of symptoms or if initial symptoms disappear.
- You can develop a gonorrheal infection of the throat by performing oral sex on an infected partner.
- The chances of contracting gonorrhea from just one sexual contact with an infected partner are about 50 percent for women and 20 to 25 percent for men.
- Untreated, gonorrhea can lead to infertility in men and women.
- Some strains of gonorrhea are resistant to penicillin.

Has your doctor ever told you that you had strep throat? Scarlet fever? Pneumonia? Bronchitis? These are but a few of the diseases that are caused by tiny, one-celled organisms called **bacteria** (singular form, bacterium), which come in various forms and shapes. While we tend to think of bacteria as harmful organisms (indeed some are), most are actually helpful rather than harmful. Bacteria are the organisms responsible for disintegrating organic waste materials. They also play vital roles in our digestive system. However, disease-causing bacteria are responsible for a host of diseases, including such STDs as gonorrhea, syphilis, chlamydia, and certain vaginal infections. This chapter focuses on gonorrhea.

▶ What Is Gonorrhea?

Gonorrhea ("the clap" or "the drip") is a bacterial infection caused by the gonococcus bacterium. Gonorrhea has been known since ancient times. The term *gonorrhea* is credited to the

Greek physician Galen, who lived in the second century A.D. Yet the bacterium responsible for the disease was not isolated until 1879, when it was first identified by Albert L. S. Neisser, after whom it was named *Neisseria gonorrhoeae*.

▶ How Widespread Is Gonorrhea?

Gonorrhea is one of the most common types of sexually transmitted diseases in our society, accounting for about 750,000 reported cases annually in the U.S.[1] Since many other cases go unreported, the actual number of cases may be as high as several million a year.

Gonorrhea strikes predominantly among young people, typically between the ages of 20 and 24.[2] If you are sexually active, you should consider yourself at risk, irrespective of your age.

▶ What Are the Symptoms of Gonorrhea?

In men, symptoms usually appear within two to five days following infection. At first, a clear penile discharge appears, which, a day or so later turns yellow to yellow-green, thickens, and becomes pusslike. Inflammation of the urethra (the tube that carries urine from the bladder out through the penis in men, or through the urinary opening in women) occurs, and urination is accompanied by a burning sensation. Thirty to 40 percent of males have swelling and tenderness in the lymph glands of the groin. Inflammation and other symptoms may become chronic if left untreated.

Gonorrhea in women primarily infects the cervix (the lower end of the uterus that adjoins the vagina), causing **cervicitis,** which is often accompanied by a yellowish pusslike discharge that inflames the genitals. Women, like men, can have burning sensations when they urinate if the infection spreads to the urethra. Although such symptoms are possible, about four women in five have no noticeable symptoms (are asymptomatic). For this reason, they are unlikely to seek treatment unless the disease advances to produce more serious symptoms. They may also innocently infect another sex partner. Although infected men are more likely to have noticeable symptoms, they too may be infected without realizing it.

Health Tips

Most women and some men who become infected with gonorrhea experience no symptoms. With or without symptoms, the infection may cause internal damage and be transmitted to others.

Even without treatment, the initial symptoms of gonorrhea, if they do occur, often abate within a few weeks. Thus, victims may think of gonorrhea as being no worse than a bad cold. The truth is that even though the early symptoms may fade, the gonococcus bacterium may continue to cause damage within the body.

Health Tips

While the initial symptoms of gonorrhea may abate, if left untreated, the infection can spread within the reproductive system, causing damage to internal organs.

▶ How Is Gonorrhea Transmitted?

The gonococcus bacterium that causes gonorrhea requires a warm, moist environment. The mucous membranes along the urinary tract in both men and women and along the cervix in women provide such an environment for the bacterium to flourish. Outside the body, the gonococcus bacterium dies in about a minute. Despite what you may have heard, there is no evidence of transmission of gonorrhea from touching toilet seats or other dry objects.[3] However, gonorrhea may be contracted by contact with a moist and warm towel or sheet used immediately beforehand by an infected person.[4] Such occurrences are rare, however. In almost all cases, gonorrhea is transmitted sexually through vaginal or anal intercourse, oral-genital sex, or from mother to newborn during delivery.[5]

Health Tips

No, you will not contract gonorrhea by touching a toilet seat. However, some other STDs, such as "crabs," can be contracted from contact with toilet seats used previously by infected persons.

Gonorrhea can also infect other parts of the body than the genitals. A person who performs oral sex (fellatio) on an infected man may contract a gonorrheal infection of the throat, called *pharyngeal gonorrhea*. Pharyngeal gonorrhea may also be transmitted, but less commonly so, by mouth-to-mouth kissing and by oral sex performed on an infected woman (cunnilingus). The eyes provide a good environment for the bacterium. Thus, a person whose hands come into contact with infected genitals and who inadvertently touches his or her eyes afterward may infect them. Infants have contracted gonorrhea of the eyes (**gonococcal ophthalmia neonatorum**) when passing through the birth canals of infected mothers. This disorder may cause blindness but has become rare because the eyes of newborns are treated routinely with antibiotic ointment toxic to gonococcal bacteria.

Gonorrhea of the pharynx and the rectum are fairly common among gay males and are spread by oral and anal intercourse, respectively. A gonorrheal infection of the cervix in a woman may be transferred to her rectum if the couple engages in anal intercourse directly following vaginal intercourse. Gonorrhea is less likely to be spread by vaginal than penile discharges. Thus, lesbians are less likely than male homosexuals to contract the disease. Still, any intimate sexual contact with an infected partner may transmit the disease.

Health Tips

Gonorrheal infections may be spread from one part of the body to another, such as from the cervix to the rectum in the case of an infected woman who engages in anal intercourse directly following vaginal intercourse.

▶ What Are the Risks of Contracting Gonorrhea?

Gonorrhea is highly contagious. Women stand a slightly greater than 50 percent chance, and men a 20 to 25 percent chance, of contracting gonorrhea after just one sexual exposure to an infected partner.[6] The risks to women are believed to be greater because women retain infected semen in the vagina following intercourse. The risk of infection increases with repeated exposure. In men, for example, the risk of infection climbs to 60 to 80 percent following four sexual encounters with one infected women, or one sexual encounter with each of four infected women.[7]

► What Are the Risks Associated with Untreated Gonorrhea?

When gonorrhea is not treated early, it may spread within the body, striking the internal reproductive organs. In men, it may result in *epididymitis* (an infection of the epididymis, the coiled tube in the back of each testicle through which sperm pass as they mature), which can cause fertility problems. Occasionally the kidneys are affected. The bacterium may spread through the cervix in women to the uterus, **fallopian tubes,** ovaries, and other parts of the abdominal cavity, causing **pelvic inflammatory disease** (PID).

Symptoms of PID include cramps, other forms of abdominal pain and tenderness, cervical tenderness and discharge, irregular menstrual cycles, coital pain, fever, nausea and vomiting. PID may also be asymptomatic. Whether or not women experience symptoms, PID can cause scarring that blocks the fallopian tubes and impairs fertility. PID is a serious illness that requires aggressive treatment with antibiotics to fight the underlying infection.[8] Surgery may also be needed to remove the infected tissue. Unfortunately, many women only become aware of a gonococcal infection when they experience the discomfort of PID.

► How Is Gonorrhea Diagnosed?

Diagnosis of gonorrhea involves clinical inspection of the genitals by a physician, followed by the culturing and examination under a microscope of a sample of genital discharge.[9] If you have any symptoms of burning urination, a yellowish, pusslike discharge from the penis or vagina, or any feelings of pelvic pain or discomfort, consult your physician.

► How Is Gonorrhea Treated?

Gonorrhea is treated effectively with antibiotics. While penicillin was once the treatment of choice, the rise of penicillin-resistant strains of *Neisseria gonorrhoeae* has led to the use of alternate antibiotics.[10] A single injection of the antibiotic *ceftriaxone,* which has an excellent response against all strains of the gonococcus bacterium,[11] is now the preferred treatment.[12] Ceftriaxone cures all forms of uncomplicated gonorrhea.[13] An alternative antibiotic such as *spectinomycin* may be used with people who cannot tolerate ceftriaxone. Successful treatment provides no protection against reinfection with gonorrhea if the person is again exposed to the bacterium. Sexual partners of persons with gonorrhea (or any other STD) should be evaluated by a physician, irrespective of whether any symptoms are present.

Health Tips

While some forms of gonorrhea are resistant to penicillin, other antibiotics are available that can cure all uncomplicated forms of gonorrhea.

Since gonorrhea and chlamydia (with or without symptoms) often occur together, persons infected with gonorrhea are usually also treated for chlamydia through the use of another antibiotic, generally *doxycycline*—or alternately *tetracycline* or *erythromycin*—administered orally over a course of seven days.[14]

Health Tips

Since the bacteria causing gonorrhea and chlamydia often travel together, if you have one, there's a good chance that you have the other. The good news is that antibiotic treatment effectively cures both.

STD FACT SHEET: GONORRHEA

What it is	A bacterial STD
What causes it	Gonococcus bacterium (*Neisseria gonorrhoeae*)
How it is transmitted	Vaginal or anal intercourse, oral-genital contact, or from mother to baby during childbirth
Signs and symptoms	In men, a yellowish, thick penile discharge, burning urination. In women, increased vaginal discharge, burning urination, irregular menstrual bleeding (most women show no early symptoms)
How it is diagnosed	Clinical inspection, culture of sample discharge
How it is treated	Antibiotics, typically ceftriaxone or spectinomycin

▶ Notes

1. CDC (1989a). *Summaries of identifiable diseases in the United States.*

2. National Center for Health Statistics. (1985). *Health: United States 1985.* Washington, D.C.: U.S. Department of Health and Human Services.

3. Calderone, M. S., & Johnson, E. W. (1989). *Family book about sexuality* (rev. ed.). New York: Harper & Row; Reinisch, J.M. (1990). *The Kinsey Institute new report on sex: What you must know to be sexually literate.* New York: St. Martin's Press.

4. Calderone & Johnson (1989).

5. Reinisch (1990).

6. Handsfield, H. (1984). Gonorrhea and uncomplicated gonococcal infection. In K. K. Holmes, et al. (Eds.), *Sexually transmitted diseases* (pp. 205–220). New York: McGraw-Hill; Platt, R., Rice, P., & McCormack, W. (1983). Risk of acquiring gonorrhea and prevalence of abnormal adrenal findings among women recently exposed to gonorrhea. *Journal of the American Medical Association, 250,* 3205–3209.

7. Reinisch (1990).

8. Reinisch (1990).

9. Ison, C. A. (1990). Laboratory methods in genitourinary medicine: Methods of diagnosing gonorrhea. *Genitourinary Medicine, 66,* 453–459; Judson, F. N. (1990). Gonorrhea. *Medical Clinics of North America, 74,* 1353–1366.

10. Goldstein, A. M., & Clark, J. H. (1990). Treatment of uncomplicated gonococcal urethritis with single-dose ceftriaxone. *Sexually Transmitted Diseases, 17,* 181–183.

11. Goldstein & Clark (1990).

12. CDC (1989b). Treatment guidelines for sexually transmitted diseases. *Morbidity and Mortality Weekly Report, 38,* No. S-8.

13. Judson (1990).

14. Moran, J. S., & Zenilman, J. M. (1990). Therapy for gonococcal infections: Options in 1989. *Reviews of Infectious Diseases,* (Suppl0. 6.) S633–S644.

What You Should Know About Syphilis

J. S. Nevid

▶ Did You Know That?

- Syphilis has been making a comeback in recent years in the U.S.
- Increased rates of syphilis in our society are linked to the increased use of cocaine.
- There is no evidence that syphilis can be picked up from a toilet seat.
- You stand a one in three chance of contracting syphilis from a single sexual contact with an infected partner.
- Syphilis does not disappear when the initial symptoms abate.
- Untreated syphilis can eventually lead to brain and heart damage and result in death.

No society wanted to be associated with **syphilis**. In Naples they called it "the French disease"; in France it was "the Neapolitan disease." Many Italians called it "the Spanish disease," but in Spain they called it "the disease of Española" (modern Haiti). But what is syphilis? What causes it? How is it spread? Why is syphilis on the rise in our society?

▶ What Is Syphilis?

Syphilis is a sexually transmitted bacterial infection. *Treponema pallidum,* the bacterium that causes syphilis, was first isolated in 1905 by the German scientist Fritz Schaudinn. The name *Treponema pallidum* (*T. pallidum,* for short), reflects Greek and Latin roots meaning a "faintly colored (pallid) turning thread"—an apt description of the corkscrewlike organism when seen under the microscope (see Figure 4-1). Because of its spiral shape, *T. pallidum* is also called a *spirochete,* from Greek roots meaning "spiral" and "hair."

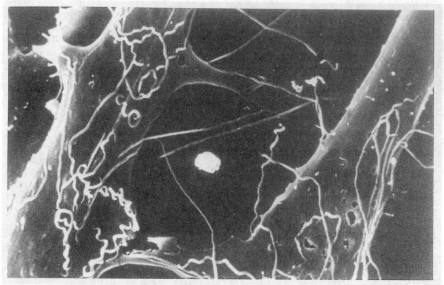

FIGURE 4-1 *Treponema Pallidum. Treponema pallidum* is the bacterium that causes syphilis. Because of the spiral shape, *T. pallidum* is also called a *spirochete.*

▶ How Widespread Is Syphilis?

The incidence of syphilis decreased in the United States with the introduction of penicillin, an antibiotic which is used to treat the infection.[1] But despite the availability of penicillin, and the recent emphasis on safer sex, syphilis has been making a comeback in recent years (see Figure 4-2).[2]

The incidence of syphilis rose 34 percent from 1981 to 1989.[3] In just one year, 1987, the number of cases of syphilis rose an astonishing 27 percent in both men and women.[4] In 1988, the rates of syphilis in the United States had reached their highest levels in 40 years.[5] By 1989, about 45,000 cases of syphilis were reported to public health agencies.[6] Many other cases go unreported.

Medical researchers suspect that the rising incidence of syphilis is linked to increased use of cocaine in our society, especially crack cocaine.[7] Cocaine users appear to be at greater risk of contracting syphilis than nonusers because they are more likely to engage in risky sexual practices, such as sex with multiple partners and with prostitutes, not because of cocaine use per se.[8] Syphilis and other STDs are often spread among drug users, prostitutes (many of whom abuse drugs themselves), and their sex partners.[9]

Syphilis has been rising fastest among minority groups in inner-city neighborhoods, largely because disadvantaged minority groups in our society are disproportionately affected by problems of drug abuse and prostitution. Syphilis remains less prevalent than gonorrhea, but it can lead to more grievous effects, including blindness, heart disease, deteriorative mental illness, and even death.

▶ How Is Syphilis Transmitted?

Syphilis is most often transmitted through vaginal or anal intercourse, or oral-genital or oral-anal contact with an infected person. Transmission usually occurs during contact between the open (infectious) lesions on the body of the infected partner and the mucous membranes or

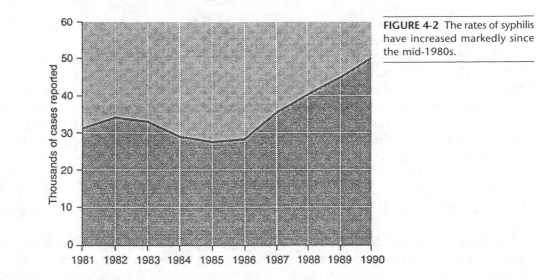

FIGURE 4-2 The rates of syphilis have increased markedly since the mid-1980s.

skin abrasions of the partner's body. The chances of contracting syphilis from one sexual contact with an infected partner is estimated at one in three.[10] While syphilis may be contracted by directly touching a **chancre**, there is no evidence that it can be transmitted by using the same toilet seat as an infected person.

Health Tips

You stand about a one in three chance of contracting syphilis from a sexual contact with an infected person.

Since the spirochete can cross the placental membrane, a pregnant woman can pass along the microbe to the fetus in-utero. Miscarriage, stillbirth, or congenital syphilis may result, causing impaired vision and hearing, or deformed bones and teeth. Diagnosis of syphilis in the mother by means of a blood test may help avoid transmission of the disease to the baby if treatment is administered early in pregnancy. The fetus will probably not be harmed if an infected mother is treated before the fourth month of pregnancy.

▶ What Are the Symptoms of Syphilis?

Syphilis progresses through several stages, each of which has characteristic symptoms. In the first or *primary stage,* a painless chancre (a hard, round, ulcerlike lesion with raised edges) appears at the site of infection two to four weeks after contact. When women are infected, the chancre usually forms on the vaginal walls or the cervix. It may also form on the external genitalia, most often on the labia (the folds of tissue that cover the vaginal opening). When men are infected, the chancre usually forms on the tip (glans) of the penis, or sometimes on the scrotum (external sac containing the testes or testicles) or penile shaft (the cylindrical body of the penis under the glans). If the mode of transmission is oral sex, the chancre may appear on the lips or tongue. If spread by anal sex, the rectum may serve as the site of the chancre. The chancre disappears within a few weeks but if the infection remains untreated, syphilis will continue to work within the body.

The *secondary stage* begins a few weeks to a few months later and is noted by the appearance of a skin rash consisting of painless, reddish raised bumps that darken after a while and burst, oozing a discharge. Other symptoms include sores in the mouth, painful swelling of joints, a sore throat, headaches, and fever, so a sufferer may wrongly assume that he or she has "the flu." A person may infect others during the primary stage, and for several years into the secondary stage. A pregnant woman, however, may pass along the infection to her newborn at any stage during the course of the infection.[11]

These symptoms soon disappear, and the infection enters the *latent stage* and may lie dormant for perhaps 1 to 40 years. But spirochetes continue to multiply during the latent stage and burrow into the circulatory system, central nervous system (brain and spinal cord), and bones.

In many cases, the disease eventually progresses to a late or *tertiary* stage. A large ulcer may form on the digestive organs, liver, lungs, skin, muscle tissue, or other organs. This destructive ulcer can often be successfully treated, but still more serious damage can occur as the infection attacks the cardiovascular system (heart and major blood vessels) or the central nervous system, in the latter case causing a condition called *neurosyphilis*. Neurosyphilis can cause brain damage, resulting in paralysis, or a deteriorating form of mental illness called **general paresis.** Damage to the cardiovascular system or central nervous system can also be fatal. The primary and secondary symptoms of syphilis inevitably disappear, so victims may be tempted to believe that they are no longer at risk. They may, therefore, fail to see a doctor. This is indeed unfortunate, because failure to eradicate the infection through proper treatment may eventually lead to the dire consequences associated with tertiary syphilis.

Health Tips

As with many other STDs, the disappearance of initial symptoms does not mean that the disease is cured. In the case of syphilis, the disease progresses through several stages if left untreated, and may eventually result in serious complications or even death.

▶ How Is Syphilis Diagnosed?

Primary-stage syphilis is diagnosed by clinical examination. When a chancre is found, fluid may be drawn from it and examined under a microscope in a procedure called a dark-field test, which makes the spirochetes more visible to the eye. The most widely used blood test is the **VDRL.** The VDRL tests for the presence of antibodies in the blood to *Treponema pallidam*. Blood tests are usually not reliable until the secondary stage begins, as it may take some time after initial infection for antibodies to the bacterium to appear in the blood.

▶ How Is Syphilis Treated?

Penicillin is the treatment of choice for syphilis. Primary and secondary syphilis, and latent syphilis of less than one year's duration, are generally treated with a single injection of penicillin (or doxycycline, tetracycline, or erythromycin for nonpregnant penicillin-allergic patients).[12] Latent stage syphilis of more than one year in duration, and neurosyphilis, are generally treated with multiple doses of injectable penicillin for two or three weeks. Like gonorrhea, successful treatment does not prevent reinfection. Also, like gonorrhea and other STDs, sex partners of persons infected with syphilis should also be evaluated by a physician.

STD FACT SHEET: SYPHILIS

What it is	A bacterial STD
What causes it	The bacterium, *Treponema pallidum* ("spirochete")
How it is transmitted	Vaginal or anal intercourse, oral-genital contact, touching an infectious sore or chancre
Signs and symptoms	Primary symptom is a hard, round painless sore (chancre) at the site of infection. If left untreated, the infection may progress through several stages.
How it is diagnosed	In its primary stage, diagnosis is by clinical examination of the chancre and microscopic examination of fluid drawn from a chancre. A blood test, the VDRL, may be used if the disease reaches the secondary stage of infection.
How it is treated	Antibiotic treatment with penicillin, or doxycycline, tetracycline, or erythromycin for nonpregnant penicillin-allergic patients.

▶ Notes

1. Zenker, P. N., & Rolfs, R. T. (1990). Treatment of syphilis, 1989. *Reviews of Infectious Diseases* (Suppl. 6), S590–S609.
2. Centers for Disease Control and Prevention. Sexually Transmitted Disease Surveillance 1995, Division of STD Prevention, September 1996.
3. American Social Health Association (1996).
4. Minkoff et al. (1990); Rolfs, R. T., Goldberg, M., & Sharrar, R. G. (1990) Risk factors for syphilis: Cocaine use and prostitution. *American Journal of Public Health, 80,* 853–857.
5. Rolfs et al. (1990).
6. Farley, A. U., Hadler, J. L., & Gunn, R. A. (1990). The syphilis epidemic in Connecticut: Relationship to drug use and prostitution. *Sexually Transmitted Diseases, 17,* 163–168.
7. Reinisch (1990).
8. Wooldridge, W. E. (1991). Syphilis: A new visit from an old enemy. *Postgraduate Medicine, 89,* 199–202.
9. CDC (1989).

Chapter 5

Viral STIs

What You Should Know About Herpes

J. S. Nevid

▶ Did You Know That?

- There are different forms of herpes caused by distinct, but related viruses.
- Some herpes infections of the genitals are actually caused by the oral herpes virus, some herpes infections of the mouth are caused by the genital herpes virus.
- Genital herpes may be contracted from sexual contact with an infected partner even during symptom-free periods.
- Although the symptoms of genital herpes disappear after an active episode, the virus remains in the body indefinitely and can cause recurrent outbreaks.
- Herpes outbreaks may be preceded by certain warning signs.
- Although oral administration of the drug acyclovir may reduce the rate of recurrent episodes of genital herpes, the long-term safety of the drug remains unclear.
- A person's attitudes play an important role in determining the emotional consequences of coping with herpes.

The hysteria that surrounded the rapid spread of herpes in the 1970s and early 80s has all but died since the world teamed to dread an even more threatening STD: AIDS. Before AIDS, it was genital herpes that many sexually active people feared the most. Herpes was feared so much because it is incurable and, at the time, essentially untreatable. Herpes still remains a very real threat. Once you get herpes, it's yours for life. After the initial attack, it remains an unwelcome guest in your body, finding a cozy place to lie low until it stirs up trouble again, causing recurrent outbreaks that usually happen at the worst times, like around final exams. Not only can you not get rid of the virus, but you can pass it along to whomever else you have sex with for the rest of your life. Ugh! Relationships, and even many prospective marriages, have been zapped when one partner learns that the other is infected. But many people learn to cope with herpes and go on with their lives and loves, adapting to it as more of an occasional nuisance or annoyance than a wholesale catastrophe.

While much of the public alarm about herpes has been overshadowed by concerns about AIDS, herpes remains a troubling and potentially even a dangerous disease, as it appears to increase the risk of cervical cancer in women. While we cannot cure it, or rid the body of the virus that causes it, progress has been made in treating the disease. Here's what you should know about herpes:

▶ What Is Herpes?

The term herpes refers to several different types of infections caused by related forms of the *herpes simplex* virus. The most common herpes virus, **herpes simplex virus type 1**, or HSV-1 virus, causes *oral herpes,* which appears as cold sores or fever blisters on the lips or mouth. Many people have recurrent "cold sores" without realizing that these are caused by a herpes virus. The oral herpes virus can also be transferred to the genitals by the hands or by oral-genital contact. It is believed that between 10 and 50 percent of the cases of genital herpes are actually caused by the HSV-1 virus (a kind of "cold sore" of the genitals).[1]

Genital herpes is caused by a related but distinct virus, the **herpes simplex virus type 2** (HSV-2). This virus produces painful shallow sores and blisters on the genitals. HSV-2 can also be transferred to the mouth through oral-genital contact. Thus either HSV-1 or HSV-2 may cause herpes outbreaks on the mouth and lips, or on the genitals. Since both viruses can be transmitted sexually, the diseases they cause can be classified as STDs. Both types of herpes viruses may also cause an infection of the throat. Oral sex is a frequent channel for transmitting the herpes virus (either HSV-1 or HSV-2) from the genitals to the throat.

▶ How Many People Have Herpes?

Physicians are not required to report cases of herpes to public health officials, so we cannot say precisely how many cases occur. Estimates are that about 30 million people in the U.S. are infected with genital herpes.[2] Researchers believe that 500,000 new cases of genital herpes occur annually.[3] More than 100 million Americans may be infected with oral herpes.

Who Is Most at Risk?

With perhaps 30 million people in the U.S. infected with genital herpes, and perhaps more than 100 million infected with oral herpes, the chances of contracting one or both forms of herpes from potential sexual partners is fairly high, especially if one has sexual contact with multiple partners. The chance of contracting genital herpes from a single sexual encounter with an infected partner during a flare-up of the disease is estimated at about 50 percent for men and 80 to 90 percent for women.[4]

Genital herpes occurs more frequently among better educated people,[5] including college students, and fears about it—especially about its effects on future relationships—are common on college campuses. Genital herpes is also more frequent in the United States among African Americans than whites.[6] Yet herpes cuts across all racial, ethnic, and educational categories.

▶ How Is Herpes Transmitted?

The herpes viruses can be transmitted through oral, anal, or vaginal sex with an infected person. Oral herpes is also easily contracted by drinking from the same cup, by kissing, and even by sharing moist towels with an infected person. Genital herpes is most often spread by vaginal or anal intercourse or by oral sex. Herpes viruses can also survive for several hours on toilet seats or other objects, where they may be transmitted by direct contact with the genitals, although this mode of transmission is probably unusual. Use of a latex condom may reduce the risk of transmitting or contracting genital herpes, especially if combined with a spermicide (a sperm killing chemical, used for contraception) containing the ingredient nonoxynol-9, which not only deactivates sperm but is toxic to the herpes virus as well as to many other STD-causing organisms. Yet transmission may occur when herpes sores (lesions) are present even with the use of condoms.[7] It may be wise to err on the side of caution and abstain from intimate genital contact during an active episode of genital herpes, at least until any herpes sores completely heal over.

Health Tips

- Since the HSV-2 virus cannot pass through a latex condom,[8] couples who are sexually active during herpes outbreaks should use a latex condom along with a spermicide that contains the ingredient nonoxynol-9, which is toxic to the herpes virus.
- However, since use of a condom is no guarantee against transmission of herpes viruses (condoms may tear or fall off, or not cover all exposed areas that may come into contact with active lesions), it would be wise to avoid genital contact until herpes sores have completely healed.

Can Genital Herpes Be Transmitted Between Flare-ups?

Unfortunately, yes. While genital herpes is most contagious during active flare-ups of the disease, alarming new evidence shows that herpes may also be transmitted from an infected partner when no symptoms (genital sores or feelings of burning or itching in the genitals) are present.[9] Some researchers suspect that *all* infected women may shed some of the virus at least some of the time they are symptom-free, making it possible for them to unknowingly infect their partners at these times.[10] The relative risks of contracting genital herpes from a symptom-free infected partner remain unclear.

Can Women Pass Along Herpes to Their Newborns?

Sadly, yes. An infected women may pass along genital herpes to her newborn as the baby makes its way through the birth canal during childbirth. Genital herpes is a potentially serious problem for a newborn, causing damage or even death.[11] To avoid the risk of the newborn becoming infected when passing through the birth canal, obstetricians usually perform Caesarean sections (C-sections) if the mother shows an active outbreak at the time of delivery. C-sections are currently recommended for women who show active lesions or warning signs of an infection at the time of delivery.[12] Unfortunately, the absence of symptoms may not guarantee the safety of the baby. In one study of some 16,000 pregnant women, a small proportion (about 3.5 women in a thousand) showed no symptoms of genital herpes but produced positive test results that indicated an active infection. They may thus have been capable of unknowingly infecting their newborns.[13]

Can Herpes Be Spread from One Part of the Body to Another?

Herpes may be spread from one part of the body to another by touching the infected area and then touching or rubbing another body part. One potentially serious result is a herpes infection of the eye—**ocular herpes**. People with active oral herpes who wear contact lenses need to be careful not to put their lenses in their mouths to wet them before inserting them into their eyes, lest they risk spreading the infection to their eyes.

Health Tips

Although thorough washing with soap and water after touching an infected area may reduce the risk of spreading the infection to other parts of the body, it is better to avoid touching the infected area altogether, especially if active sores are present.

▶ Health Risks Associated with Genital Herpes

While herpes sores heal naturally, researchers find that herpes may lead to serious complications, especially in women. The miscarriage rate among herpes sufferers is more than three times higher than the rate for the general population.[14] Herpes also appears to place women at greater risk of genital cancers, such as cervical cancer, a potential killer.[15] All women, not just herpes sufferers, are advised to have regular pelvic examinations, including Pap smears for early detection of cervical cancer.

▶ What Are the Symptoms of Genital Herpes?

Genital herpes is characterized by the appearance of genital lesions or sores, which appear about six to eight days after infection. At first they appear as reddish, painful bumps, or papules (pimples) along the penis in the man or the external genitalia in the woman. The papules may also appear on the thigh or buttocks in men or women, or in the vagina or on the cervix in women. These papules turn into groups of small blisters that are filled with fluid containing infectious viral particles. The blisters are attacked by the body's immune system (white blood cells). They become filled with pus and break open, becoming extremely painful, shallow sores, or ulcers, that are surrounded by a red ring. The person is especially infectious at this time, as the ulcers shed millions of viral particles. Other symptoms may include headaches and muscle aches, swollen lymph glands, fever, burning on urination, and a vaginal discharge in women. The blisters crust over and heal in one to three weeks. Internal sores in the vagina or on the cervix may take ten days longer than external (labial) sores to completely heal, so physicians advise infected women to avoid unprotected intercourse for at least 10 days following the healing of external sores.

Health Tips

Treat any appearance of a sore or blister around the genitals as a warning sign. Check it out with a physician.

Women with herpes should avoid unprotected intercourse for at least ten days following the healing of external sores, just in case there are any internal sores that take longer to heal.

Is Genital Herpes Cured If the Sores Heal on Their Own?

Although the symptoms of genital herpes disappear on their own within a few days or weeks, the disease does not. The virus remains in the body permanently, burrowing into nerve cells in the base of the spine, where it may lie dormant for years, or even a lifetime. The infected person is least contagious during this dormant stage. For reasons that remain unclear, the virus becomes reactivated and gives rise to symptoms in 30 to 70 percent of cases.[16]

What Factors Might Prompt Recurrences?

While the causal factors explaining recurrences are not entirely clear, scientists suspect that recurrences may be related to such factors as infections (as in a cold), stress, depression, exposure to the sun, and hormonal changes, such as those that occur during pregnancy or menstruation.[17] Yet not all researchers have been able to link emotional stress to herpes flare-ups.[18] Recurrences tend to occur within three to twelve months of the initial episode and to affect the same part of the body. They tend to be milder, and briefer in duration, than initial episodes, lasting from about three days to two weeks, and are often asymptomatic. Both initial and recurrent episodes of genital herpes tend to produce more severe symptoms in women, such as painful genital lesions.[19] Recurrences often decrease in frequency over time and may eventually disappear. Flare-ups sometimes continue to recur, however, with annoying frequency over the course of a lifetime.

Health Tips

To reduce the risk of recurrent herpes:
- Maintain regular sleeping habits.
- Avoid unnecessary stress.
- Learn to manage the stress you can't avoid.
- Avoid excessive exposure to the sun.
- Take good care of your general health.
- Take good care of your mental health and well-being.

Are There Warning Signs of an Impending Outbreak?

About 50 percent of people with recurrent genital herpes experience warning signs (called prodromal symptoms) before an active outbreak.[20] These may include feelings of burning, itching, pain, tingling, or tenderness in the affected area. These symptoms may be accompanied by sharp pains in the lower extremities, groin, or buttocks. Herpes sufferers may be more infectious when prodromal symptoms appear and should avoid unprotected sex until the flare-up is resolved. Infectiousness escalates with the appearance of active sores. Sometimes the symptoms are so mild as to go unnoticed, so that people are unaware of being infectious.

Health Tips

To reduce the risk of infecting their sexual partners, people with herpes should avoid unprotected sex beginning with the first appearance of any warning signs of an impending recurrence and lasting through the course of an active episode.

▶ What Are the Symptoms of Oral Herpes?

The symptoms of oral herpes include sores or "fever blisters" on the lips, the inside of the mouth, the tongue, or the throat. Fever and feelings of sickness may occur. The gums may become red and swollen. The sores heal over in about two weeks, and the virus retreats into nerve cells at the base of the neck, where it lies dormant between flare-ups. About 90 percent of oral herpes sufferers experience recurrences, and about half of these have five or more recurrences during the first two years after the initial outbreak.[21]

▶ How Is Herpes Diagnosed?

Herpes is first diagnosed by clinical inspection of the herpes sores or ulcers in the mouth or on the genitals. In the case of genital herpes, a sample of fluid may be taken from the base of a genital sore and cultured in the laboratory to detect the growth of the virus.[22]

▶ How Is Herpes Treated?

There is no cure nor safe and effective vaccine for herpes. Viruses, unlike the bacteria that cause gonorrhea or syphilis, do not respond to antibiotics. A recently introduced antiviral drug *acyclovir* (Brand name *Zovirax*) can help relieve pain, speed healing, and reduce the duration of viral shedding (the period of time during which the virus is found in vaginal secretions and semen) in genital herpes when applied directly in ointment form to the herpes sores. Acyclovir must be administered orally, in pill form, to be effective against internal lesions in the vagina or on the cervix. Oral administration of acyclovir may reduce the severity of the initial episode and, if taken regularly, the frequency and duration of recurrent attacks of genital herpes.[23] In one study of 525 genital herpes sufferers over a three-year period, regular use of oral acyclovir reduced the frequency of outbreaks from an average of 12 per year to only 1 or 2 per year.[24] Yet the safety of long-term use of acyclovir needs further study. Nor has the safety of using acyclovir during pregnancy been established.[25]

Health Tips

People with recurrent herpes infections should discuss with their physicians the advisability of taking the antiviral drug acyclovir to help ward off recurrent attacks.

▶ What Should You Do If You Suspect You Have Contracted Genital Herpes?

First, see your physician. Treatment with acyclovir or other medication may help during acute outbreaks. While outbreaks resolve naturally, acyclovir may speed healing. Do not engage in unprotected sexual relations from the moment that lesions first appear, or earlier if warning signs precede the outbreak of the infection. You may also wish to ask your physician about the advisability of taking oral acyclovir routinely to reduce the risk of future recurrences. Warm baths, loose fitting clothing, aspirin, and cold, wet compresses may relieve pain during flare-ups of genital herpes. Many herpes sufferers find that subsequent episodes occur less frequently and are milder than initial episodes. Some people go for years or even a lifetime without a recurrence.

Health Tips

If you develop herpes:
- See your physician.
- Avoid unprotected genital sex from the moment that sores first appear, or earlier if warning signs precede the infection.
- Wearing loose fitting clothing, taking warm baths, using aspirin or other pain relievers, and applying cold, wet compresses may help relieve pain during active episodes.

▶ Coping with the Emotional Consequences of Genital Herpes

The psychological consequences of coping with genital herpes can be more distressing than the physical effects of the disease. The prospects of a lifetime of recurrences and worries about infecting one's sex partners compound the emotional impact of herpes. Feelings of anger, depression, isolation, and shame—even self-perceptions of being tainted, ugly, or dangerous—are common features of the emotional reaction to genital herpes.[26] Herpes sufferers may avoid sexual relations for a long time. Some even restrict their choice of partners to other herpes sufferers.[27] Most herpes sufferers, however, do become sexually active again and learn to lower the risk of infecting their partners by avoiding sexual contact during active episodes. Most also learn to cope with the emotional consequences of herpes.

Attitudes play an important role in a person's ability to cope with herpes. Perceiving herpes as a manageable problem, rather than as a medical disaster or character deficit, may help a person adjust to living with the disease, as this comment from a young woman with herpes suggests:[28]

> Herpes is an inconvenience and a pain, but it's something you learn to live with. I think of it as an imbalance. Since I know it's related to stress, I keep myself in as good physical condition as possible and try not to get too upset about it.

Herpes sufferers may also benefit from participating in herpes support groups, which provide opportunities for people to share their feelings about living with herpes with other herpes sufferers and to exchange information about ways of living with the disease.[29] For information about herpes support groups and other resources that can help you cope with herpes, contact the National Herpes Hotline at (919) 361–8488.

STD FACT SHEET: HERPES

What it is	A viral infection caused by related strains of the *Herpes simplex* virus.
What causes it	Oral herpes is caused by *herpes simplex virus-type 1 (HSV-1)*; genital herpes is caused by *herpes simplex virus-type 2 (HSV-2)*.
How it is transmitted	Oral, anal, or vaginal sex with an infected partner; oral herpes may also be transmitted by using the same cup, by kissing, or even by sharing a moist towel used by an infected person. Genital contact with objects, such as toilet seats, used by an infected person may—but probably infrequently—transmit herpes viruses. Genital herpes is almost always spread by sexual contact.
Signs and symptoms	Genital herpes is characterized by the appearance of genital sores or lesions, or which may also appear on the thigh or buttocks in both sexes or in the vagina or on the cervix in women. Oral herpes involves the appearance of sores or "fever blisters" on the lips, inside the mouth, on the tongue or in the throat.
How it is diagnosed	Clinical examination of sores or lesions; culturing and examination of fluid drawn from a sore.
How it is treated	Although not a cure, the antiviral drug acyclovir promotes healing of herpetic sores and when given in oral form may reduce the frequency of recurrence.

▶ Notes

1. Braude et al. (1986); Kunz, J. R. M., & Finkel, A. J. (1987) (Eds.) *The American Medical Association family medical guide: Revised and updated.* New York: Random House.

2. American Social Health Association (1996).

3. American Social Health Association (1996).

4. Straus, S. E. (1985). Herpes simplex virus infections: Biology, treatment, and prevention. *Annals of Internal Medicine, 103,* 404–419.

5. Corey, L. (1990). Genital herpes. In K. K. Holmes, et al. (Eds.), *Sexually transmitted diseases* (2nd ed.) (pp. 391–414). New York: McGraw-Hill, Inc.

6. Brody, J.E. (1992b, August 12). Genital herpes thrives on ignorance and secrecy. *The New York Times,* p. C12; Fox, M. (1985, December). Interfering with herpes. *Today's Health,* 22.

7. Peterman, T., Cates, W., & Curran, J. (1988). The challenge of human immunodeficiency virus (HIV) and acquired immunodeficiency syndrome (AIDS) in women and children. *Fertility and Sterility, 49,* 571–581.

8. Brock, B. V., et al. (1990). Frequency of asymptomatic shedding of herpes simplex virus in women with genital herpes. *The Journal of the American Medical Association, 263,* 418–420; Dawkins, B. J. (1990). Genital herpes simplex infections. *Primary Care: Clinics in Office Practice,* 17, 95–113; Rooney, J., et al. (1986). Acquisition of genital herpes from an asymptomatic sexual partner. *New England Journal of Medicine,* 314, 1561–1564.

9. Brock et al. (1990).

10. Whitley, R., et al. (1991). Predictors of morbidity and mortality in infants with herpes simplex virus infections. *The New England Journal of Medicine, 324,* 450–454.

11. Dawkins (1990); Osborne, N. G., & Adelson, M. D. (1990). Herpes simplex and human papillomavirus genital infections: Controversy over obstetric management. *Clinical Obstetrics and Gynecology, 33,* 801–811.

12. Brown, Z. A., et al. (1991). Neonatal herpes simplex virus infection in relation to asymptomatic maternal infection at the time of labor. *The New England Journal of Medicine, 324,* 1247–1252.

13. Campbell, C. E., & Herten, R. J. (1981). VD to STD: Redefining venereal disease. *American Journal of Nursing, 81,* 1629–1635.

14. Graham, S. et al. (1982). Sex patterns and herpes simplex virus type 2 in the epidemiology of cancer of the cervix. *American Journal of Epidemiology, 115,* 729–735; Hatcher et al. (1990).

15. Straus, S. E., et al. (1984a). Suppression of frequently recurring genital herpes: A placebo controlled double-blind trial of oral acyclovir. *New England Journal of Medicine, 310,* 1545–1550.

16. Brody (1992b).

17. Kemeny, M. E., Cohen, F., Zegans, L. S., & Conant, M. A. (1989). Psychological and immunological predictors of genital herpes recurrence. *Psychosomatic Medicine, 51,* 195–208; Kunz & Finkel (1987); Longo, D. J., & Clum, G. A. (1989). Psychosocial factors affecting genital herpes recurrences: Linear vs. mediating models. *Journal of Psychosomatic Research, 33,* 161–166.

18. Rand, K. H., et al. (1990). Daily stress and recurrence of genital herpes simplex. *Archives of Internal Medicine, 150,* 1889–1893.

19. Corey (1990).

20. Reinisch (1990).

21. Reinisch (1990).

22. Mertz, G. J. (1990). Genital herpes simplex virus infections. *Medical Clinics of North America, 74,* 1433–1454.

23. Gold, D., et al. (1988). Chronic-dose acyclovir to suppress frequently recurring genital herpes simplex virus infection: Effect on antibody response to herpes simplex virus type 2 proteins. *Journal of Infectious Diseases, 158,* 1227–1234; Goldberg, L. H., et al. (1993). Longterm suppression of recurrent genital herpes with acyclovir. *Archives of Dermatology, 129,* 582–587.

24. Brody (1993e); Goldberg et al. (1993).

25. Kaplowitz, L. G., et al. (1991). Prolonged continuous acyclovir treatment of normal adults with frequently recurring genital herpes simplex virus infection. *Journal of the American Medical Association, 265,* 747–751.

26. Hatcher et al. (1990); Stone, K. M., & Whittington, W. L. (1990). Treatment of genital herpes. *Reviews of Infectious Diseases* (Suppl. 6), 5633–S644.

27. Levy et al. (1987); Mirotznik, J., et al. (1987). Genital herpes: An investigation of its attitudinal and behavioral correlates. *Journal of Sex Research, 23,* 266–272.

28. Mirotznik et al. (1987).

29. Boston Women's Health Book Collective (1984), *The New Our Bodies, Ourselves,* p. 277.

30. Laskin, D. (1982, February 21). The herpes syndrome. *The New York Times Sunday Magazine,* pp. 94–108.

Fact Sheet: Hepatitis

National Institute of Allergy and Infectious Diseases, (NIH)

Hepatitis is an inflammation of the liver caused by certain viruses and other factors, such as alcohol abuse, some medications, and trauma. Its various forms affect millions of Americans. Although many cases of hepatitis are not a serious threat to health, the disease can become chronic (long-lasting) and can sometimes lead to liver failure and death.

► Cause

There are four major types of viral hepatitis:

- *Hepatitis A,* caused by infection with the hepatitis A virus, is usually a mild disease that does not become chronic. The virus is sometimes passed on through sexual practices involving oral-anal contact. It is most commonly spread by food and water contamination

- *Hepatitis B,* caused by infection with the hepatitis B virus (HBV), may be mild or severe, acute or chronic. HBV is most commonly passed on to a sexual partner during intercourse, especially during anal sex. Because the disease is not easily spread, persons with HBV should not worry about spreading it through casual contact such as shaking hands or sharing a workspace or bathroom facility.

  Each year, an estimated 300,000 persons in the United States become infected with HBV. Hepatitis B is most commonly transmitted by sharing drug needles, by engaging in high-risk sexual behavior, from a mother to her newborn, and in the health care setting.

- *Non-A, non-B hepatitis* is primarily caused by the hepatitis C virus (HCV). Although generally a mild condition, it is much more likely than hepatitis B to lead to chronic liver disease. HCV appears to be spread through sexual contact as well as through sharing drug needles. Sexual spread, however, is inefficient and much less than that for HBV or the AIDS virus (HIV). With the advent of new tests to screen blood donors, a very small percentage of persons with HCV currently become infected through blood transfusions.

The hepatitis E virus causes another type of non A, non-B hepatitis. This virus is principally spread through contaminated water in areas with poor sanitation. This form of hepatitis does not occur in the U.S. and is not known to be passed on through sexual contact.

- *Delta hepatitis* occurs only in people who already are infected with HBV. A potentially severe disease, it is caused by a virus (HDV) that can produce disease only when HBV is also present.

  Most cases occur among people who are frequently exposed to blood and blood products, such as people with hemophilia. Small-scale epidemics have occurred among injection drug users who share contaminated needles.

  Experts believe that HDV may be sexually transmitted, but further research is needed to provide more specific evidence.

► Transmission

HBV, HCV, and HDV can be spread in the following ways:

- Having sexual intercourse with an infected person without using a condom.
- Sharing drug needles among users of injected street drugs.
- Needle-stick accidents among health-care workers.
- Mother-to-child transmission of HBV during birth.
- Transfusions. Until recently, blood transfusions were the most frequent cause of hepatitis C. Blood banks in the United States now screen donated blood for HBV and HCV and discard any blood that appears to be infected. Therefore, the risk of acquiring hepatitis from these viruses is very low in the U.S. and in other countries where blood is similarly tested. Tests to screen blood for HBV will also screen out HDV.
- Personal contact with an infected person. HBV, HCV, and HDV sometimes spread when household members unknowingly come in contact with virus-infected blood or body fluids—most probably through cuts and scrapes or by sharing personal items such as razors and toothbrushes. While it is possible to become infected by contact with saliva, blood and semen remain the major sources of infection.

► Symptoms

Many people infected with viral hepatitis have no symptoms. For example, about one-third of people infected with HBV have a completely "silent" disease. When symptoms are present, they may be mild or severe. The most common early symptoms are mild fever, headache, muscle aches, fatigue, loss of appetite, nausea, vomiting, or diarrhea. Later symptoms may include dark and foamy urine and pale feces; abdominal pain; and yellowing of the skin and whites of the eyes (jaundice).

About 15 to 20 percent of patients develop short-term arthritis-like problems as part of a more severe case of hepatitis B. Another one-third of those with hepatitis B develop only mild flu-like symptoms without jaundice. Very severe (fulminant) hepatitis B is rare, but life-threatening. Early signs of fulminant hepatitis, such as personality changes and agitated behavior, require immediate medical attention.

Some people infected with HBV or HCV become chronic carriers of the virus, although they may have no symptoms. There are an estimated 1.5 million HBV carriers in the U.S. and 300 million carriers worldwide. Children are at greatest risk. About 90 percent of babies who become infected at birth with HBV, and up to half of youngsters who are infected before age 5, become chronic carriers. It is estimated that there are between 2 and 5 million HCV chronic carriers. At least half of all HCV carriers will develop chronic liver disease, regardless of whether or not they have symptoms.

▶ Diagnosis

Hepatitis B. Several types of blood tests can detect signs of HBV even before symptoms develop. These tests measure liver function and identify HBV antigens (proteins of the virus) or antibodies (proteins produced by the body in response to the virus) in the blood.

Tests for hepatitis B include:

- *Hepatitis B Surface Antigen (HbsAg).* Most people with acute hepatitis B have HBsAg in their blood before symptoms develop. As a person recovers from the illness, HBsAg disappears. If it is still present 6 months after infection, it may indicate that a person has developed chronic hepatitis or may be a symptomless carrier of the virus. HBsAg can be detected by a number of laboratory tests such as radioimmunoassay or enzyme-linked immunosorbent assay (ELISA). Antibody to the surface antigen (anti-HBs) persists for many years. This antibody usually appears as the acute illness improves, providing protection against future HBV infections.
- *Hepatitis B Core Antigen (HBcAg).* The HBV core protein can be identified only after the surface antigen has been stripped away using special techniques. Commercially available blood tests cannot detect HBcAg in blood, but antibody to the core antigen (anti-HBc) can be detected during acute illness. High levels of anti-HBc are present at the start of illness, and they gradually decrease over time in most people. In contrast, chronic carriers of HBV have high levels of anti-HBc in their blood that may persist throughout life.
- *E Antigen HbeAg.* The presence of E antigen indicates that a person infected with HBV is highly infectious. An HbsAg-positive pregnant woman whose blood contains e antigen is likely to transmit the virus to her newborn. By contrast, antibody to the a antigen (anti-HBe) may point to a lower degree of infectivity and a reduced likelihood of becoming a carrier. Laboratory blood tests can detect e antigen as well as anti-HBe.
- *Liver Function Tests.* A number of blood tests can be performed to determine how well a person's liver is functioning, and these results can aid in diagnosing hepatitis B infection. High levels of the liver enzymes aspartate transferase (AST) and alanine transferase (ALT) are of particular importance. (These were formerly called SGOT and SGPT.)

Delta hepatitis. Until recently, delta hepatitis could be diagnosed only by liver biopsy in which a tiny piece of the liver is removed and examined. Scientists supported by the NIAID have developed a procedure to detect part of the genetic material of the virus in a patient's blood, which will allow easier, faster diagnosis. A blood test is also now available to detect antibody to delta antigen (a protein found inside the delta hepatitis virus).

Hepatitis C. A new test is now available to detect hepatitis C. The test identifies antibody to HCV, which is present in more than 50 percent of persons with acute hepatitis C and in almost all with chronic hepatitis.

▶ Treatment

At present, there are no specific treatments for the acute symptoms of viral hepatitis. Doctors recommend bed rest, a healthy diet, and avoidance of alcoholic beverages.

A genetically engineered form of a naturally occurring protein, interferon alpha, is used to treat people with chronic hepatitis C. NIH-supported studies led to the approval of interferon alpha for the treatment of those with chronic HBV as well. The drug improves liver function in some people with hepatitis and diminishes symptoms, although it may cause side effects such as headache, fever, and other flu-like symptoms. Some patients do not respond to interferon alpha, and in others its beneficial effects lessen over time. Scientists are evaluating a number of experimental therapies that may be more effective and less toxic.

▶ Possible Complications

Most patients with mild to severe acute hepatitis begin to feel better in 2 to 3 weeks and recover completely within 4 to 8 weeks. People with acute HBV infection who develop an HCV infection at the same time may be at particular risk for developing severe, life-threatening acute hepatitis.

Many chronic carriers remain symptom free or develop only a mild condition, chronic persistent hepatitis. However, a small percentage go on to develop the most serious complications of viral hepatitis: cirrhosis of the liver, liver cancer, and immune system disorders. Chronic carriers of HBV who become infected with HDV may develop severe acute hepatitis. They also have a high risk of becoming carriers of HDV.

▶ Prevention

The most effective means of preventing viral hepatitis is to avoid contact with the blood, saliva, semen, or vaginal secretions of infected individuals. People who have acute or chronic viral hepatitis should:

- Avoid sharing items that could infect others, such as razors or toothbrushes.
- Protect sex partners from exposure to their semen, vaginal fluids, or blood. Properly used condoms may be effective in preventing sexual transmission.

There are several vaccines available to prevent hepatitis B. People at high risk of infection should consider vaccination: male homosexuals and heterosexuals with multiple partners, people who receive hemodialysis or blood products, household and sexual contacts of HBV carriers, and users of intravenous street drugs who share needles. Regulations now require health care and laboratory workers who handle blood and other body fluids to be vaccinated. People who have come into direct contact with the blood or body fluids of an HBV carrier may receive one or more injections of hepatitis B immune globulin, sometimes in combination with hepatitis B vaccine. Immune globulin offers temporary protection, while the vaccine provides a longer-lasting immunity.

In an effort to eliminate chronic carriers, the U.S. Centers for Disease Control recommends that all newborn babies be vaccinated. Other groups have recommended that pregnant women be screened for HBsAg as part of their routine prenatal care. If they are infected, their babies can be given hepatitis B immune globulin as well as vaccine immediately after birth.

No vaccines yet exist for HCV or HDV; however, HBV vaccine will prevent delta hepatitis as well.

▶ Research

NIAID supported scientists are attacking hepatitis infection from several fronts. Work is under way to evaluate the potential of antiviral drugs to treat people already infected with HBV, HCV, and HDV. Vaccines and drugs are being tested in the woodchuck, an animal that develops a disease similar to HBV infection in humans. This animal also can be a chronic carrier of HDV, making it a valuable model for studying these viruses and helping scientists understand hepatitis infection.

In addition to testing their effectiveness, scientists are studying how to make antiviral drugs less toxic and how to deliver them to their appropriate targets in the body.

By studying the immune response to hepatitis viruses, scientists hope to identify the precise mechanisms that lead to either recovery or chronic disease. Knowledge is being gained from studies with transgenic mice (mice that carry human genes for HBV). By modifying viral genes and inoculating pregnant women, it may be possible to boost the immune response of babies to HBV. This approach could reduce a large number of chronic carriers and stem the spread of the disease to future generations.

National Digestive Diseases
Information Clearinghouse
2 Information Way
Bethesda, MD 20892-3570
1-800-891-5389
nddic@info.niddle.nih.gov

Fact Sheet: Human Papillomavirus and Genital Warts

▶ What Is Human Papillomavirus?

Human papillomavirus (HPV) is one of the most common causes of sexually transmitted infection (STI) in the world. More than 100 different types of HPV exist, most of which are harmless. About 30 types are spread through sexual contact. Some types of HPV cause genital warts—single or multiple bumps that appear in the genital areas of men and women including the vagina, cervix, vulva (area outside of the vagina), penis, and rectum. Many people infected with HPV have no symptoms.

There are high-risk and low-risk types of HPV. High-risk HPV may cause abnormal Pap smear results, and could lead to cancers of the cervix, vulva, vagina, anus, or penis. Low-risk HPV also may cause abnormal Pap results or genital warts.

Health experts estimate there are more cases of genital HPV infection than any other STI in the United States. According to the American Social Health Association, approximately 5.5 million new cases of sexually transmitted HPV infections are reported every year. At least 20 million people in this country are already infected.

▶ What Are Genital Warts?

Genital warts (sometimes called condylomata acuminata or venereal warts) are the most easily recognized sign of genital HPV infection. Many people, however, have a genital HPV infection without genital warts.

Genital warts are soft, moist, or flesh colored and appear in the genital area within weeks or months after infection. They sometimes appear in clusters that resemble cauliflower-like bumps, and are either raised or flat, small or large. Genital warts can show up in women on the vulva and cervix, and inside and surrounding the vagina and anus. In men, genital warts can appear on the scrotum or penis. There are cases where genital warts have been found on the thigh and groin.

▶ Can HPV Cause Other Kinds of Warts?

Some types of HPV cause common skin warts, such as those found on the hands and soles of the feet. These types of HPV do not cause genital warts.

▶ How Are Genital Warts Spread?

Genital warts are very contagious and are spread during oral, vaginal, or anal sex with an infected partner. They are transmitted by skin-to-skin contact during vaginal, anal, or (rarely) oral sex with someone who is infected. About two-thirds of people who have sexual contact with a partner with genital warts will develop warts, usually within 3 months of contact.

In women, the warts occur on the outside and inside of the vagina, on the opening to the uterus (cervix), or around the anus.

In men, genital warts are less common. If present, they usually are seen on the tip of the penis. They also may be found on the shaft of the penis, on the scrotum, or around the anus.

Rarely, genital warts also can develop in your mouth or throat if you have oral sex with an infected person.

Like many STIs, genital HPV infections often do not have signs and symptoms that can be seen or felt. One study sponsored by the National Institute of Allergy and Infectious Diseases (NIAID) reported that almost half of women infected with HPV had no obvious symptoms. If you are infected but have no symptoms, you can still spread HPV to your sexual partner and/or develop complications from the virus.

▶ How Are HPV and Genital Warts Diagnosed?

Your health care provider usually diagnoses genital warts by seeing them. If you are a woman with genital warts, you also should be examined for possible HPV infection of the cervix.

Your provider may be able to identify some otherwise invisible warts in your genital tissue by applying vinegar (acetic acid) to areas of your body that might be infected. This solution causes infected areas to whiten, which makes them more visible. In some cases, a health care provider will take a small piece of tissue from the cervix and examine it under the microscope.

If you have an abnormal Pap smear result, it may indicate the possible presence of cervical HPV infection. A laboratory worker will examine cells scraped from your cervix under a microscope to see if they are cancerous.

▶ How Are HPV and Genital Warts Treated?

HPV has no known cure. There are treatments for genital warts, though they often disappear even without treatment. There is no way to predict whether the warts will grow or disappear. Therefore, if you suspect you have genital warts, you should be examined and treated, if necessary.

Depending on factors such as the size and location of your genital warts, your health care provider will offer you one of several ways to treat them.

- Imiquimod cream
- 20 percent podophyllin antimitotic solution

- 0.5 percent podofilox solution
- 5 percent 5-fluorouracil cream
- Trichloroacetic acid (TCA)

If you are pregnant, you should not use podophyllin or podofilox because they are absorbed by your skin and may cause birth defects in your baby. In addition, you should not use 5-fluorouracil cream if you are expecting.

If you have small warts, your health care provider can remove them by one of three methods.

- freezing (cryosurgery)
- burning (electrocautery)
- laser treatment

If you have large warts that have not responded to other treatment, you may have to have surgery to remove them.

Some health care providers use the antiviral drug alpha interferon, which they inject directly into the warts, to treat warts that have returned after removal by traditional means. The drug is expensive, however, and does not reduce the rate that the genital warts return.

Although treatments can get rid of the warts, none get rid of the virus. Because the virus is still present in your body, warts often come back after treatment.

▶ How Can HPV Infection Be Prevented?

The only way you can prevent getting an HPV infection is to avoid direct contact with the virus, which is transmitted by skin-to-skin contact. If you or your sexual partner has warts that are visible in the genital area, you should avoid any sexual contact until the warts are treated.

Research studies have not confirmed that male latex condoms prevent transmission of HPV, but studies do suggest that using condoms may reduce your risk of developing diseases linked to HPV, such as genital warts and cervical cancer. Unfortunately, many people who don't have symptoms don't know that they can spread the virus to an uninfected partner.

▶ Possible Complications of HPV and Genital Warts

Cancer

Some types of HPV can cause cervical cancer. Other types are associated with vulvar cancer, anal cancer, and cancer of the penis (a rare cancer).

Most HPV infections do not progress to cervical cancer. If you are a woman with abnormal cervical cells, a Pap test will detect them. If you have abnormal cervical cells, it is particularly important for you to have regular pelvic exams and Pap tests so you can be treated early, if necessary.

Pregnancy and Childbirth

Genital warts may cause a number of problems during pregnancy. Sometimes they get larger during pregnancy, making it difficult to urinate. If the warts are in the vagina, they can make the vagina less elastic and cause obstruction during delivery.

Rarely, infants born to women with genital warts develop warts in their throats (laryngeal papillomatosis). Although uncommon, it is a potentially life-threatening condition for the child, requiring frequent laser surgery to prevent obstruction of the breathing passages. Research on the use of interferon therapy with laser surgery indicates that this drug may show promise in slowing the course of the disease.

▶ Research

Scientists are doing research on two types of HPV vaccines. One type would be used to prevent infection or disease (warts or pre-cancerous tissue changes). The other type would be used to treat cervical cancers. Researchers are testing both types of vaccines in people.

▶ More Information

National Library of Medicine
MedlinePlus
8600 Rockville Pike
Bethesda, MD 20894
1-800-338-7657
http://medlineplus.gov

Centers for Disease Control and Prevention
1600 Clifton Road
Atlanta, GA 30333
1-888-232-3228
http://www.cdc.gov

CDC National STD and AIDS Hotline
1-800-227-8922 or 1-800-342-2437
http://www.ashastd.org/nah

American Social Health Association
P.O. Box 13827
Research Triangle Park, NC 27709-9940
919-361-8400
http://www.ashastd.org

NIAID is a component of the National Institutes of Health, an agency of the U.S. Department of Health and Human Services. NIAID supports basic and applied research to prevent, diagnose and treat infectious diseases such as HIV/AIDS and other sexually transmitted infections, influenza, tuberculosis, malaria and illness from potential agents of bioterrorism. NIAID also supports research on transplantation and immune-related illnesses, including autoimmune disorders, asthma and allergies.

Press releases, fact sheets and other NIAID-related materials are available on the NIAID Web site at http://www.niaid.nih.gov.

Prepared by:
Office of Communications and Public Liaison
National Institute of Allergy and Infectious Diseases
National Institutes of Health
Bethesda, MD 20892

U.S. Department of Health and Human Services

HIV as an STD

Sten H. Vermund, Sibylle Kristensen, Madhav P. Bhatta

HIV can be spread via infected blood or blood products, and from mother to child, either peripartum or via breast-feeding. These routes of transmission can be controlled.[1,2] However, the dominant route of HIV spread throughout the world is sexual. The straightforward statement that HIV is a sexually transmitted infection has proven controversial when traditional sexually transmitted disease (STD) control measures are proposed. This chapter places the HIV epidemic in a historical content, reviews the biological interaction of HIV with other STDs, and discusses the use of efficient STD-related public health measures to limit HIV spread.

▶ Historical Perspectives on STD Control and HIV

Eighteenth and nineteenth century efforts to control STDs focused on female prostitution, considered the principal nidus of infection by the male-dominated political leadership.[3] European cities such as Paris and Berlin enacted laws requiring regular medical inspection and registration of female prostitutes and the reporting of all cases of syphilis and gonorrhea.[4] STDs were especially common among men in the armed forces.[5] The threat to military efficiency posed by the high incidence of syphilis and gonorrhea was apparent to political leaders, which led the English Parliament to require the registration and examination of prostitutes when STDs were found.[6] In St. Louis and Cincinnati, mandatory physical examination and segregation of infected prostitutes[4] proved more successful than similar measures in California, New York, Pennsylvania, and the District of Columbia.[7–9] Despite substantial legislation regulating prostitution on both sides of the Atlantic, these approaches had no measurable impact on the incidence of STDs.[10–12]

Notable advances were made in the field of venereology in the first decade of the 20th century. In 1905, German scientists Fritz Schaudinn and Erich Hoffmann identified *Treponema pallidum* as the causative agent of syphilis.[13] In 1909, immunologist Paul Ehrlich discovered salvarsan, an arsenical compound capable of killing the treponeme, and August Wassermann and his colleagues Neisser and Bruck developed the first good serologic test for syphilis.[14]

Scientific progress was accompanied by social and public health reform.[9] The Social Hygiene Movement (also known as the Purity Crusade) was a US coalition of physicians, public health and welfare workers, "purity" crusaders, and women's rights advocates who recognized that STDs were prevalent in the general population.[5] Their approach included improved medical and public health care, legislative changes, and a massive social hygiene educational campaign focused on increasing the public's fear of STD infection.[5] The social hygienists argued that unless people had basic knowledge about STDs, their modes of transmission, and their prevention, it would not be possible to reduce STD incidence. While the educational campaigns may have raised fear of infection, the stigma associated with STDs may likewise have been exacerbated, discouraging many persons from seeking care.[9]

By World War I (WWI), STDs were a major public health problem.[10] Deaths due to congenital syphilis in 1917 were 1 in 500 live births.[13] STDs were the leading cause of rejection from active duty in the military; one million men were rejected by the draft in 1918 for having syphilis.[6] Incapacitation of troops by STD symptoms was more common than war-related injury. The entry of the United States in WWI resulted in a major shift in the public and government attitude towards STDs and their control. Public concern about military readiness was strong enough to override opposition towards STD control efforts.[9] In 1917, the United States Public Health Service (USPHS) initiated a cooperative venereal disease (VD) control program in partnership with state and local health departments and with the private sector, including medical practitioners, hospitals, and voluntary agencies.[15] Since STDs in the military could not be controlled unless they were reduced in the general population as well, Congress created the Venereal Disease Control Division within the USPHS, appropriating funds for research and for administration of state treatment programs.[5] Its essential elements included case reporting, widespread availability of testing, the provision of arsphenamine, promotion of condom prophylaxis, establishment of treatment facilities, and public education programs conducted at the level of state and local health departments.[5]

After WWI, public and political interest in STD control diminished in the United States, and the US Congress cut funding in half.[6] In 1922, Congress discontinued altogether the appropriation for diagnosis and treatment clinics, and VD control programs were neglected for more than a decade.[5]

Rising STD rates were recognized as a health menace by leaders in the public health and medical communities.[13] In 1936, the Surgeon General of USPHS, Dr. Thomas Parran, revitalized the VD control programs, including such measures as:[9]

- a trained public health staff
- case finding through serological testing or Gram stain for gonorrhea
- premarital and prenatal serodiagnostic testing
- establishment of diagnostic services
- availability of treatment services
- distribution of drugs for treatment
- routine serodiagnostic testing
- a scientific information program including public education

Enough political support was obtained by Parran to permit launching key elements of the control effort. The high rejection rates among World War II (WW II) draftees due to syphilis and the increased absenteeism resulting among military personnel from syphilis and gonorrhea led to intensified STD control efforts.[13] Once again, STDs incapacitated many more troops than did war-related injuries.

The military STD control program combined massive education programs, condom advocacy and distribution, and prompt diagnosis and treatment without punitive measures.[13] The USPHS working with the Conference of State and Territorial Health Officers planned and implemented a nationwide civilian VD program. As in WW I, cooperative agreements were set up between the USPHS and the US military.[15] The control measures taken during WW II contributed to a decrease in the prevalence of syphilis from 271/100,000 in 1946, to 197/100,000 in 1949.[9]

Paradoxically, the discovery of the one-shot penicillin treatment for syphilis and the success of WW II control programs in both military and civilian sectors minimized the significance of STDs as a public health priority in the minds of the public and politicians.[14] While syphilis reached a nadir of 76 cases per 100 000 persons in 1955, the decline in STD rates was short-lived.[16] Between 1965 and 1975, cases of gonorrhea increased three-fold, rising to over 1 million per year.[16] Similarly, from the mid 1950s to the mid 1970s, cases of syphilis more than quadrupled.[17] Although some observers attribute this rise to the three Ps of the 1960s—permissiveness, promiscuity, and the Pill—little evidence suggests that any of these factors affected STD incidence.[9] However, when government spending on VD control programs peaked in the early 1950s, the rate of infections dropped to their lowest point.[14] Cutbacks in government funding for STD programs in late 1950s and early 1960s was reflected by the rise in the rates of reported STDs.[13]

STD rates continued to rise in the mid to late 1970s, particularly among men having sex with men (MSM).[18] The emergence of gay and bisexual men from the shadows of society in this time period was accompanied by a relaxed sexual standard, particularly in larger cities where there was safety and comfort in numbers.[18,19] The Castro district in San Francisco, parts of West Los Angeles and Hollywood, and Greenwich Village in New York City were but a few well-known neighborhoods where men felt at ease with their sexual orientation.[18] Similarly, in other cities around the world, MSM felt disinhibited from their repressed sexuality of decades past, and this relaxation was accompanied by an increase in STDs.[18–20] The incidence of intestinal parasites such as *Giardia lamblia* and *Entamoeba histolytica*, viral infections such as hepatitis B and herpes simplex virus type II, bacterial infections such as syphilis, anal and oral gonorrhea, and chlamydia, and even unknown conditions rose markedly. The most lethal of these was HIV.

▶ Overview of HIV Epidemic

As described in Chapter 1, HIV has been demonstrated to be a zoonosis of higher primate origin.[21] With economic and political disruptions, large-scale migrations from rural to urban Africa brought HIV to new locations where sexual behaviors were not limited by traditional taboos and family or tribal customs. High partner exchange rates are not uncommon in settings where men are working or fighting in wars far from their families and where female prostitutes (ie, commercial sex workers, professional sex workers) are available. The rapid spread of HIV to Europe, the Caribbean, and North America in the 1970s with the explosive incidence among persons with high risk exposure (MSM, high risk women, blood and blood product recipients, intravenous drug users [IDUs], and infants born to HIV-infected mothers) all occurred in the context of high partner exchange rates, particularly among MSM and IDUs.[24]

In the 1980s, HIV spread virtually unchecked in Africa resulted in the world's highest urban and rural HIV rates, with rising rates of death,[25,26] orphans,[27] and economic chaos from loss of economically productive age groups.[28] In the late 1980s, the pandemic had spread to

Asia, where it spread at a rate similar to that in Africa a decade earlier. The highest rates in the Americas were reported from Haiti and Guyana, the poorest nations in the Western Hemisphere.[29] Industrialized nations experienced large HIV epidemics compared with neighboring countries, including Brazil, the United States, Spain, and Italy.[26]

By the 1990s, the epidemic had leveled somewhat in many countries, in part due to the impact of prevention messages and programs, many promulgated by community-based organizations in peer education formats. Thailand turned the corner on its massive epidemic with programs targeting sex workers and sexual behaviors among young men, advocating 100% condom use in brothels.[30] In Uganda, educational programs likewise reduced reported seroincidence in both urban Kampala and rural areas.[31] In a clinical trial in northwest Tanzania, the control of STDs was shown clearly to reduce HIV transmission.[32] In Rwanda, the use of counseling and testing among couples whose infection status was discordant seemed to cut HIV transmission rates in half.[33]

Lessons learned worldwide in HIV control include relearning tried and true measures of STD control. Availability of STD preventive and curative services correlated inversely with degree of risk for HIV seroconversion in Zaire.[34] Active contact tracing in North Carolina worked much better than a passive partner-referral approach to inform sexual contacts that they had been exposed to HIV, with the former permitting counseling, testing, and, when needed, early treatment.[35] Colorado used contact tracing for HIV and HIV reporting in the 1980s, which correlated with the epidemic being kept to a minimum.[36] Other reports from around the world suggested that peer outreach education, STD control measures (including partner reduction and condom use), protection of the blood supply, use of sterile syringes and needles for medical use and among substance abusers, drug and alcohol treatment programs, and, in some settings, counseling and testing (particularly of discordant couples) all helped to reduce HIV seroincidence.[37,38]

Based on the past 20 years of epidemic spread, projections can be made for trends worldwide. The incipient epidemic of HIV in Eastern Europe will expand from IDUs to their sexual contacts and to infants of pregnant women, expanding the HIV problem into the general population. Tuberculosis, already on the rise in parts of Eastern Europe and Russia, will extend its reach, including multiple drug-resistant strains, in parallel with the spread of HIV. The African epidemic will continue at the highest seroprevalence in the world, replenished by young people entering the at-risk pool. The Asian epidemic will continue to expand with spread into subgroups that experience high-risk exposure but have not demonstrated many HIV cases to date, including Nepal, Bangladesh, Pakistan, and parts of India and Sri Lanka.[38–40] Based on rising STD rates, China and Mongolia will also experience a heavier HIV burden.[41–45] The epidemic in Latin America will continue to expand, particularly into areas with high STD rates, such as parts of Central America and the Amazon Basin.[45]

Governments where HIV is not a burden will continue to fund other priorities until AIDS is clearly a problem. Given the long incubation period of AIDS, this means substantial action will be taken only after many years of HIV spread. HIV in Europe and North America will continue to diminish in many communities while expanding in others; the advent of Highly Active Antiviral Therapy (HAART) may diminish the infectiousness of infected persons, but may also discourage high-risk sexual practices.[46] Given the equilibrium established in HIV seroprevalence in most Western countries, new cases will occur largely among young people.[47,48]

Despite the ongoing spread of HIV, politicians and policy makers stubbornly avoid investing in prevention. One exception is in northern Europe, where the Swedes have nearly wiped out incident, autochthonous STDs.[49,50] Despite the lessons of STD control learned in the late

19th and early 20th centuries, the current lack of insight and political courage to promote control of STDs, including HIV, has contributed directly to the magnitude of the world HIV pandemic. This links directly with the difficulty that Americans and others worldwide have with sexual issues. Progress and even success in global eradication of diseases like smallpox, dracunculiasis, and polio show what can be accomplished when public health control measures are supported, and worldwide political and economic commitments are made. Even when eradication is biologically implausible, global control measures like oral rehydration for infant diarrhea can result in measurable impact. However, many governments continue to treat STDs, including HIV, as a topic unworthy of such substantial attention.

▶ Interaction of HIV and Other STDs

Unprotected sexual contact in the presence of other sexually transmitted infections (STIs) enhances the probability of HIV transmission.[34,51–53] Sexual transmission of HIV may be greatly enhanced by several additional cofactors, including the HIV load in the infectious partner, the phenotype of the HIV isolate, the immunogenetic profile of the exposed person, the interface of virus type with secondary and primary cell receptors of HIV, and the activation state of the immune system during and after the infectious event (see Chapter 3 for details).[54–56] The increased HIV risk associated with STIs is due to damage that these infections produce in the integrity of the epithelial lining of the cervix, vagina, urethra, vulva, penis, and anus.[34,57–59] The efficiency of HIV transmission increases with STI co-infection of either ulcerative or inflammatory type.[58] Mucosal ulceration, inflammation, or exudation is likely to increase the frequency of viral contact with target cells through macroscopic or microscopic breaks in mucosal integrity and to recruit immune cells that are readily infected (eg, dendritic cells, macrophages, CD4+ lymphocytes) into the genitourinary tract.[60] Lack of male circumcision may exacerbate the risks.

STIs not only increase susceptibility in the uninfected, exposed individual but also increase the infectiousness of HIV-infected persons who are co-infected with other STIs.[55,60] Viral load in genital secretions rises markedly with co-existing urethritis/STIs. In both semen and vaginal secretions, HIV load is higher with co-existing gonococcal and chlamydia infections. In women with a cervical or vaginal ulcer, HIV is higher in genital secretions. Most notably, treatment of these STDs results in a decrease of genital shedding.[55,61] The concentration of HIV in genital secretions is likely to be a key determinant of the efficiency of HIV transmission in many parts of the world; treatment with antibiotics among persons with STIs can reduce genital shedding of HIV, a finding with marked implications for HIV-prevention programs.[62]

Sexual transmission of HIV can be diminished by STI treatment and restoration of the integrity of the normal mucosal barriers. It is postulated that the restoration of a normal vaginal ecology dominated by hydrogen peroxide–producing lactobacilli may also inhibit the sexual spread of HIV. Similarly, mother-to-child HIV transmission may be reduced with antibiotic treatment of mothers who have bacterial vaginosis.[63] This concept is based on the association of lower genital tract bacterial vaginosis with risk of histologic chorioamnionitis and the increased risk of HIV transmission among mothers with chorioamnionitis. Bacterial vaginosis has been associated with HIV, suggesting this causal pathway to be plausible and worthy of investigation for both sexual and perinatal transmission reduction.[64]

Ulcerative STDs have the strongest association with seroconversion,[34,57,58] with relative risk estimates in the 5- to 10-fold excess risk range in cross-sectional studies.[60] Frank genital ulcers are common with chancroid, herpes, syphilis, genital ulcer diseases, and genital warts.[34,57,58] Ulcerative STDs disrupt the integrity of the epithelial mucosa, facilitate HIV contact with the lymphatic and circulatory systems and recruit CD4+ lymphocytes and macrophages to the site of injury/infection,[60] aiding sexual transmission of HIV.[59]

Non-ulcerative STDs are also important risk factors for sexual transmission of HIV.[34,54,65] Relative risk estimates for HIV with non-ulcerogenic STDs have been in the 2- to 5-fold range.[60] Inflammatory and exudative reproductive tract infections such as gonorrhea, chlamydia, trichomoniasis, bacterial vaginosis, or candidiasis are less disruptive of the epithelial tissues than ulcerative STDs. However, the exudate may recruit large volumes of cervical or urethral discharge filled with susceptible cells. Inflammation may result in micro-ulcerations and superficial capillaries, thus facilitating virus-cell contact with vulnerable cells in the mucosal epithelia of the rectum, cervix, vagina, or oral cavity.[60,66] Furthermore, the recruitment of infectious lymphocytes, macrophages, or other cells into seminal or vaginal secretions may increase transmissibility.[66]

The population burden of HIV that can be attributed to STIs differs from the relative risk or risk ratio (RR) of the association. For example, smoking kills about as many people per year from heart disease (RR=1.5) as from lung cancer (RR>12) merely because heart disease is much more common than lung cancer. Similarly, more people are likely infected with HIV each year due to the mucosal disruption of an inflammatory STI than due to an ulcerogenic one because the former is far more common than frank ulcers. The public health implications of this observation must be highlighted: ulcerogenic STDs, despite having the strongest association with HIV seroconversion,[54] should not be the sole target of intervention. Instead, all STIs, including the common inflammatory and exudative conditions, should be targets of public health control in the service of HIV prevention and in the reduction of adverse reproductive consequences of STDs themselves.

Co-infection with systemic viruses, many of which are transmitted sexually, may activate the immune system. An activated immune system is easier to infect with HIV than a quiescent one, with up-regulated primary and secondary target molecules presented to infectious particles. In addition, systemic co-infection may stimulate higher HIV production, thus increasing infectiousness.[60] Organisms studied for such effects include STIs such as cytomegalovirus, Epstein-Barr virus, HTLV types I and II, and human herpes viruses types 6, 7, and 8. While in vitro studies and case reports are often intriguing, epidemiologic data are much less convincing with *Mycoplasma fermentans*.[67] In addition, co-infection may reflect the duration of risk behavior and HIV infection. For example, an HIV-infected sex worker infected 15 years ago with HIV and 12 years ago with HTLV-I can expect to be sicker than a sex-worker infected with HIV alone for 2 years.

The interactions between STIs and HIV have contributed to the AIDS epidemic, particularly when HIV prevalence is low.[66] Among high-risk populations such as STD patients who commonly report high-risk activities and high-risk partners, HIV transmission can be quite efficient.[66] In simulations of the initial 10-year period of the HIV epidemic (1981–1990), more than 90% of HIV infection worldwide was attributed to STD co-infections.[68] Even given more conservative assumptions about the prevalence of STDs and about their enhancing effects on HIV transmission, STDs can be shown to play a critical role in the rapid and extensive spread of HIV infection in diverse settings.[69] The identification and treatment of STDs as risk factors for HIV transmission must be a crucial factor in the prevention of HIV.[66,68,69]

One topic linked to sexual risk in as yet undetermined ways is the association of cervical ectopy with HIV risk.[70] Cervical ectopy is the exocervical exposure of the normally endocervically located columnar epithelium. The result of this condition is the exposure of the transformation zone (point at which the columnar epithelium transitions to squamous epithelium) to the vagina, where sperm and potential pathogens can bathe it in high concentrations. Since the transformation zone is more susceptible to STD/HIV infection than the squamous or columnar epithelia (both of which have physical and vascular protective features, respectively), cervical ectopy may also increase HIV susceptibility in the uninfected.[60] Bleeding during intercourse occurs more often among young women with cervical ectopy; hence, an HIV-infected woman with cervical ectopy may be more infectious than one without this normal cervical variant. An outstanding question is whether oral or injectable contraceptive hormones increase HIV risk since they are thought to increase cervical ectopy.[60] Unfortunately, we are largely ignorant of the risk factors for cervical ectopy, other than young age (adolescence). Since it is thought that frequent and early exposure to semen may accelerate squamous metaplastic changes in the cervix with the consequent involution of the transformation zone into the endocervix, these relationships of sexual risk behavior, age, contraception, and STDs with HIV risk may prove to be quite complex.[60,66]

▶ Public Health Measures to Reduce HIV Sexual Spread

In the absence of affordable treatment and an effective vaccine against HIV, prevention is the only hope for controlling the worldwide HIV pandemic. Influencing personal behavior is not easy, but established strategies have succeeded in controlling STDs and HIV. Knowledge about the HIV infection levels and transmission patterns in a given population, and awareness of local attitudes towards infection and protection can guide design of public health programs to promulgate safer sexual practices.[37]

▶ Behavior Change

Some politicians and religious populists advocate that strict monogamy or abstinence and drug-free lifestyles are the only acceptable behavioral goals, arguing that working towards "half measures" validates the high-risk lifestyle.[71] This point of view opposes needle exchange for infection drug users and condom provision for adolescents. Abstinence and mutual monogamy are realistic goals for a large segment of the population, particularly when it comes to maintaining these behaviors among persons already practicing these lifestyles. Among younger, sexually naive adolescents, abstinence-oriented education is the appropriate strategy, while risk reduction is the best approach for youth who are already sexually active and unmotivated to abandon their sexual relationships.[60] For a heterosexual or homosexual couple, faithfulness to one another will reduce risk of STD/HIV. However, changing human sexual behavior toward mutual monogamy or celibacy can be difficult as many persons are not motivated to achieve these goals.[72]

The promotion of condom use, partner reduction, and careful partner selection should not be discarded for a more limited message of abstinence and mutual monogamy, though this approach is being legislated in the United States to qualify for federal support. Reliance on abstinence campaigns is deemed the only moral option by some while being perceived as ineffectual by others. Provision of public health services, including condom distribution, is seen as encouraging promiscuity by some and as life-saving by others. Recurrent debates about school-based sexual education and preventive health services for adolescents epitomize these strategic differences.[73] Our failure to pursue aggressively more effective risk reduction has likely contributed to the high proportion of recent HIV seroconversions estimated to occur in America's youth.[47] Both approaches of risk reduction and risk elimination should be highlighted, taking into account community risks and norms.

Most behavioral scientists and public health professionals recognize that considerable progress in prevention can be made among persons who are not ready to give up their high-risk behaviors all at once. The Trans-theoretical or Stages of Change model of prevention science holds that persons may be able to change high-risk behavior in increments, reducing their risks of acquiring or transmitting HIV/STD even when they do not live a risk-free lifestyle.[74–76] This is analogous to a doctor helping a smoker reduce the daily number of cigarettes smoked or choose lower tar and nicotine tobacco at a time when the smoker cannot or will not quit tobacco use altogether. While tobacco risk reduction is seen as desirable to reduce risk even when risk is not being eliminated, this tolerance of risk reduction is rarely extended by public policy makers and moralists to sexual or illicit drug use activities.[71] US policy makers would do well to consider progress in northern Europe, which promulgates sexual and drug use-related risk reduction messages and has lower HIV seroprevalence.[50]

Persons engaged in high-risk behaviors are often motivated to learn about HIV. However, knowledge does not correlate with reduced-risk behavior in all circumstances.[76–78] Informed persons in denial may continue to engage in high-risk activity, underscoring the need to go beyond increasing HIV awareness through conventional educational efforts and implement novel public health measures to foster and maintain behavior change. Creative social marketing could employ the same media and style of advertisement used by commercial clients.[37] Peer counseling and sustained outreach support can also be exercised to sustain behavior change over time.[37] Insights from psychological theory and social marketing experience have led to the rational design of programs that encourage safer sexual practices and overall risk reduction.[79] Safer sex efforts include education for reduction in the number of sexual partners, selection of lower risk partners, use of condoms, prompt recognition and treatment of STDs, and reduction in drug and alcohol use.[60]

The potential for STD/HIV reduction is greatest among young women, who are at increased risk for STD and HIV infection due to both behavioral and biological mechanisms.[60] Younger women are at comparatively higher risk of HIV infection over a given number of exposures. Immature vaginal mucosa in adolescents, with large cervical ectopy zones, may be more susceptible to trauma during sexual relations and may be especially prone to infection with STDs due to the large transformation zone and exposed columnar epithelia. HIV transmission may be facilitated by sexual activity at times when blood exposure is expected (eg, menses, rape, or first coital experience).[60]

Special attention should be given to this highly neglected group of patients, many of whom are adolescents, in terms of comprehensive reproductive health education and delivery of services. Recent interest in integrating STD services in family planning and maternal and child health may work well for older women, but unmarried adolescents often do not feel welcome and often make little use of such facilities. Offering a non-judgmental and accessible service to vulnerable populations such as sex workers and adolescents could have a considerable impact on HIV prevention.[80,81] Among the innovative approaches already being used with some success in the United States and internationally are peer education, social marketing, school-based sexual education for youth, community-based programs to reduce drug experimentation in adolescents, programs for alcohol risk reduction in high-risk groups (including the military), risk reduction for active sex workers, and street outreach for runaways and the homeless, targeting populations at highest HIV risk.[82–85] Chapter 6 offers additional suggestions for developing interventions capable of reaching vulnerable women at high risk for HIV infection.

Behavioral and community-based educational and co-factor reduction efforts can be successful. In Thailand, condom promotion has been successful, especially in the sex work industry.[86,87] In Tanzania, community-based STD control has achieved short-term reductions in HIV seroincidence.[88–90] Long-term impact of STD control on HIV is unknown, but the 2-year follow-up data reveal that a relatively straightforward syndromic management approach, without use of laboratory diagnostics, reduced HIV seroincidence by 42%. In Zaire, STD and condom services for sex workers reduced HIV risk in proportion to the frequency with which the services were utilized.[34] Comprehensive services for drug users has lowered risk in the Netherlands.[93] In the United States, peer counseling among gay men and intensive counseling among runaway adolescents have proved effective in reducing high-risk behavior.[91,92] In addition, needle exchange programs to reduce contaminated injections among IDUs demonstrate efficacy and can be expected, in turn, to affect sexual transmission from IDUs to their sexual partners and offspring.[94]

▶ Barrier Methods

Male condoms are highly effective in preventing HIV transmission, both by blocking HIV and by reducing the transmission of other STDS.[95,96] In Rwanda, HIV testing and counseling, AIDS education, and free condoms and spermicides distributed to women of childbearing age had significant effects on condom use and HIV seroconversion rates prior to the 1994 genocide.[33,97] Thailand launched a nationwide campaign to reach a goal of 100% condom use among commercial sex workers.[30,86] The campaign included condom distribution in brothels and a mass advertising campaign promoting condom use.[86,87] As a result, condom use dramatically increased (more than 90%) among commercial sex workers, STD prevalence was lowered, and HIV prevalence declined among several groups with high rates of partner change.[30,86,87,98–100] Similar success have been achieved in programs involving commercial sex workers in Kenya[101,102] and in Bolivia.[103]

In Kinshasa, Laga et al. suggested that the willingness of the male clients to use condoms would need to be raised to ensure the success of any such program.[34] Although condom use increased markedly among female sex workers, condom use with all clients never exceeded more than 60%. The main obstacle cited was the male client's refusal to use a condom.[34] This illustrates the urgent need for additional chemical or physical barrier methods that are under women's control.[104] It also highlights the need to address male behavior and risk reduction as has been done in Thailand. In Thailand, the growing use of condoms among commercial sex workers prior to the large-scale condom programs is attributed to awareness in government and military circles of the high prevalence of HIV in this population.[99,100] In the United States, an increase in condom use among young adults in the 1980s was attributed to the growing perceived risks of acquiring HIV, reflecting a growing awareness of the impact of the HIV epidemic and the messages of HIV prevention programs.[105] Absolute numbers do not tell the whole story, however, since the lowest condom uptake is often among the highest risk persons.

A controlled clinical trial of condom use for HIV prevention is not feasible for ethical reasons, though available data nonetheless demonstrate that regular condom use protects against HIV infection.[106] In the United States, use of condoms in the heterosexual population remains relatively low, especially among adolescents, but is increasing in some surveys.[105] Thus, promotion of condoms as a means of safe sex practice should form an essential component of any public health measure for HIV prevention. Public awareness of the risks of HIV and of the protective benefits of condoms is not yet sufficient to convince persons at highest risk to use them. Factors inhibiting the use of condoms include their price, potential inconvenience, embarrassment resulting from their purchase and use, and perceived reduced sexual pleasure. Policies that overcome these barriers by lowering the price of condoms, improving their availability, and increasing their social acceptability could increase condom use and reduce HIV transmission.[91]

Some studies suggest that condom use is associated with higher HIV seroconversion risk. In fact, high-risk men and women may use condoms more often than mutually monogamous married persons. However, sporadic condom use by high-risk persons with repetitive exposures merely reduces the transmission efficiency for the given encounter in which the condom is used. Studies that ensure 100% condom use, as occurred in studies of spouses of men with hemophilia, prove that condom efficacy is high.[106]

Unfortunately, available female-controlled barriers (eg, female condoms, spermicides) do not have convincing data showing that these modalities are successful.[104,107] These innovative and important tools for potential HIV control could empower women to protect themselves without the cooperation of their sexual partners[108] and should remain the topic of intense research investigation as to their efficacy. Definitive field trials of microbicide and female condom must be designed and implemented quickly.[104,107]

▶ STD Control

The causal link between classic STDs and HIV transmission has been demonstrated through in vitro, clinical, and epidemiologic studies.[51,66] The increase in STD prevalence has implications for the evolution of the HIV epidemic and should be addressed effectively by strengthening STD control programs. Evidence clearly shows that interventions targeting vulnerable persons at the individual or at the community level can produce substantial reductions in high-risk sexual behaviors and reduce HIV transmission. In addition, "classic" STD control approaches such as partner notification can be helpful in reaching persons at risk.[35,109]

Despite our knowledge of the impact of STDs on HIV, STD control remains limited by several issues, including cost of diagnosis and treatment in settings with poor access to health care.[96] Syndromic management refers to the treatment of possible associated STDs based on the symptoms displayed by the patient, with or without laboratory confirmation. Syndromic management is a more feasible STD control strategy in resource-poor settings and has been endorsed by the World Health Organization (WHO) and United Nations AIDS (UN AIDS).[96] Disadvantages include the cost and risk of over-treatment with antibiotics and suboptimal identification of chlamydial and gonococcal cervical infection in women with vaginal discharge. Nonetheless, syndromic approaches offer a marked improvement over current practices for treating symptomatic STDs in most parts of the developing world.[110] In many settings, training of health care workers in STD syndromic management, making available effective antibiotics for STDs, and promoting health care-seeking behavior can decrease STD/HIV incidence.[111]

In Rakai, Uganda, a rural region near Lake Victoria, a periodic population "sweep" with curative antibiotics, independent of individual diagnosis, was implemented in the hopes it might be a cost-effective approach to HIV control.[112] This approach failed to control HIV.[112,113] In a carefully designed and conducted study, the investigators could find no HIV-related benefits for the mass chemotherapy program, though other health benefits were noted.[112] Perhaps treating STDs every tenth month was insufficient to prevent transmission compared with immediately available syndromic management as in Mwanza. Alternatively, the HIV epidemic may have been so mature that a suboptimal STD control campaign did little to change transmission dynamics.[113] The lesson learned may be that "STD control can help prevent HIV, though the techniques and the intensity of the STD control program must be adequate to alter HIV transmission dynamics in a given setting."[113]

HIV-infected persons with untreated genitourinary tract infections are likely to be far more infectious than those receiving treatment for such infections.[51] Treatment of the HIV infection itself with antiretroviral chemotherapy reduces HIV plasma virus load and almost certainly reduces genital tract viral load as well.[114] While a treated individual is less infectious early in the course of antiretroviral chemotherapy, the prolonged survival in a relatively healthy AIDS-free state may permit a longer span of high-risk sexual activity. The population consequences of widespread antiviral chemoprophylaxis and chemotherapy—net benefits to society in reduced transmission from reduced infectiousness or net increased transmission due to longer lifespan of infected individuals—remains unknown.[115,116] This issue highlights the urgency of effective behavior change programs focused on HIV-infected persons.[46]

▶ Conclusions

It is encouraging to see successful pilot projects and progress where sound public health policy has overcome political objections in an effort to reduce transmission by all reasonable and feasible routes. Converting these individual successes into sustained worldwide disease control remains elusive.[28] Given the rapid recognition of the modes of transmission of HIV (risky behavior was a recognized factor prior the discovery of HIV in 1983), the failure of subsequent control activities serves as a discouraging reminder of the difficulties faced in translating knowledge into practice. Treatment-oriented health care systems have little incentive to invest money in prevention; effective prevention targets the highest risk groups in community-based programs rather than in the health care system settings per se.

In the realm of public policy and behavior change, the AIDS epidemic requires political and community leaders to take risks within their leadership positions to educate and advocate for effective though sometimes controversial strategies for control of HIV transmission. Development and testing of novel, female-controlled barrier methods ranks among the highest research priorities. Assessment of the impact of STD control in reducing HIV should be emphasized in both industrialized and developing nations. Rapid, cheap STD diagnostics, low-cost broad-spectrum antibiotics effective against all STDs in single dose regimens, and STD vaccines are likewise needed.

A partially effective HIV vaccine could be helpful if coupled with other prevention strategies.[117] Drug abuse and risk reduction among drug users remains among the highest priorities in the United States, Europe, and parts of Asia. This topic is integrally linked to STDs as drug users often support their addiction with sexual services. The impact of alcohol and recreational drugs on sexual disinhibition further heightens HIV/STD risk (see Chapter 7 for an in-depth review).

Success in reducing perinatal transmission will depend fully on our approach to universal testing of pregnant women to permit them to choose antiretroviral chemoprophylaxis if they are seropositive (see Chapter 10 for discussion of universal testing and privacy issues). Novel approaches to perinatal risk reduction are needed to complement drugs, particularly in parts of the world where drugs and HIV testing are very costly in the local economy. These approaches include STI control in pregnant women.[63]

Finally, creativity in behavioral interventions must be highlighted. Sophisticated marketing techniques sell concepts and encourage consumption. These same strategies could be used to address social concerns and could work even better if left unshackled by political constraints.

▶ Summary Points

- The straightforward statement that HIV is a sexually transmitted infection has proven controversial when traditional STD control measures are proposed.
- Historical efforts to control STDs have focused on female prostitution and the threat of STDs to military efficiency during world wars.
- In the United States, the Venereal Disease Control Division focused on case reporting, contact tracing, widespread availability of testing, promotion of condom prophylaxis, establishment of treatment facilities, and public education programs conducted at the level of state and local health departments.
- Lessons learned worldwide in HIV control include relearning these tried and true measures of STD control. Additional measures include peer education, protection of the blood supply, use of sterile syringes and needles (medical use and for IDUs), testing of pregnant women, and partner counseling. Both approaches of risk reduction and risk elimination should be highlighted, taking into account community risks and norms.
- Sexually transmitted infections both increase the probability of HIV transmission and increase the infectiousness of HIV-infected persons. Sexual transmission of HIV can be diminished by treating the infection and restoring the integrity of the normal mucosal barriers.
- Co-infection with systemic viruses may activate the immune system, which in turn is more easily infected with HIV. In addition, systemic co-infection may stimulate higher HIV production, thus increasing infectiousness.

Chapter
6

Fungal STIs and Other STIs

What You Should Know About Vaginal Infections

J. S. Nevid

▶ Did You Know That?

- Men, too, can be infected by the organisms causing vaginal infections in women.
- Vaginitis is often caused by an overgrowth of infectious organisms that normally reside in the vagina.
- Vaginal yeast infections are actually caused by a fungus.
- According to a recent study, recurrent vaginal yeast infections can be reduced by eating a pint a day of yogurt that contains active bacterial cultures.
- The fungus that causes vaginal yeast infections may be transmitted by contact with a moist towel used by an infected woman.
- Three of four men whose partners have "trich" are found to be infected themselves, many unknowingly.
- Both partners with "trich" should be treated simultaneously, even if they have no symptoms, so as to avoid bouncing the infection back and forth between them.

Men may think that this chapter doesn't concern them and be tempted to start turning the pages at this point. While it is true that only women can suffer from vaginal infections, the microbes that cause these annoying infections may infect the male's urethral tract and be passed back and forth between sexual partners. So men, please, stay tuned. The information contained here concerns you as well.

Health Tips

While only women can have vaginal infections (naturally, since only women have vaginas), the microbes causing these infections may also cause problems for men.

▶ What Is Vaginitis?

Vaginitis is a general term that refers to any type of vaginal inflammation or infection. Different types of vaginitis are caused by different microorganisms. Most cases of vaginitis,[1] perhaps as many as 90 percent,[2] involve bacterial vaginosis (formerly called *nonspecific vaginitis*), candidiasis (commonly called a "yeast" infection), or trichomoniasis ("trich"). Some cases involve combinations of the three. Bacterial vaginosis is the most common form of vaginitis, followed by candidiasis, then by trichomoniasis.[3]

▶ What Causes Vaginitis?

Some cases of vaginitis are caused by infectious organisms that are spread by sexual contact. But other cases of vaginitis result from an allergic reaction or sensitivity to certain chemicals, rather than sexual transmission. In still other cases, organisms that ordinarily reside in the vagina without causing problems become infectious when changes in the vaginal environment allow them to multiply and overgrow.

Factors That Increase the Risk of Vaginal Infections

The environmental balance of the vagina may be upset and increase the chances of a vaginal infection due to such factors as excessive douching, dietary changes, use of antibiotics or birth control pills, lowered resistance (perhaps from fatigue or poor diet), changes in the natural body chemistry, or even wearing pantyhose or nylon underwear.

Health Tips

Various factors may be involved in changing the natural flora of the vagina, leading to an overgrowth of infectious organisms that may result in vaginitis.

▶ What Is Bacterial Vaginosis (BV)?

Bacterial vaginosis (BV) is caused by various bacteria, most commonly the bacterium *Gardnerella vaginalis*.[4] The infection arises when the bacteria causing bacterial vaginosis grow in place of the bacterial flora that normally reside in the vagina.[5]

What Are the Symptoms of BV?

The most prominent symptom in women is a thin, foul-smelling vaginal discharge. Yet many cases occur without symptoms. Besides causing troublesome symptoms in some cases, medical authorities have raised the possibility that BV may increase the risk of various gynecological problems, including infections of the reproductive tract.[6]

Health Tips

Bacterial vaginosis is not merely annoying, but may be linked to more serious problems. Women should report any noticeable symptoms to their doctors.

How Is BV Transmitted?

The bacterium is often transmitted sexually between partners, usually during sexual intercourse. Men may harbor *Gardnerella vaginalis* in their urethras (the tube from the bladder through the penis through which urine passes) which they presumably contracted from sexual contact with infected female partners.[7]

How Is BV Diagnosed?

An accurate diagnosis depends on culturing and identifying the bacteria in the laboratory.[8]

▶ What Is Candidiasis?

Candidiasis or *monilias,* which is more commonly referred to as a vaginal yeast infection, is a vaginal infection caused by *candida albicans,* a yeast-like fungus. The fungus is normally found in small quantities in the vagina. It usually causes no symptoms when the vaginal environment is normally balanced, but becomes infectious when the normal balance of the vaginal environment is upset, allowing an overgrowth of the fungus to occur. Yeast infections can also occur in the mouth in both men and women and in the penis in men. Estimates suggest that about three in four women will experience a vaginal yeast infection during their lives and perhaps 40 to 50 percent of women who do will encounter at least one recurrence.[9]

Health Tips

Vaginal yeast infections are exceedingly common, affecting perhaps three in four women at one time or another. They also frequently recur, although women may take certain precautions that can reduce the risk of recurrent infections.

What Are the Symptoms of Vaginal Yeast Infections?

Candidiasis commonly produces soreness, inflammation, and intense (sometimes maddening!) itching in the genitals that is accompanied by a white, thick, curdy vaginal discharge.

How Is a Yeast Infection Diagnosed?

Diagnosis is usually made on the basis of symptoms. A microscopic examination of vaginal fluids may be used to detect the presence of yeast cells. Culturing a sample of vaginal secretions is a yet more sensitive means of detecting yeast cells.[10]

What Factors Lead to an Overgrowth of "Yeast"?

The use of antibiotics or birth control pills, pregnancy, and diabetes are frequently implicated as factors accounting for changes in the vaginal balance that allow the fungus that causes yeast infections to proliferate. So, too, is wearing tight-fitting, restrictive, and poorly ventilated clothing or nylon underwear.

Health Tips

Factors that may increase the risk of vaginal yeast infections include:
- Use of antibiotics
- Use of birth control pills
- Pregnancy
- Diabetes
- Wearing constricting, tight-fitting clothing or nylon underwear

Does Diet Play a Role? There is increasing evidence that diet may play a role in recurrent yeast infections.[11] Researchers have recently reported that daily ingestion of one pint of yogurt containing active bacterial *(Lactobacillus acidophilus)* cultures may reduce the rate of recurrent infections.[12]

Health Tips

Research evidence shows that eating one pint a day of yogurt with active bacterial cultures may reduce the risk of recurrent vaginal yeast infections.

Can the Fungus That Causes Yeast Infections Be Passed Back and Forth Between Sexual Partners?

Yes, the fungus that causes yeast infections may be transmitted sexually during sexual intercourse, or even passed back and forth between sex partners. However, the role of sexual contact in spreading the infection is believed to be limited.[13] (Most infections in women are believed to be caused by an overgrowth of "yeast" normally found in the vagina, not by sexual transmission).

Can a Yeast Infection Be Transmitted Nonsexually?

Yes, the fungus that causes yeast infections may also be passed nonsexually, such as by sharing a moist towel or washcloth with an infected woman.[14]

Health Tips

Never share a towel with a person who has a vaginal yeast infection. For that matter, since you can never know who is carrying an STD, it's prudent to avoid sharing towels or other personal articles with anyone. Period.

Can Men Become Infected by the Organism That Causes Vaginal Yeast Infections in Women?

Yes, *candida albicans,* the organism responsible for vaginal yeast infections, can cause urinary infections in men. *Candida* can be found in fluid extracted from the penises of about one in five male sexual partners of women with recurrent yeast infections. While most men with *candida* are asymptomatic,[15] some may develop NGU or a genital thrush which is accompanied by sensations of itching and burning during urination, or a reddening of the penis.[16]

Health Tips

Men may become infected with *candida albicans,* the organism causing vaginal yeast infections in women. In men, the infection often takes the form of NGU, genital thrush, or a reddening of the penis.

Can Candidiasis Be Spread to the Mouth or Anus?

Yes, oral and anal sex can be the means of transmission of candidiasis from the genitals of one partner to the mouth and anus of the other, respectively, in either gender.

Health Tips

Candidiasis may appear in other parts of the body than the genitals, such as the mouth and anus, as the result of oral-genital and anal-genital contact, respectively.

► What Is Trichomoniasis?

Trichomoniasis or "trich" (pronounced *trick*) is caused by a protozoan (one-celled organism) type of parasite called *Trichomonas vaginalis.* About 8 million cases of trich in women occur annually in the U.S.[17] "Trich" in the female is characterized by burning or itching in the genitals and the appearance of a foamy whitish to yellowish-green discharge that is often odorous. Lower abdominal pain is reported by 5 to 12 percent of infected women.[18] Upwards of half of infected women experience a mild degree of pain during sexual intercourse or upon urination.[19] Many women notice symptoms appearing or worsening during, or just following, their menstrual periods.[20]

How Is "Trich" Diagnosed?

Examination under a microscope of a smear of vaginal secretions may be used to confirm a diagnosis in the doctor's office.[21] Yet a more sensitive method of confirming a diagnosis is based on examination of cultures grown from a sample of the woman's vaginal secretions.[22]

Can Men Get "Trich"?

In the male, *Trichomonas vaginalis* can lead to NGU, which may be noticeable by the appearance of a slight penile discharge (usually only upon first urination following morning awakening). The urethra may become slightly irritated, leading to sensations of itching or tingling along the urethral tract. However, most infected men are asymptomatic.[23] Evidence shows that three or four of ten male partners of women with "trich" harbor the infectious organism in their urinary tract,[24] in many cases unknowingly.

Can "Trich" Occur without Symptoms in Women Too?

Yes, "trich" occurs without symptoms in about one woman in two.[25] Regardless of symptoms, the infection can be passed along to one's sexual partners. "Trich" often occurs together with other STDs, such as gonorrhea, so it is important for a person with "trich" to be checked out for other STDs as well.[26]

Health Tips

Most of the men, and about half of the women, infected with "trich" experience no symptoms. Frequently, men and women pass the infection back and forth without realizing it.

Can "Trich" Be Transmitted Nonsexually?

In relatively few cases, "trich" may be transmitted by nonsexual means. Since the organism can survive for a few hours in bodily fluids deposited outside the body, it may be passed along in semen, vaginal secretions, or urine found on damp towels,washcloths, or bedclothes. There is a slight possibility that "trich" may be contracted from contact with a toilet seat used by an infected person, but only if the organism makes direct contact with the woman's genitals or the man's penis.[27]

▶ What You Should Know about Treating Vaginal Infections

How Is Bacterial Vaginosis (BV) Treated?

The drug metronidazole (brand name Flagyl) is effective in treating bacterial vaginosis; however, the drug should not be used with women during the first trimester of pregnancy.[28] The medication is administered orally, typically over the course of seven days.[29] It remains unclear whether a man whose partner is infected with bacterial vaginosis should also be treated. Most men harbor the bacterium in their urethral tract without any symptoms.[30] Lacking symptoms, they may unknowingly transmit the bacterium to their sexual partners. Yet firm evidence is lacking to show that treatment of the male partner reduces the risk of recurrence in the female[31] Nonetheless, women who suffer from bacterial vaginosis should consult with their physicians about the advisability of treating their sexual partners.

How Are Vaginal Yeast Infections Treated?

The drugs miconazole (brand name Monistat), clotrimazole (brand names Lotrimin and Mycelex), and terconazole (brand name Terazol) are effective in treating vaginal yeast infections.[32] Some of these medications are now available without a prescription. Even so, it would be wise for women who encounter any vaginal complaints to consult a physician before starting any medication to ensure that they receive the appropriate diagnosis and treatment.

Vaginal infections are frequently recurrent. Successful treatment of vaginal infections does not bestow immunity and recurrences occur commonly. Nor is there evidence showing that treatment of the male partner prevents recurrence in the female partner.[33]

How Is "Trich" Treated?

Metronidazole (Flagyl) is also effective in treating trichomoniasis. Because "trich" may pass back and forth between sexual partners, both partners should be treated simultaneously, whether or not they report symptoms. Treatment is 90 to 100 percent effective when both sex partners are treated simultaneously.[34]

Health Tips

While some medications for treating vaginal yeast infections are available without a prescription, women who suspect they are infected should consult a physician to ensure that they receive the proper diagnosis and treatment.

▶ How to Reduce the Risk of Vaginitis

The Boston Women's Health Book Collective offers the following advice to women to help them reduce the risks of developing vaginitis:[35]

1. Wash your vulva and anus regularly with mild soap. Pat dry, being careful not to touch the vulva after dabbing the anus.
2. Wear cotton panties instead of nylon underwear since nylon retains heat and moisture that cause harmful bacteria to flourish.
3. Avoid pants that are tight in the crotch.
4. Be certain that sexual partners are well-washed. Use of condoms may also reduce the spread of infection from one's sexual partner.
5. Use a sterile, water-soluble jelly like K-Y jelly if artificial lubrication is needed for intercourse—not *Vaseline*. Birth control jellies can also be used for lubrication.
6. Avoid intercourse that is painful or abrasive to the vagina.
7. Avoid diets high in sugar and refined carbohydrates since they may alter the normal acidity of the vagina.
8. Women who are prone to vaginal infections may find it helpful to occasionally douche with plain water, a solution of 1 or 2 tablespoons of vinegar in a quart of warm water, or a solution of baking soda and water. Douches consisting of unpasteurized plain (unflavored) yogurt may help replenish the "good" bacteria that is normally found in the vagina and that may be destroyed by use of antibiotics. Be careful when douching, and do not douche when pregnant or when you suspect you may be pregnant. Let us also add that you should consult your physician before douching or applying any preparations to the vagina.
9. Remember to take care of your general health. Eating poorly or getting insufficient rest will reduce your resistance to infection.

STD FACT SHEET: VAGINITIS

What it is	A general term that applies to any type of vaginal infections. The major types are bacterial vaginosis, candidias (yeast infection), and trichomoniasis ("trich").
What causes it	Bacterial vaginosis: *Gardnerella vaginalis* and other bacteria. Candidiasis: the yeast-like fungus *Candida albicans.* Trichomoniasis: the parasite *Trichomonas vaginalis.*
How it is transmitted	May result from an allergic reaction, a change in the vaginal flora that allows an overgrowth of infectious organisms, or by sexual contact. Yeast infections may also be passed from one woman to another through the sharing of damp towels or washcloths.
Signs and symptoms	Various signs, consisting mostly of irritation and itching of the genitals and by a foul-smelling vaginal discharge. Men infected with these agents may notice some itching and burning sensations during urination or perhaps a reddening or inflammation of the penis. Bacterial vaginosis and trichomoniasis are often asymptomatic in both men and women.
How it is diagnosed	Clinical inspection of symptoms, which may be followed by microscopic examination of a cultured vaginal smear.
How it is treated	Oral administration of the drug metronidazole (flagyl) for bacterial vaginosis and trichomoniasis; vaginal creams, suppositories or tablets containing the drugs miconazole, clotrimazole, or terconazole for candidiasis.

▶ Notes

1. Sobel, J. D. (1990). Vaginal infections in adult women. *Medical Clinics of North America, 74,* 1573–1602.

2. Friedrich, E. (1985). Vaginitis. *American Journal of Obstetrics and Gynecology, 152,* 247–251.

3. Reinisch (1990).

4. Briselden, A. M., & Hillier, S. L. (1990). Longitudinal study of the biotypes of Gardnerella vaginalis. *Journal of Clinical Microbiology, 28,* 2761–2764; Platz-Christensen, J., et al. (1989). Detection of bacterial vaginosis in Papanicolaou smears. *American Journal of Obstetrics and Gynecology, 160,* 132–133.

5. Hillier, S., & Holmes, K. K. (1990). Bacterial vaginosis. In K. K. Holmes, P. Mardh, P. F. Sparling, & P. J. Wiesner (Eds.). *Sexually transmitted diseases* (2nd Ed.). (pp. 547–560). New York: McGraw-Hill.

6. Hillier & Holmes (1990).

7. Hillier & Holmes (1990).

8. Reinisch (1990).

9. Sobel (1990).

10. Vaginal yeast infection can be an HIV warning. (1992, November 24). *New York Newsday,* p. 51.

11. Sobel (1990).

12. Friedrich (1985).

13. Hilton, E., et al. (1992). Ingestion of yogurt containing Lactobacillus acidophilus as prophylaxis for candidal vaginitis. *Annals of Internal Medicine, 116,* 353–357.

14. Sobel (1990).

15. Levy, M. R., Dignan, M., & Shirreffs, J. H. (1987). *Life and health* (5th ed.). New York: Random House.

16. Sobel (1990).

17. Levy et al. (1987) .

18. Levine, G. I. (1991). Sexually transmitted parasitic diseases. *Primary Care: Clinics in Office Practice,* 18, 101–128.

19. Martens, M., & Faro, S. (1989, January). Update on trichomoniasis: Detection and management. *Medical Aspects of Human Sexuality,* 73–79.

20. Rein, M. F., & Müller, M. (1990). *Trichomonas vaginalis* and trichomoniasis. In K. K. Holmes, P. Mardh, P. F. Sparling, & P. J. Wiesner (Eds.). *Sexually transmitted diseases* (2nd Ed.) (pp. 481–492). New York: McGraw-Hill.

21. Rein & Müller (1990).

22. Rein & Müller (1990).

23. Grodstein, F., Goldman, M. G., & Cramer, D. W. (1993). Relation of tubal infertility to history of sexually transmitted diseases. *American Journal of Epidemiology,* 137, 577–584.

24. Levine (1991).

25. Thomason, J. L., & Gelbart, S. M. (1989). Trichomonas vaginalis. *Obstetrics and Gynecology,* 74, 536–541.

26. Rein & Müller (1990).

27. Reinisch (1990).

28. Reinisch (1990).

29. Rein & Müller (1990).

30. Reinisch (1990).

31. CDC (1989b).

32. CDC (1989b).

33. Reinisch (1990).

34. CDC (1989b); Moi, H., et al. (1989). Should male consorts of women with bacterial vaginosis be treated? *Genitourinary Medicine,* 65, 263–268; Hillier & Holmes (1990).

35. CDC (1989b).

36. Sobel (1990).

37. Reinisch (1990); Thomason & Gelbart (1989).

38. Boston Women's Health Book Collective (1984), p. 518; adapted from Rathus et al. (1993).

Chapter

7

Global Prevalence and Incidence for Selected STIs

Global Prevalence and Incidence of Selected Curable Sexually Transmitted Infections Overview and Estimates

World Health Organization

Department of Communicable Disease Surveillance and Response

Contents

List of Boxes

List of Tables

List of Figures

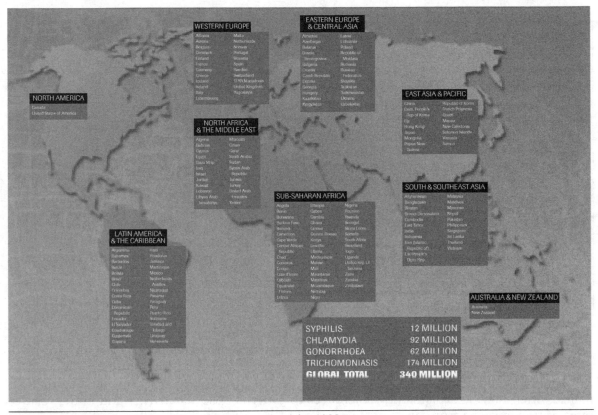

FIGURE 7-1 Estimated new cases of curable STIs among adults, 1999

▶ Introduction

Sexually transmitted infections (STIs) are a major global cause of acute illness, infertility, long term disability and death, with severe medical and psychological consequences for millions of men, women and infants.

WHO estimated that 340 million new cases of syphilis, gonorrhoea, chlamydia and trichomoniasis have occurred throughout the world in 1999 in men and women aged 15–49 years.

In 1990, WHO estimated that over 250 million new cases of STIs had occurred that year.[1] The estimation was based in a modified Delphi technique, which was chosen due the limited information on incidence and prevalence of STI available at that time from many regions including sub-Saharan Africa and some parts of Asia.

In 1995, using a revised methodology described below, the number of new cases of STIs was estimated to be 333 million.[2] The estimation for 1999 is made using the same methodology that in 1995. Data for the estimation were collected by searching published and unpublished information on prevalence and incidence, both in the literature and in the WHO country files for STIs.

The WHO estimates, although based on a comprehensive survey of the available information, are affected by the quantity and quality of prevalence and incidence data from the different regions, and our knowledge of the duration of infection.

BOX 7.1

METHODOLOGY

- Collection and compilation of database of published and unpublished prevalence data.
- Regional prevalence estimates for gonorrhoea, chlamydia and syphilis was calculated using the median prevalence rate from all countries in the region and mid year UN population estimates for adults of 15–49 years of age.
- Regional prevalence estimates for trichomoniasis in women was calculated as being two times chlamydia prevalence. For men it was calculated as one tenth of the prevalence in women.
- Regional incidence estimates were calculated by dividing prevalence by the duration of disease.
- Estimates for duration of infection was made for symptomatic, asymptomatic, treated and untreated adjusted for sex and region.

A more complete description of the methodology is available upon request from WHO.

Interpreting the data form prevalence studies and comparing results is further complicated by the nature of the populations studied. Few studies are community-based and the majority of data come from studies carried out in specific populations, such as STI or antenatal clinic attendees. Other limitations are the small samples sizes, the different diagnostic approaches and study designs used.

Data from epidemiological surveys show that within countries and between countries in the same region, the prevalence and incidence of STIs may vary widely, between urban and rural population, and even in similar population groups.

These differences reflect a variety of social, cultural, and economic factors, as illustrated by the HIV epidemic, and also differences in the access to appropriate treatment. In general, the prevalence of STIs tends to be higher in urban residents, in unmarried individuals, and in young adults. STIs tend to occur at a younger age in females than in males, which may be explained by differences in patterns of sexual activity and in the relative rates of transmission from one sex to the other.

At the population level, the spread of an STI depends upon the average number of new cases of infection generated by an infected person. This can be described in terms of the basic or case-reproduction ratio (Ro) which, for an STI, depends upon the efficiency of transmission (b), the mean rate of sexual partners change (c) and the average duration of infectiousness (D), as expressed in the form

$$Ro = b * c * D$$

The higher the value of Ro the greater the potential for the spread of the infection

▶ Background

There are more than 20 pathogens that are transmissible through sexual intercourse. Many of them are curable by appropriate antimicrobial treatment. However, in spite of the availability of effective treatment, bacterial STIs are still a major public health concern in both industrialised and developing countries.

The exact magnitude of the STIs burden is frequently unknown. Although passive STIs surveillance systems exist in some countries, the data is not always reliable or complete. The quality and completeness of the available data and estimates depend on the quality of STIs services, the extent to which patients seek health care, the intensity of case finding and diagnosis and the quality of reporting.

The completeness is further affected by the STIs natural history, since a large number of infections are asymptomatic. Moreover, only part of the symptomatic population seeks health care and even a smaller number of cases are reported. The social stigma that usually is associated with STIs may result in people seeking care from alternative providers or not seeking care at all. As a result, report-based STI surveillance systems tend to underestimate substantially the total number of new cases.

Curable STIs are not only a concern due to the discomfort resulting from the acute infection. Both symptomatic and asymptomatic infections can lead to the development of serious complications with severe consequences for the individuals and for the community. The most serious complications and long term consequences of untreated STIs tend to be in women and new-born babies.

In developing countries, STIs and their complications are amongst the top five disease categories for which adults seek health care. In women of childbearing age, STIs (excluding HIV) are second only to maternal factors as causes of disease, death and healthy life lost.[3]

Apart from being serious diseases in their own right, STIs enhance the sexual transmission of HIV infection. The presence of an untreated STD (ulcerative or non-ulcerative) increase the risk of both acquisition and transmission of HIV by a factor of up to 10. Moreover, the improvement in the management of STIs can reduced the incidence of HIV-1 infection in the general population by about 40%.[4] STIs prevention and treatment are, therefore, an important component in HIV prevention strategy.

The highest rates of STIs are generally found in urban men and women in their sexually most active years, that is, between the ages of 15 and 35. On average, women become infected at a younger age than men.

Over and Piot[5] have shown the economic implication of early detection and treatment of STIs. They have estimated that the cure or prevention of 100 initial cases of gonorrhoea in the non-core groups prevents a total of 426 future cases of gonorrhoea in the next 10 years. If the 100 cases prevented are extracted from the core group, the number of cases averted rises to 4278.

BOX 7.2

COMPLICATIONS OF STIs

In adults	*In children*
Pelvic inflammatory disease	Congenital syphilis
Ectopic pregnancy	Pneumonia
Infertility	Prematurity, low birth weight
Cervical cancer	Blindness
Spontaneous abortion	Stillbirth

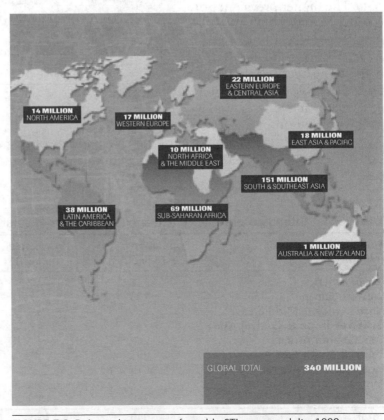

FIGURE 7-2 Estimated new cases of curable STI among adults, 1999

▶ Global Estimates

WHO estimates that 340 million new cases of STIs have occurred worldwide in 1999. The largest number of new infections occurred in the region of South and Southeast Asia, followed by sub-Saharan Africa and Latin America and the Caribbean. However, the highest rate of new cases per 1000 population has occurred in sub Saharan Africa.

▶ Chlamydia

Chlamydia is a common cause of pelvic inflammatory disease with subsequent risk for infertility. The higher prevalence of chlamydia observed amongst female adolescents (24.1%–27%),[6,7] and the association with young age[8] highlight the important role that screening of sexually active female play in the prevention of infertility.

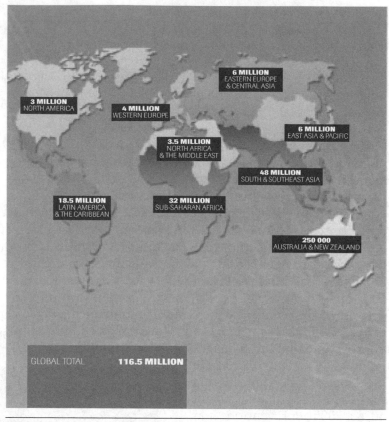

FIGURE 7-3 Estimated prevalence of curable STI among adults, 1999

In 1996 genital chlamydial infection was the most commonly reported notifiable infectious disease in the United States with an annual point estimates of approximately 3 million cases.[9]

TABLE 7.1 Estimated prevalence and annual incidence of curable STIs by region

Region (million)	Population 15–49 (million)	Prevalence (million)	Prevalence per/1000	Annual Incidence (million)
North America	156	3	19	14
Western Europe	203	4	20	17
North Africa & Middle East	165	3.5	21	10
Eastern Europe & Central Asia	205	6	29	22
Sub Saharan Africa	269	32	119	69
South & South East Asia	955	48	50	151
East Asia & Pacific	815	6	7	18
Australia & New Zealand	11	0.3	27	1
Latin America & Caribbean	260	18.5	71	38
Total	3040	116.5		340

In Western Pacific, studies amongst pregnant women have shown a prevalence rate that ranges from of 5.7% in Thailand[10] up to 17% in India.[11] One study in a rural population in Papua New Guinea showed a prevalence rate of 26%.[12]

In Australia, number of STI notified in 1998 was higher than in 1997. Chlamydia infection was the most common STI notified and the third highest for all notifiable diseases.[13]

In Europe, prevalence of chlamydia infection amongst pregnant women ranges from 2.7% in Italy to 8% in Iceland, with low prevalence and incidence rates in the Nordic countries, following a wide scale screening programmes in the 1970s (Figure 7-5).[14,15,16,17,18,19,20]

Prevalence studies from Latin America and Caribbean, show rates from 1.9% amongst

_____ BOX 7.3 _____

BASIC FACTS ABOUT CHLAMYDIA

- 70–75% of women infected with Chlamydia trachomatis are symptom free. Even in men, the rate of asymptomatic chlamydia infection is higher than the rate of asymptomatic gonorrhoea infection.

- Clinical manifestations: mucosal inflammation of the urogenital tract, throat or rectum in both males and females. Neonatal eye infection and pneumonia.

- Complications: in women, pelvis sepsis leading to abscess formation, chronic and recurrent pelvic inflammatory disease, ectopic pregnancy, infertility and chronic pelvic pain. In men, chronic genital tract infection, possibly resulting in infertility. In children, pneumonia and eye infection.

- Diagnosis: Requires sophisticated equipment, is costly and not always available in developing country laboratories.

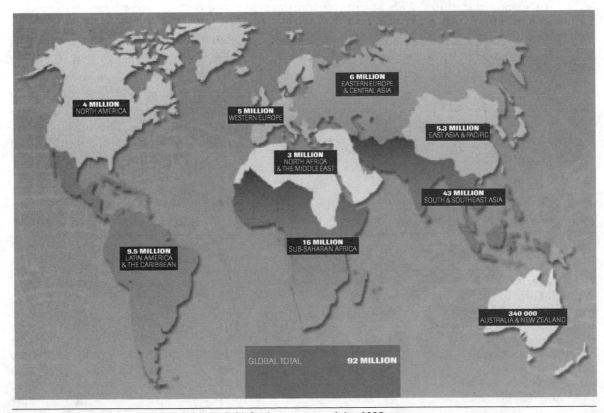

FIGURE 7-4 Estimated new cases of chlamydial infections among adults, 1999

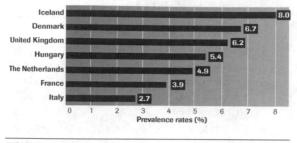
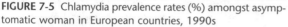

FIGURE 7-5 Chlamydia prevalence rates (%) amongst asymptomatic woman in European countries, 1990s

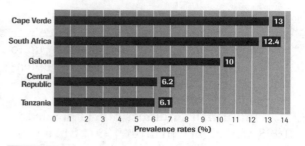
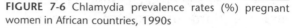

FIGURE 7-6 Chlamydia prevalence rates (%) pregnant women in African countries, 1990s

teenager in Chile,[21] 2.1% amongst pregnant women in Brazil,[22] and 12.2% amongst attendees to family planning clinics in Jamaica.[23]

In Africa, studies amongst pregnant women have revealed a prevalence rate from about 6% in Tanzania to 13% in Cape Verde, (Figure 7-6).[24,25,26,27,28]

► Gonorrhoea

In Western Europe, a significant decline of incidence of gonorrhoea has been observed during the years 1980–91 down to below 20 per 100 000 for gonorrhoea.[29]

However, since mid 1990s, an increase in cases of gonorrhoea has been observed in England and Wales, with a 35% increase in male cases and a 32% rise in female cases between 1995–97.[30] Significant increases in diagnoses of uncomplicated gonorrhoea were seen in most age groups between 1995 and 1998, with the largest average annual increases in the 16 to 19 years old of both sexes, and those over 34 years of age.[31]

In Sweden, trends in the incidence of gonorrhoea showed a steady decline with a incidence of 2.4 per 100 000 inhabitants in 1996. However, in 1997 the number of new cases was 17% higher than in 1996, which represents the first increase since 1976. The upward trend has persisted in 1998. The ratio male: female has been unchanged since 1995, with 80% of cases amongst male.[32]

TABLE 7.2 Estimated new cases of chlamydial infections (in million) among adults, 1995 and 1999

Region	1995			1999		
	Female	Male	Total	Female	Male	Total
North America	2.34	1.64	**3.99**	2.16	1.77	**3.93**
Western Europe	3.20	2.30	**5.50**	2.94	2.28	**5.22**
North Africa & Middle East	1.28	1.67	**2.95**	1.44	1.71	**3.15**
Eastern Europe & Central Asia	2.92	2.15	**5.07**	3.25	2.72	**5.97**
Sub Saharan Africa	8.44	6.96	**15.40**	8.24	7.65	**15.89**
South & South East Asia	20.28	20.20	**40.48**	23.96	18.93	**42.89**
East Asia & Pacific	2.63	2.70	**5.33**	2.74	2.56	**5.30**
Australia & New Zealand	0.17	0.12	**0.30**	0.17	0.14	**0.30**
Latin America & Caribbean	5.12	5.01	**10.13**	5.12	4.19	**9.31**
Total	**46.38**	**42.77**	**89.15**	**50.03**	**41.95**	**91.98**

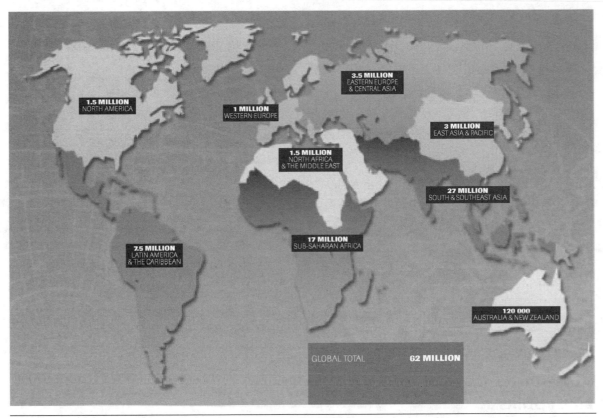

FIGURE 7-7 Estimated new cases of gonorrhoea among adults, 1999

In USA, between 1981 and 1996 the incidence of reported gonorrhoea decreased 71.3%, from 431.5 to 124.0 cases per 100 000. Rates amongst blacks were 35% times higher than among whites in 1996, compare with 11 times higher in 1981. Among women the highest rates was observed in the 15–19 years old group and in men in the 20 to 24 year olds.[33]

An important increased in gonorrhoea rates has been seen in Eastern Europe, in the newly independent states of the former soviet union, with the highest rate in Estonia, Russia and Belarus (111, 139 and 125 per 100 000 respectively).

In the Baltic countries, the average age of patients suffering from STI is decreasing as shown in a study looking the epidemiological situation in the Baltic countries for the period 1990–94.[34]

_____ **BOX 7.4**_____

BASIC FACTS ABOUT GONORRHOEA

Gonorrhoea is a common STIs, although up to 80% of women and 10% of men are asymptomatic.

- Clinical manifestations: inflammation of the mucous membranes of the urogenital tract, throat or rectum. Neonatal eye infection

- Complications: In women, pelvic infection leading to infertility, ectopic pregnancy, chronic pelvic inflammatory disease, chronic pelvic pain in women. In men, urethral strictures. In both sex, septicaemia, arthritis, endocarditis and meningitis. In new-born infant, eye infection can lead to blindness.

- Diagnosis: Needs sophisticated equipment, is costly and not always available in developing country laboratories.

In the Western Pacific the highest estimated prevalence rates for gonorrhoea (3% or greater) are found in Cambodia and Papua New Guinea. In other countries, estimated rates are below 1%[35] (Figure 7-8).

In Australia, notification of gonococcal infection doubled since 1991.[36]

In Africa, prevalence rates of gonorrhoea have shown rates amongst pregnant women as low as 0.02 in Gabon,[37] 3.1% in Central African Republic[38] and 7.8% in South Africa.[39]

Studies conducted amongst patients with urethral/vaginal discharge or dysuria showed a prevalence rate for gonorrhoea of 5.7% in Benin,[40] 8.4% in Tanzania[41] and 17.1% in Malawi.[42]

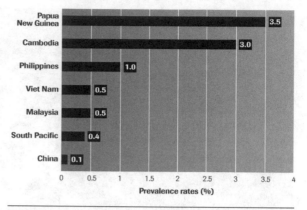

FIGURE 7-8 Estimated gonorrhoea prevalence rate (%) in adults over 15 years of age, 1990s

Amongst symptomatic patients, the prevalence rate for gonorrhoea in African countries have ranged from 5.7% in Benin to 17.1 in Malawi.

In children, untreated gonococcal ophthalmia can cause blindness. According to historical data, around 3% of new-borns with gonococcal ophthalmia will develop complete blindness if untreated, and 20% will have corneal damage of some degree.

▶ Syphilis

In Western Europe, syphilis prevalence has declined substantially since the peak after the second World War, with incidence rates below 5 per 100 000 in the majority of countries.[42,43,44]

In the USA, trends of congenital syphilis began to decline in 1992 after an increase that follow a national syphilis epidemic in 1980s early 1990s. Rates of congenital syphilis declined from 78.2 in 1992 to 20.6 per 100 000 live births in 1998, with high rate in the south-eastern United States and among minority racial/ethnic populations. The trend observed is parallel with the trend for primary and secondary syphilis.[46]

TABLE 7.3   Estimated new cases of gonorrhoea infections (in million) in adults, 1995 and 1999

Region	1995 Female	Male	Total	1999 Female	Male	Total
North America	0.92	0.83	**1.75**	0.84	0.72	**1.56**
Western Europe	0.63	0.60	**1.23**	0.63	0.49	**1.11**
North Africa & Middle East	0.77	0.77	**1.54**	0.68	0.79	**1.47**
Eastern Europe & Central Asia	1.16	1.17	**2.32**	1.81	1.50	**3.31**
Sub Saharan Africa	8.38	7.30	**15.67**	8.84	8.19	**17.03**
South & South East Asia	14.55	14.56	**29.11**	15.09	12.12	**27.20**
East Asia & Pacific	1.47	1.80	**3.27**	1.68	1.59	**3.27**
Australia & New Zealand	0.07	0.06	**0.13**	0.06	0.06	**0.12**
Latin America & Caribbean	3.67	3.045	**7.12**	4.01	3.26	**7.27**
Total	**31.61**	**30.54**	**62.15**	**33.65**	**28.70**	**62.35**

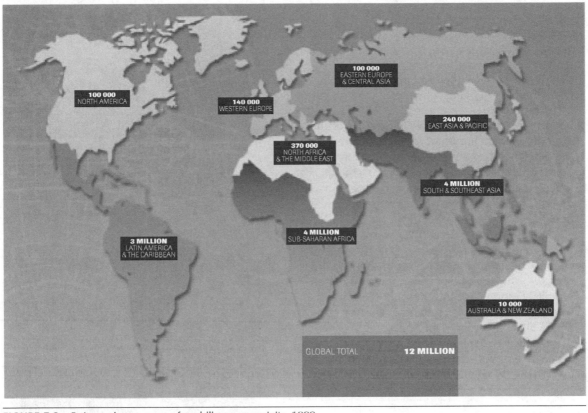

FIGURE 7-9 Estimated new cases of syphilis among adults, 1999

In contrast with the decline in rates observed in Western Europe, since 1989 there has been an alarming increased of the rates in the newly independent states of the former Soviet Union. Syphilis incidence has increased from 5–15 per 100 000 observed in 1990 to as high as 120–170 per 100 000 of population in 1996[47] (Figure 7-10 and 7-11).[48]

In the Western Pacific, relatively high syphilis prevalence rates are found in Cambodia (4%), Papua New Guinea (3.5%) and the South Pacific (8%).[49]

In Mongolia, syphilis rates showed a decreasing trend during 1983–93 from 70 to 18 cases per 100 000 population, followed by an increase to 32 cases per 100 000 in 1995, with a 1.5 – 3.0 fold higher rate amongst the 15–24 age group.[50]

In the eastern Mediterranean Region, in 1997, the highest syphilis prevalence rate amongst pregnant women was reported by Djibouti (3.1%), followed by Morocco (3.0%) and Sudan (2.4%). Amongst blood donors, the highest prevalence was seen in Morocco (1.3%), followed by Qatar (1.1%).[51]

In Africa, syphilis prevalence rates amongst pregnant women varies from 2.5% in Burkina Faso to 17.4% in Cameroon (Figure 7-12).[52,53,54,55]

Prenatal screening and treatment of pregnant women for syphilis is cost-effective, even in areas of prevalence as low as 0.1% in South Africa, peri-natal death was 19.4 times more likely if incomplete treatment or no treatment at all was received.[56]

BOX 7.5

BASIC FACTS ABOUT SYPHILIS

Syphilis is the classic example of a STI that can be successfully controlled by public health measures due to the availability of a highly sensitive diagnostic test and a highly effective and affordable treatment.

Clinical manifestations: ulceration of the uro-genital tract, mouth or rectum. If untreated, this is followed by a more generalised infection which is usually characterised by disseminated muco-cutaneous lesions. There may be fever and general malaise, as well as hair loss and mild hepatitis.

Complications: pregnancy wastage (abortion, premature delivery, and stillbirth) neonatal or congenital syphilis that occurs in about a third of new-born babies of women with untreated syphilis. Disorders of the musculo-skeletal, cardiovascular and nervous systems in the final stage of the disease (tertiary syphilis)

Diagnosis: Screening test is simple and relatively cheap but not always available in developing country laboratories.

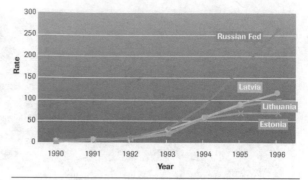
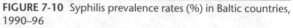

FIGURE 7-10 Syphilis prevalence rates (%) in Baltic countries, 1990–96

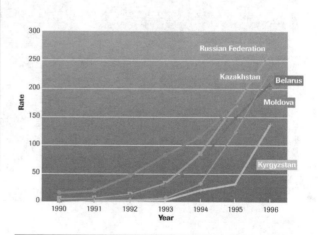

FIGURE 7-11 Syphilis prevalence rates (%) in former Soviet Union countries, 1990–96

TABLE 7.4   Estimated new cases of syphilis (in million) amongst adults, 1995 and 1999

Region	1995 Female	1995 Male	Total	1999 Female	1999 Male	Total
North America	0.07	0.07	0.14	0.054	0.053	0.107
Western Europe	0.10	0.10	0.20	0.069	0.066	0.136
North Africa & Middle East	0.28	0.33	0.62	0.167	0.197	0.364
Eastern Europe & Central Asia	0.05	0.05	0.10	0.053	0.052	0.105
Sub-Saharan Africa	1.56	1.97	3.53	1.683	2.144	3.828
South & South East Asia	2.66	3.13	5.79	1.851	2.187	4.038
East Asia & Pacific	0.26	0.30	0.56	0.112	0.132	0.244
Australia	0.01	0.01	0.01	0.004	0.004	0.008
Latin America and Caribbean	0.56	0.70	1.26	1.294	1.634	2.928
Total	5.55	6.67	12.22	5.29	6.47	11.76

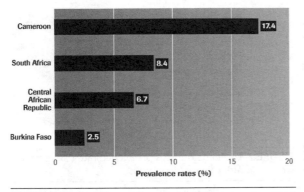

FIGURE 7-12 Syphilis prevalence rates (%), pregnant women in Africa, 1990s

▶ Trichomoniasis

In spite of the fact that trichomononiasis is the most common of STIs, data on prevalence and incidence are limited.

Vaginal trichomoniasis has been associated with increased HIV virus seroconversion in women.[57] Additionally, trichomoniasis is associated with adverse birth outcomes as premature delivery or rupture of the membranes and low birth weight.[58]

Recently, a study conducted in the Democratic Republic of Congo amongst HIV positive and negative pregnant women, show that trichomona vaginalis was isolated twice as often in HIV sero-positive women. In addition trichomoniasis was associated with low birth weight in the group of HIV sero-negative women.[59]

Trichomoniasis prevalence rates amongst pregnant women in Latin America and Caribbean in the 1990s ranges from 2.1% in Brazil,[60] 3.6% in Barbados,[61] 8% in Nicaragua[62] and 27.5% in Chile.[63]

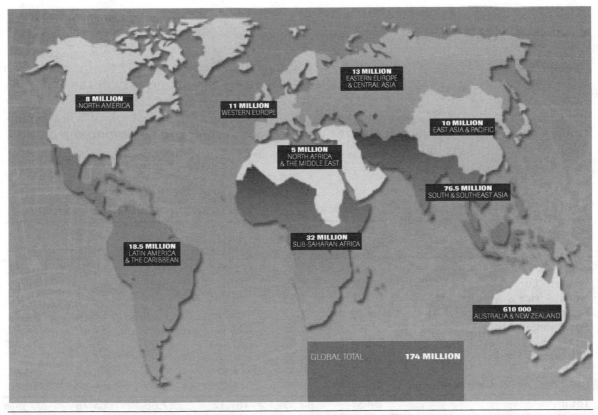

FIGURE 7-13 Estimated new cases of trichomoniasis among adults, 1999

_____ BOX 7.6 _____

BASIC FACTS ABOUT TRICHONIONIASIS

It is the most common STI worldwide. It causes symptoms in approximately 50% of infected women. In men, infection is usually urethral and of short duration, but men easily transmit the parasite to women during the short period when they are infected.

Clinical manifestations: vaginitis and occasionally male urethritis

Complications: trichomonas infections have no systemic complications but there is evidence that vaginal trichomonas infection facilitates the spread of HIV infection

Diagnosis: Test not always available in developing country laboratories

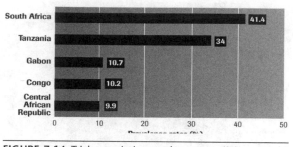
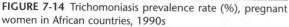

FIGURE 7-14 Trichomoniasis prevalence rate (%), pregnant women in African countries, 1990s

Prevalence studies amongst pregnant women in Africa show rates from 9.9% in Central African Republic to 41.4 in South Africa (Figure 7-14).[64,65,66,67,68]

Few prevalence studies have been conducted amongst men. Recently, a study in Malawi shows a prevalence of 20.8% with symptomatic men and 12.2% with asymptomatic.[69] Another study amongst male patients with urethral discharges in Egypt shows a prevalence rate of 28.8% and 8.2% with men suffering from impotence and infertility.[70]

▶ Prevention of STIs

The scale of the STI problem is to great to be dealt with in specialised STD centres alone, and steps must be taken to expand and integrate STI management in primary health and other health facilities.

The objectives of STI prevention and care are to reduce the prevalence of STI by interrupting their transmission, reducing the duration of infection and preventing the development of complications in those infected.

TABLE 7.5 Estimated new cases of trichomoniasis (in million) among adults, 1995 and 1999

Region	1995 Female	1995 Male	1995 Total	1999 Female	1999 Male	1999 Total
North America	3.78	4.23	8.01	3.90	4.29	8.18
Western Europe	5.30	5.76	11.06	5.09	5.52	10.62
North Africa & Middle East	2.32	2.22	4.54	2.35	2.25	4.60
Eastern Europe & Central Asia	4.90	5.17	10.07	6.36	6.75	13.11
Sub-Saharan Africa	15.07	15.35	30.42	15.93	16.19	32.12
South & South East Asia	39.56	35.87	75.43	40.06	36.36	76.42
East Asia & Pacific	4.83	4.53	9.36	4.91	4.61	9.51
Australia	0.29	0.32	0.61	0.29	0.32	0.61
Latin America & Caribbean	8.52	9.10	17.62	8.79	9.50	18.30
Total	84.57	82.55	167.12	87.68	85.78	173.46

Neisseria Gonorrhoea and Antibiotic Resistance

Genital tract gonorrhoea can be treated successfully by single dose therapy if the causative organism is susceptible to the antibiotic used. The capacity of Neisseria gonorrhoea to develop resistance is, however, one barrier to the use of effective treatment, so that treatment regimens must be tailored to the prevalence of antimicrobial resistance in each country.

Worldwide the major trends in antimicrobial resistance are related to the penicillin and quinolones. There are areas with high proportion of high-level resistance to tetracycline, an antibiotic frequently used in developing country, even if a not recommended therapy for gonorrhoea. There have been sporadic reports of isolates resistant to spectinomicin as well as of decreasing susceptibility to third generation cephalosporins.

_____ **BOX 7.7** _____

PREVENTION OF STIs

Primary prevention

- Health education and promotion of safer sex and risk reduction
- Information campaigns on the association between HIV and other STIs
- Promotion of condoms

Secondary prevention

Aim to reduce the prevalence by shortening the duration of disease by:

- Promotion of early health care seeking behaviour
- Accessible, effective and acceptable care
- Education and counselling
- Early detection and treatment of asymptomatic infections through case finding and screening

The data collected during seven-year from the regional surveillance programme in Western Pacific WHO Region (GASP), even if with significant interregional differences, show that the proportion of quinolone-resistant gonococci is in a continuing trend in 11 of 13 countries in which quinolone resistance was assessed. The increase in resistance has been substantial in some countries: in Hong Kong a rise from 3.3% in 1994 to 49% in 1998, in Singapore from 0.3% in 1993 to 7% and in Australia from < 0.1% in 1993 to 5.6% in 1997. The widespread resistance of gonococcus to penicillin, still remains at high level, while the percentage of isolate high-resistant to tetracycline is particularly elevated (70%) in Singapore and Solomon Islands.[71]

Significant increasing trend of ciprofloxacin resistance was also found in India and Japan, where a low level of penicillin resistance was detected.[72,73]

In the USA the gonococcal isolate surveillance programme (GISP) report for 1997 recorded, overall, the presence of 33.4% of strains resistant to the penicillin, tetracycline, or both. Resistance to fluoroquinolones, one of the currently recommended treatments for gonorrhoea, is rare with the exception of Ohio State in which decreased susceptibility persists at 16%.[74] A higher prevalence in penicillin and tetracycline was noted in south American countries and Caribbean with low level of quinolone resistance.

The data from national surveillance programmes in Western Europe indicate a decreased prevalence of penicillin resistant gonococci in the last years (31% in Sweden, 8% in Netherlands, 13% France, 19% Denmark, 6% Finland, 0.8% Scotland). In contrast the number of fluoroquinolone resistant gonococci is increasing: ciprofloxacin resistance was detected in 3.2% of strains in Netherlands, 3% in France, 9% in Denmark, 1% in Finland, 0.8% in Scotland. Tetracycline resistance was observed in a high proportion of strains. Resistant gonococcal strains are often isolated from imported case.[75,76,77,78,79,80]

Studies from a number of African countries on small samples indicate that penicillin resistance is broadly diffused among isolates; data on fluoroquinolone resistance are scantly, because of the inconstant use of these drugs. The majority of isolates exhibit resistance to tetracycline including high-level resistance.[81]

▶ References

1. World Health Organization. WHO Features No 152, WHO Geneva, 1990.
2. WHO. *Global prevalence and incidence of selected curable sexually transmitted diseases: overview and estimates*. World Health Organization, Geneva (1995).
3. World Bank. *World Development report: Investing in Health*. Washington, 1993.
4. Gilson L, Mkanje R, Grosskurth H, Mosha F, Picar J, Gavyole A, Todd J, Mayaud P, Swai R, Fransen L, Mabey D, Mills, A, Hayes R. Cost-effectiveness of improved treatment services for sexually transmitted diseases in preventing HIV-1 infection in Mwanza Region, Tanzania. *Lancet* 1997, 350: 1805–09.
5. Over M, Piot P. Human Immunodeficiency Virus infection and other sexually transmitted diseases in developing countries: public health importance and priorities for resource allocation. *Journal of Infectious Diseases* 1996, 174 (Suppl 23) S 162–75.
6. Bunnell RE, Dahlberg L, Rolfs R, Ramsonm R, Gershman K, Farshy C, Newhall WiJ, Schmid S, Stone K, St Lous M. High prevalence and incidence of sexually transmitted diseases in urban adolescent females despite moderate risk behaviour. *Journal of Infectious Diseases*. 180(5): 1624–31, 1999.
7. Burstein GR, Gaydos CA, Diner-West M, Howell MR, Zenilman JM, Quinn TC. Incident Chlamydia trachomatis Infections among inner-city adolescent females. *JAMA* 280(6): 521–6, 1998.
8. Cook RL, St George K, Lassak M, Tran N, Anhalt JP, Rinaldo CR. Screening for Chlamydia trachomatis infection in college women with a polymerase chain reaction assay. *Clinical infectious Diseases*. 28(5): 1002–7, 1999.
9. Center for Disease Control and Prevention. Summary of notifiable diseases. United States. 1996. *Morbidity and Mortality Weekly Report* 1996; 45: 4–6.
10. Kilmarx PH, Black CM, Limpakarnjanarat K, Shaffer N, Yanpaisarn S, Chaisilwattana P, Siriwasin W, Young NL, Farshy CE, Mastro TD, St Louis ME. Rapid assessment of sexually transmitted diseases in a sentinel population in Thailand: prevalence of chlamydia Infection, gonorrhoea, and syphilis among pregnant women, 1996. *Sexually Transmitted Infections* 74(3): 189–93, 1998 Jun.
11. Paul VK, Singh M, Gupta U, Buckshee K, Bhargava VL, Takkar D, Nag VL, Bhan MK, Deorari AK. Chlamydia trachomatis infection among pregnant women: prevalence an oprenatal importance. *National Medical Journal of India* 12(1): 11–4, 1999 Jan–Feb.
12. Passey M, Mgone CS, Lupiwa S, Suve N, Tiwara S, Lupiwa T. Clegg A, Alpers MP. Community based study of sexually transmitted diseases in rural women in the highlands of Papua New Guinea: prevalence and risk factors. *Sexually Transmitted Infections*. 74(2): 120–7, 1998 Apr.
13. Thomson J, Lin M, Halliday L, Preston G, Mcintyre P, Gidding H, Amin J, Roberts L, Higgins K, Brooke F, Milton A, O'Brien E, Witteveen D, Crerar S. (1999) Australia's notifiable diseases status, 1998. *Annual report of the National Notifiable Diseases Surveillance System. Communicable Diseases Intelligence*. 23(11): 277–305.

14. Jonsdottir K, Geirsson RT, Steingrimsson O, Olafsson JH, Stefansdottir S. Reduced prevalence of cervical Chlamydia Infection among women requesting termination. *Acta Obstetricia et Gynecologica Scandinavica*. 76(5): 438–41, 1997.

15. Munk C, Morre SA, Kjaer SK, Poll Pa, Bock JE, Meijer CJ, vand den Brule AJ. PCR detected chlamydia trachomatis infections from the uterine cervix of young women from the general population: prevalence and risk determinants. *Sexually Transmitted Diseases* 26(6): 325–8m 1999 Jul.

16. Kirkwood K, Horn K, Glasier A, Sutherland S, Young H, Patrizio C. Non-invasive screening of teenagers for Chlamydia trachomatis in a family planning setting. *British Journal of Family Planning* 25(1):11–2, 1999 Apr.

17. Deak J, Nagy E, Vereb I, Meszarons G, Kovaos L, Nyari T, Berbik I. Prevalence of Chlamydia trachomatis infection in a low-risk population in Hungary. *Sexually Transmitted Diseases*. 24 (9): 538–42, 1997 Oct.

18. Van de Hoek JA, Mulder-Folkerts DK, Coutinho RA, Dukers NH, Buimer M, van Doornum GJ. Opportunistio screening for genital infections with Chlamydia trachomatis among the sexually active population of Amsterdam. *Nederlands Tijdschrift voor Geneeskunde*. 143(13): 668–72, 1999, Mar 27.

19. Malkin JE, Prazuck T, Bogard M, Blanchi A, Cessot G, De Fanti AS, Baldin A, Bohbot JM, Halioua B, Lafaix C. Screening of Chlamydia trachomatis genital infection in a young Parisian population. *Sexually Transmitted Infections* 75(3):188–9, 1999 Jun.

20. Bavastrelli M, Midulla M, Rossi D, Salzano M, Calzolari E, Midulla C, Sanguigni S, Torre A, Giardini O. Sexually active adolescents and young adults: a high risk group for Chlamydia trachomatis infection. *Journal of Travel Medicine* 5(2): 57–60, 1998 Jun.

21. Gaete MV, Prado VE, Altamirano PD, Martinez JB, Urrejola P, Pinto JM. Prevalence of Chlamydia trachomatis and Neisseria gonorrhoea in Chilean asymptomatic adolescent males determined by urine sample. *Sexually Transmitted Infections*, 75(1):67–8, 1999 Feb.

22. Simoes JA, Giraldo PC, Faundes A. Prevalence of cervicovaginal infections using gestation and accuracy of clinical diagnosis. *Infectious Diseases in Obstetrics and Gynaecology* 6(3):129–33, 1998.

23. Behets FM, Ward E, Fox L, Reed R, Spruyt A, Bennett L, Johnson L, Hoffman I, Figueroa JP. Sexually transmitted diseases are common in women attending Jamaican family planning ollncis and appropriate detection tools are lacking. *Sexually Transmitted Infections*, 74 Suppl 1: S123–7, 1998 Jun.

24. Wessel HF, Herrmann B, Dupret A, Moniz F, Brito C, Berstrom S. Genital infections among antenatal care attendees in Cape Verde, *African Journal of Reproductive Health*, 2(1): 32–40, 1998.

25. Sturm AW, Vilkinson D, Ndovela N, Bowen S, Connolly C. Pregnant women as a reservoir of undetected sexually transmitted diseases in rural South Africa: implications for disease control. *American Journal of Public Health*, 88(8): 1243–5, 1998.

26. Bourgeois A, Henzel D, Dibanga G, Malonga-Mouelet G, Peeters M, Coulaud JP, Fransen L, Delaporte E. Prospective evaluation of a flow chart using a risk assessment for the diagnosis of STDs in primary healthcare centres in Libreville, Gabon. *Sexually Transmitted Infections* 74 Suppl 1:S128–32, 1998.

27. Blankhart D, Muller O, Gresenguet G, Weis P. Sexually transmitted infections in young pregnant women in Bangui, Central African Republic. *International Journal of STD & AIDS*, 10(9): 609–14, 1999.

28. Mayaud P, ka-Gina G, Cornelissen J, Todd J, Kaatano G, West B, Uledi E, Rwakatare M, Kopwe L, Manoko D, Laga M, Grosskurth H, Hayes R, Mabey D. Validation of a WHO algorithm with

risk assessment for the clinical management of vaginal discharge in Mwanza, Tanzania, *Sexually Transmitted Infections* 74 Suppl 1: S77–84, 1998.

29. De Schryver A, Meheus A. Epidemiology of sexually transmitted diseases: the global picture. *WHO Bulletin OMS* 68: 639–53, 1990.

30. Anonymous. The incidence of gonorrhoea in England and Wales is rising. *Communicable disease Report. CDR Weekly* 7(25): 217–20, 1997.

31. Lamagni TL, Hughes G, Rogers PA, Paine T, Catchpole M. New cases seen at genitourinary medicine clinics: England 1998. *CDR Communicable Disease Report CDR* Supp 6 (9): S2–12, 1999.

32. Berglund T, Fredlund H, Ramstedt K. Reemergence of gonorrhea in Sweden. *Sexually Transmitted Disease* 26(7):390–1, 1999.

33. Fox KK, Whittington WL, Levine WC, Moran JS, Zaidi AA, Nakashima AK. Gonorrhea in the United States, 1981–1996: Demographic and Geographic trends. *Sexually Transmitted Diseases* 25(7): 386–93, 1998.

34. Lacdane G, Bukovskis M. Epidemiology of sexually transmitted diseases in the Baltic countries. *Acta Obstetricia et Gynecologica Scandinavica*, supp 164: 128–31, 1997.

35. World Health Organization, Regional Office for the Western Pacific. *STI/HIV Status and trends of STI, HIV and AIDS at the end of the Millennium*, Western Pacific Region, 1999.

36. Thompson J et al. Ibid 13.

37. Blankhart D. Ibid 27.

38. Bourgeous A. Ibid 26.

39. Sturm AW. Ibid 25.

40. Alary M, Baganizi E, Guedeme A, Padonou F, Davo N, Adjovi C, van Dyck E, Germain M, Joly J, Mahony JB. Evaluation of clinical algorithms for the diagnosis of gonococcal and chlamydial infections among men with urethral discharge and dysuria an women with vaginal discharge in Benin. *Sexually Transmitted Infections*. 74 Supp 1: S 44–9, 1998.

41. Mayaud P et al. Ibid 28.

42. Costello DC, Wangel AM, Hoffman IF, Canner JK, Lule GS, Lema VM, Liomba VM, Liomba NG, Dallabetta GA. Validation of the WHO diagnostic algorithm and development of an alternative scoring system for the management of women presenting with vaginal discharge in Malawi. *Sexually Transmitted Infection*. 74 Supp 1: S50–8, 1998.

43. Garcia-Lechuz JM, Rivera M, Catalan P, Sanchez Carillo C, Rodriguez-Creixems M, Bouza E. Differences in curable STDs between HIV and non-HIV population in Spain. *Aids Patient Care & STDs*. 13(3): 175–7, 1999.

44. Paget WJ, Zimmermann HP. Surveillance of sexually transmitted diseases in Switzerland, 1973–1994: evidence of declining trends i gonorrhoea and syphilis. *Sozial and Praventivmedizin*, 42(1): 30–6, 1997.

45. Lamagni TL et al. Ibid 31.

46. Anonymous. Congenital syphilis, United States, 1998. MMWR Morbidity and Mortality Weekly Report, 48(340): 757–61, 1999.

47. WHO/EURO *Epidemic of sexually transmitted diseases in Eastern Europe*. Report on a Who Meeting, Copenhagen, Denmark 13–15 May 1996.

48. Renton AM, Borisenko KK, Meheus A, Gramyko A. Epidemic of syphilis in the newly independent states of the former Soviet Union. *Sexually Transmitted Infections* 74(3): 165–66, 1998.

49. World Health Organization, Regional Office for the Western Pacific. *STI/HIV status and trends of STI, HIV and AIDS at the end of the Millennium*, WHO/WPO, 1999.

50. Purewdawa E, Moon T, Baigalmaa C, Davaajav K, Smith M, Vermund S. Rise in sexually transmitted diseases during democratization and economic crisis in Mongolia. *STD & AIDS*; 8(6): 398–401, 1997.

51. WHO/EM, *Report on the Intercountry workshop on STD prevalence study*, Amman, Jordan, 12–15 October 1998.

52. Meda N, Sangare L, Lankoande S, Compaore IP, Catraye J, Sanou PT, Van Dyck E, Cartoux M, Soudre RB. The HIV epidemic in Burkina Faso: current status and the knowledge level of the population about AIDS, 1994–95. *Revue d'Epidemiologie et de Santé Publique*, 46(1): 14–23, 1998.

53. Blankhart D et al. Ibid 27.

54. Sturm AW et al. Ibid 25.

55. Mbopl Keou FX, Mbu R, Mauclere P, Andela A, Tetanye E, Leke R, Chaouat G, Barre-Sinoussi F, Martin P, Belec L. Antenatal HIV prevalence in Yaounde, Cameroon. *International Journal of STD & AIDS* 9 (7): 400–2, 1998.

56. Wilkinson D, Malme S, Connolly C. Epidemiology of syphilis in pregnancy in rural South Africa: opportunities for control. *Tropical Medicine and International Health*, 21(1) 1997, 57–62.

57. Laga M, Manoka A, Kivuvu M, Malele B, Tuliza M, Nzila N. Nonulcerative sexually transmitted diseases as risk factors for HIV-1 transmission in women: results from a cohort study. *AIDS* 7: 95–102, 1993.

58. Cothc MF, Pastorek JG, Nugent RP, Hillier SL, Gibbs RS, Martin DH et al. Trichomonas vaginalis associated with low birth weight and pre-term delivery. *Sexually Transmitted Diseases* 24: 353–60, 1997.

59. Sutton MY, Sternberg M, Nsuami M, Behets F, Nelson AM, St Louis ME. Trichomoniasis in pregnant human immunodeficiency virus-infected and human immunodeficiency virus-uninfected congoiese women: prevalence, risk factors, and association with low birth weight. *American Journal of Obstetrics & Gynecology* 181(3): 656–62, 1999.

60. Simoes JA, Giraldo PC, Ribbeiro Filho AD et al. Prevalencia e fatores de risco associados as infeccoes cervico-vaginais durante a gestacao. *Rev Bras Ginecol Obstet* 18 (6): 459–67, 1996.

61. Levett PN, Taravinga M, Maheswaran K et al. Genital tract infections in sexually active women in Barbados. *West Indian Medical Journal* 44: 128, 1995.

62. Espinoza E, Egger M, Herrmann B, Isler M, Voken K, Davey Smith G. STD in Nicaragua: population rate estimates and health seeking behaviour. IX International Conference on AIDS (ICAIDS). Abstract NOo PO C06 2702, 1993.

63. Franjola R, Anazco R, Puente R et al. Trichomonas vaginalis infection in pregnant women and newborn infants. Rev Med Chil 117(2): 142–145.

64. Blankhart et al. Ib 27.

65. Wessel et al. Ib 24.

66. Bourgeois et al. Ibid 26.

67. Mayaud et al. Ibid 28.

68. Sturm et al. Ibid 25.

69. Hobbs MM, Kazembe P, Reed AW, Miller WC, Nkata E, Zimba D, Daly CC, Chakraborty H, Cohen MS, Hoffman I. Trichomonas vaginaleis as a cause of urethritis in Malawian men. *Sexually Transmitted Diseases*. 26(7): 381–7, 1999.

70. el Seoud SF, Abbas MM, Habib FS. Study of trichomoniasis among Egyptian male patients. *Journal of the Egyptian Society of Parasitology,* 28(1): 263–70, 1998.

71. WHO Ibid 35.
72. Ray K, Bala M, Kumar J, Misra RS. Trend of antimicrobial resistance in Neisseria gonorrhoeae at New Delhi, India, Int J STD AIDS 2000; 11: 115–118.
73. Tanaka M, Nakayama H, Haraoka M, Saika T, Kobayashi I, Naito S. Antimicrobial resistance of Neisseria gonorrhoeae and high prevalence of ciprofloxacin-resistant isolates in Japan, 1993 to 1998. *J Clin Microbiol* 2000; 38: 521–525.
74. Fox KK et al. Ibid 33.
75. Berglund T et al. Ibid 32.
76. Anonymous. Gonorrhoea 1998 EPI-NEWS n. 25, 1999. Tove Ronne Ed.
77. Nissinen A, Jarvinen H, Liimatainen O, Jahkola M, Huovinen P, and the Finnish Group for Antimicrobial Resistance. Antimicrobial resistance in Neisseria gonorrhoeae in Finland, 1976 to 1995. *Sex Transm dis 1997*; 24: 576–581.
78. Young H. Epidemiology and treatment outcome of infection with antibiotic resistant strains of Neisseria gonorrhoeae in Scotland. Communicable Disease and public health 1999; 2: 198–202.
79. Anonymous. Les gonococcies en France en 1997. Réseau RENAGO.
80. De Neeling AJ, Van Santen-Verheuvel M, Peerbooms PGH, Willelms, RJL. Emerging resistance to ciprofloxacin in Neisseria gonorrhoeae in the Netherlands. C183.
81. Lind I. Antimicrobial resistance in Neisseria gonorrhoeae. *CID* 1997; 24S: S93–97.

Chapter 8

Social Implications of STIs

Policy and Practice

▶ Ensuring Access to HPV Vaccines through Integrated Services: A Reproductive Health Perspective

Amy E. Pollack,[a] Miranda Balkin,[b] Lindsay Edouard,[c] Felicity Cutts[d] & Nathalie Broutet[e] on behalf of the WHO/ UNFPA Working Group on Sexual and Reproductive Health and HPV Vaccines

Abstract In 2006, a quadrivalent human papillomavirus (HPV) vaccine was licensed, and another vaccine may be licensed soon. Little is known about the practical considerations involved in designing and implementing cervical cancer prevention programmes that include vaccination as a primary means of prevention. Although the vaccine may ultimately be indicated for both males and females, young girls, or girls and women aged 9–25 years, will be the initial candidates for the vaccine. This paper describes avenues for service delivery of HPV vaccines and critical information gaps that must be bridged in order to inform future sexual and reproductive health programming. It proposes the role that the sexual and reproductive health community, together with immunization and cancer control programmes, could have in supporting the introduction of HPV vaccines within the context of current health systems.

Bulletin of the World Health Organization 2007;85:57–63.

Voir page 196 le résumé en français.

[a]Columbia University Mailman School of Public Health, New York, NY, USA.

[b]Global Health Strategies, New York, NY, USA.

[c]United Nations Population Fund, New York, NY, USA.

[d]Department of Immunization, Vaccines and Biologicals, WHO, Geneva, Switzerland.

[e]Department of Reproductive Health and Research, WHO, 1211 Geneva 27, Switzerland. Correspondence to this author (email: broutetn@who.int).

Ref. No. 06-034397

(Submitted: 6 July 2006–Final revised version received: 5 October 2006–Accepted: 24 October 2006)

▶ Introduction

Cervical cancer is a gender-specific disease that disproportionately affects women in the lowest socioeconomic classes throughout the world. A meta-analysis of 57 studies revealed that there was an estimated 100% increased risk of invasive cervical cancer for women in low social class categories when compared with those in high social class categories; this difference reflects a lack of access to screening and treatment services.[1] Likewise, these differences also occur between developed and developing countries, translating inequity in access to inequity in the quality services.

In 2004, the 57th World Health Assembly adopted WHO's global reproductive health strategy, which identified five priority areas including "combating sexually transmitted infections"; the strategy also specifically addressed cervical cancer prevention.[2] In addition, a resolution on cancer prevention and control was adopted by WHO's Member States, and a new vision and strategy for global immunization that aims to ensure equal access to immunization for every child, adolescent and adult was endorsed during the 58th World Health Assembly in 2005. With the upcoming introduction of a vaccine to prevent human papillomavirus (HPV) infection, a comprehensive approach to preventing cervical cancer—which incorporates vaccination, screening and early treatment—opens up new opportunities for strengthening reproductive health services and building interdisciplinary links.

▶ Cervical Cancer: Burden of Disease

Cervical cancer remains the second most common cancer in women worldwide and the primary cause of cancer-related deaths among women in developing countries.[3] Screening programmes have successfully reduced disease rates in developed countries that support cytology-based services; these services are too complex for most developing countries to implement. More than 80% of the estimated 500 000 incident cases annually and more than 90% of the 257 000 deaths caused by cervical cancer occur in developing countries (Figure 8-1).[4] This disparity is due in large part to the fact that a majority of women in these countries have never been screened for cervical cancer.

▶ HPV Infection

HPV is a sexually transmitted infection, recognized as the necessary cause of 99% of all cervical cancers. More than 100 types of HPV have been identified, including at least 13 types that may cause cervical cancer: these are termed "high-risk" types. Of these, HPV types 16 and 18 cause approximately 70% of cervical cancer worldwide.[5] There is geographical and country-specific variability; in sub-Saharan Africa and Latin America types 16 and 18 account for only 65% of invasive cancers. Other, "low-risk" types, mainly 6 and 11, cause genital warts in men and women but not cervical cancer. In most studies, the age-specific peak prevalence of HPV infection occurs among those aged < 25 years, and the peak incidence of cervical cancer occurs at around age 50.[6] Although 90% of all HPV infections are cleared, persistent infection in some women leads to the development of cancer 20 or 30 years later. This prolonged latent phase allows for screening of the cervix to detect precancerous abnormalities.

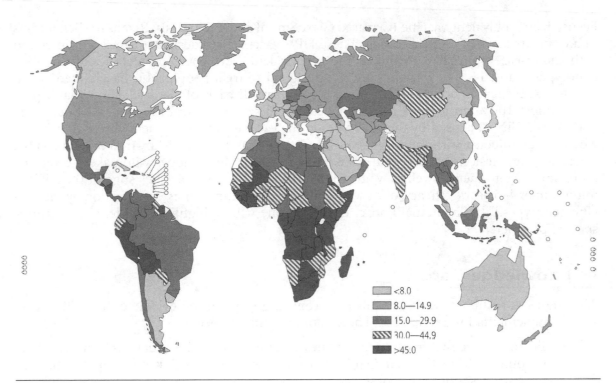

FIGURE 8-1 Worldwide incidences of cervical cancer per 100,000 females (all ages), age-standardized to the WHO standard population, 2005.[4]

▶ Cervical Cancer Screening: Secondary Prevention

Cervical cancer prevention programmes have been cytology-based, but their success depends upon having high rates of coverage of women in the right age group, implementing repeated quality-controlled screening and developing excellent recall services for treating pre-cancerous abnormalities. In low-resource settings, the capacity to implement this complex, high-resource protocol to cover entire populations has been limited.

Alternative cost-effective screening and management options include visual inspection with acetic acid (VIA), with immediate cryotherapy of visible cervical lesions, and testing for HPV DNA;[7,8] these options also improve efficiency by limiting the steps a woman needs to take to access treatment.[9] When compared with cervical smear methods, the DNA screening test appears to be cost-effective, is more objective and less labour-intensive, and has high sensitivity and specificity.[10] Although the current DNA test is too expensive for use in developing countries, lower-cost tests are being developed.

▶ HPV Vaccines

HPV vaccines are prepared from virus-like particles produced by recombinant technology. The quadrivalent vaccine (Gardasil, Merck and Co., Whitehouse Station, NJ, USA) has recently been licensed, and a bivalent vaccine (Cervarix, GlaxoSmithKline Biologicals, Rixensart, Belgium) is in advanced stages of clinical testing. These HPV vaccines are designed to prevent infection with and disease from HPV 16 and 18; the quadrivalent vaccine also protects against low-risk genotypes 6 and 11. The vaccines are not designed to treat people who have already been infected with these genotypes. The results from phase III trials of Gardasil, show that it provides almost 100% protection against moderate and severe cervical intraepithelial neoplasia (CIN 2 and CIN 3) caused by the genotypes in the vaccine among women who have not previously been infected with these genotypes.[11] Gardasil has also been shown to protect against external genital lesions caused by types 6 and 11, which Merck hopes will make the vaccine more attractive to men as well as women.[11, 12] Trial data for both vaccines suggest they offer a minimum of 4–5 years' efficacy, of close to 100%, in preventing persistent infection by the vaccine genotypes.[13,14] The actual impact of the vaccine will be highly dependent on country-specific parameters.[15]

► Knowledge Gaps

Although the results of vaccine trials are promising, gaps in the evidence that will inform service implementation remain.[16,17] These gaps are outlined below.

- **Performance in Africa.** Both vaccines lack safety and efficacy data from Africa where chronic malnutrition, HIV and other infectious diseases that may compromise the immune response are widespread.
- **Duration of action.** Data showing that antibodies persist at levels as high as, or higher than, those seen in natural infection extend to almost 5 years' post-vaccination; antibody levels plateau after 18 months.[13] As further data accrue from extended follow-up of clinical trials, the need for a booster dose can be evaluated.
- **Data on different immunization schedules.** Evaluation is required of the degree of flexibility in intervals between doses and the possibility of two doses being sufficient.
- **Data on infants and young children.** Lack of safety and immunogenicity studies in infants or young children will hinder the integration of vaccines into the traditional Expanded Programme on Immunization (EPI) schedule, which is tailored to childhood vaccination.
- **Cross-protection.** Data on Cervarix indicate there is a high level of cross-protection against new infections with HPV type 45 and a moderate level of protection against type 31,[13] which together are responsible for a further 10% of cervical cancers globally. For the quadrivalent vaccine, antibodies capable of neutralizing both vaccine-type and HPV types 31 and 45 have been demonstrated.[18] Studies on both vaccines continue to evaluate cross-protection against clinical disease associated with these types.
- **Potential replacement infection.** Increases in the prevalence of infection with other types of HPV that develop to fill the "ecological niche" of persistent infection—once infection by types included in the vaccines no longer have that role—will become apparent only during post-introduction surveillance.
- **Vaccine compatibility.** For the quadrivalent vaccine, immunogenicity data show no interference when hepatitis B vaccine is administered simultaneously.[11] Administration of HPV vaccine in combination with other vaccines has not been tested nor have the vaccines been tested in people who are on long-term drug therapy. Bridging studies should address these issues.

▶ Critical Programmatic Issues for Introducing HPV Vaccines

Advocacy, Information and Education

International public health advocacy at the highest level was instrumental in obtaining a purchasing commitment from the GAVI Alliance (formerly the Global Alliance for Vaccines and Immunization) for hepatitis B vaccine as well as a ranking scheme that assisted donors in their decision-making about financial support.[19] In the case of cervical cancer prevention, advocacy must come from those who understand the disease and its societal and population-based burden. Surveys have indicated that knowledge about HPV and cervical cancer among women, men and even health professionals is relatively low.[20] Health professionals at all levels and policy-makers have the greatest opportunity to generate political will and, therefore, need to be well informed.[21]

Since HPV is sexually transmitted, culturally appropriate information must be developed to avoid a negative reaction against vaccination or sexual and reproductive health services, particularly since young girls will be the ones who are vaccinated. It is also important to avoid the risk of a girl-only focus; even if only women and girls receive the vaccine, information must also be given to men and boys about cervical cancer and behavioural interventions to reduce HPV transmission. Targeted and adapted information will help to avoid discrimination or other kinds of misunderstanding. Several studies have demonstrated that if parents understand the benefits of vaccination their apprehension about discussing issues of sexual health or acknowledging that their child may be, or may become, sexually active can be overcome.[22]

Evidence-based standardized informational materials should be developed or identified for wide distribution by health professionals. The significant role of the sexual and reproductive health community in nurturing advocates to campaign for the adequate allocation of resources, nationally and internationally, must not be underestimated. Comprehensive prevention programmes that offer screening and early treatment alongside new vaccine programmes would allow an opportunity to provide community-based education regarding sexual and reproductive health in broader terms.[23]

Target Populations

Adolescent Girls

Data indicate that for greatest impact the vaccine will need to target girls before they initiate sexual activity (that is, before sexual debut), beginning, for example, at the age of 9 years, possibly with additional catch-up vaccination of young women up to the age of 25 years, where resources permit. Infection with high-risk HPV types is consistently high among almost all adolescent female populations tested. Although efficacy trials did not include girls aged < 15 years,[24] bridging studies have established that antibody responses in girls and boys aged 9–15 years are higher than in older people.[25,26]

Providing a vaccine "against cancer" to adolescent girls raises several challenges. For the vaccine to be acceptable, parents will need to have a better understanding of cervical cancer and the reasons for vaccinating young girls to prevent a disease from occurring decades later. A sobering lesson may be gleaned from past efforts to eradicate poliomyelitis that were complicated by misinformation or rumors.[27] Although European studies report high acceptability rates for HPV vaccine,[28,29] there is a clear lack of understanding of the causes of cervical cancer across class and national lines.

Many young unmarried girls and women face significant challenges in accessing the health care necessary to meet their sexual and reproductive health needs. While neither national immunization programmes nor sexual and reproductive health programmes are ideal for providing services to young adolescents, a package of health services should be developed to offer girls an HPV vaccine and other interventions that could have a broader impact on their reproductive health.

Boys and Men

HPV prevalence is lower in men than in women, although it is still frequent; it is not known whether men clear such infections more quickly or are less likely to be infected.[30] Although one of the vaccines may be licensed for use in males, modelling studies suggest this will reduce cervical cancer only marginally when coverage in women is very high.[31] There are, however, other reasons to consider male vaccination.

Gardasil, and possibly later-generation vaccines, will provide protection against genital warts and other external genital lesions[11,32] that affect both women and men. HIV infection is associated with an increased prevalence of genital warts, and giant condyloma (Buschke–Löwenstein tumours) have also been observed in HIV-positive patients who have histological evidence of invasion without metastases.[33]

Both men and women who practice receptive anal sex are at risk of developing anal intraepithelial neoplasia, the precursor to anal cancer, which is also linked to HPV infection.[34] HIV-positive men with HPV are twice as likely to develop anal cancer as men who are HIV-negative.[30]

Studies suggest that education and information actively designed to inform men about cervical cancer have an impact on their female partners' willingness or ability to access services.[35] Ultimately, resources should be directed first towards the targeted age and sex of the population; however, the involvement of both males and females in vaccination efforts might increase acceptability, both directly and indirectly.

Potential Delivery Strategies

National Immunization Programmes

Despite the successes of EPI there are several programmatic challenges in introducing HPV vaccines as part of the programme in many countries.[16] It may seem attractive to link HPV vaccine to tetanus toxoid administration because both target young adult women, have a schedule requiring three or more doses, and have similar intervals between doses. However, coverage of tetanus toxoid through routine services reaches only around 50% globally, and much of the vaccine is given to parous women.[16] Tetanus toxoid is also given to school-aged children, but can be given at the time the child starts school since the duration of immunity is known. Given the limited data on the duration of protection of the HPV vaccines, and absence of clinical trials in children aged < 9 years old, school entry would be too early for co-administration.

School-based Vaccination

Where enrolment rates are high, school-based vaccination may be extremely successful in eliminating disease.[36] Parents usually trust health-care recommendations made in a school setting, especially when they are endorsed by professionals involved in the setting, such as teachers.[37] In countries where education is mandatory and/or accessible to all children, laws mandating vaccination before enrolment may increase vaccination rates by as much as four-fold.[38] School-based vaccination may be cost-efficient because children are already gathered in one place and accounted for.[39]

However, in many countries, by the age of 9 years only a minority of girls are still in school.[40] Poor enrolment rates, limited school facilities in rural areas, migration and school fees are obstacles that prevent many girls from remaining in school until an age appropriate for HPV vaccination.[41] For countries with low school attendance among girls aged ≥ 9 years, the most practical delivery method may be through annual immunization campaigns. However, delivering HPV vaccines through such campaigns would require evaluation of a schedule with a longer interval between the second and third doses than has been administered in trials.

Sexual and Reproductive Health Services for Adolescents

Sexual and reproductive health services, and family planning services in particular, are almost exclusively accessed by women during or following a first pregnancy and access is motivated by a desire to space births rather than to delay early childbearing.[42] Young women aged 9–25, and especially unmarried women in that age range, have particular difficulty overcoming social and political barriers to gaining access to reproductive health services.[43,44] The time between early childhood and sexual debut defines one of the most difficult cohorts to reach for health care.

Adolescent health programmes are developing user-friendly services that aim to provide counselling on sexual health that focuses on the prevention of pregnancy and sexually transmitted infections including HIV. The presence of a new intervention, such as an HPV vaccine, could extend the scope of these services and help to integrate other interventions, thereby making them more attractive to young people.

Role of Sexual and Reproductive Health Services

Existing sexual and reproductive health programmes can have an important strategic role in integrating primary and secondary prevention services. As a sexually transmitted disease that causes cervical cancer, HPV has significant implications for reproductive health. Consequently, the context of vaccine delivery and the target populations may be different from the traditional EPI milieu. Young women who may have initiated sexual activity only recently, or who are seeking family planning after childbirth, represent target populations for catch-up for both primary and secondary prevention for the following reasons:

- a positive experience with vaccination among this group will be a natural entry point towards the eventual vaccination of adolescents or pre-adolescents, especially this group's children;
- sexual and reproductive health programmes provide a broad range of services within a comprehensive approach to sexual and general health;
- sexual and reproductive health initiatives that reach out to older adolescents should address cervical cancer prevention;
- this group is the target of other interventions addressing sexually transmitted infections and most of the voluntary counselling and testing programmes for HIV; and
- nursing staff caring for this group are oriented towards preventing cervical cancer and most are trained in counselling.

It may be possible to implement simplified screening and vaccination programmes as part of an integrated reproductive health strategy to reach girls and women if a coordinated effort is made by all stakeholders. This would require synchronization with and timely inputs from programmes with experience in vaccine delivery, in sexual and reproductive health and in cancer control.

Health Systems and Policies

Considerations for Introduction

The introduction of HPV vaccine into a national health-care system will raise questions for all countries. They will need to: use evidence to determine the age cohort to target, develop a service-delivery strategy, address the training needs of health professionals and other issues related to human-resource development, forecast the demand and supply of the vaccine, develop product-financing mechanisms and mechanisms for procurement and supply-chain management, and implement monitoring and evaluation programmes.

Evaluation of potential product financing and procurement mechanisms should be considered in the context of existing mechanisms used by organizations such as UNICEF, the GAVI Alliance, and the International Financing Facility for Immunization. The Global Immunization Vision and Strategy provides opportunities for engagement because it highlights the importance of introducing new vaccines, extending them to other age groups and linking vaccines with other interventions.[45] Because global financing mechanisms for an HPV vaccine will depend on the cost of the vaccines, financing and procurement-related issues must be considered as soon as possible.

The Role of Supply and Demand in Ensuring Equitable Access

Manufacturing limitations for HPV vaccines are unclear. Without 5-year estimates of purchasing demand, the industry is unlikely to invest in building manufacturing capacity or move towards cost structures that include lower profit margins. A business case for HPV vaccine production and procurement that is specific to developing countries must be developed. Demonstration projects that will both inform industry using demand forecasting and provide models for introduction that maximize acceptability and access based on country-specific assessments are being implemented (J. Sherris, personal communication, 2006).

During negotiations on pricing structures, ministers of finance and purchasing agencies must not lose sight of the costs of service delivery. Ancillary costs, such as transportation and human resources (providers, educators and so forth), must be accounted for. Estimating these ancillary costs for cost–effectiveness models has proven difficult because they are country-specific. Countries must consider their pre-existing screening services, already functional school-based and/or expanded EPI programmes, and the comparable costs of other priority health interventions.

▶ Conclusion

Cervical cancer is a unique public health challenge. It is gender specific, caused by a sexually transmitted virus, and primary and secondary prevention target opposite ends of a wide age spectrum. The natural history of cervical cancer has been studied in depth, and screening programmes that identify pre-cancerous lesions have been successful in significantly reducing incidence and mortality, albeit at a significant cost. Taken together, early vaccination of adolescents with screening and adequate evidence-based treatment could be components of a comprehensive strategy with the long-term goal of eliminating cervical cancer.

However, several knowledge gaps need to be bridged before HPV vaccine programmes can be introduced on a large scale, particularly in developing countries. Furthermore, even if the vaccines are introduced rapidly, screening and early treatment programmes will continue to be needed throughout the next several decades to prevent disease in women already infected or those who become infected with oncogenic HPV types not included in the vaccines.

There are critical issues of equity associated with introducing these new vaccines. International organizations, national governments and private foundations must address, at the highest level, how to minimize delays in accessing the vaccines in poor countries and to ensure access is equitable. Public spending on health is so low in those countries that have the greatest disease burden that external finance mechanisms to subsidize the purchase of vaccines will be necessary. These mechanisms may include advanced market commitments and long-term fund pledges through the International Financing Facility for Immunizations. Additional support from the GAVI Alliance to strengthen health systems should be garnered to facilitate introduction.[46]

We understand enough of the science and about the social issues to generate realistic prevention strategies. However, the challenge of delivering a vaccine that prevents both a sexually transmitted infection and cancer to an adolescent population will make it necessary to inform and educate not only adolescents but also their parents and the health-care providers who inform them. This must be seen as an opportunity, especially for the sexual and reproductive health community, given the need to educate adolescents early about risk-taking and general health. Health workers accustomed to wrestling with reproductive health concerns, both social and medical, are best prepared to be advocates for the HPV vaccine. Ultimately, each country will have to determine which parts of its health system have the capacity to implement effective and maximally efficient services.

Current adolescent vaccination programmes usually provide only single-dose boosters, for example, of tetanus toxoid and diphtheria-containing vaccines, and the three-dose HPV vaccination series represents a challenge; but it is also an opportunity to strengthen adolescent vaccination services. The HIV/AIDS community recognizes that introducing an HPV vaccine may provide a platform for the introduction of an AIDS vaccine in the future, given the probable need to vaccinate the same target population of adolescents. Introducing the HPV vaccine will also provide a test case for acceptability and a unique opportunity to reach out with important health messages to an often neglected demographic cohort.

The challenge for policy-makers and opinion-leaders is to acknowledge lessons learned from prior initiatives to introduce vaccines, and to ensure that this gender-specific disease has the necessary priority on the global public health agenda. High-level advocacy and a partnership among immunization, cancer-control and the reproductive health sectors must emerge to ensure that the right initiatives are implemented rapidly to prevent this disease that characterizes health inequity today.

▶ Acknowledgements

The members of the WHO/UNFPA working group on sexual and reproductive health and HPV vaccines are: Paul Blumenthal, Nathalie Broutet, Venkatraman Chandra-Mouli, Patricia Claeys,

Felicity Cutts, Catherine d'Arcangues, Lindsay Edouard, Peter Fajans, Peter Hall, Dale Huntington, Patrick Kadama, Arletty Pinel, Andreas Ullrich, Paul Van Look.

Funding: Funds were provided by the United Nations Population Fund under Project RHB5R241, Special Programme of Research, Development and Research Training in Human Reproduction.

Competing interests: none declared.

Résumé

Garantir l'accès aux vaccins HPV grâce à un système de services intégrés: point de vue de la santé génésique

En 2006, un vaccin quadrivalent contre le papillomavirus humain (HPV) a été homologué et un autre vaccin de ce type pourrait l'être aussi prochainement. On sait encore peu de choses sur les aspects pratiques qui devront être pris en compte dans la conception et la mise en œuvre des programmes de prévention du cancer de l'utérus intégrant la vaccination comme moyen de prévention primaire. Bien que ce vaccin puisse à terme être indiqué pour les individus des deux sexes, les jeunes filles, c'est-à-dire les filles et les femmes de 9 à 25 ans, seront les premières candidates pour la vaccination. Ce document présente les canaux de délivrance des vaccins HPV et les lacunes dans les connaissances critiques et devant être comblées pour que l'on dispose d'un support pour l'élaboration des futurs programmes de santé sexuelle et génésique. Il expose le rôle de soutien que la communauté des professionnels de la santé sexuelle et génésique, en collaboration avec les programmes de vaccination et de lutte anticancéreuse, pourrait avoir dans l'introduction des vaccins HPV dans le contexte des systèmes de santé actuels.

▶ References

1. Parikh S, Brennan P, Boffeta P. Meta-analysis of social inequality and the risk of cervical cancer. *Int J Cancer* 2003;105:687–91.

2. *Reproductive health strategy to accelerate progress towards the attainment of international development goals and targets.* Geneva: WHO; 2005.

3. Parkin DM, Bray F, Ferlay J, Pisani P. Global cancer statistics 2002. *CA Cancer J Clin* 2005;55:74–108.

4. *Projections of mortality and burden of disease to 2030,* 2005. Available from: http://www.who.int/healthinfo/statistics/bodprojections2030/en/index.html

5. Muñoz N, Bosch FX, Castellsague X, Diaz M, de Sanjose S, Hammouda D, et al. Against which human papillomavirus types shall we vaccinate and screen? *The international perspective. Int J Cancer* 2004;111:278–85.

6. Muñoz N, Mendez F, Posso H, Molano M, van den Brule AJ, Ronderos M, et al. Incidence, duration, and determinants of cervical human papillomavirus infection in a cohort of Colombian women with normal cytological results. *J Infect Dis* 2004;190:2077–87.

7. Goldie SJ, Gaffikin L, Goldhaber-Fiebert JD, Gordillo-Tobar A, Levin C, Mahe C, et al. Cost effectiveness of cervical cancer screening in five developing countries. *N Engl J Med* 2005;353:2158–68.

8. Denny L, Kuhn L, de Souza M, Pollack AE, Dupree W, Wright TC. Screen-and-treat approaches for cervical cancer prevention in low–resource settings. *JAMA* 2005;294:2173–81.

9. Denny L. The prevention of cervical cancer in developing countries. *BJOG* 2005;112:1204–12.

10. Goldie SJ, Kuhn L, Denny L, Pollack AE, Wright TC. Policy analysis of cervical cancer screening strategies in low-resource settings: clinical benefits and cost-effectiveness. *JAMA* 2001;285:3107–15.

11. US Food and Drug Administration. *Quadrivalent human papillomavirus (types 6, 11, 16, 18) recombinant vaccine,* 2006 (product approval information: licensing action). Available from: http://www.fda.gov/cber/products/hpvmer060806.htm

12. Villa LL, Costa RL, Petta CA, Andrade RP, Ault KA, Giuliano AR, et al. Prophylactic quadrivalent human papillomavirus (types 6, 11, 16, 18) L1 virus-like particle vaccine in young women: a randomized double-blind placebo-controlled multicentre phase II efficacy trial. *Lancet Oncol* 2005; 6:271–8.

13. Harper DM, Franco EL, Wheeler CM, Moscicki AB, Romanowski B, Roteli-Martins CM, et al. Sustained efficacy up to 4–5 years of a bivalent L1 virus-like particle vaccine against human papillomavirus types 16 and 18: follow-up from a randomised control trial. *Lancet* 2006;367:1247–55.

14. Goldie SJ, Grima D, Kohli M, Wright TC, Weinstein M, Franco E. A comprehensive natural history model of HPV infection and cervical cancer to estimate the clinical impact of a prophylactic HPV 16/18 vaccine. *Int J Cancer* 2003;106:896–904.

15. Lowndes CM, Gill ON. Cervical cancer, human papillomavirus and vaccination. *BMJ* 2005;331:915–6.

16. *Report of the Consultation on Human Papillomavirus Vaccines,* 2005. Available from: http://www.who.int/entity/vaccine_research/documents/816%20%20HPV%20meeting.pdf

17. WHO consultation on human papillomavirus vaccines. *Wkly Epidemiol Rec* 2005;35:299–302.

18. Smith JF, Brownlow MK, Brown MJ, Esser MT, Ruiz W, Brown DR. *Gardasil™ antibodies cross-neutralize pseudovirion infection of vaccine-related HPV types,* 2006. Available from: http://www.abstracts2view.com/ipv/ (abstract no. PL 1–6).

19. Mahoney RT, Maynard JE. The introduction of new vaccines into developing countries. *Vaccine* 1999;17:646–52.

20. Sherris J, Agurto I, Arrossi S, Dzuba I, Gaffikin L, Herdman C. Advocating for cervical cancer prevention. *Int J Gynecol Obstet* 2005;89 Suppl 2:S46–54.

21. Kahn JA, Zimet GD, Bernstein DI, Riedesel JM, Lan D, Huang B, et al. Pediatrician's intention to administer human papillomavirus vaccine: the role of practice characteristics, knowledge and attitudes. *J Adolesc Health* 2005;37:502–10.

22. Zimet GD. Understanding and overcoming barriers to human Papillomavirus vaccine acceptance. *Curr Opin Obstet Gynecol* 2006:18 Suppl 11: S23–8.

23. Agurto I, Arrossi S, White S, Coffey P, Dzuba I, Bingham A, et al. Involving the community in cervical cancer prevention programs. *Int J Gynecol Obstet* 2005;89 Suppl 2:S38–45.

24. Mao C, Koutsky LA, Ault KA, Wheeler CM, Brown DR, Wiley DJ, et al. Efficacy of human papillomavirus-16 vaccine to prevent cervical intraepithelial neoplasia: a randomized controlled trial. *Obstet Gynecol* 2006;107:18–27.

25. Villa LL, Ault KA, Giuliano AR, Costa RLR, Petta CA, Andrade RP, et al. Immunologic responses following administration of a vaccine targeting human papillomavirus types 6, 11, 16, and 18. *Vaccine* 2006;24:5571–83.

26. Henry J. Kaiser Family Health Foundation. *GSK HPV vaccine produces stronger immune response in girls ages 10–14 than in older women,* 2005. Available from: http://www.kaisernetwork .org/daily_reports/rep_index.cfm?hint=2&DR_ID=34384

27. Soares C. Polio postponed: politics slow polio's eradication—and cause it to spread. *Sci Am* 2005;292:8–9.

28. Paavonen J, Halttunen M, Hansson BG, Nieminen P, Rostila T, Lehtinen M. Prerequisites for human papillomavirus vaccine trial: results of feasibility studies. *J Clin Virol* 2000;19:25–30.

29. Gudmundsdottir T, Tryggvadottir L, Allende M, Mast TC, Briem H, Sigurdsson K. Eligibility and willingness of young Icelandic women to participate in a HPV vaccination trial. *Acta Obstet Gynecol Scand* 2003;82:345–50.

30. Partridge JM, Koutsky LA. Genital human papillomavirus infection in men. *Lancet Infect Dis* 2006;6:21–31.

31. Barnabas RV, Laukkanen P, Koskela P, Kontula O, Lehtinen M, Garnett GP. Epidemiology of HPV 16 and cervical cancer in Finland and the potential impact of vaccination: mathematical modelling analyses. *PLoS Med* 2006; 3:e138.

32. Villa LL. Prophylactic HPV vaccines: reducing the burden of HPV-related diseases. *Vaccine* 2006;24 Suppl 1:S23–8.

33. Chin-Hong PV, Vittinghoff E, Cranston RD, Browne L, Buchbinder S, Colfax G, et al. Age-related prevalence of anal cancer precursors in homosexual men: the EXPLORE study. *J Natl Cancer Inst* 2005;97:896–905.

34. Daling JR, Madeleine MM, Johnson LG, Schwartz SM, Shera KA, Wurscher MA, et al. Human papillomavirus, smoking, and sexual practices in the etiology of anal cancer. *Cancer* 2004;101:270–80.

35. Bradley J, Barone M, Mahe C, Lewis R, Luciani S. Delivering cervical cancer prevention services in low-resource settings. *Int J Gynecol Obstet* 2005;89: S21–9.

36. Khalil MK, Al-Mazrou YY, AlHowasi MN, Al-Jeffri M. Measles in Saudi Arabia: from control to elimination. *Ann Saudi Med* 2005;25:324–8.

37. Tung CS, Middleman AB. An evaluation of school-level factors used in a successful school-based hepatitis B immunization initiative. *J Adolesc Health* 2005;37:61–8.

38. Wilson TR, Fishbein DB, Ellis PA, Edlavitch SA. The impact of a school entry law on adolescent immunization rates. *J Adolesc Health* 2005;37:511–6.

39. Wallace LA, Young D, Brown A, Cameron JC, Ahmed S, Duff R, et al. Costs of running a universal adolescent hepatitis B vaccination programme. *Vaccine* 2005;23:5624–31.

40. United Nations Educational, Scientific and Cultural Organization (UNESCO). *Primary education: girls,* 2006. Available from: http://portal.unesco.org/education/en/ev.php-URL_ID= 30870&URL_DO=DO_TOPIC&URL_SECTION=201.html

41. Yameogo KR, Perry RT, Yameogo A, Kambire C, Konde MK, Nshimiriman D, et al. Migration as a risk factor for measles after a mass vaccination campaign, Burkina Faso, 2002. *Int J Epidemiol* 2005;34:556–64.

42. United Nations Population Fund (UNFPA). *The world reaffirms Cairo: official outcomes of the ICPD at ten review,* 2006. Available from: http://www.unfpa.org/publications/detail.cfm?ID=226

43. International Conference on Population and Development (ICPD). *Summary of the ICPD programme of action. Chapter IV: gender equality, equity and empowerment of women,* 1995. Available from: http://www.unfpa.org/icpd/summary.htm#chapter4

44. Mathur S, Mehta M, Malhotra A. *Youth reproductive health in Nepal: is participation the answer?* 2004. Available from: http://www.engenderhealth.org/ia/foc/pdf/yrh-nepal.pdf

45. Bilous J, Eggers R, Gasse F, Jarrett S, Lydon P, Magan A, et al. A new global immunization vision and strategy. *Lancet* 2006;367:1464–6.

46. Churchwell C. *Funding R&D for neglected diseases,* 2005. Available from: http://hbswk.hbs.edu/item.jhtml?id=4665&t=globalization

Syndemics, Sex and the City: Understanding Sexually Transmitted Diseases in Social and Cultural Context

Merrill C. Singer[a],*, Pamela I. Erickson[b], Louise Badiane[b], Rosemary Diaz[b], Dugeidy Ortiz[b], Traci Abraham[b], Anna Marie Nicolaysen[b,c]

[a]Hispanic Health Center, 175 Main Street, Hartford, CT 06106, USA
[b]University of Connecticut, CT, USA
[c]Hispanic Health Council, Hartford, CT, USA

Available online 16 June 2006

Abstract

This paper employs syndemics theory to explain high rates of sexually transmitted disease among inner city African American and Puerto Rican heterosexual young adults in Hartford, CT, USA. Syndemic theory helps to elucidate the tendency for multiple co-terminus and interacting epidemics to develop under conditions of health and social disparity. Based on enhanced focus group and in-depth interview data, the paper argues that respondents employed a cultural logic of risk assessment which put them at high risk for STD infection. This cultural logic was shaped by their experiences of growing up in the inner city which included: coming of age in an impoverished family, living in a broken home, experiencing domestic violence, limited expectations of the future, limited exposure to positive role models, lack of expectation of the dependency of others, and fear of intimacy.
© 2006 Elsevier Ltd. All rights reserved.

Keywords: Syndemics; Sexually transmitted diseases; Young adults; African American; Puerto Rican; Political economy

*Corresponding author. Tel.: +1860 527 0856; fax: +1860 724 0437.
E-mail addresses: anthro8566@aol.com (M. C. Singer), pamela.erickson@uconn.edu (P. I. Erickson).

► Introduction

This paper reports the findings of a multi-method qualitative study of sexual ideas, attitudes, and behaviors among African American and Puerto Rican young adults (18–25 years of age) in Harford, CT, USA. These findings are of note because of the ongoing intertwined epidemics in Hartford (and elsewhere) of two sexually transmitted diseases (STDs) in the study's target age and ethnic groups as well as a third disease, AIDS, for which sexual contact is a primary route of transmission. Findings from this Centers for Disease Control (CDC) funded study, entitled Project PHRESH.comm (Philadelphia and Hartford Research Effort on Sexual Health and Communication), suggest key cultural and contextual factors underlying the spread of these STDs in the city. The analysis presented is framed by syndemic theory (Freudenberg, Fahs, Galea, & Greenberg, 2006; Singer, 1996; Singer & Clair, 2003), which seeks to elucidate the tendency for multiple, co-terminus and interacting epidemics to develop under conditions of health and social disparity. As Easton (2004, p. 211) notes, "The concept of syndemics is useful for understanding how sociocultural, historical, and geographical, realities in urban areas interact with and compound the adverse consequences of disease."

► Syndemics Theory

The traditional biomedical approach to disease is characterized by an effort to treat diseases as if they were distinct entities in nature, separate from other diseases, and independent of the social contexts in which they are found. This approach proved useful historically in focusing medical attention on the immediate causes and expressions of disease and contributed to the emergence of modern biomedical treatments, some of which have been enormously successful. However, as the compendium of knowledge has advanced, it has become increasingly clear that diseases do not necessarily exist in isolation from other diseases and conditions, that disease interactions are of considerable importance to disease course and consequence, and that the social conditions of disease sufferers are critical to understanding health impacts at the individual and population levels. Rather than existing as discrete conditions, multiple life-threatening diseases often are concentrated in particular populations.

Beyond disease clustering, there is growing evidence of important interactions among comorbid diseases (Wasserheit, 1992). One such interaction has been found, for example, between type 2 diabetes mellitus and various infections, such as hepatitis C viral infection in women (O'Connor, West, Lorntz, Vinicor, & Jorgensen, 2004). The worldwide prevalence of type 2 diabetes has been increasing and now impacts the lives of millions of women around the globe. Various factors are recognized as contributing to the onset of type 2 diabetes, including obesity and aging. The role of infection, however, is only beginning to be recognized. Already it is clear that risk for serious infections of various kinds increases significantly with poor diabetes control, but appreciation of more complex relationships between infection and type 2 diabetes is now emerging as well (Soule et al., 2005; Visnegarwala, Chen, Raghavan, & Tedaldi, 2005). The NHANES III study found that type 2 diabetes increases among people who have been infected with the hepatitis C virus. (O'Connor et al., 2004). Similarly, several health reports note that diabetes is present in as many as 37% of those who are critically ill with severe acute respiratory syndrome (SARS) (Booth et al., 2003; Fowler et al., 2003). These examples suggest the importance of dynamic diabetes-infection linkages. It is disease interactions of this sort that are a central element in syndemics. Syndemic theory seeks to draw attention to and provide a framework for the analysis of these interactions.

Various syndemics (although not always labeled as such) have been described in the literature already, including the SAVA syndemic (substance abuse, violence and AIDS) (Singer, 1996), the hookworm, malaria and HIV/AIDS syndemic (Hotez, 2003), the Chagas disease, rheumatic heart disease and congestive heart failure syndemic (Cubillos-Garzon, Casas, Morillo, & Bautista, 2004), the asthma and infectious disease syndemic (Johnson & Martin, 2005), the malnutrition and depression syndemic (Heflin, Siefert, & Williams, 2005), and the mental health and HIV/AIDS syndemic (Stall et al., 2003). Additionally, several syndemics have been identified that involve STDs (Chesson, Heffelfinger, Voigt, & Collins, 2005; Craib, Meddings, & Strathdee, 1995; Otten, Zaidi, Peterman, Rolfs, & Witte, 1994). Here too, researchers report interactions between comorbid STDs and other diseases (Nusbaum, Wallace, Slatt, & Kondrad, 2004).

Beyond disease clustering and interaction, the term syndemic also points to the importance of social conditions in disease concentrations, interactions and consequences. In syndemics, the interaction of diseases or other health problems (e.g., malnutrition) commonly arises because of adverse social conditions (e.g., poverty, stigmatization, oppressive social relationships) that put socially devalued groups at heightened risk. As Farmer (1999) argues with reference to TB, it is impossible to understand its persistence in poor countries as well as its recent resurgence among the poor in industrialized countries without assessing how social forces, such as political violence and racism, come to be embodied and expressed as individual pathology.

An examination of STDs in Connecticut generally, and Hartford specifically, presented below, suggests the existence of an STD syndemic (STDS) involving several co-morbid diseases rooted in the social conditions of poverty and racial discrimination.

▶ STDs in Connecticut

In Connecticut, physicians are required to report new cases of five STDs: syphilis, gonorrhea, chlamydia, chancroid, and neonatal herpes. In recent years, there have been no new cases of either chancroid or neonatal herpes reported, and few new cases of syphilis had been reported until recently (Farley, Hadler, & Gunn, 1990; Connecticut Department of Public Health, 2000, 2004). By contrast gonorrhea and chlamydia already have become significant epidemics in the state's population.

In 2003, there were approximately 3000 cases of gonorrhea reported in Connecticut; 61.5% of these cases were among women, 40.5% were among African Americans, and 55% were among youth and young adults 15–24 years of age. (Connecticut Department of Public Health, 2004). Of these cases statewide, 47% were in Hartford. In fact, it is believed that gonorrhea is much more common than these statistics would suggest. It is estimated that at least half of all cases go unreported. Risk factors for gonorrhea infection include having vaginal, oral or anal sex with multiple sex partners, having a sex partner with a past history of any STD, and having sex without the use of a condom.

Currently, chlamydia is the most commonly diagnosed STD in Connecticut. Each year since 1999 there have been 5000–7000 new cases reported in the state, primarily among women

(Connecticut Department of Public Health, 2004). About 16% of chlamydia cases diagnosed in the state are from Hartford.

In addition to these two epidemics, AIDS continues to be a significant epidemic in Hartford. Disproportionately, AIDS cases have been concentrated in ethnic minority populations in the city. By 1999, African Americans and Latinos comprised 42% and 44% of AIDS cases, respectively in Hartford, while accounting for 36% and 41%, respectively of the city's total population. Of the three principal routes of HIV transmission—injection drug use, men having sex with men, and heterosexual sex—injection drug use has consistently been the most prevalent reported route of infection among Hartford's AIDS cases (Connecticut Department of Public Health, 2000). The distribution of AIDS cases, however, is not tightly predicted by injection drug use, suggesting the importance of other factors such as sexual transmission even among injection drug users (IDUs).

Notably, as the percentage of AIDS cases among IDUs in the city declined in the last few years of the 20th century, the percentage attributed to heterosexual transmission rose from fewer than 10% of cases during the late 1980s and early 1990s to 16% of new cases through 1999. At the same time, the percentage of new cases among females increased from 18% to 30% between 1990 and 1999, and women were reported with AIDS at a younger age than men (e.g., 20.8% vs. 12.6% in the 13–29-yearold age group) (Hartford Community Health Partnership, 2003). These data indicate the growing importance of sexual transmission of HIV in Hartford, especially among ethnic minority populations. Co-infection with another STD—which increases the ability of HIV to be transmitted during sexual contact—and having multiple sexual partners have been suggested as key factors in accounting for higher rates of HIV among ethnic minorities in the city (Singer, Jia, Schensul, Weeks, & Page, 1992). This interpretation is supported by a review of findings from PHRESH.comm.

▶ Methods

The data we use in this paper come from the Hartford, CT component of the larger study using the first two of seven research methods from a 5-year qualitative and quantitative study of communication and negotiation about barrier contraceptive use for STD and pregnancy prevention among low income, inner city African American and Puerto Rican self-identified heterosexual young adults (age 18–25) in Hartford and Philadelphia. The major goal of this project is to understand strategies and patterns of communication and negotiation surrounding condom and other barrier contraceptive use in these sexually active at-risk populations. The study weaves together a variety of qualitative and quantitative methods, including focus group discussions, systematic cultural assessment techniques (Bernard, 2001), in-depth individual sexual and romantic life history interviews, sexual behavior diaries, scenario drama discussions, and structured interviews staged over 4 years of data collection (2004–2008). The aim of this design is to collect a variety of data that will be triangulated to yield a detailed and contextualized understanding of sexual and romantic relationships in light of social and cultural factors, and to use these data to inform the development of targeted risk-reduction strategies.

Participants for all methods are recruited through street outreach at two kinds of venues: general street settings and specialized activity sites. The first of these includes places with heavy pedestrian traffic in areas identified through prior research. The latter refers to the local community college, adult education centers, youth and young adult programs, and park and recreation sites. To recruit participants, project outreach workers approach individuals who appear to meet inclusion criteria and engage them in conversation about the goals of the project, screen for inclusion criteria, and invite participation.

In this paper, we use data from the first two methods: focus group discussions (FGDs) and in-depth, individual sexual and romantic life histories (SRIs). These two methods elicited data on the socio-cultural context of relationships, the local terms used by participants in discussing sexual and romantic relationships and sexual behavior (FGDs), and the natural history of sexual and romantic relationships (SRIs). Participants in the FGDs were allowed to participate in the SRIs, as the former method collected group-level and the latter collected individual-level data. Eight percent of SRI participants were also FGD participants. While we will report some difference across gender, for the issues of concern to this analysis ethnicity did not appear to be a significant factor.

The FGDs included free listing and ranking of salient terms and a guided discussion surrounding six domains of interest: (1) types of sexual and romantic relationships; (2) types of sexual behavior and understandings/thoughts/ideas about monogamy and abstinence; (3) understanding of birth control methods, condoms, and safer sex; (4) factors considered when contemplating initiation of a new sexual relationship; (5) the physical and emotional risks of involvement in heterosexual relationships; and (6) the socio-cultural and economic factors that affect sexual and reproductive behavior. In Hartford, eight FGDs were convened with African American and Puerto Rican males and females (i.e., two groups within each ethnic/gender group of interest). A total of 61 people participated in the eight, 5–6 hour FGDs. Unusually long FGDs were used as a means of gathering rich data that would assist in the development of subsequent methods such as the SRIs. Participants received $60 for their time.[1]

The SRIs were open-ended interviews with 60 individuals at each site (i.e., 15 each African America and Puerto Rican males and females). Interviewers used a written guide to elicit a detailed history of each respondent's self-determined most important romantic and sexual relationships. The goal was not to obtain data about contraceptive use/risk reduction strategies in the past, but rather to understand the range of sexual and romantic relationships that are meaningful to inner city young adults and the patterning of entry into and exiting relationships over time as well as a general sense of risk prevention behaviors. The SRI interviews lasted about 2 hours and participants were paid $30.

In many ways, the in-depth, personal SRI interviews provided a counterpoint to the FGDs in that they elicited information about relationships (from purely sexual to committed) and their personal, emotional meaning to the participant. While the FGDs provided a "universe" of relationship types and sexual behaviors in which participants engage, as well as what they think about and how they decide about potential relationships, the SRIs provided knowledge of what is important with respect to feelings and emotional attachment in relationships at the individual level. Together, these methods provide an emic or insider view of sexual and romantic relationships.

Each participant also completed a form that collected basic demographic information. Table 8.1 provides the sociodemographic characteristics of the study participants for the focus groups and sexual and romantic history interviews in Hartford.

The research protocol for all methods in the study was approved by the Institutional Review Boards (IRB) at the CDC, the University of Connecticut, the Hispanic Health Council in Hartford, and the Family Planning Council of Philadelphia. Written informed consent was obtained from each participant.

TABLE 8.1   Sociodemographic characteristics of participants

(FGD)	Focus Group Discussions Interviews (SRI)	Sexual and Romantic History
Number of participants	65	60
Mean age (years)	20.4	21.2
Less than High School Education (%)	40	38
Employed in last 6 months (%)	63	59
Employed currently (%)	34	38
Never married (%)	93	91
Have children (%)	41	48
Lives with parents (%)	47	40

Participants in the two samples were quite similar across all of the characteristics reported in Table 8.1. The mean age of participants was just slightly over 20 years. While a majority of the individuals in both groups had graduated from high school, a sizeable percent in each group (40%) had dropped out of high school or earlier. While very few of the participants in either group had ever been married, over 40% of both groups had children. Large percentages of both groups continued to live with parents. The majority of participants in both groups had been employed at least some of the time during the last 6 months; however, only a minority was employed at the time of their interview.

▶ Findings on STD Risk in Hartford

Sexual and Romantic Relationships

From the total 16 FGDs at the Hartford and Philadelphia sites, we elicited 146 terms for different kinds of sexual and romantic relationships in the free list exercise. Findings indicate a wide range of relationship types from purely casual one-night stands to emotionally committed live-in arrangements, but with a particularly large number of relationships at the casual end of the spectrum.

From these free list data from the two sites, we selected the 30 relationships that were mentioned in three or more FGDs on the assumption that frequency of mention was an indication of saliency (see Table 8.2).[2] These terms were used for a free pile sort in which the 60 SRI participants sorted relationship types into meaningful groups of their own construction. Cluster analysis (using Anthropac 4.98, Borgatti, 1996) documented two distinct groupings—relationships that were primarily sexual and those that were primarily romantic and emotionally meaningful, which we hereafter call sexual and serious relationships following terminology used by the participants (see Table 8.2). Forcing more categories in the cluster analyses (using Anthropac's hierarchical tabu search forcing 15 clusters) revealed three clusters (two with definite sub-clusters) that suggested a more nuanced understanding of kinds of relationships in which participants engage, their potential for developing into something more lasting, and the stages in relationship development.

TABLE 8.2 Four main groups and subtypes of sexual and romantic relationships

**Relationships That Are Not Committed
or Expected to Be Monogamous**

Booty calls	Someone to call when you have sexual needs
Chicken-head	Someone who gives oral sex without commitment
Creep shots/Creepin'/Creeps	A purely sexual relationship one is embarrassed to admit
Friend/friendship	Someone you are checking out
Head doctor/Head game/Head nurse	Someone who prefers oral sex to intercourse,
Hit & run/hittin' & skippin' it/hit it & split it	A purely sexual, brief relationship
One night stand	A single event sexual relationship
Shag/Shag Partner/Shaggin	Someone you have sex with periodically
Shorty	A girlfriend, but may be less than serious
Thang thang'Thing on the side/Little thing	A relationship on the side, not main partner

Sexual and Monetary/Commodity Exchange

Ho/Whore	A prostitute
Jump/Jump off	Someone willing to have sex with little wooing
Sugar daddy	A man who gives presents or money

Romantic But Not Committed

Dating	Someone you are seeing
Boyfriend	A guy you are romantically involved with
Boo/Boo-butt	A boyfriend
Girlfriend	A girl you are romantically involved with
Freaky/Freaky ones	Someone who will do anything sexual

Committed/Expected to Be Monogamous

Committed	A monogamous relationship
Monogamous	A monogamous relationship
Husband	Legally married
Marriage	A convention legal marriage
Hubby	Common-law, can imply the burdens of monogamy
My man	The man a woman is most involved with
Parent of your child	Someone who remains in your heart because you have a child together
Baby mama/Baby's mother	Mother of your child, can imply an intrusive, enduring, and interfering but still someone with whom you share something important
Baby daddy/Baby's father	Father of your child (same as above)

This interpretation was further supported by multi-dimensional scaling (Anthropac's MDS) of the pile sort data that suggested three groups of relationships. We identified the domains underlying these groupings from the labels participants assigned to their sorted piles. The first group, *sexual relationships,* included the two subgroups *casual sexual relationships just for sex* (e.g., "purely sexual", "these are just fucking and you leave", "sex friends") or as *exchange for resources* ("person that helps you out, gives you things financially," "friends who provide money and stuff"). Half (15) of the relationship types were purely sexual (e.g., "booty call," "thang thang") and three implied an exchange of sex for access to resources (i.e., "jump," "ho," "sugar daddy"). These purely sexual relationships can be short-term, never proceeding to a romantic stage by definition (e.g., "ho," "one night stand"). Alternately, they can be longer term but still purely sexual relationships (e.g., "friends with benefits", "shorty") in which the partners can be quite attached to each other as friends; these usually do not develop into romantic relationships. Purely sexual relationships may involve types of sexual behavior (e.g., oral sex, kinky sex) that are different from those in more romantic or committed relationships.

Although serious relationships might involve some of these more specialized sexual behaviors, they are not likely to be defined by them or limited to them. Indeed, seeking a certain type of sexual gratification may play a significant role in the persistence of secondary sexual relationships during a serious relationship.

In the kinds of relationships in which sex is exchanged for resources like money or material items such as clothes, shoes, cell phones, or car tires, this is not considered commercial sex work by participants, but rather as a more general form of economic support or exchange of services.

> *Participant 1:* A jump takes care of you.
> *Facilitator:* You mean just sexually?
> *Participant 2:* Monetary! Financial wise.
> *Participant 1:* I need my tires fixed; can I get some tires? And if he say no, he got to go!
> *Participant 3:* You got to make it clear. You's not my man, you just my side partner. (African American Females, FGD)

Separate from the sexual relationships are those serious relationships in which people can "catch feelings" for each other, the participants' way of talking about becoming emotionally and romantically involved with another. The second grouping in the MDS analysis involved this stage ("girlfriends and boyfriends that are dating," "getting to know person/talk about feelings"). Six of the relationships fell into this group and were considered romantic but not yet completely committed (e.g., dating, boyfriend/girlfriend). Getting to know a person in whom one is interested sexually and romantically is called "talking." "Feeling the person" (understand/empathize with/care about) means that the couple is transitioning to a socially recognized couple or boyfriend/girlfriend stage.

The final stage is a serious, usually long-term relationship in which catching feelings (i.e., romantic love, attachment, and commitment) and longevity are the main themes. This is the third MDS grouping comprised of *serious relationships with a current partner* ("you're going to be together for a long time," "you are with this person and no one else," "love") or *with your baby's father/mother* ("they are people you have to deal with all your life because you have a child together"). Seven of the relationship types were serious relationships that were ideally monogamous (e.g., "hubby/wifey") and two indicated the parent of your child (i.e., "baby mama/baby daddy")—forty-one percent of FGD and 47% of SRI participants already had children although most (over 90%) had never been married. The often-used phrase "baby mama/daddy drama" suggests the intrusive nature and kind of influence that baby mamas/daddies can have on subsequent serious relationships to the point that how many baby mamas/daddies a person has becomes a factor in deliberations about whether to become involved in a relationship with them.

In the FGDs, participants talked freely about the normalcy of multiple relationships among people in their age group, even among those in supposedly serious relationships. Several of the sexual relationship terms refer explicitly to a partner on the side of a more serious relationship (e.g., "creep shots," "thing on the side") although any of them can be side partners. These participants summarize the ubiquity of the norm of multiple relationships:

Participant 1: That's the point. You never know. What, you never sit around and then think: "He's cheating on me?" In all, he really is. 'Cause you really don't care, because you got to not care 'cause he'll do it anyway. You can't be like that's my man and I'm the only one, not in 2004 you're not. Trust! Everybody got somebody extra.

Participant 2: Even if you say that you the wifey, like how we say we got a hubby, we still got our man on the side. Just like you the wifey, he still got the other girl on the side. You ain't goin' to never know.

Participant 3: Somebody always got some better coochie than the next person, so it's going to happen. That's life. I'm telling you. I don't believe in that faithful committed junk. That junk don't live here. (African American Females, FGD)

Since multiple partners are the rule, it is not very surprising that participants indicated a fundamental lack of trust between current partners and those entering new relationships. In fact, catching feelings is considered dangerous and there is a sense that emotional involvement is risky.

So all that just boils down to the whole big word, fear. That's what it is, fear of being in a relationship. (African American Male, FGD)

In sum, in the FGDs, we found a generalized fear of commitment and a sense of certainty about sexual infidelity even in committed relationships that may be fueled to some extent by the fact that some sexual relationships, especially secondary relationships, are driven by the need for access to resources. Although the terms differ, there are parallels to findings of Lichtenstein and Schwebke (in press) from a study of STDS and sexuality among African American men.

Data from the SRIs support the key findings from the FGDs. Both male and female participants indicated that catching feelings and entering into a serious relationship were risky. The SRI data document the natural history of young people's serious relationships, which numbered between one and six, and their non-serious, but nevertheless memorable, relationships which numbered between one and 15. Life history data document the ubiquity of multiple relationships even during serious relationships, which are supposed to be sexually exclusive. In fact, less than 5% of participants had ever been in a serious relationship in which neither they nor their partner had side partners. The majority (72%), both males (69%) and females (76%), had a secondary partner during one or more of their serious relationships, or had a serious partner who they thought had cheated on them (males 79%, females 86%). In addition, many said that they were already talking to someone else before ending a serious relationship, serving as a catalyst for ending a current relationship when the partner finds out or as a motivating factor to move on once the current relationship grows stale or becomes otherwise unappealing (e.g., controlling behavior by the partner, violence, interference from the baby mama/daddy)—in either case, hedging bets against being alone.

Participant: Um, when I was with Carlos, me and Carlos broke up when we were up here, so we broke up for like a couple of weeks or whatever, because, you know he just keeps, he kept playing me [seeing other women] . . . we always would break up and get back together and stuff like that and while we were broken up I was messing with Jamal. (Puerto Rican Female, SRI)

Condom Use in Relationships

The participants in FGDs and SRIs indicated a high awareness of the need for STI/HIV prevention through condom use with casual sexual partners.

You know what Russian roulette is? That's having unprotected sex with somebody. You are having sex with every hundreds of thousands of people that they have been with, if you are unprotected. (African American Female, FGD)

Agreement was virtually unanimous that it was the norm to use condoms with a casual sexual partner for both men and women.

Participant 1: If you don't want no STDs you go and use a condom.
Participant 2: Or else you go to a clinic and get checked up at the same time, you and your broad. Like, if you wanna have kids. (African American Male, FGD)

Actual use, however, was subject to the immediate context of the event, the longevity of the relationship, and the level of feeling and commitment attached to it. In casual relationships where condoms are most socially acceptable and likely to be used, situational factors like the lack of availability of a condom in the heat of the moment or impairment by drugs or alcohol can lead to an unprotected sexual encounter.

Participant 1: Sometimes, you get in a sexual act, and sometimes you protect yourself and sometimes you don't. Some people just get caught up in the moment. Like, Raul is conscientious about the way he goes about doing things, but some people get caught up in the heat of the moment. (Puerto Rican Male, FGD)

Participants made it clear that condom use was likely to be only a temporary strategy because men prefer to "hit it raw" (i.e., have skin-to-skin contact while having sex):

When you do it like raw, you feeling the best way. That the best shit in the world. But when you got condoms it's like nothing, it's nothing . . . raw is better. It's natural. (Puerto Rican Male, FGD)

When feelings are involved and relationships become more serious, condoms are quickly abandoned both because people like raw sex and because condoms signify a lack of trust.

Participant 1: Yeah, like when at first I'm going with her, I use a condom. But now after that, I just turn that shit off like, man, fuck it.
Facilitator: So then, why do you take off the condom?
Participant 1: Because that's the female I'm gonna be fucking for a while.
Participant 2: Cause you feel safe with her . . . feel comfortable with her.
(African American Males, FGD)

Women indicate that sometimes fear of losing a partner makes them reluctant to ask for condom use.

Participant 1: 'Cause you so wrapped up into what this guy is telling you, you not actually thinking about yourself. Damn, he love me, he want to be with me. Damn, what if I tell him to put a condom on? Will he leave me? You got some people that think like that and they don't realize the consequences 'til it's done. (Puerto Rican Females, FGD)

The last participant is telling the group that her relationship has become more serious, and she no longer expects to use condoms precisely because they indicate a lack of trust. It is also important to note that relationships develop quickly and condom abandonment often takes place within quite a short period of time, usually one or two months.

The Cultural Logic of Sexual Decision-Making, Risk Assessment, and Condom Use

Analysis of FGD data suggests that participants employ a cultural logic system borne of their life experiences. Elements of this logic system were elicited using a free list exercise in which the participants told us all the things young people consider before having sex with someone new. Their responses are summarized below and include the following considerations:

(1) Your knowledge about the Other, especially: (a) are they a "psycho"; (b) do they have sex with many others; (c) have you had sex with them before; (d) do they fit the folk category of "clean" (hygienic and disease-free);
(2) Your knowledge of the Other's family (do they come from good people, respectable people);
(3) Information provided to you by friends or family about the Other;
(4) The Other's "street rep" (based on continuum from "clean" to "scallywag/ho");
(5) The current status of your relationship with the Other (brand new or a month old or more);
(6) The kind of relationship you have or want to have with the Other (e.g., "a jump" vs. a "wifey");
(7) Situational factors at the moment of potential sexual interaction (e.g., availability of a condom);
(8) Visible or olfactory indications of health vs. disease/dirty;
(9) How attractive you find the Other person physically and sexually; and
(10) The Other's assets (e.g., car, own apartment, job, etc.) and liabilities (e.g., how many baby mamas/daddies, criminal background, abusive, use/sell drugs).

In sum, the kinds of things that young adults in our sample consider tend to center around their assessment of how attractive their prospective partner is and how sexually pleasing the relationship will be, how stable he/she is emotionally and financially, whether or not he/she already has children, and finally, how "safe" the potential partner is with respect to STDs/HIV. The kinds of information used to assess this last factor include the person's street reputation—whether a man is a "player," or a "scallywag" (i.e., has had a lot of sexual partners without attention to prevention) and whether a woman is a "ho" or a "chicken head" (i.e., has sex for material gain or just because she likes to give head [oral sex]). Stated a female participant:

Smooth talker. Umm . . . he was my sweet. He was like a ladies' man, like basically . . . I think the reason that I went out with him is because like I hear these girls talking about him so I'm like . . . you know, curious [laughs]. So I'm like: "There must be something that's going on." (African American Female, SRI)

Also of importance is his/her appearance and hygiene—if they smell bad, have dirty clothes, are missing teeth, look "dusty" (poorly dressed and unhygienic), or if the woman has a foul vaginal odor (determined by what is referred to as "the finger test"):

Participant 1: I used to do something, like I'm not trying to be perverted or nothing. I used to, like, when I would finger her. . . .
Participant 2: . . .and then you go [sniffs finger], well, if you smell [it], then you know. If you smell it from here, good-bye.
(Puerto Rican Males, FGD)

In deciding about a new partner, men tended to emphasize the importance of physical appearance and the potential for sexual satisfaction more than women, who also mentioned these factors but tended to put more emphasis on assets and liabilities and the potential for a longer term relationship. Further, males were found to be less likely to think about risk in relationships than were females, and often had to be prompted by FGD facilitators to give examples of the kinds of risks that are encountered in relationships. Females, by contrast, were much more likely to have a ready list of risk factors that they associated with romantic and sexual relationships. Both males and females, however, mentioned the same basic domains of risk: reproductive issues, violence, interaction with ex-partners (especially baby mama/daddy), drama (i.e., intense interpersonal interchanges—anger, shouting, mind games, etc.), fear of falling in love and losing control, and emotional vulnerability, pain, and heartbreak. Men, however, particularly emphasized vulnerability, losing control, getting hurt (e.g., falling in love, betrayal, heartbreak, loneliness, anger), having to deal with partners who were "psycho" or intrusive (including ex-partners and/or baby daddies of a new partner), and physical risk of STDs, violence, and incarceration.

For women, risks included physical and emotional abuse, rape, pregnancy, STDs, dealing with ex-girlfriends and baby mamas, and a litany of emotional risks—heartbreak, betrayal, dependence, depression, anger, jealousy, loneliness, fear, stress, and loss of control. In general, women began their lists with physical vulnerability and men with emotional vulnerability. Men thought less about risk in relationships, but women were keenly attuned to risk, perhaps because of their greater perceived physical vulnerability to pregnancy, physical and sexual abuse, and the greater importance attached to their good reputations than for men. Those labeled "Hos," they know, are not girlfriend material.

Even with this greater vulnerability, women tended to value having a relationship more than they valued being risk-free; hence even if they wanted a man to use a condom, they might not risk upsetting him by asking him to use one. Moreover, even if condoms were used at the beginning of a relationship, their use was often curtailed before very long because increasing familiarity tends to breed trust in the Other and confidence in his/her safety. Within a month or two, condom use was often abandoned because the Other was now familiar and appeared to be clean. The fact that one had not already gotten sick (i.e., exhibited symptoms) was taken as proof that the Other was safe.

An important aspect of this cultural model of risk assessment is that both women and men tend to think in terms of "who is safe" rather than "which behaviors are risky." In other words, riskiness is an attribute of particular people, not of particular actions in which anyone might engage. Participants tend not to be aware of asymptomatic disease; hence, if they feel fine, they believe they are fine or if someone looks "clean" they are clean. Similarly, someone from a good family is likely to be "safe." If someone were deemed on the basis of appearance or family background to be safe then there was no need to use a condom to avoid disease as no disease would be present. Even if someone were not deemed to be completely safe, condom availability still strongly influenced whether or not condoms were used in all kinds of relationships. Thus, lack of condom availability tends not to be a strong barrier to having sex.

One consequence of the cultural logic model employed by the participants in our study is that it puts them at high risk for STD infection. Notably, 22% SRI participants and 11% of FGD participants reported that they had ever been told by a doctor or nurse that they had an STD. Females were much more likely to report having had an STD (35% of SRI and 15% of FGD female participants) than male participants (5% of SRI and 13% of FGD male participants). These high rates of infection are noteworthy. Rates of STD infection in equivalent age general samples reported by the CDC (1999) include 5% diagnosed with chlamydia among 20–24-year-old female family planning clinic patients in Connecticut and 3% and 8% diagnosed with gonorrhea and chlamydia respectively among 16–24-year-old women entering the U.S. Job Corp in Massachusetts.

Socio-Political Context of Inner City Families

The patterns of sexual behavior and condom use within relationships among inner city youth in Hartford, and the cultural logic that informs these behaviors, did not emerge in a vacuum; rather they have been shaped by their experiences growing up in the inner city (or relocating there after growing up in another, but often socio-economically similar, locale). In the focus groups and one-on-one interviews, participants cited a number of key features of their psychosocial life experiences that have shaped their views, attitudes, understandings, and behaviors. These include the following:

- Coming of age in an impoverished family,
- Living in a broken home,
- Experiencing domestic violence,
- Having limited expectations about one's future, lack of hope about significant improvements,
- Having limited exposure to positive relationship role models,
- Having a lack of expectation about living a long life (feeling old early, especially men),
- Having a low level of expectation about the dependability of others (i.e., limited ability to trust), and
- Fear of intimacy as dangerous because it makes one vulnerable.

It is within this psychosocial milieu of threat and uncertainty that the sentiments, beliefs, decisionmaking and sexual behaviors of participants regarding multiple concurrent relationships, lack of relationship trust, patterns of condom use and disuse, and fear of attachment become understandable. Collectively, the factors cited above appear to mitigate against strict and prolonged adherence to risk reduction strategies, which are predicated on being able to realistically engage in long-term planning for a healthy life.

▶ Discussion

Findings from Project PHRESH reveal the social and cultural contexts of sexual behaviors among our participants while suggesting key conceptual, attitudinal, and behavioral factors that may help explain high rates of STDs in the communities and age groups of concern. Study participants have learned to be cautious about commitment in romantic relationships and tend to hedge their bets by having multiple partners and various kinds of relationships. Moreover, four contextual factors appear to be critical in limiting condom use: (1) condoms are not always available when passions run high; lack of a condom is often not a barrier to having sex; (2) the decision to use a condom flows from a culturally informed assessment of a partner's presumed level of risk rather than from a public health understanding of risky behaviors; (3) emotional involvement in relationships runs counter to continued condom use; the decision to curtail condom use is made quickly; and (4) relationships in which condoms are not used are multiple, overlapping and sequential. The result is a high level of risk for STD. This risk is not random or meaningless; it is conditioned by socioeconomic factors that press participants to focus on short-term pleasure and emotional and material gains rather than on long-term planning and monogamous partnerships. It is, in short, a rational response to social disparity. The results of our investigation, however, lead us towards pessimistic conclusions regarding STD prevention and risk reduction behaviors with current methods. While existing prevention efforts have succeeded in teaching participants about condoms, the context of their utilization creates multiple opportunities for sexual disease transmission.

▶ Conclusion

Disease discriminates. Some groups in society get more of it than others. Consistently research has shown that especially concentrated and chronic social disadvantage across multiple spheres of life, enduring discrimination in access to quality health care, and relative poverty, are significantly detrimental to the health not just of individuals but of whole social groups (Budrys, 2003; Hayward, Crimmins, Miles, & Yang, 2000). What have been found to be of greatest importance in the relationship between social inequality and poorer health are structurally imposed "ecosocial" and "psychosocial factors" (Bosman, Schrijvers, & Mackenback, 1999; Kawachi, Kennedy, & Wilkinson, 1999). Kreiger (2001) introduced the term ecosocial to label a configuration of local social environmental conditions (e.g., the social deprivation of living in an impoverished neighborhood) that are the products of class and ethnic inequality. Psychosocial factors of note include a set of interrelated experiences linked to health, such as internalized racism, stigmatization or other social discrimination, living in fear and uncertainty (because of a prevalence of crime and violence in the local social environment), having a low locus of control borne of repeated exposure to discrimination, and feelings of hopelessness about the future.

It is the set of social, psychological, and economic factors experienced by our participants that appear to underlie the set of sexual ideas, attitudes and behaviors, and sexual behavior decisions described in this paper. These beliefs and actions are responses to the uncertainties, threats, and emotional injuries concentrated in the local social environment as a result of significant and increasing socioeconomic inequality. These conditions, and the beliefs and behaviors they give rise to in turn, help drive the spread of multiple and potentially interacting STDs, a phenomenon that is termed here the STDS. The STDS in Hartford is reflected in the comparatively high rates of HIV and other STD infections in the low-income, inner city ethnic minority neighborhoods from which study participants were recruited and the comparatively high rates of STD diagnoses reported by study participants. As this discussion suggests, the analysis of syndemic spread must take into account cultural and behavioral patterns in the social context. While syndemics reflect social conditions and unequal social relationships, their diffusion is mediated by the beliefs and behaviors of involved communities, and these, in turn, reflect human responses to the life experiences of injustice and social suffering.

Finally, the findings and conclusions of this study have intervention and policy implications. Certainly they should reduce trust in approaches that see individual irresponsibility, damaged family values, or lack of morality as the key causes of STDSs. Community attitudes and behaviors are complex and attentive to social conditions, including, especially, the ecosocial and psychosocial factors that shape day-to-day experiences. Social policies and interventions should be no less attentive to such factors if they are to make a difference in overcoming health inequalities. At the same time, knowing through research what people actually believe and do, and hearing their voices about such matters, presents a firmer foundation on which to construct prevention messages and effective prevention (Singer et al., 2005).

▶ Acknowledgements

Funding for this study was provided for by the Centers for Disease Control and Prevention, grant #U58/CCU123064, Pamela Erickson and Linda Hock-Long, PIs. Our sister site in this cooperative agreement, the Family Planning Council of Philadelphia is implementing the same research protocol with a similar population of 18–25 year-old young adults in Philadelphia. All names are pseudonyms.

▶ References

Bernard, R. (2001). *Research methods in anthropology: Qualitative and quantitative approaches* (3rd ed). Walnut Creek, CA: Altamira.

Booth, C., Matukas, L., Tomlinson, G., Rachlis, A., Rose, D., & Dwosh, H. (2003). Clinical features and short-term outcomes of 144 patients with SARS in the greater Toronto area. *Journal of the American Medical Association, 289,* 2801–2809.

Borgatti, S. (1996). *Anthropac 4.98.* Chestnut Hill, MA: Analytic Technologies.

Bosman, H., Schrijvers, C., & Mackenback, J. (1999). Socioeconomic inequalities in mortality and importance of perceived control: Cohort Study. *British Medical Journal,* 319, 1469–1470.

Budrys, G. (2003). *Unequal health: How inequality contributes to health or illness.* Roman & Lanham, MD: Littlefield Publishers.

Centers for Disease Control (CDC). (1999). *Sexually transmitted disease surveillance report: STDS in adolescents and young adults.* Atlanta, Ga: CDC.

Chesson, H., Heffelfinger, J., Voigt, R., & Collins, D. (2005). Estimates of primary and secondary syphilis rates in persons with HIV in the United States, 2002. *Sexually Transmitted Disease, 32*(5), 265–269.

Connecticut Department of Public Health. (2000). *HIV/AIDS Surveillance Report, Year-end Edition. HIV/AIDS Surveillance Program.* Hartford, CT.

Connecticut Department of Public Health. (2004). *Sexually transmitted diseases. Connecticut STD Control Program* at site: http://www.dph.state.ct.us/BCH/infectiousdise/STD_2003/std_gc_table10.htm accessed 5/12/05.

Craib, K., Meddings, D., & Strathdee, S. (1995). Rectal Gonorrhoea as an independent risk factor for HIV infection in a cohort of homosexual men. *Genitourinary Medicine, 71,* 150–154.

Cubillos-Garzon, L., Casas, J., Morillo, C., & Bautista, L. (2004). Congestive heart failure in Latin America: The next epidemic. *American Heart Journal, 47*(3), 386–389.

Easton, D. (2004). *The urban poor: Health issues. Encyclopedia of medical anthropology,* Vol. 1 (pp. 207–213).

Farley, T., Hadler, J., & Gunn, R. (1990). The syphilis epidemic in Connecticut: Relationship to drug use and prostitution. *Sexually Transmitted Diseases, 17*(4), 163–168.

Farmer, P. (1999). *Infections and inequality: The modern plagues.* Berkeley, CA: University of California Press.

Fowler, R., Lapinsky, S., Hallett, D., Detsky, A., Sibbald, W., & Slutsky, A. (2003). Critically ill patients with severe acute respiratory syndrome. *Journal of the American Medical Association, 290,* 367–373.

Freudenberg, N., Fahs, M., Galea, S., & Greenberg, A. (2006). The impact of New York City's 1975 fiscal crisis on the tuberculosis, HIV, and homicide syndemic. *American Journal of Public Health, 96*(3), 424–434.

Hartford Community Health Partnership. (2003). *HIV/AIDS Surveillance report.* Hartford: City of Hartford Health Department.

Hayward, M., Crimmins, E., Miles, T., & Yang, Y. (2000). The significance of socioeconomic status in explaining the racial gap in chronic health conditions. *American Sociological Review, 65,* 910–930.

Heflin, C., Siefert, K., & Williams, D. (2005). Food insufficiency and women's mental health: Findings from a 3-year panel of welfare recipients. *Social Science & Medicine, 61*(9), 1971–1982.

Hotez, P. (2003). *The hookworm vaccine initiative.* Washington, D.C.: Sabin Vaccine Institute, Georgetown University.

Johnson, S., & Martin, R. (2005). Chlamydophila pneumoniae and Mycoplasma pneumoniae: A role in asthma pathogenesis. *American Journal of Respiratory and Critical Care Medicine, 172*(9), 1078–1089.

Kawachi, I., Kennedy, B., & Wilkinson, R. (1999). *The social and population health reader,* Vol. 1. New York: The New Press.

Kreiger, N. (2001). Theories for social epidemiology in the 21st century: An ecosocial perspective. *International Journal of Epidemiology, 30,* 668–677.

Lichtenstein, B., & Schwebke, J. (in press). Partner notification methods for African American men being treated for trichomoniasis: A consideration of main men, second hitters and third players. *Medical Anthropology Quarterly,* 19(4), 383–401.

Nusbaum, M., Wallace, R., Slatt, L., & Kondrad, E. (2004). Sexually transmitted infections and increased risk of co-infection with human immunodeficiency virus. *Journal of the American Osteopathic Association, 104*(12), 527–535.

O'Connor, S., West, S., Lorntz, B., Vinicor, F., & Jorgensen, C. (2004). Women and infectious disease—Chronic disease interactions [conference summary]. *Emerging Infectious Diseases* [serial on the Internet]. At: http://www.cdc.gov/ncidod/EID/vol10no11/04-0623_14.htm. Accessed May 18, 2005.

Otten, M., Zaidi, A., Peterman, T., Rolfs, R., & Witte, J. (1994). High rate of HIV Seroconversion among patients attending urban sexually transmitted disease clinics. *AIDS, 8,* 549–553.

Singer, M. (1996). A dose of drugs, a touch of violence, a case of AIDS: Conceptualizing the SAVA Syndemic. *Free Inquiry in Creative Sociology, 24*(2), 99–110.

Singer, M., & Clair, S. (2003). Syndemics and public health: Reconceptualizing disease in bio-social context. *Medical Anthropology Quarterly, 17*(4), 423–441.

Singer, M., Jia, Z., Schensul, J., Weeks, & Page, J. (1992). AIDS and the IV drug user: The local context in prevention efforts. *Medical Anthropology, 14,* 285–306.

Singer, M., Stopka, T., Shaw, S., Santilices, C., Buchanan, D., Teng, W., et al. (2005). Lessons from the field: From research to application in the fight against AIDS among injection drug users in three New England Cities. *Human Organization, 64*(2), 179–191.

Soule, J., Olyaei, A., Boslaugh, T., Busch, A., Schwartz, J., Morehouse, S., et al. (2005). Hepatitis C infection increases the risk of new-onset diabetes after transplantation in liver allograft recipients. *American Journal of Surgery, 189*(5), 552–557.

Stall, R., Mills, T. C., Williamson, J., Hart, T., Greenwood, G., Paul, J., et al. (2003). Association of co-occurring psychosocial health problems and increased vulnerability to HIV/AIDS among urban men who have sex with men. *American Journal of Public Health, 93*(6), 949–954.

Visnegarwala, F., Chen, L., Raghavan, S., & Tedaldi, E. (2005). Prevalence of diabetes mellitus and dyslipidemia among antiretroviral naive patients co-infected with hepatitis C virus (HCV) and HIV-1 compared to patients without co-infection. *Journal of Infection, 50*(4), 331–337.

Wasserheit, J. (1992). Epidemiological synergy. Interrelationships between human immunodeficiency virus infection and other sexually transmitted diseases. *Sexually Transmitted Diseases, 19,* 61–77.

▶ Notes

1. Compensation for participant time was calculated roughly at $15/hour. Informed consent and preliminary instruction for FGDs required about an hour and actual data collection from 3 to 5 hours. Participants had one break with refreshments during the FGDs. Facilitators reported that, while ultimately successful, the FGDs were very long and exhausting for both themselves and the participants. Some of the participants indicated to the facilitators that this was the first time they had ever talked to anyone or thought about their sexual experiences and behavior in this way and that it had been an important learning experience for them. Despite the length of the sessions, many participants expressed interest in having subsequent sessions.

2. There were only four terms that were absent or rare in the Hartford FGDs. Only one term in the list was not mentioned at all in Hartford ("hit and run") and three others that were mentioned in only one Hartford group. Most of the terms (26) were mentioned in two or more groups at both sites (see Table 8.2). What is more notable about the terms in use is the dominance of African American youth culture, language, and modes of speaking among all the participants.

► Suggested Readings and Resources for Part 2

NIAID Fact Sheet on Chlamydia August 2006
http://www.niaid.nih.gov/factsheets/stdclam.htm

CDC Fact Sheet on Chlamydia April 2006
http://www.cdc.gov/std/chlamydia/STDFact-Chlamydia.htm

The National Women's Health Information Center, Chlamydia, May 2005
http://www.womenshealth.gov/faq/stdchlam.htm

The National Women's Health Information Center, Gonorrhea, May 2005
http://www.womenshealth.gov/faq/stdgonor.htm

NIAID Fact Sheet on Gonorrhea August 2006
http://www.niaid.nih.gov/factsheets/stdgon.htm

CDC Fact Sheet on Chlamydia April 2006
http://www.cdc.gov/std/Gonorrhea/STDFact-gonorrhea.htm

CDC Fact Sheet on Syphilis May 2004
http://www.cdc.gov/std/syphilis/STDFact-Syphilis.htm

NIAID Fact Sheet on Syphilis, December 2005
http://www.niaid.nih.gov/factsheets/stdsyph.htm

The National Women's Health Information Center, Syphilis, May 2005
http://www.4woman.gov/faq/stdsyph.htm

CDC Fact Sheet on Bacterial Vaginosis, May 2004
http://www.cdc.gov/std/bv/STDFact-Bacterial-Vaginosis.htm

NIAID Fact Sheet: October 2004: Bacterial Vaginosis
http://www.niaid.nih.gov/factsheets/vaginitis.htm

Women's Health Information Center, Bacterial Vaginosis, May 2005
http://www.4woman.gov/faq/stdbv.htm

NIAID Fact Sheet on Herpes October 2005
http://www.niaid.nih.gov/factsheets/stdherp.htm

CDC Fact Sheet on Herpes May 2004
http://www.cdc.gov/std/Herpes/STDFact-Herpes.htm

The National Women's Health Information Center, Herpes, May 2005
http://www.4woman.gov/faq/stdherpe.htm

CDC Fact Sheet on HPV May 2004
http://www.cdc.gov/std/HPV/STDFact-HPV.htm

NIAID Fact Sheet on HPV August 2006
http://www.niaid.nih.gov/factsheets/stdhpv.htm

The National Women's Health Information Center, HPV, June 2006
http://www.4woman.gov/faq/stdhpv.htm

CDC Fact Sheet on Hepatitis, December 2006
http://www.cdc.gov/ncidod/diseases/hepatitis/b/faqb.htm

Women's Health Information Center, Hepatitis, January 2005
http://www.4woman.gov/faq/hepatitis.htm

Women's Health Information Center, HIV/AIDS December 2006
http://www.4woman.gov/hiv/what/

NIAID Fact Sheet on HIV/AIDS, March 2005
http://www.niaid.nih.gov/factsheets/hivinf.htm

Women's Health Information Center Trichomoniasis May 2005
http://www.4woman.gov/faq/stdtrich.htm

CDC Fact Sheet Trichomoniasis May 2004
http://www.cdc.gov/std/Trichomonas/STDFact-Trichomoniasis.htm

NIAID Fact Sheet: October 2004: Trichomoniasis and Vaginal Yeast Infection
http:/www.niaid.nih.gov/factsheets/vaginitis.htm

Women's Health Information Center, Vaginal Yeast Infections, April 2006
http://www.4woman.gov/faq/yeastinfect.htm

CDC Factsheet on Scabies February 2005
http://www.cdc.gov/ncidod/dpd/parasites/scabies/factsht_scabies.htm

Mayo Clinic, Scabies, March 2006
http://www.mayoclinic.com/health/scabies/DS00451

CDC Fact Sheet on Pubic Lice August 2005
http://www.cdc.gov/ncidod/dpd/parasites/lice/factsht_pubic_lice.htm

National Library of Medicine, Pubic Lice, October 2006
http://www.nlm.nih.gov/medlineplus/ency/article/000841.htm

Global Prevalence and Incidence of Selected STIs
http://www.who.int/docstore/hiv/GRSTI/index.htm

Levine, R. (2007). Preventing HIV/AIDS and STIs in Thailand. *Case Studies in Global Health.* Jones and Bartlett Publishers.

CDC HPV Vaccine Fact sheet August 2006
http://www.cdc.gov/std/hpv/STDFact-HPV-vaccine.htm

Syndromic Management Training: Paving the Way for the Adoption of Sexually Transmitted Infection Treatment Norms in the Dominican Republic FHI/UNAIDS Best Practices in HIV/AIDS Prevention
http://www.fhi.org/en/HIVAIDS/pub/guide/bestpractices.htm

Lesedi: Services for Women at High Risk Help Reduce Sexually Transmitted Infection (STI) Prevalence in a South African Mining Community FHI/UNAIDS Best Practices in HIV/AIDS Prevention
http://www.fhi.org/en/HIVAIDS/pub/guide/bestpractices.htm

▶ Part 2

Critical Thinking

1. Do you believe the HPV vaccine should become a mandatory vaccination? Why or why not?
2. Are some types of STIs more stigmatized than others? Why or why not?

Discussion Questions

1. What are the different types of bacterial STIs?
2. How are bacterial STIs transmitted? How are they treated?
3. What are the different types of viral STIs?
4. How are the viral STIs transmitted? How are they treated?
5. What are the different types of vaginal infections? How are they transmitted?
6. What are some of the knowledge gaps surrounding the HPV vaccine?

PART THREE

HIV/AIDS

Chapter 9

Immunology of HIV/AIDS

Understanding the Immune System: How It Works

▶ Introduction

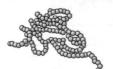

Bacteria:
streptococci

Virus:
herpes virus

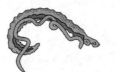

Parasite:
schistosome

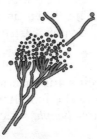

Fungus:
penicillium mold

The immune system is a network of cells, *tissues,* and organs that work together to defend the body against attacks by "foreign" invaders. These are primarily *microbes* (germs)—tiny, infection-causing *organisms* such as *bacteria, viruses, parasites,* and *fungi.* Because the human body provides an ideal environment for many microbes, they try to break in. It is the immune system's job to keep them out or, failing that, to seek out and destroy them.

When the immune system hits the wrong target or is crippled, however, it can unleash a torrent of diseases, including *allergy,* arthritis, or *AIDS.*

The immune system is amazingly complex. It can recognize and remember millions of different enemies, and it can produce secretions and cells to match up with and wipe out each one of them.

The secret to its success is an elaborate and dynamic communications network. Millions and millions of cells, organized into sets and subsets, gather like clouds of bees swarming around a hive and pass information back and forth. Once immune cells receive the alarm, they undergo tactical changes and begin to produce powerful chemicals. These substances allow the cells to regulate their own growth and behavior, enlist their fellows, and direct new recruits to trouble spots.

▶ Self and Nonself

The key to a healthy immune system is its remarkable ability to distinguish between the body's own cells—self—and foreign cells—nonself. The body's immune defenses normally coexist peacefully with cells that carry distinctive "self" marker *molecules.* But when immune defenders encounter cells or organisms carrying markers that say "foreign," they quickly launch an attack.

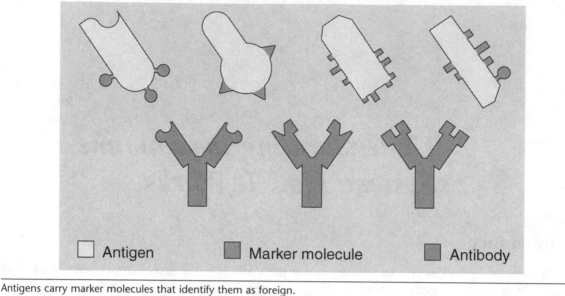

| Antigen | Marker molecule | Antibody |

Antigens carry marker molecules that identify them as foreign.

Anything that can trigger this *immune response* is called an *antigen*. An antigen can be a microbe such as a virus, or even a part of a microbe. Tissues or cells from another person (except an identical twin) also carry nonself markers and act as antigens. This explains why tissue transplants may be rejected.

In abnormal situations, the immune system can mistake self for nonself and launch an attack against the body's own cells or tissues. The result is called an *autoimmune disease*. Some forms of arthritis and diabetes are autoimmune diseases. In other cases, the immune system responds to a seemingly harmless foreign substance such as ragweed pollen. The result is allergy, and this kind of antigen is called an *allergen*.

▶ The Structure of the Immune System

The organs of the immune system are positioned throughout the body. They are called *lymphoid organs* because they are home to *lymphocytes,* small white blood cells that are the key players in the immune system.

Bone marrow, the soft tissue in the hollow center of bones, is the ultimate source of all blood cells, including white blood cells destined to become immune cells. The *thymus* is an organ that lies behind the breastbone; lymphocytes known as *T lymphocytes,* or just *"T cells,"* mature in the thymus.

Lymphocytes can travel throughout the body using the *blood vessels.* The cells can also travel through a system of *lymphatic vessels* that closely parallels the body's veins and arteries. Cells and fluids are exchanged between blood and lymphatic vessels, enabling the lymphatic system to monitor the body for invading microbes. The lymphatic vessels carry *lymph,* a clear fluid that bathes the body's tissues.

Small, bean-shaped *lymph nodes* are laced along the lymphatic vessels, with clusters in the neck, armpits, abdomen, and groin. Each lymph node contains specialized compartments where immune cells congregate, and where they can encounter antigens.

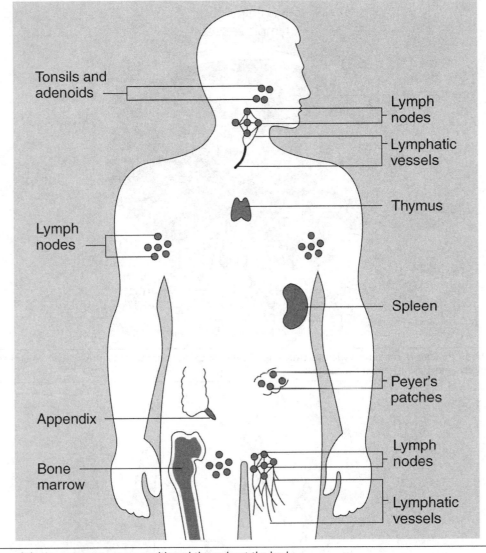

The organs of the immune system are positioned throughout the body.

Immune cells and foreign particles enter the lymph nodes via incoming lymphatic vessels or the lymph nodes' tiny blood vessels. All lymphocytes exit lymph nodes through outgoing lymphatic vessels. Once in the bloodstream, they are transported to tissues throughout the body. They patrol everywhere for foreign antigens, then gradually drift back into the lymphatic system, to begin the cycle all over again.

The *spleen* is a flattened organ at the upper left of the abdomen. Like the lymph nodes, the spleen contains specialized compartments where immune cells gather and work, and serves as a meeting ground where immune defenses confront antigens.

Clumps of lymphoid tissue are found in many parts of the body, especially in the linings of the digestive tract and the airways and lungs—territories that serve as gateways to the body. These tissues include the *tonsils, adenoids,* and *appendix.*

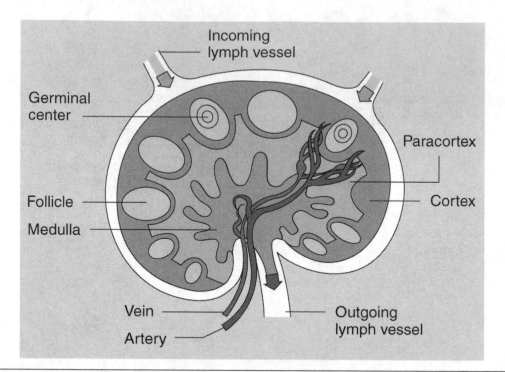

The lymph node contains numerous specialized structures. T cells concentrate in the paracortex, B cells in and around the germinal centers, and plasma cells in the medulla.

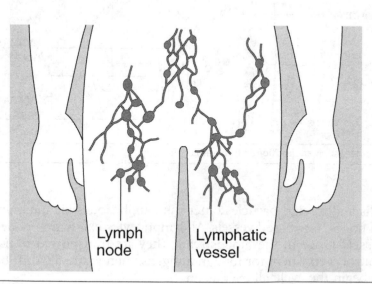

Immune cells and foreign particles enter the lymph nodes via incoming lymphatic vessels or the lymph nodes' tiny blood vessels.

▶ Immune Cells and Their Products

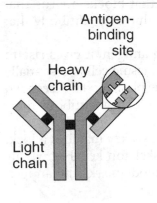

An antibody is made up of two heavy chains and two light chains. The variable region, which differs from one antibody to the next, allows an antibody to recognize its matching antigen.

The immune system stockpiles a huge arsenal of cells, not only lymphocytes but also cell-devouring *phagocytes* and their relatives. Some immune cells take on all comers, while others are trained on highly specific targets. To work effectively, most immune cells need the cooperation of their comrades. Sometimes immune cells communicate by direct physical contact, sometimes by releasing chemical messengers.

The immune system stores just a few of each kind of the different cells needed to recognize millions of possible enemies. When an antigen appears, those few matching cells multiply into a full-scale army. After their job is done, they fade away, leaving sentries behind to watch for future attacks.

All immune cells begin as immature *stem cells* in the bone marrow. They respond to different *cytokines* and other signals to grow into specific immune cell types, such as T cells, *B cells,* or phagocytes. Because stem cells have not yet committed to a particular future, they are an interesting possibility for treating some immune system disorders. Researchers currently are investigating if a person's own stem cells can be used to regenerate damaged immune responses in autoimmune diseases and immune deficiency diseases.

B Lymphocytes

B cells and T cells are the main types of lymphocytes.

B cells work chiefly by secreting substances called *antibodies* into the body's fluids. Antibodies ambush antigens circulating the bloodstream. They are powerless, however, to penetrate cells. The job of attacking target cells—either cells that have been infected by viruses or cells that have been distorted by cancer—is left to T cells or other immune cells (described below).

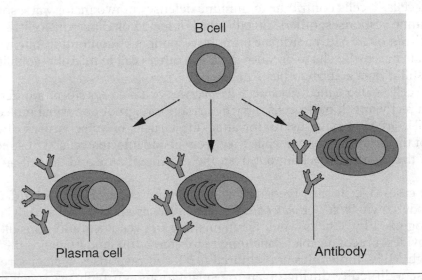

B cells mature into plasma cells that produce antibodies.

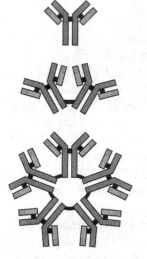

Immunoglobulins

Each B cell is programmed to make one specific antibody. For example, one B cell will make an antibody that blocks a virus that causes the common cold, while another produces an antibody that attacks a bacterium that causes pneumonia.

When a B cell encounters its triggering antigen, it gives rise to many large cells known as *plasma cells*. Every plasma cell is essentially a factory for producing an antibody. Each of the plasma cells descended from a given B cell manufactures millions of identical antibody molecules and pours them into the bloodstream.

An antigen matches an antibody much as a key matches a lock. Some match exactly; others fit more like a skeleton key. But whenever antigen and antibody interlock, the antibody marks the antigen for destruction.

Antibodies belong to a family of large molecules known as *immunoglobulins*. Different types play different roles in the immune defense strategy.

- Immunoglobulin G, or IgG, works efficiently to coat microbes, speeding their uptake by other cells in the immune system.
- IgM is very effective at killing bacteria.
- IgA concentrates in body fluids—tears, saliva, the secretions of the respiratory tract and the digestive tract—guarding the entrances to the body.
- IgE, whose natural job probably is to protect against parasitic infections, is the villain responsible for the symptoms of allergy.
- IgD remains attached to B cells and plays a key role in initiating early B-cell response.

T Cells

Unlike B cells, T cells do not recognize free-floating antigens. Rather, their surfaces contain specialized antibody-like receptors that see fragments of antigens on the surfaces of infected or cancerous cells. T cells contribute to immune defenses in two major ways: some direct and regulate immune responses; others directly attack infected or cancerous cells.

Helper T cells, or *Th cells,* coordinate immune responses by communicating with other cells. Some stimulate nearby B cells to produce antibody, others call in microbe-gobbling cells called phagocytes, still others activate other T cells.

Killer T cells—also called *cytotoxic T lymphocytes* or *CTLs*—perform a different function. These cells directly attack other cells carrying certain foreign or abnormal molecules on their surfaces. CTLs are especially useful for attacking viruses because viruses often hide from other parts of the immune system while they grow inside infected cells. CTLs recognize small fragments of these viruses peeking out from the cell membrane and launch an attack to kill the cell.

In most cases, T cells only recognize an antigen if it is carried on the surface of a cell by one of the body's own *MHC,* or *major histocompatibility complex,* molecules. MHC molecules are proteins recognized by T cells when distinguishing between self and nonself. A self MHC molecule provides a recognizable scaffolding to present a foreign antigen to the T cell.

Although MHC molecules are required for T-cell responses against foreign invaders, they also pose a difficulty during organ transplantations. Virtually every cell in the body is

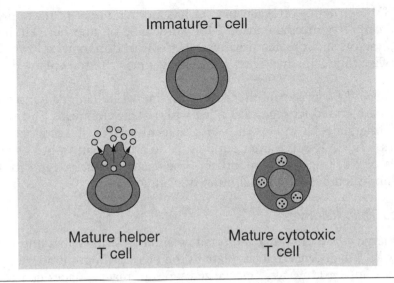

Some T cells are helper cells, others are killer cells.

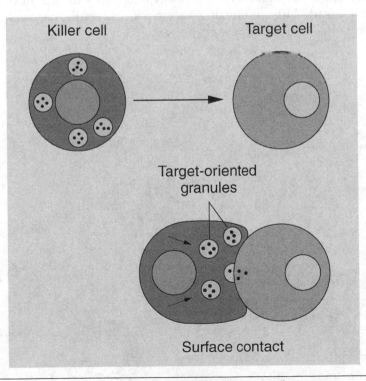

Killer cell makes contact with target cell, trains its weapons on the target, then strikes.

covered with MHC proteins, but each person has a different set of these proteins on his or her cells. If a T cell recognizes a nonself MHC molecule on another cell, it will destroy the cell. Therefore, doctors must match organ recipients with donors who have the closest MHC makeup. Otherwise the recipient's T cells will likely attack the transplanted organ, leading to *graft rejection.*

Natural killer (NK) cells are another kind of lethal white cell, or lymphocyte. Like killer T cells, NK cells are armed with *granules* filled with potent chemicals. But while killer T cells look for antigen fragments bound to self-MHC molecules, NK cells recognize cells lacking self-MHC molecules. Thus NK cells have the potential to attack many types of foreign cells.

Both kinds of killer cells slay on contact. The deadly assassins bind to their targets, aim their weapons, and then deliver a lethal burst of chemicals.

Phagocytes and Their Relatives

Phagocytes are large white cells that can swallow and digest microbes and other foreign particles. *Monocytes* are phagocytes that circulate in the blood. When monocytes migrate into tissues, they develop into *macrophages.* Specialized types of macrophages can be found in many organs, including lungs, kidneys, brain, and liver.

Macrophages play many roles. As scavengers, they rid the body of worn-out cells and other debris. They display bits of foreign antigen in a way that draws the attention of matching lymphocytes. And they churn out an amazing variety of powerful chemical signals, known as *monokines,* which are vital to the immune responses.

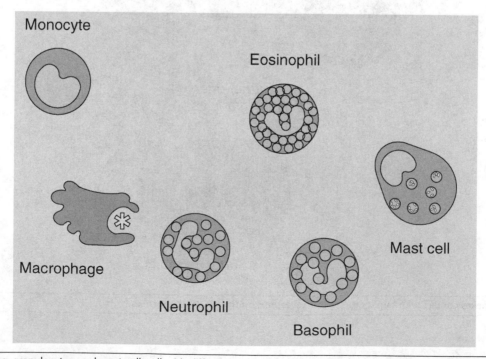

Phagocytes, granulocytes, and mast cells, all with different methods of attack, demonstrate the immune system's versatility.

Granulocytes are another kind of immune cell. They contain granules filled with potent chemicals, which allow the granulocytes to destroy *microorganisms*. Some of these chemicals, such as histamine, also contribute to inflammation and allergy.

One type of granulocyte, the *neutrophil*, is also a phagocyte; it uses its prepackaged chemicals to break down the microbes it ingests. *Eosinophils* and *basophils* are granulocytes that "degranulate," spraying their chemicals onto harmful cells or microbes nearby.

The *mast cell* is a twin of the basophil, except that it is not a blood cell. Rather, it is found in the lungs, skin, tongue, and linings of the nose and intestinal tract, where it is responsible for the symptoms of allergy.

A related structure, the blood *platelet,* is a cell fragment. Platelets, too, contain granules. In addition to promoting blood clotting and wound repair, platelets activate some of the immune defenses.

Cytokines

Components of the immune system communicate with one another by exchanging chemical messengers called cytokines. These proteins are secreted by cells and act on other cells to coordinate an appropriate immune response. Cytokines include a diverse assortment of *interleukins, interferons,* and *growth factors.*

Some cytokines are chemical switches that turn certain immune cell types on and off.

One cytokine, interleukin 2 (IL-2), triggers the immune system to produce T cells. IL-2's immunity-boosting properties have traditionally made it a promising treatment for several illnesses. Clinical studies are ongoing to test its benefits in other diseases such as cancer, hepatitis C, and *HIV* infection and AIDS. Other cytokines also are being studied for their potential clinical benefit.

Other cytokines chemically attract specific cell types. These so-called *chemokines* are released by cells at a site of injury or infection and call other immune cells to the region to help repair the damage or fight off the invader. Chemokines often play a key role in inflammation and are a promising target for new drugs to help regulate immune responses.

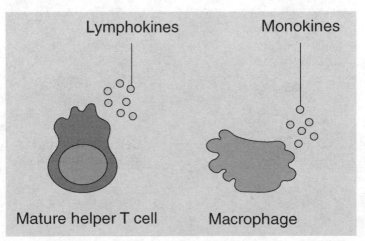

Cytokines include lymphokines, produced by lymphocytes, and monokines, made by monocytes and macrophages.

Complement

The *complement* system is made up of about 25 proteins that work together to "complement" the action of antibodies in destroying bacteria. Complement also helps to rid the body of antibody-coated antigens (antigen-antibody complexes). Complement proteins, which cause blood vessels to become dilated and then leaky, contribute to the redness, warmth, swelling, pain, and loss of function that characterize an *inflammatory response*.

Complement proteins circulate in the blood in an inactive form. When the first protein in the complement series is activated—typically by antibody that has locked onto an antigen—it sets in motion a domino effect. Each component takes its turn in a precise chain of steps known as the *complement cascade*. The end product is a cylinder inserted into—and punc-

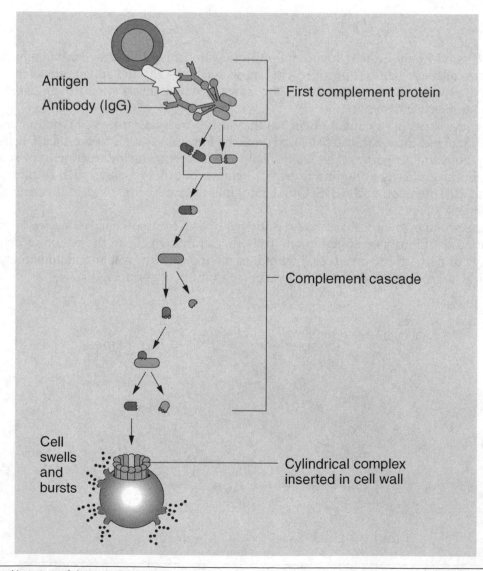

Antigen ——— First complement protein

Antibody (IgG) ———

Complement cascade

Cell swells and bursts

Cylindrical complex inserted in cell wall

The interlocking steps of the complement cascade end in cell death.

turing a hole in—the cell's wall. With fluids and molecules flowing in and out, the cell swells and bursts. Other components of the complement system make bacteria more susceptible to *phagocytosis* or beckon other cells to the area.

▶ Mounting an Immune Response

Infections are the most common cause of human disease. They range from the common cold to debilitating conditions like chronic hepatitis to life-threatening diseases such as AIDS. Disease-causing microbes *(pathogens)* attempting to get into the body must first move past the body's external armor, usually the skin or cells lining the body's internal passageways.

The skin provides an imposing barrier to invading microbes. It is generally penetrable only through cuts or tiny abrasions. The digestive and respiratory tracts—both portals of entry for a number of microbes—also have their own levels of protection. Microbes entering the nose often cause the nasal surfaces to secrete more protective mucus, and attempts to enter the nose or lungs can trigger a sneeze or cough reflex to force microbial invaders out of the respiratory passageways. The stomach contains a strong acid that destroys many pathogens that are swallowed with food.

If microbes survive the body's front-line defenses, they still have to find a way through the walls of the digestive, respiratory, or urogenital passageways to the underlying cells. These passageways are lined with tightly packed *epithelial cells* covered in a layer of mucus, effectively blocking the transport of many organisms. Mucosal surfaces also secrete a special class of

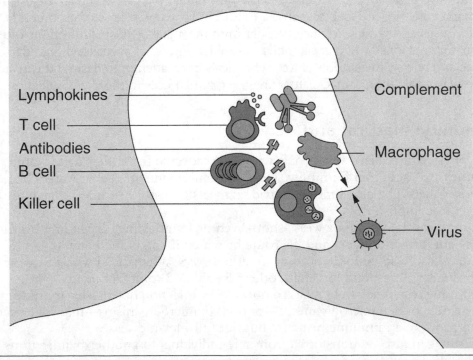

When challenged, the immune system has many weapons to choose.

antibody called IgA, which in many cases is the first type of antibody to encounter an invading microbe. Underneath the epithelial layer a number of cells, including macrophages, B cells, and T cells, lie in wait for any germ that might bypass the barriers at the surface.

Next, invaders must escape a series of general defenses, which are ready to attack, without regard for specific antigen markers. These include patrolling phagocytes, NK cells, and complement.

Microbes that cross the general barriers then confront specific weapons tailored just for them. Specific weapons, which include both antibodies and T cells, are equipped with singular receptor structures that allow them to recognize and interact with their designated targets.

Bacteria, Viruses, and Parasites

The most common disease-causing microbes are bacteria, viruses, and parasites. Each uses a different tactic to infect a person, and, therefore, each is thwarted by a different part of the immune system.

Most bacteria live in the spaces between cells and are readily attacked by antibodies. When antibodies attach to a bacterium, they send signals to complement proteins and phagocytic cells to destroy the bound microbes. Some bacteria are eaten directly by phagocytes, which signal to certain T cells to join the attack.

All viruses, plus a few types of bacteria and parasites, must enter cells to survive, requiring a different approach. Infected cells use their MHC molecules to put pieces of the invading microbes on the cell's surface, flagging down cytotoxic T lymphocytes to destroy the infected cell. Antibodies also can assist in the immune response, attaching to and clearing viruses before they have a chance to enter the cell.

Parasites live either inside or outside cells. Intracellular parasites such as the organism that causes malaria can trigger T-cell responses. Extracellular parasites are often much larger than bacteria or viruses and require a much broader immune attack. Parasitic infections often trigger an inflammatory response when eosinophils, basophils, and other specialized granular cells rush to the scene and release their stores of toxic chemicals in an attempt to destroy the invader. Antibodies also play a role in this attack, attracting the granular cells to the site of infection.

▶ Immunity: Natural and Acquired

Long ago, physicians realized that people who had recovered from the plague would never get it again—they had acquired immunity. This is because some of the activated T and B cells become *memory cells*. The next time an individual meets up with the same antigen, the immune system is set to demolish it.

Immunity can be strong or weak, short-lived or long-lasting, depending on the type of antigen, the amount of antigen, and the route by which it enters the body.

Immunity can also be influenced by inherited *genes*. When faced with the same antigen, some individuals will respond forcefully, others feebly, and some not at all.

An immune response can be sparked not only by infection but also by immunization with *vaccines*. Vaccines contain microorganisms—or parts of microorganisms—that have been treated so they can provoke an immune response but not full-blown disease.

Immunity can also be transferred from one individual to another by injections of *serum* rich in antibodies against a particular microbe *(antiserum)*.

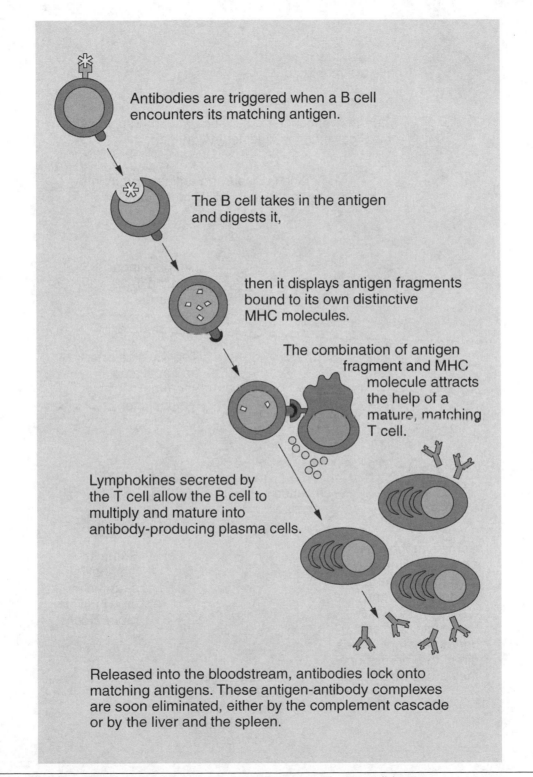

Antibodies are triggered when a B cell encounters its matching antigen.

The B cell takes in the antigen and digests it,

then it displays antigen fragments bound to its own distinctive MHC molecules.

The combination of antigen fragment and MHC molecule attracts the help of a mature, matching T cell.

Lymphokines secreted by the T cell allow the B cell to multiply and mature into antibody-producing plasma cells.

Released into the bloodstream, antibodies lock onto matching antigens. These antigen-antibody complexes are soon eliminated, either by the complement cascade or by the liver and the spleen.

Misguided T cells can attack insulin-producing cells of the pancreas, contributing to diabetes.

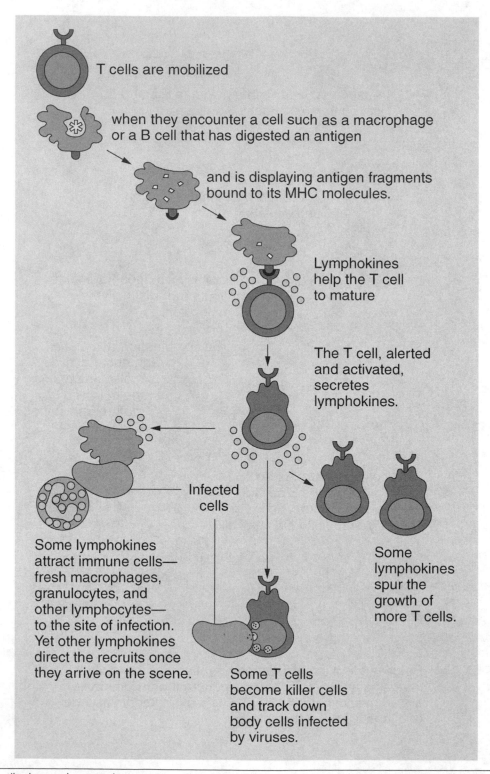

T cells are mobilized

when they encounter a cell such as a macrophage or a B cell that has digested an antigen

and is displaying antigen fragments bound to its MHC molecules.

Lymphokines help the T cell to mature

The T cell, alerted and activated, secretes lymphokines.

Infected cells

Some lymphokines attract immune cells— fresh macrophages, granulocytes, and other lymphocytes— to the site of infection. Yet other lymphokines direct the recruits once they arrive on the scene.

Some lymphokines spur the growth of more T cells.

Some T cells become killer cells and track down body cells infected by viruses.

Antigen-antibody complexes can become trapped in, and damage, the kidneys and other organs.

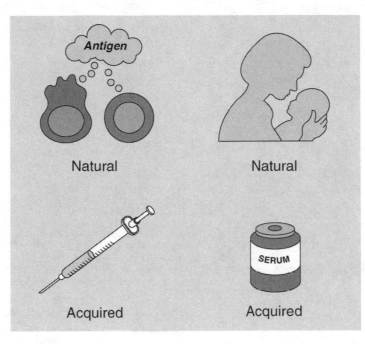

For example, immune serum is sometimes given to protect travelers to countries where hepatitis A is widespread. Such *passive immunity* typically lasts only a few weeks or months.

Infants are born with weak immune responses but are protected for the first few months of life by antibodies received from their mothers before birth. Babies who are nursed can also receive some antibodies from breast milk that help to protect their digestive tracts.

Immune Tolerance

Immune *tolerance* is the tendency of T or B lymphocytes to ignore the body's own tissues. Maintaining tolerance is important because it prevents the immune system from attacking its fellow cells. Scientists are hard at work trying to understand how the immune system knows when to respond and when to ignore.

Tolerance occurs in at least two ways. Central tolerance occurs during lymphocyte development. Very early in each immune cell's life, it is exposed to many of the self molecules in the body. If it encounters these molecules before it has fully matured, the encounter activates an internal self-destruct pathway and the immune cell dies. This process, called clonal deletion, helps ensure that self-reactive T cells and B cells do not mature and attack healthy tissues.

Because maturing lymphocytes do not encounter every molecule in the body, they must also learn to ignore mature cells and tissues. In peripheral tolerance, circulating lymphocytes might recognize a self molecule but cannot respond because some of the chemical signals required to activate the T or B cell are absent. So-called clonal energy, therefore, keeps potentially harmful lymphocytes switched off. Peripheral tolerance may also be imposed by a special class of regulatory T cells that inhibits helper or cytotoxic T-cell activation by self antigens.

The Disease and Its Epidemiology

Tony Barnett and Alan Whiteside

HIV/AIDS is not the first global epidemic, and it certainly won't be the last: it is a disease that is changing human history. HIV/AIDS shows up global inequalities. Its presence and impacts are felt most profoundly in poor countries and communities. Here we look at its origins, how it is transmitted and the particular characteristics which make consideration of its social and economic roots and impacts necessary. Because of its scale and the international and local concern it evokes, we are confronted by quantities of information that may threaten to overwhelm us. Thus, in the last part of the chapter we look at data: what we know about AIDS and HIV, and how we know it, and how those data are used to construct particular accounts of the epidemic process.

Communicable diseases have been responsible for past epidemics and pandemics. They played an important role in human history and we had few defences against them. Bubonic plague, which spread from the Mediterranean ports of southern Europe in 1347, changed the course of European, and thus of world, history.

> Most historians now accept the plague's role in destroying feudal barriers to economic growth, and creating an instant demand for labour which had to be satisfied from a drastically reduced work force. In effect, the fourteenth century bubonic plague intensified the action of powerful structural forces which were turning Europe toward modernity. (McGrew, 1985, p. 40)

During the first outbreak of plague in Europe from 1347 to 1351, mortality varied at between one-eighth and two-thirds of the population. Overall, three out of ten Europeans may have died, some 24 million people (Watts, 1999 in Cook, 1999). Some historians have argued that consequent labour scarcity led to technical, social and religious innovation, and ultimately to capitalism.

While Europe was affected by epidemics, they devastated other regions of the world. From the middle of the last millennium contact between Europe, the Americas,

_____ BOX 9.1 _____

DEFINITIONS

An epidemic is a rate of disease that reaches unexpectedly high levels, affecting a large number of people in a relatively short time. Epidemic is a relative concept: a small absolute number of cases of a disease is considered an epidemic if the disease incidence is usually very low. In contrast, a disease (such as malaria) is considered endemic if it is continuously present in a population but at low or moderate levels, while a pandemic describes epidemics of worldwide proportions, such as influenza in 1918 or HIV/AIDS today (Barfield, 1997, p. 150).

Australasia and parts of Africa proved disastrous for immunologically naive indigenous populations. Lacking defences against common European diseases such as smallpox, typhus, measles and influenza, these populations fell ill faster and diseases were more virulent. Diseases spread easily and mortality rates were very high. The result was massive depopulation: whole peoples disappeared; others were so seriously depleted as to have been written out of history.

Documentation of this process begins with Columbus's landfall on the Caribbean island of Hispaniola. In 1492 at the time of his arrival, there were at least a million Taino people. A disease akin to smallpox appeared in 1519 and by 1550 the Taino were extinct (Watts 1997, p. 88). This pattern of devastation was repeated throughout the Caribbean islands. The Aztec and Inca kingdoms of mainland South and Central America were next. The troops of the Spanish conquistador Hernán Cortès brought smallpox. It is estimated that the population of Mexico fell from 25.2 million in 1518 to 1.1 million in 1605. Similarly affected were the Inca to the south and Native American populations to the north. There, Spanish explorers had encountered a vibrant culture with towns and temples in the Mississippi valley. By the early 1700s this had vanished along with most of the people.

The role of disease in human history has been charted by a number of authors: initially by McNeil (1976) and most recently by Diamond (1999). McNeil began by posing the question, 'How did Cortès and his tiny band of less than 600 Spaniards conquer the mighty Aztec empire, whose subjects numbered many millions?' (McNeil, 1976, p. 1). Diamond's perspective is informed by a question posed by a Papua New Guinean: 'Why is it that you white people developed so much cargo and brought it to New Guinea, but we black people had little cargo of our own?' (Diamond, 1999, p. 14). For McNeil the disease was the key. Diamond, however, saw disease as part of a broader geographical determinism.

By the end of the nineteenth century the principles of disease transmission were generally known in Europe. The first well-known public health intervention was in 1854 when Dr John Snow tracked the source of an outbreak of cholera in London to a water pump in Broad Street. Closing the public pump brought the outbreak under control. However it was not until 1883 that Robert Koch identified the cholera bacillus. The first identified 'germs' or disease-causing organisms were the bacilli of anthrax and tuberculosis discovered by Louis Pasteur in the 1870s. In the latter part of the nineteenth century a flurry of activity (often associated with expansion of European empires) led to the identification of more 'germs' and linked them with specific diseases. Thus began scientifically based public health interventions.

Among these was the US-funded Yellow Fever Commission, which in 1900 identified the mosquito as the vector for disease transmission. In Havana anti-mosquito measures reduced the number of cases from 1,400 in 1900 to none in 1902. Public health interventions were being developed and seen to work.

Medical advances lead to the development of vaccines initially for polio, and by the 1960s for most other major childhood illnesses. Global smallpox vaccination resulted in eradication of the virus; the last case was reported in Somalia in 1977. By the mid-twentieth century, drug and vaccine development suggested to many that the world might be entering a period when the battle against infectious disease could be won. The next challenge was viral disease.

Prior to the emergence of HIV/AIDS, the last global epidemic had been influenza in 1918–19, so long ago that there was little 'institutional memory' of global epidemics. In the wealthy world there was also little memory of any killer epidemics. Poliomyelitis ceased to be a major concern with the introduction of a vaccine in 1955. Between 1946 and 1955 in the US there were on average 32,890 cases per year and 1,742 deaths. After the introduction of vaccination the number of cases fell to 5,749 and deaths to 268 (Oldstone, 1998, p. 109). In the rich world preventable diseases are generally prevented. Most people have clean water, heat, decent housing, nutritious diets and access to health care. The diseases that kill the rich are diseases of affluence such as heart disease. Outside of the rich world there have been major successes in immunisation against childhood diseases, although large numbers of children are still not reached and they die.

Where epidemics do emerge, scientific and medical responses are mobilised and emergencies are contained. However all is not well. Public health systems are underfunded; politically they attract few votes, and in parts of the world they are close to collapse. For the moment, there is only a mere intimation of any system of *global* public health.

Neither public health nor clinical medicine pays sufficient attention to what does improve health—escaping from poverty, access to good food, clean water, sanitation, shelter, education and preventative care. Clinical medicine has only marginal effects on people's long-term health. In the US—which spends the largest proportion of GNP on medical care of any country— 'less than 4% of the total improvements in life expectancy can be credited to twentieth century advances in medical care' (Garrett, 2000, p. 10). Preventive medicine is often piecemeal. For example, measles immunisation may be undertaken in slums where diarrhoeal disease is rife. Social and economic conditions negate many gains made by any particular intervention. Health is not only about confronting individual diseases. Well-being, of which health is a part, is a reflection of general social and economic conditions.

The 1990s has seen the recognition of many 'emergent' diseases—Ebola, Lassa fever, Marburg fever are well known and hit the headlines. More serious is multi-drug resistant TB. Also of concern are the rise of antibiotic resistant bacteria, new strains of salmonella and most recently bovine spongiform encephalopathy and the related human form, new variant Creuzfeld-Jakob Disease (nvCJD).

HIV/AIDS has emerged into this setting. It is the first global epidemic for 60 years. Working from past experience, many hoped that the solutions lay in a quick technical fix—drugs or a vaccine. But there has been no medical-scientific solution. With the exception of its first manifestations in the US, this disease is linked to poverty and inequality and the ways that globalisation exacerbates these. Its consequences will be felt for decades to come, and its origins lie far back in time and deep within the structures of social, economic and cultural life. The epidemic is not just about medicine or even public health.

▶ The Emergence of the New Epidemic: The Discovery of AIDS and HIV

The story of HIV/AIDS begins in 1979 and 1980 when doctors in the US observed clusters of previously extremely rare diseases. These included a type of pneumonia carried by birds (*pneumocystis carinii*) and a cancer called Kaposi's sarcoma. The phenomenon was first reported in the *Morbidity and Mortality Weekly Report* (*MMWR*) of 5 June 1981, published by the US Center for Disease Control in Atlanta. The *MMWR* recorded five cases of *pneumocystis carinii*. A month later it reported a clustering of cases of Kaposi's sarcoma in New York. Subsequently, the number of cases of both diseases—which were mainly centered around New York and San Francisco—rose rapidly, and scientists realised that they were dealing with something new.

The first cases were among homosexual men. As a result the disease was called Gay-Related Immune Deficiency Syndrome (GRID). American epidemiologists began to see cases among other groups, initially mainly haemophiliacs and recipients of blood transfusions. Subsequently the syndrome was identified among injecting drug users, and infants born to mothers who used drugs. It was apparent that this was not a 'gay' disease. It was renamed 'Acquired Immunodeficiency Syndrome', shortened to the acronym AIDS:

- The 'A' stands for Acquired. This means that the virus is not spread through casual or inadvertent contact like flu or chickenpox. In order to be infected, a person has do something (or have something done to him or her) which exposes him or her to the virus.
- 'I' and 'D' stand for Immunodeficiency. The virus attacks a person's immune system and makes it less capable of fighting infections. Thus, the immune system becomes deficient.
- 'S' is for Syndrome. AIDS is not one disease but rather presents itself as a number of diseases that come about as the immune system fails. Hence, it is regarded as a syndrome.

The illness was seen simultaneously in a number of locations outside the US. In Zambia, Dr. Anne Bayley, Professor of Surgery at the University Teaching Hospital in Lusaka, reported a significant rise in the number of Kaposi's sarcoma cases (Bayley, 1984). In 1982, reports of a significant wave of deaths in the south of the country began to reach the Ugandan Ministry of Health. In 1983 the ministry sent a team to investigate this new disease in the Lake Victoria fishing village of Kasensero. They concluded that it was AIDS (Kaleeba et al., 2000; Hooper, 1990). Hooper (1999) documents similar recognition of the disease in Tanzania, Congo and Rwanda.

In October 1983 a team of American and European doctors travelled to Kigali and Zaire where they identified and described cases of AIDS. Of course many hundreds of African doctors were well aware that a new disease was killing their patients. However these frontline health care workers do not write for learned journals such as the *Lancet* or *Science and Nature*, so the cases and the disease remained unreported.

Outside Africa AIDS cases were identified in all Western countries and in Australia, New Zealand and some Latin American countries—most notably Brazil and Mexico. From 1981 there was global recognition of the syndrome; clinicians and others now knew what to look for and that it could be given a name. Immediately there was a question of where HIV/AIDS was seen, by whom and what it meant. What it meant and how it was represented in the press and the popular consciousness was of the greatest significance for people affected by a disease linking sex, sexuality, death, ethnicity and status. Inevitably it became a vehicle for stigma (Farmer, 1992).

Once the new syndrome had been identified, the pace of scientific and epidemiological activity to identify the cause of the disease increased. In 1983 a team lead by French scientist Luc Montagnier identified the virus we now know as HIV-1 (the Human Immunodeficiency Virus). In 1985, a second Human Immunodeficiency Virus, HIV-2, was identified. This is more difficult to transmit and is slower acting and less virulent than HIV-1. Initially HIV-2 was found in west Africa with the greatest number of infections outside this area in Angola, Mozambique, France and Portugal. 'Overall, the most striking feature about the global epidemiology of HIV-2 is its lack of epidemic spread internationally' (De Cock and Brun-Vézinet, 1996).

Viruses have been defined as 'a piece of nucleic acid surrounded by bad news' (Oldstone, 1998, p. 8). They are genetic material covered with a coat of protein molecules. They do not have cell walls, are parasitic, and can only replicate by entering host cells. The genetic material of viruses is commonly DNA, or less frequently RNA. Viruses have few genes compared with other organisms: HIV has fewer than 10 genes (as does Ebola and measles); smallpox has between 200 and 400 genes. The smallest bacteria has 5,000–10,000 genes (Oldstone, 1998, p. 9). Humans have between 30,000 and 80,000 (Ridley, 2000, p. 5).

HIV belongs in the family of viruses known as retroviruses, scientifically called *Retroviridae*. The first retroviruses were only identified in the 1970s. All members of this family have the ability to produce latent infections. HIV is in a virus group called the lentiviruses. These develop over a long period, producing diseases, many of which affect the immune system and brain (Schoub, 1999). The viruses have a unique enzyme, reverse transcriptase. Outside the cells they infect, they consist of two strands of RNA. Once they infect a cell they make DNA copies of their own RNA and are able to reproduce. It is this feature as well as the ability of the virus to mutate rapidly which makes it hard to develop pharmaceutical responses.

▶ How HIV Works

For infection to occur, the virus has to enter the body and attach itself to host cells (see Figure 9-1). HIV attacks a particular set of cells in the human immune system known as CD4 cells. There are two main types of CD4 cells. The first type are CD4 positive T cells which organise the body's overall immune response to foreign bodies and infections. These T helper cells are the prime target of HIV. For a person to become infected, virus particles must enter the body and attach themselves to the CD4 cells. HIV also attacks immune cells called macrophages. These cells engulf foreign invaders and ensure that the body's immune system will recognise them in the future.

Once the virus has penetrated the wall of the CD4 cell it is safe from the immune system because it copies the cell's DNA, and therefore cannot be identified and destroyed by the body's defence mechanisms. Virus particles lurk in the cells until their replication is triggered. Once this happens they make new virus particles that bud from the surface of the host cell in vast numbers, destroying that cell as they do so. These viruses then go on to infect more CD4 cells.

When a person is infected a battle commences between the virus and the immune system. There is an initial burst of activity during which many cells are infected, but the immune system fights back, manufacturing immense numbers of antibodies. This period is marked by an unseen and unfelt war in a person's body. The viral load

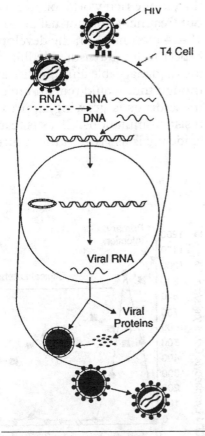

FIGURE 9-1 The virus in action
Source: Whiteside and Sunter (2000), p. 7.

is high, the immune system is taking a knock, and the person's HIV status cannot be detected using standard tests. This is commonly called 'the window period' and lasts from several weeks to several months. At this stage a person is highly infectious as his or her viral load (the number of viral particles they are carrying) is considerable. This fact is of epidemiological importance. The more people there are in the early stage of infection, the greater the chance of effective transmission between people. An infected person will usually experience an episode of illness at the end of the window period—but this will often resemble flu and will not be seen as a marker for HIV.

The window period is followed by the long incubation stage. During this phase, the viruses and the cells they attack are reproducing rapidly and being destroyed as quickly by each other. Up to 5% of the body's CD4 cells (about 2,000 million cells) may be destroyed each day by the billions of virus particles (Schoub, 1999, p. 85). Eventually, the virus is able to destroy the immune cells more quickly than they can be replaced and slowly the number of CD4 cells falls. In a healthy person there are 1,200 CD4 cells per microlitre of blood. As infection progresses, the number will fall. When the CD4 cell count falls below 200, opportunistic infections begin to occur and a person is said to have AIDS. Infections will increase in frequency, severity and duration until the person dies. It is these opportunistic infections that cause the syndrome referred to as AIDS.

The period from HIV infection to illness and death is crucial. It was generally believed that, in the rich world, on average people lived for ten years before they began to fall ill. Without treatment, the normal period from the onset of AIDS to death was thought to be a further 12–24 months. With the development of effective anti-retroviral therapies, infected people can expect to live a reasonable life for a longer time. Indeed, it is hoped that AIDS can be turned into a manageable chronic disease like diabetes. In this event, people could expect to live longer though they would remain infected. However, recent evidence suggests that viral resistance to these drugs is growing, approximately 20% of new HIV diagnoses in the UK are of drug resistant mutations.[1] If, as is feared, this phenomenon is generalised, then the threat from the epidemic is as great in the future as it is in the present.

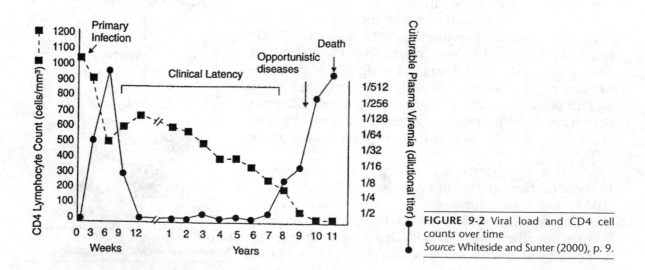

FIGURE 9-2 Viral load and CD4 cell counts over time
Source: Whiteside and Sunter (2000), p. 9.

Development and use of anti-retroviral therapies creates new problems:

- the virus mutates, there are over 120 sites in its structures which can mutate, and 'with hundreds of millions of virus particles being produced daily, it is not difficult to see how readily mutations occur which give rise to a wide range of biological variants even within the same individual' (Schoub, 1999, p. 87). This gives rise to drug resistance.
- if people perceive AIDS as 'just' a chronic manageable condition they may be less inclined to take precautions against infection.

The incubation period in the developing world was thought to be shorter—between six and eight years. This was based on the assumption that people in the poor world had more challenges to their immune systems, poorer nutrition, and less access to health care. It seemed inevitable that they would progress to symptomatic AIDS faster. However of six African studies reported in 1996, four suggested progression rates similar to those in the industrial world, and two found shorter periods. Data then were 'scanty and are limited to sub-Saharan Africa' (Mulder, 1996, p. 15). Schoub (1999) notes, 'little is known as yet about the rate of progression in African patients where the prognosis appears to be considerably worse (than among homosexual men in Western countries)' (Schoub, 1999, p. 42; parentheses added).

One recent study found that the time from HIV illness to death is shorter for untreated patients in Uganda than in the rich world, and the spectrum of HIV/AIDS related disease is different. However the period from infection to illness did not seem to vary. This suggests that tropical diseases and infections such as TB or sexually transmitted infections do not hasten the progression of HIV to AIDS in Uganda (French et al., 1999, p. 509).

The issue of how long a period a person has between infection and illness is crucial for planning for the epidemic's economic and social impact. There is no one easy answer: time from infection to illness and from illness to death appears to be linked to disease environment, availability of health care and other factors. The period from onset of symptoms to death is shorter in poor countries. This has been borne out by a number of studies, most recently French et al. (1999) who speculate that it is because patients do not receive early and appropriate treatment—an obvious issue in resource-constrained environments.

The differences between the poor and rich worlds also apply to the rich and the poor worldwide, and come down to the following: people who are able to eat enough nutritious food, who lead stress-free lives and who are not exposed to multiple infections will stay healthy and live longer. This is true generally and does not apply just to those who are HIV infected. However HIV infection throws inequality into even starker relief. 'Extreme poverty deprives people of almost all means of managing risk themselves' (World Bank, *World Development Report*, 2000/01, p. 146). For the poor, HIV is more likely to be a death sentence than for those who can care for themselves and afford treatment.

Detecting HIV and Describing AIDS

HIV was hard to locate because it is a retrovirus, hiding itself in the body's immune system. The first tests detected the *antibodies* to the virus rather than the virus itself. These might be compared to foot-prints on a sandy beach: they show a person has been there even though that person cannot be seen. Antibodies show that a person has been (and in the case of HIV, is) infected. Even today, most screening and diagnostic tests are based on discovery of antibodies rather than the virus. These tests have a high degree of sensitivity (which means that they do not miss positive results—if the person is infected then the tests will show this) and specificity (which means that they do not miss negative results—if the person is not infected the tests will not suggest that they are). The most advanced tests have reduced the window period to about three weeks. People are said to be HIV positive when the HIV antibodies are detected in their blood.

It is more difficult to define AIDS. In areas where CD4 counts and viral loads can be measured, people are regarded as having AIDS when their CD4 count falls below 200. In most settings, however, the capacity to carry out such sophisticated tests does not exist. In such places AIDS is defined clinically by examining the patient and making an assessment of his or her condition. A number of opportunistic infections, some of which are common in HIV infected people, take particular advantage of a depleted immune system. TB is one of these. Complicating matters further, new drug therapies make it possible for people to move from a state of AIDS, when they are very sick, to one of being HIV positive and leading a fairly normal life.

▶ The Origin of HIV

HIV derives from a virus that crossed the species barrier into humans. It is closely related to a number of Simian (monkey) Immunodeficiency Viruses (SIVs) found in Africa. The evolution of the virus over time is traced through a 'family tree' as shown in Figure 9-3. This differs from the more familiar family tree because to read it you must start near the middle. In this case, the proximity of the different types of virus is an indication of how closely they are related. For example, HIV-1 is clearly related to chimpanzee SIV and HIV-2 to macaque SIV.

How did HIV enter the human population? Here we need to make a brief diversion to look at some other diseases. An important starting point is that the spread of diseases from animals to humans is not unique to HIV. Indeed we know that human diseases also spread to animals—but animals do not have access to science and the media, thus this goes unrealised and unremarked by most people. The influenza virus evolves in birds—waterfowl to be exact.[2] Virologists describe these birds as 'reservoirs' of infection. They carry nearly all known types of influenza, with no ill-effects, and spread them to the rest of the animal kingdom through their feces. Hence, many kinds of animals can get flu—horses, ferrets, seals, pigs—as well as human beings.

However, viruses can only infect and take over a cell if it has a proper 'receptor'. Human cells do not

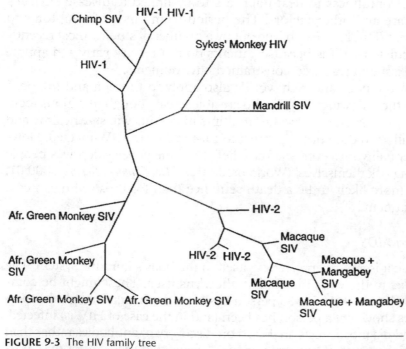

FIGURE 9-3 The HIV family tree
Source: Wills (1996)

have a receptor enabling them to contract avian flu directly. For human infection to occur another species must act as an intermediary; it can play this role by having a receptor for avian flu and humans in turn having a receptor for its flu. Pigs are one such species. The process can be as simple as a flu-contaminated duck dropping feces into the dirt in which a pig then rolls. The pig is then infected and passes the virus on to a farmer. It can also be more complex. It is possible for a pig to be infected with one kind of flu, say human flu, only to contract another avian flu. The pig then has two types of flu simultaneously. When the pig re-infects the human, it passes on a pig-bird-human influenza. The Hong Kong flu, for example, held seven genes from a human virus and one gene from a duck virus: these met inside a pig, producing a new hybrid.

It is not just different viruses that can combine to create new and possibly more deadly diseases in the host. Viruses, and indeed all diseases, also replicate themselves within the host. This gives rise to variants of the virus within one person. These may in turn recombine to create new variants, some of which may be more virulent or drug resistant.

The speed with which HIV-1 replicates makes it a formidable enemy. There are two major strains of HIV-1. Group M causes over 99% of the world's HIV/AIDS infections. Groups O and the newly discovered N cause the remainder (Stine, 2001). Group M is divided into eleven sub-types or clades (A to K). The ability of the virus to mutate rapidly has significance in the quest for both a cure and a vaccine.

The question of when and how HIV entered human populations has been a source of great debate. We know that at some point the virus entered the blood of humans and then spread through sexual contact from person to person. In west Africa the less virulent HIV-2 spread from macaque monkeys. HIV-1 spread from chimpanzees into humans in central Africa. Four lines of evidence have been used to substantiate the zoonotic (transmission of a disease from one species to another) origin of AIDS:

1. similarities in organisation of the viral genome
2. phylogenic[3] relatedness of a particular HIV strain to that of SIV in the natural host
3. geographical coincidence between the SIV and particular HIV strains
4. plausible routes of transmission (Van Rensburg, 2000).

How did HIV cross the species barrier? We know that it is not an easily transmittable disease. It is carried in body fluids, with the highest concentration in blood, semen and vaginal secretions. For transmission to occur it had to enter the human body and reach the infectable cells. It thus had to breach the skin or mucosal barriers. There are a number of hypotheses as to how this might have happened:

- *Bush meat.* It is not hard to imagine a hunter killing, or someone butchering, an infected monkey and in the process contaminating a cut on his hand with the monkey's blood.
- *Contaminated vaccine.* This is most elegantly (and lengthily) argued by Hooper (1999). He suggests that experimental polio vaccination campaigns in central Africa in the 1950s, using vaccine cultivated on chimpanzee kidneys, may have provided the opportunity for the virus to cross the species barrier.
- *Contaminated needles.* The arguments above may explain how the virus crossed into humankind but they do not explain the rapid spread. It has been suggested that vaccine campaigns and poorly equipped clinics in rural Africa may have contributed to this through the use of unsterilised needles on one patient after another.

- *Ritual behaviour*. Finally, it has been suggested that use of monkey blood in certain rituals might have caused transmission. This hypothesis reflects a high degree of ethnographic ignorance and no little prejudice, as no one has described these rituals or given any examples as to where they take place.

The second and third hypotheses place the beginnings of the epidemic in the twentieth century. Hooper suggests that the polio campaigns of the late 1950s in Congo and Rwanda were the spark that ignited the fire. The cut hunter view has been used to suggest that the epidemic originated in infection across the species barrier in the 1930s.[4] Interestingly, in this case the transfer of the virus from an animal into a human may have happened on a number of previous occasions. However, because on those occasions each infected person did not in turn infect more than one other person, the potential epidemic petered out. There could have been a pool (or pools) of infection among isolated peoples in some parts of Africa for many years. What was different about the crossing of the species barriers in the 1930s (and the subsequent pattern of the epidemic) was the environment into which the virus was introduced. The upheavals of the colonial and post-colonial periods and development of modern transport infrastructure allowed HIV to spread quickly into the global community.

When all is said and done, the debate about the exact manner of zoonotic transmission is largely irrelevant. What matters today and in the future is that the virus has infected humans and is spreading fast.

▶ Modes of Infection

Fortunately for humankind, HIV is not a robust virus and it is hard to transmit. Unlike many diseases it can only be transmitted through contaminated body fluids. For a person to be infected, the virus has to enter the body in sufficient quantities. It must pass through an entry point in the skin and/or mucous membranes into the bloodstream. The main modes of transmission, in order of importance, are:

- unsafe sex
- transmission from infected mother to child
- use of infected blood or blood products
- intravenous drug use with contaminated needles
- other modes of transmission involving blood; for example, bleeding wounds.

Sexual Transmission

The vast majority of HIV infections are the result of sexual transmission. Initially most cases were discovered among homosexual men. This was because HIV was first identified in this group in the West. Moreover, the chances of infection are higher during anal intercourse than vaginal sex. The relative probability of HIV infection per type of exposure is shown in Table 9.1. There is a small chance that HIV can be transmitted through oral sex, especially if a person has abrasions in the mouth or gum disease.

The presence of sexually transmitted diseases (STDs), particularly those involving ulcers or discharges, will greatly increase the odds of HIV infection. An STD means that there is more chance of broken skin or membranes allowing the virus to enter the body. Furthermore, the very same cells that the virus is seeking to infect will be concentrated at the site of the STD because these cells are fighting the infection.

TABLE 9.1 Probability of HIV-1 infection per exposure

Mode of Transmission	Infections per 1000 Exposures
Female-to-male, unprotected vaginal sex	0.33–1
Male-to-female, unprotected vaginal sex	1–2
Male-to-male, unprotected anal sex	5–30
Needle stick	3
Mother-to-child transmission	130–480
Exposure to contaminated blood products	900–1000

Source: World Bank (1997a), p. 59.

Mother-to-child Transmission

After sexual transmission, the next most important cause of HIV infection is mother-to-child transmission (MTCT). It is known that the child can be infected with HIV prenatally, at the time of delivery, or postnatally through breastfeeding. Infection at delivery is the most common mode of transmission. A number of factors influence the risk of infection, particularly the viral load of the mother at birth—the higher the load, the higher the risk. A low CD4 count is also associated with increased risk. Anti-retroviral drugs may decrease the viral load and inhibit viral reproduction in the infant, thus decreasing the risk of MTCT. A number of studies of the use of anti-retroviral drugs to combat MTCT have shown that the chance of this transmission can be greatly reduced at a relatively low cost and using fairly simple treatment regimes.

An important issue requiring clarification is the role of breastfeeding. On the one hand, formula feeding reduces the risk of MTCT; on the other hand, it increases the risk of children dying of other causes, particularly when they live in poverty. Breastfeeding has been promoted in developing countries for many years as part of child health and survival strategies. There are many problems with formula feeding, including the cost and availability of the product in the short and long term, access to clean water, the means and fuel to boil the water and prepare the feed, and knowledge of how to mix the feed. The formula approach also means that women can be 'labeled' as being HIV positive, by virtue of their using replacement feed. Recent work suggests that the key to reducing risk is consistency in either breastfeeding or formula feeding an infant. Mixing the two is the most risky approach. 'A baby who is fed both the breast-milk of an HIV-positive mother and poorly made-up formula feeds is "getting the worst of both worlds" ' (Chinnock, 1996, p. 15).

Infection Through Blood and Blood Products

Use of contaminated blood or blood products is the most effective way of transmitting the virus as it introduces the virus directly into the bloodstream. This is one of the reasons why so many haemophiliacs were infected during the early years of the epidemic: they received unscreened blood products. It also accounts for early infections among recipients of blood transfusions. Fortunately, in most countries, the risks of transmission through this route are now minimal. Blood banks seek to discourage those who might be infected from donating blood, and the technology is available to test all donations. However, because of the window period when people are infected but the antibodies are not detectable, the risk of infection cannot be entirely eliminated. The problem is greatest where blood is sold by donors and this gave the initial impetus to the epidemic in a number of Asian countries.

Intravenous Drug Use

Drug users who share needles are at risk of infection. If the equipment or drugs are contaminated, then the virus will be introduced directly into the body. This has driven the epidemic in Eastern Europe, the former Soviet Union and parts of Asia.

Other Modes of Transmission

There is a possibility that HIV may be transmitted in other ways. Medical or other instruments that are contaminated can transmit the virus. Examples include dental equipment, syringes and tattoo needles. Sterilisation procedures should ensure that this does not happen. Accidents through needlestick injury or during surgery are a concern for medical staff. Standard precautions, use of gloves and sterilising equipment, will protect doctors and nurses against HIV transmission from patients, and vice versa.

▶ Responding to the Disease

First prize with any disease is to prevent it. If prevention programmes had been successful, there would be no story to tell around HIV and AIDS. Unfortunately prevention programmes have not been successful in many parts of the world, and, where the epidemic has been controlled, no one is quite sure what actually worked.

Prevention

The principle of successful prevention is ensuring that people are not exposed to the disease or, if they are, that they are not susceptible to infection. Vaccines provide the latter form of protection but are not yet available for HIV. Preventing infections through blood transfusion depends on screening all donations and discouraging potentially infected donors from donating their blood. Occupational exposure can be reduced through adopting universally accepted precautions regarding safety and sterility. In the event that a health care worker is exposed, immediate treatment with anti-retroviral therapy can greatly reduce the risk of infection. In the case of injecting drug users, simple procedures such as the use of sterilised needles and needle exchange programmes have been very successful in some countries.

Preventing Sexual Transmission

As sex is the main mode of transmission, prevention strategies are most important here. One of the first responses to the epidemic was to call for the isolation of HIV infected people. This was seen by many as impractical, oppressive and discriminatory. The one exception is Cuba. In the 1980s the authorities tested the entire population, isolating those found to be HIV positive in 'sanatoria'. This has contributed to the low level of HIV infection seen to date in that country. At the end of 1997, it was estimated that there were only 1,400 infected Cubans (UNAIDS/Pan American Health Organisation/WHO, 1998). However, for this approach to work, a high degree of governmental control is necessary, people entering the country who might be infected and/or spread the disease have to be tested, and there has to be good border control. In addition, there needs to be a programme of regular repeat testing. This was never an option for most countries and certainly not for poorer countries. Apart from the expense and difficulty of implementing such a programme, some argue that it is a violation of human rights.

To prevent sexual transmission there is a limited but potentially effective range of interventions. The first set of interventions is 'biomedical'; these aim to reduce sexual transmission. Good sexual health is paramount. This means that STDs should be treated immediately, and the availability of STD treatment in the rich world has probably played a major role in controlling HIV. Sexual practices that increase risk can be discouraged or made safer: a southern African example is 'dry sex' where a woman may use a drying agent in her vagina to increase friction during intercourse. This practice increases the risk of tears and abrasions, and can therefore facilitate the entry of the virus. The Filipino practice of inserting small metal balls into the penis, also in the belief that these *bolitas* increase pleasure, can create a portal for infection.

The most available biomedical intervention is the use of condoms. These provide a barrier to the virus and, if properly used, are effective. Both male and female condoms are available, but female condoms are more expensive and more difficult to use.

The second set of interventions seeks to prevent exposure to HIV by altering sexual behaviour; these are the Knowledge, Attitude and Practices and Behaviour (KAPB) interventions. First, people need to have *knowledge*, then they need to change their *attitudes* and finally alter their *practices* and *behaviour*. People are encouraged to stick to one partner, to delay first sexual intercourse, and to use condoms if they have more than one partner. This is the classic ABC message: A—abstain; B—be faithful; C—condom if necessary. The problem is that even if people have the knowledge, they may not have the incentive or the power to change their behaviour. If prevention is to move beyond knowledge to action, we must look at the socio-economic causes of the epidemic and intervene there too.

Treatment[5]

Enormous resources have gone into the search for a cure and a vaccine. Neither has yet been developed. However, there have been major advances in clinical treatment.

Developments in treatment have resulted in declining mortality rates from HIV among the rich. There are three stages in the treatment of HIV positive people. The first is when they are infected, but CD4 cell counts are high. At this point, the emphasis is on 'positive living'—staying healthy, eating the correct food, and so on. The second stage is when the CD4 cell count begins to drop. At this stage, prophylactic treatment to prevent TB and other common infections commences. The third stage is the use of anti-retroviral drugs to fight HIV directly.

Since the first anti-retroviral drugs were developed, many new generations of drugs have become available. At the moment anti-retroviral drugs may be used in single therapies (just one drug), double therapies (a combination of two drugs) or triple therapies (three drugs). The way the drugs act is shown in Figure 9-4. Single drug therapy is no longer used much because it causes fairly swift mutation of the virus into drug resistant strains. Dual therapy is cheaper than triple therapy, but the antiviral effect is less immediate as the viral load falls slowly and the viral control may be of a limited duration. Highly Active Anti-Retroviral Therapy (HAART) is any anti-retroviral regimen capable of suppressing HIV for many months and perhaps years in a significant number of individuals. Such is the case with triple therapy. It usually involves the use of two reverse transcriptase inhibitors and one protease inhibitor. Although not a cure, such treatments are effective in rapidly reducing the viral load to undetectable levels, thereby prolonging survival.

When to introduce a HAART regimen is of importance. Early treatment prevents damage to the body caused by high and prolonged viral loads—but it does use up the big guns sooner, which can decrease subsequent options if resistance builds up. That is why some clinicians prefer to step up the treatment gradually starting with single drug therapy. Cost is also a factor.

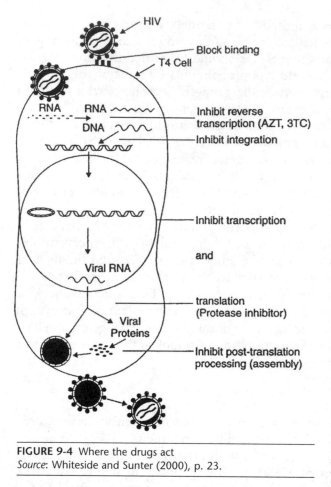

FIGURE 9-4 Where the drugs act
Source: Whiteside and Sunter (2000), p. 23.

The cost of anti-retroviral AIDS treatment in the rich world ranges between US$10,000 and US$20,000 per patient per year, although it can go much higher. Effective treatment of HIV/AIDS involves more than merely prescribing drugs: patients need regular consultations, testing for viral load and CD4 cell counts and, if treatment fails, testing for drug resistance. All this adds to costs.

Some Latin American countries (such as Brazil and Argentina) have been able to negotiate down the costs of the drugs. Argentina pays US$0.33 for AZT pills that previously cost US$2. Donations or subsidisation of drugs by the large pharmaceutical companies can reduce the costs of treatments. For example, in Senegal discounted drugs enable patients to have access to a range of therapeutic options costing between US$1,000 and US$1,800 per year (Gellman, 2000). It is not clear if the other costs are included.

The cheapest price on offer for the most advanced triple therapy at the beginning of 2001 was from drug company Cipla Ltd of Bombay who offered to sell drugs for US$600 per patient per year to the South African government and US$350 to non-governmental organisations (NGOs) (Swarms, 2001). The difference in cost may be based on whether the cost of observing patents is included or not. This is illustrated by comparing the costs of Flucanzole (used to treat AIDS-related meningitis) in Thailand (which does not observe patents), where the drug costs US$0.30 and Kenya (which does observe patents), where it costs US$18 (Kimani, 2000).

One study (Voelker, 2000) determined that for treatments to be affordable, HAART would need to be available at a monthly cost per person of US$10 for Zambia, US$20 for Botswana and US$45 for Mozambique. These figures assumed that it would be reasonable to spend 15% of the total health budget to treat 25% of the HIV positive population.

Anti-retroviral therapies are used when patient CD4 counts fall and their immune systems fail. Before this happens most HIV infected people will experience infection from other treatable diseases. These include candidiasis, meningitis and TB. In most of the poor world drugs to treat these infections are not available or are too expensive.

Of course, for the majority of AIDS sufferers all these treatments are out of reach because pharmaceutical companies are unprepared to make the drugs available at affordable prices. Furthermore most countries do not have the infrastructure to deliver the therapies.

Patient adherence is a real problem. Some triple drug therapies involve taking 18 pills a day in a particular sequence. Yet adherence to prescribed anti-HIV drug regimens is crucial for long-term success. Missing a single dose of medication may allow drug concentration in blood and tissues to drop below that needed for full HIV suppression. This decrease allows HIV replication to occur in the optimum environment for selection of drug resistant mutant strains. Combination pills are at present being developed to make adherence easier.

Vaccines

Intensive research is being carried out to develop a vaccine, so far with limited success. More than 15 years have passed since the first efforts, but as yet a vaccine remains elusive. Unfortunately the amount of money spent on researching AIDS vaccines is small (US$300–600 million a year) and is focused on strains found mainly in the US and Western Europe. The World Bank and the European Union, among others, have been involved in the search for new mechanisms and incentives to increase research and development of vaccines for developing countries. The International AIDS Vaccine Initiative (IAVI), based in New York, plays an increasingly important role in mustering resources and facilitating development.

▶ HIV and Other Diseases

As their immune systems are progressively suppressed, other diseases will affect HIV positive people. Most of these are not a threat to uninfected people. But people with HIV are very much more likely to develop active TB.[6] In the absence of HIV, the chance of developing TB is low. In the event that a person is co-infected with HIV, the chance rises greatly. It is estimated that 40–50% of people with TB in South Africa are co-infected with HIV, and one-third of people with HIV are expected to contract TB. This has to be seen against a general background of high TB infection in South Africa. The annual incidence there in 1998 was 254 per 100,000 people—in Europe it is 19; in China, 113, and in India, 187.

TB can be treated. For instance, the DOTS regime (Directly Observed Treatment, short course) has dramatically raised cure rates. But this is for all patients. Prophylactic treatment for HIV positive people is far more costly and problematic. Not for nothing are HIV and TB variously referred to as 'the terrible twins' and 'Bonnie and Clyde'.

New evidence suggests that there are links between HIV and malaria. It is possible that people with HIV contract malaria more easily and certainly have a poorer prognosis.

So far we have described disease and processes in the individual body as a result of this particular virus. Disease is of social and economic significance. It causes groups of people to become infected, fall ill and die. HIV/AIDS is unique. The disease is sexually transmitted, therefore it affects prime-age adults; it is fatal and it is widespread. It is unusual for this group (prime-age adults) to be the target of any disease. This is why it has profound social and economic consequences. To understand the aggregate nature of disease, as a precursor to looking at these consequences, we need to understand something about HIV/AIDS epidemiology and epidemiology in general.

▶ Epidemiology

Epidemiology has been defined as 'the study of the distribution and determinants of health-related conditions and events in populations, and the application of this study to the control of health problems' (Katzenellenbogen et al., 1997, p. 5).

Epidemiology examines patterns of disease in aggregate. It describes the social and geographical distribution and dynamics of disease. However, as we shall see, this is not at all straightforward, especially with regard to HIV/AIDS, because:

- data can be confusing, often people do not distinguish between HIV and AIDS
- data quality is variable
- data are *constructed* according to a variety of implicit or explicit assumptions
- data may be *interpreted* according to biases which people bring depending on their discipline, politics or paymaster.

Data are important. We need to know where the epidemic is located and where it might spread if we are to design effective prevention interventions. If we want to consider the potential social and economic impact of an HIV/AIDS epidemic, we need to have some idea of the numbers of people who are infected with the virus, and who and where they are. We need to be able to predict how many people will fall ill and die and when this will happen. For example, an education department needs to know how pupil numbers will change and what effects the epidemic will have on teacher availability and training needs. In this section we are concerned with how we know about the epidemic, how we obtain data on the disease, how we understand it and interpret it and the policy implications of this understanding.

Epidemiology provides only some of the required information. In later chapters we shall add to what epidemiology has to tell us by reviewing another set of questions about *why* epidemics take different forms in different societies. Our argument is that there are social and economic characteristics which make an epidemic grow more or less rapidly. They determine whether the epidemic is concentrated in a few 'high risk' or 'core' groups or whether it becomes generalised to the wider population. These determinants, which make a society more or less *susceptible* to epidemic spread, are closely tied to the characteristics which make that society more likely to suffer adverse consequences resulting from increased illness and death. We use the term *vulnerability* to talk about this greater or lesser likelihood of adverse impact.

Epidemic Curves

A key concept is the epidemic curve. HIV—indeed, any disease—will move through a susceptible population, infecting some and missing others. Epidemics follow an 'S' curve, as shown in Figure 9-5. They start slowly and gradually. At a certain stage, a critical mass of infected people is reached and the growth of new infections accelerates thereafter. The epidemic then spreads through the population until many of those who are susceptible to infection have been infected. Some are lucky because even though they are susceptible, they never come into contact with an infectious person. With modern transport networks there are few instances of isolated communities. Hence, epidemics can rapidly go global. The large and rising global population also means that many more people will be infected.

In the final phase of an epidemic—where the 'S' flattens off at the top and turns down—people are either getting better or deaths outnumber new cases so that the total number alive and infected passes its peak and begins to decline. With most diseases the curve will decline rapidly. HIV and AIDS are different.

What sets HIV and AIDS apart from other epidemics is that there are two curves, as shown in Figure 9-5. With most other diseases, infection is followed by illness within a few days or, at most, weeks. In the case of HIV the infection curve precedes the AIDS curve by between five and eight years. This reflects the long incubation period between infection and the onset of illness. This is why HIV/AIDS is in some ways such a lethal epidemic compared to, say, Ebola fever. In the latter case, victims of the disease quickly and visibly fall ill, putting the general population and public health professionals on their guard. The community takes precautions to halt spread and the infected person is rapidly immobilised, reducing his or her infective potential.

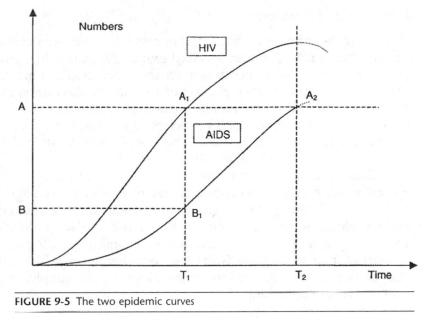

FIGURE 9-5 The two epidemic curves

HIV infection moves through a population giving little sign of its presence. It is only later, when substantial numbers are infected, that AIDS deaths begin to rise. People do not leave the infected pool by getting better because there is no cure. They leave by dying (of AIDS or other causes). The effect of life-prolonging ARTs is, ironically, to increase the pool of infected people.

Figure 9-5 illustrates this point clearly. The vertical axis represents numbers of infections or cases of illness and the horizontal represents axis time. At time T_1, when the level of HIV is at A_1, the number of AIDS cases will be very much lower, at B_1. AIDS cases will only reach A_2 (that is, the same level as A_1) at time T_2. By then years will have passed and the numbers of people who are infected with HIV will have risen even higher.

Figure 9-5 also shows that while prevention efforts may aim to lower the number of new infections, the reality is that without affordable and effective treatment, AIDS case numbers and deaths will continue to increase after the HIV tide has been turned.

Beyond the point T_2, the lines are dotted. This is because we do not know how either the HIV or the AIDS curves will proceed. In only two poorer countries, Uganda and Thailand, does national HIV prevalence (and incidence—see below) appear to have peaked and turned down.

Figure 9-5 shows an epidemic curve. But a national epidemic is made up of many sub-epidemics, with different gradients and peaks. These sub-epidemics vary geographically and in terms of their distribution among social or economic groups. In many countries in the poor world HIV spread first among drug users and commercial sex workers (CSWs). From there it moved into other groups: mobile populations, men who visited sex workers, and eventually into the broader population. One common feature in both the rich and poor world is that HIV spreads among people at the margins of society, the poor and dispossessed.

Incidence and Prevalence

Incidence is the number of new infections which occur over a time period. The *incidence rate* is the number of infections per specified unit of population in a given time period. Rates can be per 1,000, per 10,000 or per million for rare diseases. The time may be per annum, but in the case of more rapidly moving infections it may be days or weeks. *Prevalence* is the absolute number of infected people in a population at a given time—it is a still photograph of current infections. The *prevalence rate* is the percentage of the population which exhibits the disease at a particular time (or averaged over a period of time). A numerical example and an illustration appear in Table 9.2 and Figure 9-6, respectively.

Data on incidence and prevalence are key statistics for tracking the course of the HIV epidemic. With HIV, prevalence rates are given as a percentage of a specific segment of the population. Commonly used groups are antenatal clinic attendees, adults aged between 15 and 65, blood donors, men with STDs, or the 'at risk' population—usually taken to mean 15- to 49-year-olds who are sexually active. Uniquely, HIV prevalence is given as a percentage rather than as a rate, as is the case for other diseases. Why this is the case is not clear; it may be because of the need to communicate figures simply, or because advocates find percentages most compelling.

TABLE 9.2   Incidence and Prevalence

Year	Population	Incidence (actual)	Incidence rate per 1000	Prevalence	Prevalence rate (%)
1	9,750	0	0	0	0
2	10,000	50	5	50	0.5
3	10,500	50	4.7	100	1.0
4	11,000	150	13.6	250	2.3
5	12,000	750	62.5	1,000	8.3

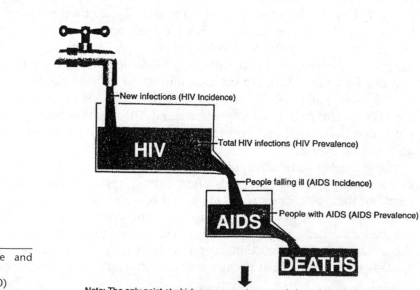

FIGURE 9-6 HIV/AIDS incidence and prevalence
Source: Whiteside and Sunter (2000)

Annual incidence is calculated by subtracting the previous year's prevalence from that of the current year. Because we don't know when people were actually infected—we only know the date on which their serostatus is ascertained—the data (incidence) which would be most helpful in measuring the impact of prevention efforts are simply not available. Moreover, high incidence may occur even when prevalence has levelled off, because those dying are being replaced by new infections.

Currently we have to use prevalence data to track how the epidemic is moving through a population, comparing one year with another. The aim of control and prevention measures is to reduce both prevalence and incidence. To achieve this the number of new infections produced by each existing infection must be reduced.

The Reproductive Rate

The gradient, final height and rate of decline of an epidemic curve is determined by the average number of secondary cases generated by one primary case in a susceptible population and the period over which this takes place. This is also known as 'the basic reproductive number' and is represented by the symbol R_0 (Anderson and May, 1992; Anderson, 1999). In order for an epidemic to be maintained, R_0 has to equal 1; in other words, each person who gets better or dies has to infect one other person. At this point the disease is endemic but stable. When $R_0 > 1$, each person infects more than one other person, the number of cases will rise. When $R_0 < 1$ then the epidemic will be disappearing. In South Africa in 2000 the R_0 for HIV was estimated at 5, while that of malaria was 100 (Whiteside and Sunter, 2000, p 10).

The percentage or number infected in a population depends on the degree of susceptibility of individuals in that population. This term is usually used in the narrow biomedical sense of transmission efficiency. 'Transmission efficiency is expressed as the probability that a contact will occur between infected and susceptible individuals multiplied by the likelihood that a contact will result in transmission' (Anderson, 1996, p 73). In this book we argue that susceptibility is far more than the result of biomedical events in the body; understanding and acting on this insight is fundamental both to reducing the rate of spread of the HIV/AIDS epidemic and to dealing with its long-term economic and social consequences.

Most epidemics are of relatively short duration. This is determined by the time from initial infection to the end (recovery or death) of the infectious period. Cholera epidemics may last only a few months in any one location. A measles epidemic with its typical two-week period from infection to illness will last between six months to a year. In the case of a disease where the gestation period is several years, the epidemic will last for decades. This is the case with HIV and it may be similar with nvCJD.

The HIV curve tells us where the epidemic has been. Projections tell us where it might go. HIV is not on its own important for understanding the social and economic impact of the epidemic. What is important is the AIDS curve (see Figure 9-5). If we are to consider impact we need to have an idea of the size of the potential AIDS epidemic which will hit a particular society.

How bad is the epidemic? How many people are infected and will die? How serious and global a crisis is it? These are all questions which are seldom posed in a precise way. Those who believe AIDS is a 'crisis' believe it is *the* major challenge facing most of the world. Thus 'Acquired immunodeficiency syndrome (AIDS) has become a major development crisis. It kills millions of adults in their prime' (General Assembly on HIV/AIDS, 2001). A memorandum issued on 2 June 1999 to World Bank staff and supporters announcing the new AIDS in Africa initiative (World Bank, *World Development Report*, 1998), stated: 'This fire is spreading. AIDS already accounts for 9% of adult deaths from infectious disease in the developing world. By 2020, that share will *quadruple* to more than 37%. The global death toll will soon surpass the worst epidemics of recorded history.'

Those who deny that there is an acute problem come in various shades: some say that there is no evidence of increased illness; others say that this can be explained by poverty, urbanisation or drug use. Even where the seriousness of the issue is recognised there is often debate over the exact figures. Effectively, people say: 'If you can't tell us exactly what is going on, why should we believe you at all?' This is a facet of denial processes which appears throughout the history of the epidemic.

Data Sources

This section looks at how data are derived. We begin with AIDS case data and then go on to look at HIV. We establish the ways in which the epidemic trajectory differs from country to country, and how social, economic and cultural situations determine this. Here we provide a background to some of the difficulties in obtaining and interpreting such data.

Key data sources include governments, non-governmental organisations, academic establishments, and in some instances the private sector. Data are of variable quality but—*and this is important to note*—all data produced by all agencies originate from the countries themselves. Thus data reflect what is available in countries and what they choose to report. Epidemiologists and statisticians may make assumptions and extrapolate, but they are dependent on the information they are given.

Two main bodies collect and compile international data. UNAIDS produces estimates of AIDS cases, HIV prevalence in various groups, numbers of deaths and orphans. These data are collected and published annually in the *Report on the Global HIV/AIDS Epidemic*. Thus we are told that in 1999, 5.4 million people were newly infected, 2.8 million died and 34.3 million were living with HIV/AIDS. UNAIDS also produces country epidemiological factsheets.[7]

The second source of data is the United States Bureau of Census which collates official data and also data from many other published and 'grey literature' sources.[8] Staff of the Bureau can be seen at all conferences of note photographing posters, collecting papers and checking findings with people on site.

AIDS Case Data

In the early years of the epidemic, AIDS case data were the main source of information. Each year or month the 'body count' rose. This was most vividly demonstrated in Randy Shilts's documentation of the first few years of the epidemic, largely in the US (Shilts, 1987). As the 1980s unfolded, AIDS cases were reported from more and more countries across the world. Graphs were produced showing exponential increases in the numbers of cases and deaths. Unfortunately there was public confusion between HIV and AIDS, aided and abetted by press reports which failed to distinguish between infection and disease.

In the poor world reporting required that someone actually took the time and trouble to notify public authorities that they were seeing AIDS patients. The question was and still is: 'Do we have a clear picture of the number of AIDS cases or deaths?' The answer is 'No', and indeed we never did.

In most countries AIDS is not a notifiable disease, which means that medical staff are not legally required to report cases. Even if they do there are serious constraints to this process:

- reporting may be very slow. It takes time for data to flow into a central point and be collated
- data may be inaccurate because of unwillingness to report cases. This may be due to stigma associated with AIDS; to potential discrimination by medical insurance companies, not paying for treatment of AIDS related conditions, and by the life insurance industry excluding claims where the cause of death is given as AIDS
- the condition from which a person dies may not be recognised as being AIDS related. Instead the patient may be recorded as having, for example, TB or meningitis
- doctors may feel that it is pointless to report cases as there is no incentive, they are too busy or they get no feedback.

Many people in poor countries are not seen by the formal medical services. Figure 9-7 shows the numbers of 'filters' a report has to go through before it becomes an official 'case'; in other words, before it is counted. The right-hand column shows the factors which can prevent this. Consider that somebody is dying in a small house, in a small village, several miles on foot from the nearest motorable road and many miles from the nearest all-weather road. There is a small clinic ten miles away but the medical orderly has not been paid for several months and has little in the way of drugs or equipment. The person's family has exhausted its resources and strength in caring for her. How is this person to become a 'case' recorded in the capital city some 300 or more kilometres away?

The fact is that no poor country has counted its AIDS cases. Indeed even in hospitals, many of which lack test kits, we cannot know how many AIDS cases there really are. What then is the value of AIDS case data? First, if they are collected consistently and in sufficient quantities, trends will be apparent. Second, they can give an indication of the scale of the problem. Finally, they can show where the epidemic is located by age, gender, mode of transmission and geographical area. Figure 9-8 illustrates the situation in Malawi in 1995. The first cluster of cases is those resulting from mother-to-child transmission. The next is for young women, peaking in the 20–24 age group, and finally there is a cluster of male deaths in the 30–34 age group.

Most social and economic statistics have political ramifications. AIDS

	AIDS case not recorded because:
Person falls ill with AIDS	
↓	
Is seen by formal medical service	→ Person visits traditional healer/does not seek care
↓	
Is correctly diagnosed	→ Is not correctly diagnosed or diagnosed with an opportunistic infection
↓	
Case recorded	→ Case not recorded
↓	
Record sent to data collection point	→ Report not forwarded/lost in post, etc.
↓	
Data collected and published	→ Report lost/not published

FIGURE 9-7 The problems of AIDS case reporting

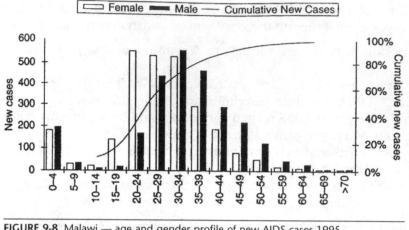

FIGURE 9-8 Malawi — age and gender profile of new AIDS cases 1995
Source: Loewenson and Whiteside (1997).

case data have always been 'political'. In the early years of the epidemic, countries were reluctant to admit to the existence of the disease because of what they felt its presence might suggest or imply about the morals and behaviour of their citizens, or what it might do to the tourist industry. This was the initial reaction in Kenya and Thailand.

Perhaps the most telling example of the politicisation of data was in Zimbabwe. The first report to the Global Programme on AIDS in Geneva was of several hundred cases in 1987. A few weeks later South Africa (then still under the apartheid regime) reported 120 cases. Within days the Zimbabwean government reduced its reported cases to 119 (*AIDS Analysis Africa*, 1990, p. 6).

The next potential data source is AIDS deaths. However, with few exceptions, there is no vital registration in poorer countries, and even where there is, information will not be collected on the cause of death by disease. Where death data are recorded information can be extracted. But we must always remember that even if AIDS cases are accurately recorded at any given time, they reflect the HIV infections of five or more years earlier.

HIV Data

HIV data tell us how many people are infected in a population, and are most frequently presented as prevalence. Ideally data would show exactly who in a population is infected and when they were infected. This would allow plans to be made for care and support of infected people and their families and human resource management. Deaths make families less able to provide for their members, the workforce less able to work, and increase demand for services such as health and welfare. Such data should also enable the epidemic to be tracked and the success (or failure) of interventions to be measured.

The ideal survey would cover an entire population. Every individual would give a blood or saliva sample for testing. Such a survey would furnish a point prevalence (the prevalence at that point in time). To track the epidemic, subsequent surveys would have to be carried out. This would be a logistical nightmare, would be costly and would raise ethical issues: do you compel people to take part? If people are identified then what do you do with them? As mentioned earlier, this type of survey has only been done in Cuba—an island with a population of 11.1 million.

Second best would be a population-based random survey which samples men and women across age groups to provide a representation of the situation in the whole population within certain calculable bounds of error. Such surveys have been done in a few places. They are expensive, require a lot of organisation, raise ethical issues and need to be repeated if they are to have value. In the past one of the major obstacles to population-based surveys was that the

HIV test required blood. Taking blood is an invasive procedure to which many people will not consent. The development of saliva tests over the past few years has made population surveys much more viable.[9]

Presently available data are drawn mainly from samples of specific population sub-groups. These are then extrapolated to larger populations. UNAIDS notes that different types of epidemic require different types of surveillance:

> In largely heterosexually driven epidemics where there is evidence that men and women in the general population have become infected with HIV in significant numbers, HIV surveillance is based . . . on pregnant women attending antenatal clinics that have been selected as sentinel surveillance sites . . . the more regular the studies, the clearer the picture of current prevalence. Where data are not available for the current year, all available data points are plotted on a curve, and an estimate for the current year is made according to what is known about the course of epidemics with predominantly heterosexual transmission. To account for differences in the spread of HIV, this is generally done separately for urban and for rural areas. (UNAIDS, 2000f, p. 116–18)

Many sub-Saharan African countries and a few in Asia and the Caribbean have conducted regular antenatal clinic HIV prevalence studies since the end of the 1980s. Antenatal clinic attenders provide a good sample because they are sexually active and adult. A major advantage is that blood is routinely taken from women attending these clinics for a number of standard tests and surveys can be repeated.

Population-based surveys were rare. However, where they have been done they show that in heterosexually driven epidemics the differences between these data and those from pregnant women are not great (Figure 9-9). Thus antenatal clinic data may be used cautiously as a proxy for the general population.

In most countries in Asia, South and Central America and Eastern Europe, the first manifestations of the disease, AIDS cases, were found in particular groups. These became subject to epidemiological surveillance. It was assumed that they represented high-risk behaviours. They included intravenous drug users; men who have sex with men, and sex workers and their clients. Here the methods for estimating HIV prevalence are different. What is needed is information on HIV prevalence in each group with high-risk behaviour, together with estimates of the size of each of these populations and the prospect of the epidemic bridging to the broader population. 'Since these behaviours are often socially unacceptable and sometimes illegal, information on both HIV prevalence levels and the size of the population affected can be much harder to come by. Consequently, uncertainties around these estimates may well be greater for countries where the epidemic is concentrated in specific

_____ **BOX 9.2** _____

ANTENATAL SURVEYS

Antenatal HIV surveys are based on a sample of women attending antenatal clinics. A portion of the blood drawn for routine testing will be marked with the woman's age, the clinic's location and possibly some other social, economic or marital status data, and then sent for testing. This testing is called *anonymous* and *unlinked*. In other words, individual women cannot be identified as the source of a particular sample.

Such surveys should be done on a regular basis, either every year or every two years. In India they were initially done every six months to give rapid, consecutive results.

There are biases: younger women will be overrepresented as they are more sexually active and likely to fall pregnant; HIV positive women will be underrepresented as HIV infection reduces fertility.

An obvious drawback is that the survey is confined solely to women attending state antenatal clinics. It does not cover those women who either do not have access to state health care or who can afford to see private practitioners.

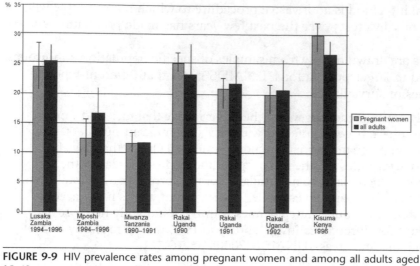

FIGURE 9-9 HIV prevalence rates among pregnant women and among all adults aged 15–49
Source: UNAIDS (2000F)

groups' (UNAIDS, 2000f, pp. 116–18). A good example of the difficulties is countries where drug possession is a capital offence. In these circumstances it is particularly hard to track the epidemic in intravenous drug users.

UNAIDS presents data in its annual reports, but it is hedged with caveats. Estimates of new HIV infections and HIV related deaths are developed through 'simple back-calculation' procedures, which are based on the 'well-known natural course of HIV infection which determines the relationship between HIV incidence, prevalence and mortality' (UNAIDS, 2000f, pp. 116–18). Estimates for mother-to-child transmission (including breastfeeding) and HIV mortality in children are calculated from countries' age-specific fertility rates and documented region-specific rates of mother-to-child transmission.

Private sector companies and organisations are beginning to collect data for their own purposes. We know that in southern Africa insurance companies are gathering such information because they routinely test people before offering cover. These data are biased to those applying for policies and are often commercially sensitive, and so they tend not to be publicly available. For companies wishing to estimate how the epidemic is going to affect their workforce, the advent of saliva and urine tests mean surveys can be carried out more easily. These tests are non-invasive and relatively cheap. In consultation with the workers, this information was collected by one major employer in Botswana and how, if it is correctly and sensitively used, it can be valuable in designing company responses to the impact of the epidemic.)

Finally it is a routine procedure to test blood donations and these data can provide a picture of what is going on in what should be a low-risk group. Blood donors may be considered a low-risk group because organisations collecting blood try to exclude HIV positive people.

HIV data are also collected and constructed according to political social and other biases. The mere act of looking for HIV in one particular group has political and social significance. A national epidemic is the construct of a particular reporting system embedded in a specific polity which filters information into data; it is the signal which is modulated out of the background noise. The polity is a part of the modulating process. It defines and enables the reporting system, and may itself be an aspect of the relative susceptibility of societies. For example, a political system that insists on classifying HIV infections by 'race' would present one perspective. A system which refused to recognise the existence of male homosexuality or widespread intravenous drug use would present another filter; and a political system which could not afford to report accurately because there was no money for test kits would produce yet another slant.

Arguments about numbers may also be politically charged. This was apparent in the correspondence pages of the *South African Medical Journal* in 2000. Four independent researchers—Dorrington, Bradshaw, Bourne and Abdool Karim (Dorrington et al., 2000)—argued that the officially stated decline in HIV prevalence from 1998 to 1999 (from 22.8% to 22.4%) was incorrect. An examination of the 1999 results showed that prevalence fell only in Mpumalanga, a province with 7% of South Africa's population. Otherwise rates of infection showed little or no change in three provinces and rose in the remaining five. Dorrington et al. (2000) therefore concluded, using population weighted methods, that national prevalence should not have fallen; rather, a small increase was to be expected. Government officials and a respondent from the South African Medical Research Council (2000) argued that the data were accurate, and castigated Dorrington et al. for their pessimism, for their failure to approach the Department of Health before writing with 'whatever suggestions they might have', and for not 'joining in an active partnership against HIV/AIDS'.

Readers may think that this debate smacks of rearranging the deckchairs on the *Titanic*. The magnitude of the crisis is not debated, just the detail. However such a discussion points to the danger of debating figures rather than focusing on what they tell us about dealing with prevention and impact mitigation. It also shows the defensiveness of some governments (Dorrington et al., 2000).

The Use of Data

Data have three key functions: advocacy, prevention and prediction.

Advocacy requires people to see and understand the potential for the epidemic to develop and the impact it may have. The problem, clear from the preceding discussion, is that AIDS data are inadequate and outdated and HIV data do not show a visible epidemic.

Prevention remains the goal of all in the field of HIV/AIDS. HIV data give a picture of where the epidemic is located, the scale of the problem and who should be targeted for prevention interventions. They help in assessing if prevention activities are working. A decline in prevalence among younger women is seen as the first sign of hope. However this needs to be treated with caution, as it is not clear if the infections are averted or simply deferred. Women may be uninfected in their late teens because they do not have sex or because they use condoms. They become infected later, when they become sexually active or decide to have children.

Lack of incidence data also means that if the prevalence plateaus, we cannot be sure whether this is because people who die are being replaced with new infections. The turnover can be considerable. An apparently stable epidemic hides many deaths and new infections. The new generation of tests—both blood and saliva—may assist in providing incidence data which will help to show whether interventions are having any effect. But few give any consideration to the question of the impact of the disease. HIV infections become AIDS cases and AIDS deaths. AIDS cases need care, and AIDS deaths cut to the core of households and societies, leaving orphans and impoverishment.

Prediction tells us about the future course of the epidemic and its possible impacts. This is done through modelling. Here we use HIV data because AIDS case data have limited value. While it is useful to know the scale of the problem facing us in the present, what is most important in planning for impact is to know what will happen in the future. How many people will fall ill? How many orphans will there be? In order to look into the future the epidemic has to be projected through a process of modelling.

Mathematical models (which are translated into computer programmes) may be used to create projections of the course of the epidemic and its impacts, and more specifically estimate their magnitude.

HIV/AIDS projection models may be used for several different purposes, such as:

- projecting HIV prevalence and numbers
- projecting future AIDS cases, AIDS related deaths and orphans
- examining the demographic impact of AIDS and addressing questions regarding the impact of AIDS on population growth rates, the population age structure, numbers of orphans,[10] and life expectancy
- simulating different intervention strategies and comparing their strengths and weaknesses
- assessing the impact of the AIDS epidemic; for example, in terms of increased health expenditure and interactions with other diseases such as tuberculosis[11]
- creating different scenarios which illustrate the effect of different assumptions on the projected outcome

All models depend on data, and the amount and type of data required will depend on the model used, the questions to be answered and the data to hand. This in turn will depend critically on whether a country is able to collect information about its epidemic. Does it have the technical, financial and political resources to do so? It is important to keep in mind that models are simply tools which may be used to guide decision making. Models are by definition a *representation* of an *aspect* of reality and they cannot possibly replicate the complexity of any real situation.

Conclusion

This chapter has described the basic science of HIV and the AIDS. It has explored the epidemiological instruments through which we 'know' or construct our knowledge about the aggregate effects of the disease.

At every point we see that data about the epidemic—including what it is, how it is defined, and how it is measured—are not neutral. Data are the outcomes of social, economic and cultural processes. Data are political: it may be that the governments do not want to admit that the epidemic exists; perhaps because they don't believe that their citizens 'behave in *these* ways', or that there are potential economic consequences. Admitting that there is an uncontrolled epidemic may also mean acknowledging that government policies have failed.

The form in which data appear depends on who is looking at information and how: doctors look among their patients, actuaries among those who form their client pool, anthropologists and sociologists in the particular group they are studying. Bias also arises from who is paying for the data—if you have an AIDS project it is not in your interest to show there is no AIDS!

Data are used to model the development and impact of the epidemic, but this, too, is not a neutral activity: models have assumptions and biases built into them according to the disciplines and beliefs of those who develop them and those who pay for them. Results will be interpreted differently according to the biases (explicit or implicit) of those who use them.

We have indicated the disease has implications far beyond the individual bodies that it destroys. It has social and economic causes and consequences.

Chapter
10

Opportunistic Infections

Opportunistic Infections and Cancers Associated with HIV Disease/AIDS

Gerald Stine

► Chapter Concepts

- Suppression of the immune system allows harmless agents to become harmful opportunistic infections (OIs).
- OIs respond well to Highly Active Antiretroviral Therapy (HAART).
- OIs in AIDS patients are caused by viruses, bacteria, fungi, and protozoa.
- In the United States, about 95% of the HIV-infected are coinfected with herpes 1 and/or 2, and hepatitis B. About 40% are coinfected with hepatitis C, and 35% are coinfected with tuberculosis.
- Human Herpes Virus-8 may be the cause of Kaposi's sarcoma.
- In the United States, 14% of AIDS patients are coinfected with tuberculosis.
- The cost of treating OIs can be very high.
- There are two types of Kaposi's sarcoma (KS): Classic and AIDS-associated.
- KS is rarely found in hemophiliacs, injection drug users, and women with AIDS.
- The clinical presentation of OIs has been impacted by the use of protease inhibitors.
- Self-evaluation/education quiz is offered.

► What Is an Opportunistic Disease?

Humans evolved in the presence of a wide range of parasites—viruses, bacteria, fungi, and protozoa that do not cause disease in people with an intact immune system. But these organisms can cause a disease in someone with a weakened immune system, such as an individual with HIV disease. The infections they cause are known as **opportunistic infections** (OIs). Thus, OIs occur after a disease-causing virus or microorganism, normally held in check by a functioning immune system, gets the opportunity to multiply and invade host tissue after the immune system has been compromised. For most of medical history, OIs were rare and almost always appeared in patients whose immunity was impaired by either cancer or genetic disease.

With improved medical technology, a steadily growing number of patients are severely immuno-suppressed because of medications and radiation used in bone marrow or organ transplantation and cancer chemotherapy. HIV disease also suppresses the immune system. Perhaps as a corollary to their increased prevalence, or because of heightened physician awareness, OIs seem to be occurring more frequently in the elderly, who may be rendered vulnerable by age-related declines in immunity. New OIs are now being diagnosed because the pool of people who can get them is so much larger, and, in addition, new techniques for identifying the causative organisms have been developed. However, most of the infections considered opportunistic are not reportable, which interferes with a clear-cut count of their growing numbers.

Although OIs are still not commonplace, they are no longer considered rare—they occur in tens of thousands of HIV/AIDS patients. But despite this increase, physicians and their patients have reasons to be optimistic about their ability to contain these infections. The reasons are: (1) In a massive federal effort, driven by the HIV/AIDS epidemic, researchers are finding drugs that can prevent or treat many of the OIs; and (2) various anti-HIV drug therapies have shown promise for warding off OIs by boosting patients' immune systems.

▶ The Prevalence of Opportunistic Diseases

The prevalence of OIs in the United States is very high. There are some 300,000 HIV-seropositive individuals with T4 or CD4+ cell counts below 200/μL of blood. Worldwide, there are over 6 million HIV infected with a T4 or CD4+ cell count of 200 or less. More than 100 microorganisms—bacteria, viruses, fungi, and protozoa—can cause disease in such individuals, even though only a fraction of these (17) are included in the current surveillance definition for clinical AIDS. In a large survey from the Centers for Disease Control and Prevention (CDC), such OIs were diagnosed in 33% of individuals at one year and in 58% at two years after documentation of a T4 cell count below 200/μL. In 1995, 1997, 1999, and 2002 the CDC presented guidelines for prevention and treatment of OIs in HIV-infected persons (*MMWR*, 2001). The new treatments for OIs have extended the survival of AIDS patients, but they have also opened new issues. With the growing proportion of longer-term AIDS survivors, new OIs have become prominent, together with concerns about cost, compliance, drug interactions, and quality of life (Laurence, 1995; *MMWR*, 1995). The six most common AIDS-related OIs are bacterial pneumonia, candidal esophagitis, pulmonary/disseminated TB, mycobacterium avium complex disease, herpes simplex reinfection, and *Pneumocystis carinii* pneumonia or PCP. The year 1997 marked the first time, since the AIDS pandemic began in the United States, that the incidence of AIDS-defining OIs among HIV-infected persons fell in number from the previous year's total.

▶ Prophylaxis Against Opportunistic Infections

In the United States

Drug prophylaxis against OIs has become a cornerstone of treatment for AIDS patients. For example, the prevalence of PCP dropped from about 80% in 1987 to about 20% by mid-1994 because of excellent drug therapy. The mortality of PCP without treatment is almost 100% (Dobkin, 1995). Researchers at the University of California, San Francisco, found that on average it costs $215,000 to extend by one year, the life of an HIV-infected patient with PCP who is treated in an intensive care unit (Laurence, 1996). That is more than twice the comparable care cost for 1988. Part of the reason given was that as people with AIDS survived longer, they were presenting with third, fourth, and fifth episodes of PCP superimposed on other chronic infections. The downside to OI prophylaxis is that it is difficult to find drugs that work without harmful side effects. In addition, viruses and organisms that cause OIs become resistant to the drugs over time. This is one of the primary reasons researchers are looking for ways in which to boost an immunosuppressed patient's immune system.

In Underdeveloped Nations

Treatment recommendations that are taken for granted in the developed world are not always applicable in Africa or other resource-limited regions and must, at times, be explored in different clinical settings. For example, cofactors such as prevalence of malaria and other parasitic infections or the geographical distribution of various microbial organisms and viruses may alter the pattern or order of clinical events that will be observed as people progress to late stage disease.

▶ Opportunistic Infections in HIV-Infected People

AIDS is a devastating human tragedy. It appears to be killing about 95% of those who demonstrate the symptoms. One well-known American surgeon said, "I would rather die of any form of cancer rather than die of AIDS." This statement was not made because of the social stigma attached to AIDS or because it is lethal. It was made in recognition of the slow, demoralizing, debilitating, painful, disfiguring, helpless, and unending struggle to stay alive.

Because of a suppressed and weakened immune system, viruses, bacteria, fungi, and protozoa that commonly and harmlessly inhabit the body become pathogenic (Figure 10-1). Prior to 1998, about 90% of deaths related to HIV infection and AIDS were caused by OIs, compared with 7% due to cancer and 3% due to other causes. Now, with the use of antiretroviral drugs, OIs cause about 50% of deaths. Liver and kidney organ failure, heart disease, and various cancers are on the increase as the cause of death in AIDS patients.

POINT OF INFORMATION 10.1

THE CHANGING SPECTRUM OF OPPORTUNISTIC INFECTIONS

Twelve years ago there was hardly any standardized use of protective agents to block the infectious complications or opportunistic infections (OIs) associated with HIV-induced immunodeficiency. Now there is an array of drugs that can be used in strategies to prevent or delay nearly all the major OIs. With this advancement has come the need to weigh the pros and cons of various strategies. Cost, antimicrobial resistance, drug interactions, and pill overload are all important considerations.

Effect of Anti-HIV Therapy on Opportunistic Infections

As presented in Chapter 4, the use of anti-HIV combination drug therapy (AIDS drug cocktails) has produced a number of unexpected results in patient response to those drugs. Soon after combination therapy began, physicians witnessed a rather confusing or unusual presentation of OIs. In some cases certain OIs improved, in others the situation deteriorated. Such changes in OIs expression are occurring now, at a time when hundreds of thousands of HIV-infected Americans are on **Highly Active Antiretroviral Therapy (HAART)**.

Treatment in the HAART Era

HAART therapy appears to scramble the human immune system. When HIV patients take retroviral medicines that control HIV replication, their immune systems begin to recuperate in ways that are puzzling and controversial. For example, patients recover immunity to some deadly opportunistic infections but appear unable to fight diseases for which they were vaccinated as children, for example, tetanus, or to target HIV itself. Collectively, such observations indicate HAART patients can only raise successful immune responses against pathogens they see regularly. For example, cytomegalovirus is an organism found in almost everybody's blood, so the immune systems of HAART patients see the pathogen constantly and generate cells and antibodies that attack it. But tetanus is something people rarely encounter, so HAART patients, unlike their HIV-negative counterparts, fail to raise immune responses against it. The ultimate irony is that HAART, when successful, destroys all but a few million HIVs that are forced into hiding.

Recent studies suggest that the incidence of esophageal condidiasis and, by inference, other forms of *Candida* infection has fallen by 60% to 70% on patients treated with HAART. The use of HAART dramatically changed the epidemiology of opportunistic infections and is clearly associated with gradual recovery of the immune system (Powderly et al., 1998; Ledergerber et al., 1999).

This information aside, when HIV is controlled with the antiretroviral drugs, immunity to infections—other than HIV—usually starts to return. As a result, some opportunistic infections go away without specific treatment; and sometimes patients can stop prophylactic treatment for certain opportunistic diseases. However, entering year 2004, it is still unclear who can stop prophylaxis safely, and who cannot.

Studies from 1998 through 2004, using protease inhibitor drugs in HAART have shown that virtually no patient whose T4 level rose to and stayed over 200 per microliter of blood (μL) developed an OI. This is the strongest evidence to date that immune reconstruction is occurring with protease inhibitor therapy, and suggests that it occurs early and with quite modest improvements in T4 cell levels. The implication is that the search for immunorestorative therapy other than with the current antiretroviral is somewhat less urgent than previously believed, though still a clear priority.

Ominous Shadows

It is now clear that sustained viral suppression is not feasible in all patients receiving HAART. A post-HAART era is projected, during which resurgence of opportunistic infections will be seen. This era may be marked by a higher rate of infection by antimicrobial-resistant microorganisms in patients with HIV infection than in the pre-HAART era of the late 1980s to the late 1990s.

Viral Load Related to Opportunistic Infections

HIV clinicians have recently looked at the predictive value of plasma HIV RNA for the development of three OIs: PCP, CMV, and MAC. Using a database of patients participating in AIDS Clinical Trial Groups (ACTG), for every 1-log increase in plasma HIV RNA level, the risk of developing one of these OIs was increased 2- to 3-fold. Plasma HIV RNA level was predictive of an increased risk of an OI independent of T4 cell count, which also predicted OI risk. This information confirms that maintaining control of viral replication may be a critical component of preventing OIs in HIV-infected patients.

HIV-Related Opportunistic Infections Vary Worldwide

The course of HIV infection tends to be similar for most patients: Infection with the virus is followed by seroconversion and progressive destruction of T4 or CD4+ cells. Yet the opportunistic infections and malignancies that largely define the symptomatic or clinical history of HIV disease vary geographically. People with HIV and their physicians in different regions confront distinct problems, mainly because of differences in exposure, in access to diagnosis and care, and in general health.

Comparisons between the data about opportunistic infections in different countries must be made with care. But most developing nations lack the facilities and trained personnel to identify opportunistic infections correctly; consequently, their prevalence may be underreported. Clinicians in developed countries can order sophisticated laboratory analyses to identify pathogens. Those in developing countries must rely on signs and symptoms to make their diagnoses. Oral candidiasis and herpes zoster are easy to diagnose without laboratory backup because the lesions are visible. While some pneumonias and types of diarrhea can be specified, others, such as extrapulmonary tuberculosis, cytomegalovirus infections, cryptococcal meningitis,

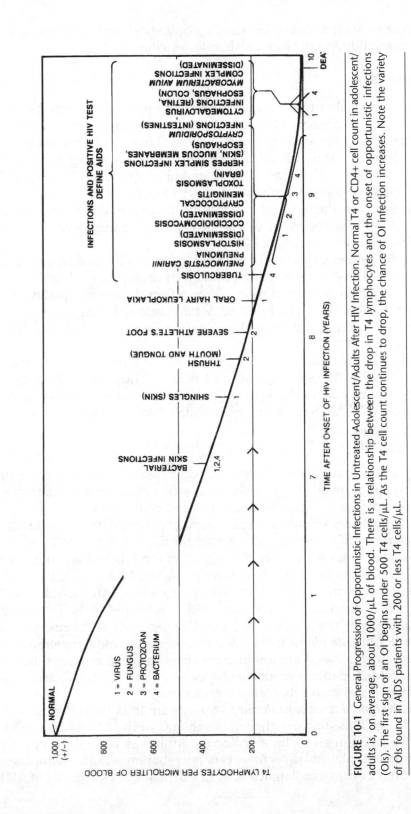

FIGURE 10-1 General Progression of Opportunistic Infections in Untreated Adolescent/Adults After HIV Infection. Normal T4 or CD4+ cell count in adolescent/adults is, on average, about 1000/μL of blood. There is a relationship between the drop in T4 lymphocytes and the onset of opportunistic infections (OIs). The first sign of an OI begins under 500 T4 cells/μL. As the T4 cell count continues to drop, the chance of OI infection increases. Note the variety of OIs found in AIDS patients with 200 or less T4 cells/μL.

and systemic infections such as histoplasmosis, toxoplasmosis, microsporidiosis, and nocardiosis, go underreported due to the lack of laboratory facilities.

Socioeconomic Factors

Geography explains much about the varying patterns of opportunistic infections, but a decisive factor is often financial capacity. On the most fundamental level, money is needed to create an infrastructure that limits exposure to pathogens. Thus, while few people with HIV in wealthy countries develop certain bacterial or protozoal infections, they are a major cause of death in poor areas that cannot provide clean water and adequate food storage facilities.

Financial resources also affect clinicians' abilities to diagnose AIDS and, when appropriate, to provide the proper medicine. AIDS patients in Africa often die of severe bacterial infections because they don't have the antibiotics or the clinical care they need. They don't survive long enough to develop diseases such as PCP.

United States, Europe, and Africa—The United States and Europe on one end, and Africa on the other, represent the global extremes of financial resources for health care. The most common opportunistic infections each region faces reflect the overall quality of health care, sanitation, and diet. For example, Thailand and Mexico belong to the large group of nations that have intermediate incomes and correspondingly intermediate patterns of HIV complications (Harvard AIDS Institute, 1994).

AIDS patients rarely have just one infection (Table 10.1). The mix of OIs may depend on lifestyle and where the HIV/AIDS patient lives or has lived. Thus, a knowledge of the person's origins and travels may be diagnostically helpful. (Note: a number of the symptoms listed in the CDC definition of HIV/AIDS can be found associated with certain of the OIs presented.)

Fungal Diseases

In general, healthy people have a high degree of innate resistance to fungi. But a different situation prevails with opportunistic fungal infections, which often present themselves as acute, life-threatening diseases in a compromised host (Medoff et al., 1991).

Because treatment seldom results in the eradication of fungal infections in AIDS patients, there is a high probability of recurrence after treatment (DeWit et al., 1991).

Fungal diseases are among the more devastating of the OIs and are most often regional in association. AIDS patients from the Ohio River basin, the Midwest, or Puerto Rico have a higher-than-normal risk of histoplasmosis (his-to-plaz-mo-sis) infection. In the Southwest, there is increased risk for coccidioidomycosis (kok-sid-e-o-do-mi-ko-sis). In the southern Gulf states, the risk is for blastomycosis. Other important OI fungi such as ***Pneumocystis carinii*** (numo-sis-tis car-in-e-i), ***Candida albicans*** (kan-di-dah al-be-cans), and ***Cryptococcus neoformans*** (krip-to-kok-us knee-o-for-mans) are found everywhere in equal numbers. Because of their importance as OIs in AIDS patients, a brief description of histoplasmosis, candidiasis, *Pneumocystis carinii* pneumonia, and cryptococcosis are presented.

Histoplasmosis (Histoplasma capsulatum)—Spores are inhaled and germinate in or on the body (Figure 10-2). This fungal pathogen is endemic in the Mississippi and Ohio River Valleys. Signs of histoplasmosis include prolonged influenza-like symptoms, shortness of breath, and possible complaints of night sweats and shaking chills. Histoplasmosis in an HIV-positive person is considered diagnostic of AIDS. In about two-thirds of AIDS patients

TABLE 10.1   Some Common Opportunistic Diseases Associated With HIV Infection

Organism/Virus	Clinical Manifestation
Protozoa	
Cryptosporidium muris	Gastroenteritis (inflammation of stomach-intestine membranes)
Isospora belli	Gastroenteritis
Toxoplasma gondii	Encephalitis (brain abscess), retinitis, disseminated
Fungi	
Candida sp.	Stomatitis (thrush), proctitis, vaginitis, esophagitis
Coccidioides immitis	Meningitis, dissemination
Cryptococcus neoformans	Meningitis (membrane inflammation of spinal cord and brain), pneumonia, encephalitis, dissemination (widespread)
Histoplasma capsulatum	Pneumonia, dissemination
Pneumocystis carinii	Pneumonia
Bacteria	
Mycobacterium avium complex (MAC)	Dissemination, pneumonia, diarrhea, weight loss, lymphadenopathy, severe gastrointestinal disease
Mycobacterium tuberculosis (TB)	Pneumonia (tuberculosis), meningitis, dissemination
Viruses	
Cytomegalovirus (CMV)	Fever, hepatitis, encephalitis, retinitis, pneumonia, colitis, esophagitis
Epstein-Barr	Oral hairy leukoplakia, B cell lymphoma
Hepatitis C (HCV)	Liver cirrhosis or cancer (major reason for liver transplants)
Herpes simplex	Mucocutaneous (mouth, genital, rectal) blisters and/or ulcers, pneumonia, esophagitis, encephalitis
Papovavirus J-C	Progressive multifocal leukoencephalopathy
Varicella-zoster	Dermatomal skin lesions (shingles), encephalitis
Cancers	
Kaposi's sarcoma	Disseminated mucocutaneous lesions often involving skin, lymph nodes, visceral organs (especially lungs and GI tract)
Primary lymphoma of the brain	Headache, palsies, seizures, hemiparesis, mental status, or personality changes
Systemic lymphomas	Fever, night sweats, weight loss, enlarged lymph nodes

Patients with compromised immune systems are at increased risk for all known cancers and infections (including bacterial, viral, and protozoal). Most infectious diseases in HIV-infected patients are the result of proliferation of organisms already present in the patient's body. Most of these opportunistic infections are not contagious to others. The notable exception to this is tuberculosis.

Disclaimer: This table was developed to provide general information only. It is not meant to be diagnostic nor to direct treatment.

(Adapted from Mountain-Plains Regional Education and Training Center HIV/AIDS Curriculum, 4th ed., 1992 updated, 1997; and from MMWR 2002.)

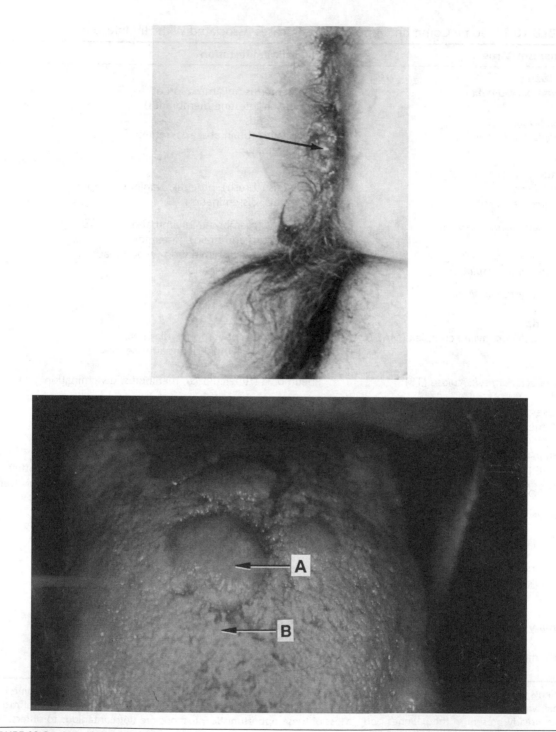

FIGURE 10-2   **A.** Anal Histoplasmosis. Histoplasmosis is caused by *Histoplasmosis capsulatum* and causes infection in immuno-compromised patients. *(Courtesy CDC, Atlanta)* **B.** AIDS patient's tongue showing multiple shiny, firm Histoplasma erythematous nodules (see arrow A) and thrush (see arrow B). *(Photograph courtesy of Marc E. Grossman, New York)*

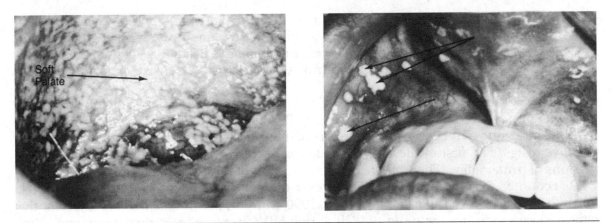

FIGURE 10-3 Thrush. **A.** An overgrowth of *Candida albicans* on the soft palate in the oral cavity of an AIDS patient. **B.** Creamy patches of candida that can be scraped off, leaving a red and sometimes bleeding mucosa. *(A., Courtesy CDC, Atlanta; B., Schiodt, Greenspan, and Greenspan 1989.* American Review of Respiratory Disease, *1989, 10:91–109. Official Journal of the American Thoracic Society. © American Lung Association)*

with histoplasmosis, it is the initial OI. Over 90% of cases have occurred in patients with T4 cell counts below 100/μL. (Wheat, 1992).

Candidiasis or Thrush (Candida albicans)— This fungus is usually associated with vaginal yeast infections. It is a fungus quite common to the body and in particular inhabits the alimentary tract. It is normally kept in check by the presence of bacteria that live on the linings of the alimentary tract. However, in immunocompromised patients, especially those who have received broad spectrum antibiotics, candida multiplies rapidly. Because of its location in the upper reaches of the alimentary tract, if unchecked, it may cause mucocutaneous candidiasis or **thrush,** an overgrowth of candida in the esophagus and in the oral cavity (Figure 10-3). Mucosal candidiasis was associated with AIDS patients from the very beginning of the AIDS pandemic (Powderly et al., 1992). In women, overgrowth of candidiasis also occur in the vaginal area.

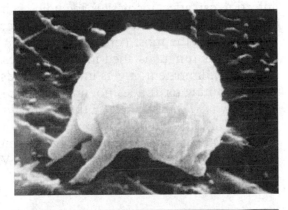

FIGURE 10-4 Scanning Electron Microscope Image of *P. carinii* Attached to Embryonic Chick Lung Cells in Culture. Note the tubular extensions through which it extracts nutrients from host lung tissue. *(Propagation of Pneumocystis carinii in Vitro,* © *Pediatric Research, 11:305–316)*

Oral or esophageal candidiasis causes thick white patches on the mucosal surface and may be the first manifestation of AIDS. Because other diseases can cause similar symptoms, candidiasis by itself is not sufficient for a diagnosis of AIDS.

Pneumocystis carinii—The life cycle and reproductive characteristics of *P. carinii* are not completely understood because the organism is difficult to culture for laboratory study. However, the molecular biology and molecular taxonomy are now being rapidly constructed (Walzer, 1993; Stringer et al., 1996). Virtually everyone in the United States by age 30 to 40 has been exposed to *P. carinii*. It lies dormant in the lungs, held in check by the immune system. Prior to the AIDS epidemic, *P. carinii* pneumonia was seen in children and adults who had a suppressed immune system as in leukemia or Hodgkin's disease and were receiving chemotherapy. In the AIDS patient, the onset of *P. carinii* pneumonia is insidious—patients may notice some shortness of breath and they cannot run as far. It causes extensive damage within the alveoli of the lungs (Figure 10-4).

Prior to 1981, fewer than 100 cases of *P. carinii* infection were reported annually in the United States; yet 80% of AIDS patients develop *P. carinii* pneumonia at some time during their illness. This is one of the few AIDS-related conditions for which there is a choice of relatively effective drugs. The first of these to be made available was the intravenous and aerosolized versions of pentamidine. There are frequent recurrences of this infection. (Montgomery, 1992). PCP accounted for a diagnosis of AIDS in over 65% of AIDS cases in 1990. In 1994 it had fallen to 20% due to available therapy (Ernst, 1990; Murphy, 1994). The triad of symptoms that almost always indicates the onset of PCP during HIV disease is fever, dry cough, and shortness of breath (Grossman et al., 1989). *P. carinii* pneumonia is unlikely to develop in people with HIV disease unless their T4 cell count drops below 200 (Phair et al., 1990).

Cryptococcosis (Cryptococcus neoformans)—Since its discovery in 1894, *C. neoformans* has been recognized as a major cause of deep-seated fungal infection in the human host. The infection can affect many sites, including skin, lung, kidney, prostate, and bone. However, symptomatic disease most often represents infection of the central nervous system. Cryptococcal meningitis is the most common form of fungal meningitis in the United States (Ennis et al., 1993). This fungus is shed in pigeon feces, the spores of which enter the lungs. If the lung does not eliminate it, it gets into the bloodstream, travels to the brain, and can cause cryptococcal meningitis. It does not appear to be spread from person to person.

C. neoformans is a fatal OI that occurs in about 13% of AIDS patients (Brooke et al., 1990). It is acquired through the respiratory tract and most commonly causes cryptococcal meningitis. In AIDS patients, *C. neoformans* causes infection of the skin, lymph nodes, and kidneys. *Cryptococcus* cannot be cured and it does recur. Which anti-fungal drugs should be used is a subject of controversy.

Viral Diseases

Hepatitis C—Hepatitis means an inflammation or swelling of the liver. Viruses can cause hepatitis. Alcohol, drugs (including prescription medications) or poisons can also cause hepatitis. In late 1999, **hepatitis C** caused by the hepatitic C virus (**HCV**) was classified as an OI because the relative risk for liver-associated death is increased 7-fold in HIV-positive patients compared to non-HIV-infected individuals. It is estimated that 200 million people worldwide are infected with the hepatitis C virus. Over 4 million of the infected live in America.

HIV/HCV Means Double Trouble

The hepatitis C virus (HCV) is now at least four times as widespread in America than HIV. It kills between 10,000 and 15,000 each year and is predicted to kill 30,000 a year by 2010. Its transmission is similar to that of HIV. About 40% of HIV-infected in America, about 400,000 people, are believed to be coinfected with the HCV. Among some groups, primarily HIV-positive current and former intravenous drug users, the coinfection rate is thought to be about 90%. According to the National Hemophilia Foundation, the coinfection rate among HIV-positive hemophiliacs is equally high. For those who become infected with HCV, the virus produces no symptoms for 10–30 years. Then symptoms like fatigue, joint and abdominal pain, nausea, and lapses in concentration begin to set in. Because doctors have not traditionally screened patients for the virus, many people do not even know they are infected until their livers show signs of serious damage. Studies now indicate that HIV can greatly speed the progression of hepatitis C. That means that many with HIV may suffer advanced liver disease (cirrhosis of the liver) after just 5 or 10 years, even as the antiretroviral drugs boost their life expectancies. Studies on HCV's effects on AIDS patients have been contradictory, but the coinfection has been associated with a higher risk of progression to HIV disease and AIDS. The antiretroviral drugs used to fight HIV, particularly the protease inhibitors, place a great strain on the liver, the organ whose function is to metabolize them. Some patients infected with both viruses find that their bodies have great difficulty tolerating many HIV/AIDS medications. As yet, there is no national policy for dealing with this virus.

Herpes Viruses

Because of a depleted T4 or CD4+ cellular component of the immune system, AIDS patients are at particularly high risk for the herpes family of viral infections: cytomegalovirus, herpes simplex virus types 1 and 2, varicella-zoster virus, and Epstein-Barr virus.

Cytomegalovirus (CMV)—This virus is a member of the human herpes virus group of viruses. CMV is the perfect parasite. It infects most people asymptomatically. When illness does occur, it is mild and nonspecific. There have been no epidemics to call attention to the virus. Yet CMV is now considered the most common infectious cause of mental retardation and congenital deafness in the United States. It is also the most common viral pathogen found in immunocompromised people (Balfour, 1995).

The virus is very unstable and survives only a few hours outside a human host. It can be found in saliva, tears, blood, stool, cervical secretions, and in especially high levels in urine and semen. Transmission occurs primarily by intimate or close contact with infected secretions. The incidence of CMV infection prior to HAART therapy beginning in 1996, varied from between 30% and 80% depending on the geographical community tested. In the 1980s, over 90% of homosexual males tested positive for CMV (Jacobson et al., 1988).

CMV infection of AIDS patients usually results in prolonged fever, anemia (too few red blood cells), leukopenia (too few white blood cells), and abnormal liver function. CMV also causes severe diarrhea and HIV-associated retinitis resulting in eventual blindness (*Emergency Medicine*, 1989; Lynch, 1989; Dobkin, 1995).

Prior to HAART therapy, 75% of AIDS patients had an eye disease, with the retina the most common site (Russell, 1990). The retina, which is a light-sensitive membrane lining the inside of the back of the eye, is also part of the brain and is nourished by blood vessels. AIDS-related damage to these vessels produces tiny retinal hemorrhages and small cotton wool spots—early indicators of disease that are often detected during a routine eye examination (Figure 10-5). Since the beginning of HAART therapy, CMV retinitis has fallen to about 5% in AIDS patients.

In unusual circumstances, the virus can produce dramatic symptoms, such as loss of vision within 72 hours. Without treatment, CMV can destroy the entire retina in three to six months after infection.

Herpes Viruses Types 1 & 2 (HSV 1 & 2)—Herpes infections are one of the most commonly diagnosed infections among the HIV/AIDS population. Almost all HIV-infected individuals (95%) are coinfected with HSV 1 and/or HSV 2. Both viruses cause *severe* and progressive eruptions of the mucous membranes. HSV 1 affects the membranes of the nose and mouth.

Also, when herpetic lesions involve the lips or throat, 80% to 90% of the time they either precede or occur simultaneously with **herpes-caused pneumonia** (Gottlieb et al., 1987). Bacterial or fungal superinfections occur in more than 50% of herpes-caused pneumonia cases and are a major contributory cause of death in AIDS patients.

Mortality from HSV pneumonia exceeds 80% (Lynch, 1989). Herpes may also cause blindness in AIDS patients. The following is from Paul Monette's *Borrowed Time:*

> I woke up shortly thereafter, and Roger told me—without a sense of panic, almost puzzled—that his vision seemed to be losing light and detail. I called Dell Steadman and made an emergency appointment, and I remember driving down the freeway, grilling Roger about what he could see. It seemed to be less and less by the minute. He could barely see the cars going by in the adjacent lanes. Twenty minutes later we were in Dell's office, and with all the urgent haste to get there we didn't really reconnoiter till we were sitting in the examining room. I asked the same question—what could he see?—and now Roger was getting more and more upset the more his vision darkened. I picked up the phone to call Jamiee, and by the time she answered the phone in Chicago he was blind. ***Total blackness, in just two hours!***
>
> The retina had detached. (An operation on retinal attachment was successful and sight was restored. The cause of the retinal detachment was a herpes infection of the eyes.)

HSV 2 also affects the membranes of the anus, causing severe perianal and rectal ulcers primarily in homosexual men with AIDS. Herpes of the skin can generally be managed with oral **acyclovir** (Zovirax), Foscavir, or Famvir.

Herpes Zoster Virus (HZV)—Like herpes simplex, this virus has the potential to cause a rapid onset of pneumonia in AIDS patients. Untreated HZV pneumonia has a mortality rate of 15% to 35%. HZV is now monitored as an early indicator that HIV-positive people are progressing toward AIDS.

Protozoal Diseases

An increasing number of infections that have not been observed in immunocompromised patients are being found in AIDS patients. Two such infections are caused by the protozoans *Toxoplasma gondii*, and *Cryptosporidium muris*.

Toxoplasma gondii—*T. gondii* is a small intracellular protozoan parasite that lives in vacuoles inside host macrophages and other nucleated cells. It appears that during and after entry, *T. gondii* produces secretory products that modify vacuole membranes so that the normal *fusion* of cell vacuoles with lysosomes containing digestive enzymes is blocked. Having blocked vacuole-lysosome fusion, *T. gondii* can successfully reproduce and cause a disease called **toxoplasmosis** (Joiner et al., 1990). It can infect any warm-blooded animal, invading and multiplying within the cytoplasm of host cells. As host immunity develops, multiplication slows and tissue cysts are formed. Sexual multiplication occurs in the intestinal cells of cats (and apparently only cats); oocysts form and are shed in the stool (Sibley, 1992). Transmission may occur transplacentally, by ingestion of raw or undercooked meat and eggs containing tissue cysts or by exposure to oocysts in cat feces (Wallace et al., 1993).

In the United States, 10% to 40% of adults are chronically infected but most are asymptomatic. *T. gondii* can enter and infect the human brain causing **encephalitis** (inflammation of the brain). Toxoplasmic encephalitis develops in over 30% of AIDS patients at some point in their illness (Figure 10-6). The signs and symptoms of cerebral toxoplasmosis in AIDS patients may include

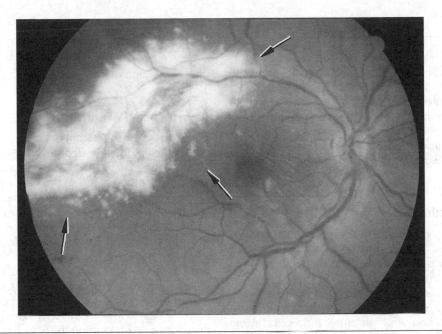

FIGURE 10-5   Cytomegalovirus Retinitis. The disease, as seen in this photograph, involves the posterior pole of the right eye. Fluffy white infiltrate **(cotton wool spots)** with a small amount of retinal hemorrhage can be seen in the distribution of the superior vascular arcade. *(Courtesy of Scott M. Whitcup, M.D., National Eye Institute, National Institutes of Health, Bethesda, Md.)*

fever, headache, confusion, sleepiness, weakness or numbness in one part of the body, seizure activity, and changes in vision. These symptoms can get worse and progress to coma and death unless toxoplasmosis is promptly diagnosed and treated. Thus, for most AIDS patients, it is believed that *T. gondii* is latent within their bodies and is reactivated by the loss of immune competence.

Cryptosporidium—*Cryptosporidium* is the cause of cryptosporidiosis, and is a member of the family of organisms that includes *Toxoplasma gondii* and *Isospora*. Its life cycle is similar to that of other organisms in the class Sporozoa. Oocysts are shed in the feces of infected animals and are immediately infectious to others. In humans, the organisms can be found throughout the GI tract. *Cryptosporidium* causes profuse watery diarrhea of 6 to 26 bowel movements per day with a loss of 1 to 17 liters of fluid (a liter is about 1 quart). It is an infrequent infection in AIDS patients, usually occurring late in the course of disease as immunological deterioration progresses.

Studies of transmission patterns have shown infection within families, nursery schools, and from person to person, probably by the fecal-oral route. The infection is particularly common in homosexual men, perhaps as a consequence of anilingus (oral-anal sex).

Bacterial Diseases

There is a long list of bacteria that cause infections in AIDS patients. These are the bacteria that normally cause infection or illness after the ingestion of contaminated food, such as species of *Salmonella*. Others, such as *Streptococci, Haemophilus*, and *Staphylococci* are common in advanced HIV disease. A number of other bacteria-caused sexually transmitted diseases such as syphilis, chancroid, gonorrhea, and chlamydial diseases are also associated with HIV disease.

_____BOX 10.1_____

A PHYSICIAN'S AGONIZING DILEMMA

Opportunistic infections are the primary threat to patients with AIDS; they are the main causes of illness and death. The cruel irony is that although there are 30 or more FDA-approved drugs to treat these infections, most cannot be used in patients receiving Zidovudine (ZDV) *because the combination drug therapy is devastatingly toxic to bone marrow.*

EXAMPLE:

Cytomegalovirus (CMV) Retinitis

CMV retinitis is one of the *worst* of the opportunistic infections (Gottlieb et al., 1987). Both the patient who contracts CMV retinitis and the treating physician confront an almost impossible dilemma: whether to continue the Zidovudine and risk blindness or to treat the retinitis and risk death from another infection. A physician recently said, "In my experience, I have never yet been able to combine Zidovudine with the experimental drug ganciclovir (DHPG), which is the only recognized treatment for CMV retinitis, because the combination destroys the bone marrow. I therefore face the virtually impossible task of asking a 25-year-old person: 'Which of these options do you prefer: to take Zidovudine and keep on living but go blind, or to preserve your sight by having retinitis treatment but risk dying?' That is a truly terrible question to ask of any patient, especially a young one." He continued, "Recently, I treated just such a young patient. He had been taking Zidovudine for AIDS when he contracted CMV retinitis. When I presented him with this agonizing choice, he told me, 'I definitely don't want to go blind. I want to be treated for this retinitis.' So he stopped taking Zidovudine and was started on DHPG treatment. He started to have seizures, which were a consequence of the toxoplasmosis brain abscess that eventually ended his life. Just before he died, he told me that the worst decision he ever made was to stop taking Zidovudine. "I should have stayed on it,' he said, 'and gone blind."' (Robert J. Awe, M.D., 1988)

Cryptococcal Meningitis

The situation for AIDS patients with cryptococcal meningitis is similarly depressing. Because of the severe bone marrow toxicity, it is virtually impossible to use amphotericin B, the effective treatment for this meningitis, at the same time as Zidovudine. Besides, the use of amphotericin B has its own side effects as can be noted from this excerpt from Paul Monette's *Borrowed Time: An AIDS Memoir:*

Amphotericin B is administered with Benadryl in order to avoid convulsions, the most serious possible side effect. It was about nine or ten when they started the drug in his veins, and I sat by the bed as nurses streamed in and out. A half hour into the slow drip, the nurse monitoring the IV walked out, saying she'd be right back, and a couple of minutes later Roger began to shake. I gripped him by the shoulders as he was jolted by what felt like waves of electric shock, staring at me horror-struck. Though Cope [the physician] would tell me later, trying to ease the torture of my memory, that "mentation" [mental activity] is all blurred during convulsions, I saw that Roger knew the horror (page 336).

When the nurse returned she looked at him in dismay: "How long has this been going on?" Then she ordered an emergency shot of morphine to counteract the horror. When at last he fell into a deep sleep they all told me to go home, saying they would try another dose of the ampho in a few hours. I was so ragged I could barely walk. So I left him there with no way of knowing how near it was [Roger's death], or maybe not brave enough to know.

Whichever option is chosen, the patient is bound to suffer, and perhaps die, either of cryptococcal meningitis or of some other infection.

One difference between AIDS and non-AIDS individuals is that bacterial diseases in AIDS patients are of greater severity and more difficult to treat. Two bacterial species, *Mycobacterium avium intracellulare* and *Mycobacterium tuberculosis* are of particular importance as agents of infection in AIDS patients (Table 10.2).

Mycobacterium avium intracellulare (MAI)—Over the past 40 years, MAI has gone from a rare, reportable infection to something that is common in most large American communi-

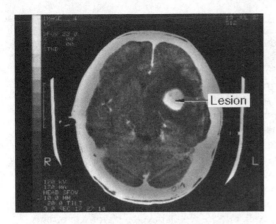

FIGURE 10-6 *Toxoplasma gondii* Lesions in the Brain. Radiographic imaging shows a deep ring-enhancing lesion located in the basal ganglia. *(By permission of Carmelita U. Tuazon, George Washington University)*

ties. Unlike tuberculosis, which is almost exclusively spread person to person, MAI is, in most instances, environmentally acquired. MAI exists in food, animals, water supplies, and soil, and enters people's lungs as an aerosol when they take showers.

The fact that MAI produced disseminated disease in AIDS cases was recognized in 1982. The epidemiology of MAI continues to evolve. MAI occurs in 18% to 43% of people with HIV disease and has been implicated as the cause of a nonspecific **wasting syndrome.** AIDS patients demonstrate **anorexia** (inability to eat), weight loss, weakness, night sweats, diarrhea, and fever. Some patients also experience abdominal pain, enlarged liver or spleen, and malabsorption. In contrast to viral infections, this bacterium rarely causes pulmonary or lung problems in AIDS patients. Among persons with AIDS, the risk of developing disseminated MAI increases progressively with time. AIDS patients surviving for 30 months had a 50% risk of developing disseminated MAI. It appears most HIV-infected persons will develop disseminated MAI if they do not first die from other OIs (Chin, 1992).

Mycobacterium tuberculosis—Tuberculosis (TB) infects one-third of the world's population, over 2 billion people, and is now the leading cause of illness and death in people infected with HIV. Tuberculosis is an infectious disease caused by the bacterium *Mycobacterium tuberculosis,* which is spread almost exclusively by airborne transmission. TB has been observed in elephants, cattle, mice, and other animal species. In 1993, TB was transmitted from an infected seal to its trainer in Australia. In the United States, monkeys are the primary source of animal-to-human transmission.

The disease can affect any site in the body, but most often affects the lungs. When persons with pulmonary TB cough, they produce tiny droplet nuclei that contain TB bacteria, which can remain suspended in the air for prolonged periods of time. (With respect to transmission, the cough to TB is like sex to HIV.) Anyone who breathes air that contains these droplet nuclei can become infected with TB. It has been suggested that there is a minimal chance of inhaling HIV in blood-tinged TB sputum (Harris, 1993).

About 10% of otherwise healthy persons who have latent tuberculosis infection will become ill with active TB at some time during their lives (*MMWR*, 1992). With HIV disease, the risk is 10% per year (Daar et al., 1993). It has been estimated that through year 2005, 16 million HIV-infected people worldwide will be coinfected with TB. HIV activates latent TB which erodes the lungs. TB in turn agitates HIV, speeding its destruction of the immune system. The result: In many countries, it is TB that most often triggers death in AIDS patients.

_____ BOX 10.2 _____

LIFE GOES ON!

by Wendi Alexis Modeste

What this epidemic has cost me is the complete faith I had in the medical profession. I was raised believing that doctors were second only to priests and God. They were never to be questioned. Whatever the doctor said was law. If a person didn't get well after seeing the doctor, somehow they (the patient) had done something wrong. This was pretty much standard thinking for middle-class African-Americans. For a variety of reasons (mainly no self-esteem) I became a drug addict, prostitute, convict, battered, homeless woman, in that order! With the exception of emergency room admissions (which are a joke and a whole 'nother story) I had no access to health care.

Now, as a PWA (person with AIDS) fortunately/unfortunately on SSI, Medicaid pays for my nine different AIDS medications, clinic visits, treatment, tests, etc. When I received the "exciting news" that I was eligible for "all" Medicaid benefits, I was still under the impression doctors were those super-intelligent, gifted, Christian, saint-like people. Girlfriend, I am here to tell you, AIDS has totally shot that Marcus Welby theory straight to hell!

Early in my diagnosis, I went to my physician because my tongue was almost completely covered with what looked like cottage cheese. There was also a horrible pink lesion dead center. The first time I showed it to my doctor he said, "Ugh," and made a face. He told me to wait a month. If nothing changed or got worse when I returned he'd have someone look at it. Being ignorant about the disease at that time, and still blindly believing in the medical profession, I waited a month, then returned. Again I showed the doctor my tongue. He asked me if I wanted him to write me a prescription for codeine and Valium. I totally freaked! By this time, I'd done some reading and realized I probably had thrush and some sort of herpes. This physician was aware of my serostatus. He also knew that I was a person with a 20-year history of drug abuse. I'd been in recovery less than a year and this jerk wanted to prescribe for me two of the most addictive and abused prescription drugs. I'd never mentioned being in pain or that I was experiencing any type of anxiety. I contacted the Executive Director of this health facility and asked to have a different doctor assigned to me. In an attempt to make me feel guilty about requesting a change, I was told about the problems doctors have in getting Medicaid reimbursement. I was neither intimidated nor impressed. A new doctor was

assigned. My new physician was very nice. After *I* told *him* what I thought my diagnosis was, he prescribed the appropriate medications. He was not trained in AIDS/HIV. I could have dealt with his ignorance because I knew he was trying. His nurse, however, was a different story. Every time she came to do my vitals she'd say the same thing: "I always get nervous when taking the temperature of you guys." She'd then force a little chuckle and go on to say, "Oh, well, I figure we all have to die of something." (I assume this was to show me what a courageous Florence Nightingale she was.)

Let me tell you, when you are burning up with a 103 degree temp. and your bowels haven't stopped running for a week, causing your butt to feel like it's on fire, it's real hard to be the patient, understanding AIDS educator. I really get crazy when the person I'm forced to educate is someone whose been privileged to more information than myself.

But life goes on!

One day I had a toothache. I go to the dentist. After waiting half the day, I'm brought into the treatment room for an X-ray. At first I thought the dental assistant had made a mistake. Surely this room had been prepared for a paint job. Everything was draped in white towels. The entire dental unit, including where my head, arms and feet went, was completely covered. The seat of the unit was securely wrapped up, as was the metal extension arm that holds the overhead dental lamp. All surfaces of the walls were also draped. When I asked the reason for this "painter preparation," I was informed it was done because I have AIDS, and they had to protect their other patients from coming into contact with my contaminated blood. Needless to say, I saw red! I knew I had to protect myself. I mean, what kind of dentistry were they practicing if they were concerned about my blood splattering that far and wide? What was even more frightening was that they'd done all this unnecessary draping and I was only having an X-ray. I filed a complaint with the Human Rights Dept.

I became a patient at the AIDS Care Center in Syracuse. My physician, a woman (need I say more?), is a caring person and well-educated about AIDS/HIV. My nurse/social worker is excellent, but as all of us living with AIDS know, shit happens. One day I awaken with enough yeast in my body to make all the baked goods in Central New York rise. My doctor isn't in. I wait a couple of days but can no longer stand the discomfort. I beg to see a doctor in the AIDS Care Unit. I'm assigned the doctor who sees the HIV-infected prisoners. (My heart and soul truly go out to those guys.) First he talks with me over the phone to find out if I can possibly wait another week when my doctor is due to return. I tell him my tongue is unrecognizable, the yeast in my esophagus is burning like a heart attack, and the Roto-Rooter service couldn't satisfy the itch caused by the yeast in my vagina. HELL NO, I can't wait another week! I go in to see him. I show him my tongue. I can't believe it, but like the first doctor, he uses that medical term, "Ugh," then says, "That does look nasty." At this point I'm ready to French kiss this idiot. But it gets worse. He won't touch me, let alone examine anything. He asks me what I think will work. I feel too badly to curse, so I tell him Mycelex, Myastatin suspension, Monistat 7. He writes the prescriptions and for good measure increases my acyclovir. For this he gets paid? He did nothing!

I'm now as educated as a lay person can be about HIV disease/AIDS. In addition to my doctor at the AIDS Care Center, I have a private primary care physician. Sometimes it's easier to get in to see this doctor. I call his office one day because there is swelling and burning on the sides of my tongue I cannot eat. My regular doctor isn't in, but one of his associates assures me if I come in to the office he'll see me right away and give me something to ease the pain so I can at least eat. As a fat person who proudly admits a genuine fondness for food, I can tell you not being able to eat registers serious panic in my soul. Nothing stops me from eating. I was probably the only overweight homeless dope addict living on the streets of NYC. Being scared is putting it mildly. I scrape up the carfare and go to the office. After waiting an unreasonably long time, Doogie Howser's twin comes in to see me and announces he's Dr. Jones, whom I spoke to on the phone. OK, I know not to judge a book by its cover. I mean, Doogie is pretty good on TV. Dr. Jones looks at my tongue and proceeds to ask a zillion questions, all of which are answered in my chart. Finally he says he's never seen an HIV-infected person or a person with AIDS, and frankly he doesn't know what to do. He then suggests I eat popsicles for a few days because the cold will soothe the pain and the sugar should help give me energy. I kid you not, this actually happened. This jerk prescribed me popsicles. I truly wished I could transmit the virus by biting at this point. He used me so he could write in his journal or resume (or somewhere) that he'd treated a person with AIDS. He could also charge Medicaid for nothing.

But this type of quackery must stop.

The last gripe I'm going to list is this patient statement I hear all the time when I get an unexplained fever or infection and no one can determine its origin. I'm told, "there hasn't been enough studies done on the paths this disease takes in women. Even less has been done on the effects of different AIDS medications on people of color." This is said to me as if it's my fault they don't know. This disease has been documented for ten years in both men and women. I know African-Americans were dying of AIDS long before the gay white community mobilized and, thank God, refused to lay down and die quietly. There is no excuse for the fact that there's no studies done on these populations.

I am thankful to Dr. Sallie Klemmens and nurse/clinician/social worker Judith Swartout at University Hospital's designated AIDS Care Center here in Syracuse. I am thankful for Dr. Barbara J. Justice who with God's help kept me alive when I lived on the streets of NYC. They are all examples of what the medical profession should be about. Dr. Justice made me feel that I counted and should be assertive about my health care. Though no longer my surgeon, she continues to be a source of inspiration and a fountain of information for me. These three are gems in a field I think is greatly overrated, overpaid, and run by capitalist male chauvinist pigs.

Though medical people wear white, that absence of color symbolizing purity and goodness, I beg you all, "Don't believe the hype!" We need a national health care system for everyone. As PWAs we must be assertive about our health care. Good health care is a right not a privilege.

As a child I cried when I learned there was no Santa Claus. When my illusion about the medical profession was shattered I got angry. I decided to fight with the only ammunition I had, education! **Knowledge gives one power.** A close friend of mine told me I shouldn't submit this article because I might offend some members of the medical profession. He also felt because I'm on Medicaid I'm not supposed to complain, I should be grateful. To his comments I respond, raised with two college-educated parents, never wanting or needing anything, I wasn't supposed to be a drug addict. Unfortunately I was. After 20 years of addiction, I wasn't supposed to be able to stop. I've been in recovery almost two years now.

I'm not supposed to be living with AIDS, but with God's help I'm happy and living large (as the kids say now).

The best things I do have always been what I'm not supposed to do!

Power to all PWAs!

Wendi Alexis Modeste, a PWA who was diagnosed in 1990, died August 25, 1994.
Source: Modeste, W.A., August 1991, Issue 68, PWA Coalition Newsline. Reprinted with permission.

Tuberculosis is not generally considered to be an OI because people with healthy immune systems contract TB. After infection with M. tuberculosis about 5% of immunocompetent individuals will develop TB (Daley, 1992). But, people with a depressed immune system are much more likely to develop the disease.

▶ TB and HIV

HIV infection is now considered to be the single most important risk factor in the expression of TB. HIV disease is associated with the reactivation of a dormant or inactive TB infection (Stanford et al., 1993).

M. tuberculosis infection occurs in about 35% of HIV-infected individuals. The CDC defines extrapulmonary TB combined with an HIV-positive test as diagnostic of AIDS.

According to the World Health Organization, TB worldwide is the leading cause of death in HIV-infected people and among adults from a single, infectious organism. TB has killed at least 200 million people since 1882, the date of the discovery of the bacterium that causes TB. Millions more die from TB each year. Globally, TB was estimated to account for 30% of AIDS-related deaths in 1999, and greater than 30% each year from 2000 through 2004. March 24 of each year is recognized as World TB Day.

In the United States, 14% of AIDS patients are also coinfected with TB. Health officials state that between 40% and 60% of those developing multidrug-resistant TB will die (Ezzell, 1993).

Other Opportunistic Infections

Other opportunistic infectious organisms and viruses and the diseases they cause and possible therapies are listed in Table 10.1. Table 10.2 separates OIs into the body parts most affected by a particular organism or virus.

From diagnosis until death, the AIDS battle is *not* just against its cause, HIV, but against those organisms and viruses that cause OIs. Opportunistic infections are severe, tend to be disseminated (spread throughout the body), and are characterized by multiplicity. Fungal, viral, protozoal, and bacterial infections may be controlled for some time but are rarely curable.

▶ Cancer or Malignancy in AIDS Patients

The word "malignancy" means a cancer. Specifically, cancer is an abnormal growth of cells that divide uncontrollably and may spread to other parts of the body. There are many kinds of cancer, which can involve just about any part of the body.

HIV infection carries with it a high susceptibility to certain cancers. Because of the severe and progressive impairment of the immune system, host defense mechanisms that normally protect against certain types of cancer are lost. Cancers develop in approximately 40% of AIDS patients. Four kinds of cancer that occur with increased frequency are: **progressive multifocal leukoencephalopathy, squamous cell carcinoma** (oral and anal), **non-Hodgkin's lymphoma,** and **HIV/AIDS-associated Kaposi's sarcoma (KS).** None of these cancers, except for KS, is considered to be an opportunistic infection because the rest are not infections. They are cancers arising from cells that have lost control of their division processes. Of the nine types of AIDS-associated cancers, KS occurs with the greatest frequency and is discussed in some detail. Lymphomas are briefly described (Table 10.3). (For a review of HIV/AIDS-related cancers read Hessol, 1998; Grulich 2000.)

TABLE 10.2 Categories of Organism and Viral Involvement in Opportunistic Diseases

Symptoms	Causative Agent	Symptoms	Causative Agent
Generally Present		Proctocolitis[a]	*Entamoeba histolytica*
Fever, weight	*Pneumocystis carinii*	(diarrhea,	Campylobacter
loss, fatigue,	Cytomegalovirus	abdominal pain,	Shigella
malaise	Epstein-Barr virus	rectal pain)	Salmonella
	Mycobacterium avium intracellulare		*Chlamydia trachomatis*
	Candida albicans		Cytomegalovirus
		Proctitis[a]	*Neisseria gonorrhoeae*
Diffuse Pneumonia		(pain during	Herpes simplex
Dyspnea, chest	*Pneumocystis carinii*	defecation,	*Chlamydia trachomatis*
pain, hypoxemia,	Cytomegalovirus	diarrhea, itching	*Treponema pallidum*
abnormal chest	*Mycobacterium tuberculosis*	and perianal	
X-ray	*Mycobacterium avium intracellulare*	ulcerations)	
	Candida albicans		
	Cryptococcus neoformans		
	Toxoplasma gondii	**Neurological Involvement**	
		Meningitis,	Cytomegalovirus
		encephalitis,	Herpes simplex
Gastrointestinal Involvement		headaches,	*Toxoplasma gondii*
Esophagitis	*Candida albicans*	seizures, dementia	*Cryptococcus neoformans*
(sore throat,	Herpes simplex		Papovavirus
dysphagia)	Cytomegalovirus (suspected)		*Mycobacterium tuberculosis*
Enteritis	*Giardia lamblia*	Retinitis	Cytomegalovirus
(diarrhea,	*Entamoeba histolytica*	(diminished	*Toxoplasma gondii*
abdominal pain,	*Isospora belli*	vision)	*Candida albicans*
weight loss)	Cryptosporidium		
	Strongyloides stercoralis		
	Mycobacterium avium intracellulare		

[a] Especially in those persons practicing anal sex.

Adapted from Amin, 1987.

For Sexual Exposures—People should use male latex condoms during every act of sexual intercourse to reduce the risk of exposure to cytomegalovirus, herpes simplex virus, and human papillomavirus, as well as to all other sexually transmitted pathogens. Use of latex condoms will help prevent the transmission of HIV to others. Avoid sexual practices that may result in oral exposure to feces (oral-anal contact) to reduce the risk of intestinal infections such as cryptosporidiosis, shigellosis, campylobacteriosis, amebiasis, giardiasis, and hepatitis A and B (*MMWR*, 2002).

TABLE 10.3   Malignancies Associated With HIV/AIDS

Kaposi's sarcoma (epidemic form)
Burkitt's lymphoma
Non-Hodgkin's lymphomas
Hodgkin's disease
Chronic lymphocytic leukemia
Carcinoma of the oropharaynx
Hepatocellular carcinoma
Adenosquamous carcinoma of the lung
Cervical cancer
Anal cancer
Squamous cell carcinoma
Progressive multifocal leukoencephalopathy
Vulva cancer

Kaposi's Sarcoma
(cap-o-seas sar-com-a)

No other HIV/AIDS-related opportunistic disease attacks and singles out one segment of the population as KS does with HIV-positive gay men. Men with KS outnumber women approximately 95% to 5%; HIV-positive homosexual men with KS outnumber heterosexual men almost as significantly. KS is extremely rare in hemophiliacs with HIV. In fact, in one major study of hemophiliacs with HIV, only 1 in 93 developed KS, and he happened to be a gay man.

HIV infection represents an overwhelming risk factor for the development of KS, which was rare in the United States (incidence less than 1/100,000/year) before the HIV epidemic. Today, KS still remains one of the most frequent diseases affecting HIV-infected individuals. It is an aggressive disease, with involvement of the gut, lung, pleura, lymph nodes and the hard and soft palates.

In the United States, Kaposi's sarcoma is at least 20,000 times more common in people with HIV/AIDS than in the general population, and 300 times more common than in other immunosuppressed groups (Beral et al., 1990).

KS was first described by Moritz Kaposi in 1877 as a cancer of the muscle and skin. Characteristic signs of early KS were bruises and birthmark-like lesions on the skin, especially on the lower extremities. KS was described as a slow-growing tumor found primarily in elderly Mediterranean men, Ashkenazi Jews, and equatorial Africans.

Kaposi's sarcoma as described by Moritz Kaposi is called classic KS and it differs markedly from the KS that occurs in AIDS patients (Figure 10-7). Classic KS has a variable prognosis (forecast), is usually slow to develop, and causes little pain (**indolent**). Patient survival in the United States ranges from 8 to 13 years with some reported cases of survival for up to 50 years (Gross et al., 1989). Symptoms of classic KS are ulcerative skin lesions, swelling (**edema**) of the legs, and secondary infection of the skin lesions.

Kaposi's Sarcoma and AIDS

The HIV/AIDS epidemic has brought a more virulent and progressive form of KS marked by painless, flat to raised, pink to purplish plaques on the skin and mucosal surfaces that may spread to the lungs, liver, spleen, lymph nodes, digestive tract, and other internal organs. In its advanced stages it may affect any area from the skull to the feet (Figure 10-8). In the mouth, the hard palate is the most common site of KS (Figure 10-9) but it may also occur on the gum line, tongue, or tonsils.

KS in AIDS patients comes on swiftly and spreads aggressively. However, there have been *no reported* AIDS deaths due to just KS. But, KS can have enormous psychological impact particularly if the lesions occur on exposed areas.

Some of the most inconvenient and uncomfortable KS targets include the soles of the feet, the nose, and the oral cavity. Lesions on the lower extremities or on the feet are often asso-

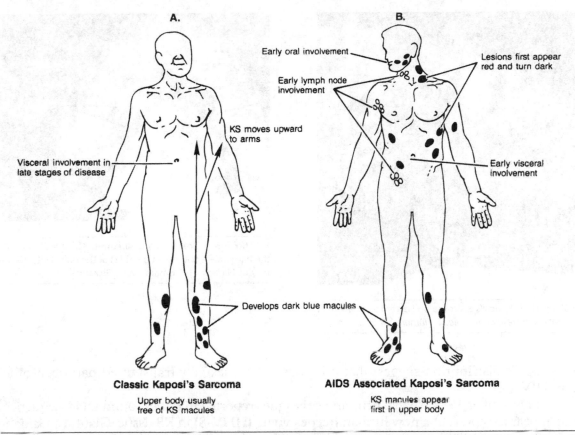

FIGURE 10-7 Classic and AIDS-Associated Kaposi's Sarcoma. **A.** Patients with classic KS (non-AIDS-related) demonstrate violet to dark blue bruises, spots, or macules on their lower legs. Gradually, the lesions enlarge into tumors and begin to form ulcers. KS lesions may, with time, spread upward to the trunk and arms. The movement of KS appears to follow the veins and involves the lymph system. In the late stages of the disease, visceral organs may become involved. **B.** For AIDS patients, initial lesions appear in greater number and are smaller than in classic KS. They first appear on the upper body (head and neck) and arms. The lesions first appear as pink or red oval bruises or macules that, with time, become dark blue and spread to the oral cavity and lower body, the legs, and feet. Visceral organs may be involved early on and the disease is aggressive. However, death is not caused by KS.

ciated with edema and swelling, causing not only severe pain but difficulty putting on shoes and walking. Swelling can be complicated by bacterial cellulitis, ulceration and skin breakdown, often with gram-negative bacterial infections. In addition to the obvious cosmetic damage, lesions on the face may be accompanied by swelling around the eyes that can sometimes progress to the point where patients literally cannot open their eyes. Finally, oral lesions can be painful and make eating and speaking problematic.

The prevalence of KS among gay men in 1981 was 77%; by 1987, it had fallen to 26% and by 2004 to less than 5% in gay men on HAART. This drop in KS among gay men is paralleled by a fall in CMV cases.

Human Herpes Virus Is the Kaposi's Virus—Most HIV/AIDS researchers now believe that HIV is not the primary pathological agent for Kaposi's sarcoma. Beral and colleagues (1990) at the Centers for Disease Control and Prevention concluded that the epidemiological data

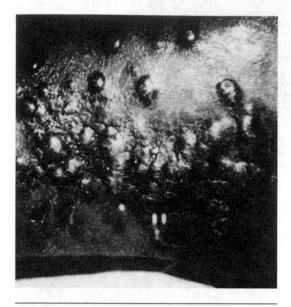

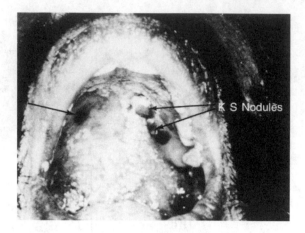

FIGURE 10-9 Oral Kaposi's Sarcoma. KS can be seen on the hard palate and down the sides of the oral cavity. (Courtesy of Nicholas J. Fiumara, M.D., Boston)

FIGURE 10-8 Kaposi's Sarcoma on Lower Leg of an AIDS Patient. *(Courtesy of Nicholas J. Fiumara, M.D., Boston)*

on Kaposi's distribution suggest that it is caused by a sexually transmitted pathogen other than HIV.

In December 1994, Yuan Chang and colleagues reported that they found DNA sequences that appear to represent a **new human herpes virus (HHV-8)** in KS tissue. Gianluca Gaidano and colleagues (1996) report that their data confirm that HHV-8 DNA sequences are found, at high frequency, with selected types of AIDS-related KS. Evidence continues to accumulate indicating that HHV-8 is the infectious agent responsible for KS (Kledal et al., 1997; Said et al., 1997).

Many research papers on whether herpes virus 8 causes KS have been published in recognized scientific/medical journals. It appears there is a cause and effect relationship; HHV-8/KS.

The work of Charles Rinaldo and colleagues (2001) reveals that healthy non-HIV-infected people who carry HHV8 have a healthy immune response and control the virus. HIV-infected persons who carry HHV8 have a poor immune response to the virus, which then becomes a precursor for the expression of KS. In 2002, Michael Cannon and colleagues reported that the risk of an HIV-positive man developing the AIDS-defining cancer Kaposi's sarcoma is linked to the amount of human herpes virus 8 (HHV-8) in peripheral blood monoculear cells (PBMC) and oral fluids, rather than the CD4+ cell count or viral load. The study found that HHV-8 is likely to be orally transmitted.

The Kaposi's virus may have entered the same population in which HIV is endemic, which would explain why the two are often transmitted together (O'Brien et al., 1999). HIV may produce the right conditions for Kaposi's development by causing growth factor production, and possibly by suppressing the body's immune defenses against cancer.

The work of Dennis Osmond and colleagues states that a KS-associated herpes virus was present in about 25% of gay males in San Francisco in 1978, several years before the CDC reported on the immune deficiency disease later called AIDS. As evidence mounts that genital herpes plays an important role in facilitating HIV acquisition, researchers are debating whether herpes screening and treatment should be considered for an HIV prevention strategy.

Lymphoma (lim-fo-mah): Cancer of the Lymph Glands

Lymphomas are the second most common cancer in HIV and are now the seventh most common cause of death for people with AIDS. A lymphoma is a neoplastic disorder (cancer) of the lymphoid tissue (Figure 10-10). B cell lymphoma occurs in about 1% of HIV-infected people, but makes up about 90% to 95% of all lymphomas found in people with HIV disease (Herndier et al., 1994; Scadden, 2002). Although it occurs most often in those demonstrating persistent generalized lymphadenopathy (swollen lymph glands), the usual site of lymphoma growth is in the brain, the heart, or the anorectal area (Brooke et al., 1990). The

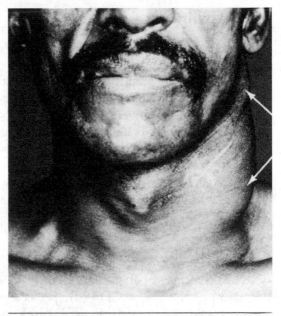

FIGURE 10-10 HIV/AIDS Patient Demonstrating a Lymphoma of the Neck. *(Courtesy CDC, Atlanta)*

most common signs and symptoms are confusion, lethargy, and memory loss. Lymphomas are increasing in incidence primarily due to the extension of the life span of AIDS patients because of medical therapy (Table 10.1).

Progressive Multifocal Leucoencephalopathy (leuco means white; encephalo means brain; pathy means disease)

Progressive multifocal leucoencephalopathy (PML) is an opportunistic infection caused by a papovavirus [Jamestown Canyon virus (JCV)] affecting 4% of AIDS patients. It is usually fatal within an average of 3.5 months and there is no treatment. In a few patients spontaneous improvement and prolonged survival have been reported. Some observations have indicated that cytosine arabinoside, a potent antiviral, may reverse the symptoms of PML. Symptoms of PML include altered mental status, speech and visual disturbances, gait difficulty, and limb incoordination (Guarino et al., 1995).

HIV Provirus: A Cancer Connection

In early 1994 AIDS investigators reported that HIV, on entering lymph cell DNA, activated nearby cancer-causing genes (oncogenes). The evidence suggests that HIV itself may trigger cancer in an otherwise normal cell.

These findings may mean that a variety of retroviruses that infect humans may also cause cancer (McGrath et al., 1994). Such findings raise concerns for developing an HIV vaccine. Using a weakened strain of HIV to make the vaccine may, when used, increase the incidence of lymphoma and other cancers.

▶ Disclaimer

This chapter is designed to present information on opportunistic infections in HIV/AIDS patients. The author does not accept any responsibility for the accuracy of the information or the consequences arising from the application, use, or misuse of any of the information contained herein, including any injury and/or damage to any person or property as a matter of product liability, negligence, or otherwise. No warranty, expressed or implied, is made in regard to the contents of this material. This material is not intended as a guide to self-medication. The reader is advised to discuss the information provided here with a doctor, pharmacist, nurse, or other authorized health-care practitioner and to check product information (including package inserts) regarding dosage, precautions, warnings, interactions, and contra-indications before administering any drug, herb, or supplement discussed herein.

▶ Summary

One of the gravest consequences of HIV infection is the immunosuppression caused by the depletion of the T4 or CD4+ helper cell population; suppressed immune systems allow for the expression of opportunistic diseases and cancers. The OI, end organ failures, and cancers kill AIDS patients, not HIV per se. It is the cumulative effect of several OIs that creates the chills, night sweats, fever, weight loss, anorexia, pain, and neurological problems.

One tragic disease that does not result from an OI is Kaposi's sarcoma (KS), characterized as a cancer that can spread to all parts of an AIDS patient's body. About 20% of AIDS patients, mostly gay men, have KS. It is not usually found in hemophiliacs, injection-drug users, or female AIDS patients.

▶ Review Questions

1. Define opportunistic infection (OI).
2. Which OI organism expresses itself in 80% of AIDS patients? Where is it located and what does it cause?
3. Which of the protozoal OI organisms causes weight loss, watery diarrhea, and severe abdominal pain?
4. Which of the bacterial OIs causes "wasting syndrome," night sweats, anorexia, and fever?
5. True or False: Kaposi's sarcoma (KS) is caused by HIV. Explain.
6. Name the two kinds of KS.
7. True or False: KS affects all AIDS patients equally. Explain.
8. True or False: Candidiasis and ulceration may be present in patients with HIV infection.
9. True or False: Oral candidiasis occurs frequently with HIV infection.
10. True or False: The use of combination anti-HIV drug therapy, especially those combinations containing a protease inhibitor, have substantially decreased the severity and number of OIs in AIDS patients.
11. Opportunistic Infections Crossword Puzzle

OPPORTUNISTIC INFECTIONS

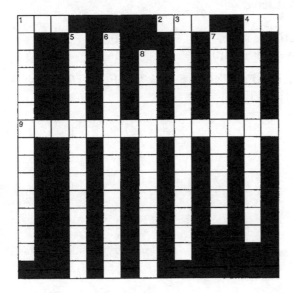

ACROSS

1. Centers for Disease Control and Prevention
2. Cytomegalovirus
4. Opportunistic infection
9. Protozoal infection

DOWN

1. Infection of the central nervous system
3. Bacteria, fungi, viruses, and protozoa
4. Pathogenic when immune system impaired
5. Fungal disease
6. To become serologically positive
7. Associated with yeast infection
8. Protozoan infection

▶ HIV/AIDS Self-Evaluation/Education Quiz

Before you begin reading, take this quiz to help determine your current knowledge about HIV infection and AIDS.

1.	HIV infects only homosexual persons.	T	F	?
2.	AIDS affects only adults.	T	F	?
3.	The agent that causes AIDS is HIV.	T	F	?
4.	HIV is a bacterial agent.	T	F	?
5.	The risk of an HIV infection from a blood transfusion is low, but it can happen.	T	F	?
6.	Patients with AIDS have reduction in T4 or CD4+ cells.	T	F	?
7.	People who have antibodies to HIV always develop AIDS.	T	F	?
8.	HIV has been found in vaginal secretions, saliva, blood, and other body fluids.	T	F	?
9.	AIDS is not a disease, but a syndrome.	T	F	?
10.	HIV is easily transmitted to people.	T	F	?
11.	The period from exposure to HIV to the expression of AIDS may be at least a year.	T	F	?
12.	There is no known cure for HIV disease.	T	F	?
13.	There is no known cure for AIDS.	T	F	?
14.	HIV carriers without signs of active disease can transmit the virus.	T	F	?
15.	All HIV-infected persons progress to AIDS.	T	F	?
16.	All persons with AIDS die prematurely.	T	F	?

17. An effective HIV vaccine will be developed by 2007.   T   F   ?
18. A person can be diagnosed with AIDS but have
    no outward symptoms.   T   F   ?
19. One can have a zero T4 cell count and still be alive.   T   F   ?
20. AIDS is considered a new disease of the twentieth century.   T   F   ?

The correct answers to these questions are: 1.F; 2.F; 3.T; 4.F; 5.T; 6.T; 7.F; 8.T; 9.T; 10.F; 11.T; 12.T; 13.T; 14.T; 15.F; 16.T; 17.?; 18.T; 19.T; 20.T.

Chapter
11

Transmission

Transmission of HIV

Darrell Ward

Scientists identified the means by which HIV was transmitted in the early days of the epidemic, well before the virus itself was discovered. No new modes of transmission have been discovered since. Throughout the world, people can contract HIV infection in three possible ways:

- Through sexual contact, either homosexual or heterosexual. Heterosexual contact is the leading means of HIV transmission worldwide, and the fastest growing mode of HIV transmission in the nation.
- Through contact with blood or other body fluids, blood products, or tissues of an infected person. This usually occurs by inoculation of HIV through needle sharing among users of illicit drugs; much more rarely, by accidental needle stick or splashes of blood on mucous membranes; and extremely rarely, through sustained contact of infected blood with breaks in the skin.
- Through transfer of the virus from an infected mother to her infant before or during birth, or shortly after birth through breast-feeding. This mother-to-infant transfer is also known as "perinatal transmission." Perinatal transmission is in rapid decline in the United States.

Transfer of a virus from mother to infant is also known as "vertical transmission," which refers to transfer of the virus from one generation to the next. This term, along with "horizontal transmission," is used often in the scientific literature. Horizontal transmission refers to transfer of the virus from one person to another in a population. Sexual transmission and blood-to-blood transmission are both examples of horizontal transmission.

Free HIV particles have been isolated from blood, semen, vaginal fluid, and breast milk. Other body fluids in which HIV is found include cerebrospinal fluid, which bathes the brain and spinal cord; synovial fluid, which bathes the surfaces of joints; pleural fluid, which occupies the narrow space between the lungs and the chest wall; and amniotic fluid, which surrounds the fetus. Researchers have also isolated HIV from saliva, tears, feces, and urine, in which it is sometimes present in very small amounts. No cases of HIV transmission through these fluids have been fully documented.

TABLE 11.1 Percentage of AIDS Cases According to Mode of Transmission: From the Beginning of the Epidemic to December 31, 1996

Mode of Transmission	United States Rates[1]	Estimated World Rates[2]
Sex between men	50	5–10
Injection drug use	26	5–10
Men who have sex with men and who inject drugs	6	*Not available*
Heterosexual intercourse	9	>70
Exposure of hemophiliacs to infected blood products	1	*Not available*
Exposure to contaminated blood or blood products during a medical procedure	1	3–5
Risk factor undetermined*	7	*Not available*

*The "Risk factor undetermined" category includes persons whose cases are still under investigation; persons unwilling to disclose high-risk information or unaware of a clear-cut exposure; persons with possible occupational exposure; and persons who were incompletely investigated upon their death, or who were lost to follow-up or declined to be interviewed.

Table 11.1 shows percentage of AIDS cases in adults and adolescents according to the mode of transmission in the United States and worldwide, from the beginning of the epidemic to December 31, 1996. It is important to realize that the leading modes of HIV transmission in the United States—sex between men and injection drug use—are different from the leading mode of transmission worldwide, which is heterosexual intercourse. Moreover, HIV transmission through heterosexual intercourse is increasing in the United States. This becomes clear when the exposure categories for AIDS cases reported in the year 1985 in the United States are compared with cases reported in 1996 (Table 11.2).

▶ **Sexual Transmission**

Sexual transmission of HIV is thought to account for 90% of AIDS cases worldwide. In the United States, Canada, and most of Europe, most cases of sexual transmission have occurred between men having sex with men, but cases due to heterosexual transmission increased more than sixfold from 1985 to 1996 (from 2% to 13%) in the United States, and that proportion will probably continue to grow. Heterosexual transmission of HIV in western Europe, for example, increased nine times from 1985 to 1990. Worldwide, vaginal intercourse has always been the predominant mode of HIV transmission.

The risk of transmission from an infected male to an uninfected female through unprotected vaginal intercourse is thought to be about 1 per 100 sexual contacts (i.e., out of 100 couples having one instance of vaginal intercourse in which the man is HIV positive and the woman HIV negative, 1 case of transmission will occur). The risk of transmission during anal intercourse is believed to be considerably higher, with an estimated transmission rate of 1 in 20 instances of unprotected anal intercourse.

TABLE 11.2 Modes of Transmission in 1985 Compared with 1996: Percentage of AIDS Cases in the United States

Mode of Transmission	Cases Reported in 1985[3]	Cases Reported in 1996[4]
Sex between men	67	40
Injection drug use	17	25
Men who have sex with men and who inject drugs	8	4
Heterosexual intercourse	2	13
Exposure of hemophiliacs to infected blood products	1	<1
Exposure to contaminated blood or blood products during a medical procedure	2	1
Risk factor undetermined	3	17*

*The "Undetermined" category for 1996 will decrease over time as investigations of these new AIDS cases are conducted.

The risk of female-to-male transmission is lower, with a rate estimated to be in the range of 1 per 1,000 infected women (i.e., out of 1,000 couples having vaginal intercourse in which the woman is HIV positive and the man HIV negative, 1 case of transmission will occur). The higher rate of male-to-female transmission is thought to be one reason why women outnumber men in cases of infection due to heterosexual transmission. The risk of female-to-female HIV transmission is lower yet.

These rates are highly variable, though, because many factors may alter an individual's susceptibility and HIV's infectiousness. These factors include the following:

- The presence of either acute HIV infection or advanced HIV disease (AIDS) in the infected partner increases the risk of sexual transmission. Although individuals with asymptomatic disease are also infectious to others, people recently infected temporarily have very high levels of virus in their blood and body fluids and secretions, as do people with advanced disease, which makes them relatively more infectious to their partners.
- The presence of genital tract infections in either partner increases the risk. The risk of transmission markedly increases if yeast infection or genital sores or ulcers are present. Such sores can be caused by ulcer-producing sexually transmitted diseases (STDs) such as syphilis, herpes, and chancroid. Sores or ulcers in the uninfected partner facilitate contact between that person's CD4 lymphocytes and macrophages and HIV from the infected partner; sores in the infected person provide additional avenues for release of HIV, exposing the uninfected partner to a greater dose of virus. Note, too, that genital ulcers in an HIV-infected person tend to increase in frequency, extent, and duration as the health of his or her immune system declines.
- STDs that do not produce ulcers, such as gonorrhea, chlamydia, and trichomoniasis, also increase the risk of acquiring HIV. This is thought to occur because these diseases cause inflammation of the mucous membranes of the genital tract. Inflammation is a

normal immune response to infection or injury, but it activates and attracts large numbers of white blood cells including monocytes, macrophages, and T lymphocytes to the inflamed area. In the HIV-infected partner this increases the amount of free virus and the number of virus-infected cells in genital secretions. In the HIV-negative partner the risk of acquiring HIV infection is increased because the inflammation of the genital tract concentrates cells susceptible to HIV infection in the genital tissues.

- Anal intercourse and, probably, intercourse during menstruation also increase the risk of sexual transmission. The rectal lining is thin, much more so than the vaginal lining, and contains many lymphocytes, macrophages, and other cells that HIV can infect. Anal intercourse also easily causes tears in the rectal lining that result in direct contact between infected semen and the blood of the receptive partner.
- Number of instances of intercourse is also related to risk. The greater the number of exposures to infected semen or vaginal secretions, the higher the risk of HIV transmission.
- Genetic characteristics of the particular HIV strain to which a person is exposed, as well as genetic characteristics of the exposed person, affect the risk of HIV transmission. A very small percentage of individuals have remained uninfected despite repeated exposure to HIV. It is now believed that certain individuals have a genetically determined natural resistance to HIV (see "Long-Term Nonprogressors"). Some strains of HIV appear to be more infectious than others. It has even been speculated that some HIV subtypes might be more infectious than others through vaginal intercourse.
- Some studies have suggested that the use of oral contraceptives, diaphrams, cervical caps, or intrauterine devices (IUDs) increases the risk of HIV transmission. This is difficult to determine because people who use these modes of contraception may be less likely to also use condoms during intercourse.
- A risk of HIV transmission exists even during safer sex; minimizing this risk requires that condoms be used consistently and correctly.

Oral Sex

The risk represented by oral sex is relatively low as compared to that of anal or vaginal sex. Data are not available to determine the probability of HIV transmission by oral-penile contact. As of 1996, however, there were ten reports involving 17 persons who were thought to have become HIV infected through oral-penile sex. Although oral sex poses a low risk of HIV transmission, the Centers for Disease Control and Prevention (CDC) guidelines have consistently recommended use of a condom during oral-penile contact and a barrier during oral-vaginal contact.

A recent study[5] in monkeys suggested that oral sex could hold a higher risk of infection than once thought. The study involved placing free simian immunodeficiency virus (SIV) particles on the back of the tongue of seven infant rhesus monkeys. Six of the monkeys became infected.

The implications of this for humans are unclear. Scientists commenting on the study pointed out that the conditions used in the experiment did not really mirror what happens in humans during oral sex. Human saliva is known to have an inhibitory effect on the infectiousness of HIV. In addition, the concentrations of the virus used in the monkey study were higher than those most humans would encounter during oral sex.

Whatever the implications of this study for the risk of HIV transmission during oral sex, it certainly in no way implies risk of transmission through casual contact. There is no evidence at all of transmission through kissing, the sharing of eating utensils, etc.

▶ Blood and Blood Products

HIV is present in blood of both asymptomatic and symptomatic people as free virus particles and in infected cells. The number of free virus particles in the blood can rise to extremely high levels during the period of acute infection. Then, within weeks, viral levels decrease and the virus nearly disappears from the blood. As the disease progresses, however, the number of CD4 cells in the blood drops and the number of free virus particles progressively rises again. In advanced HIV disease (i.e., AIDS), there might be as many as a million free virus particles per milliliter of blood, as a large proportion of CD4 cells are infected, each of which can produce thousands of virus particles daily.

Transmission by blood and body fluids can occur very efficiently through the sharing of needles and other equipment used to inject drugs, or through transfusion of HIV-contaminated blood or blood products. Although such cases have been very rare, media reports have periodically raised the public's concern about HIV transmission from HIV-infected patients to health-care workers, and from HIV-infected health-care workers to patients (see below).

Needle Sharing and Drug Use

Transmission of HIV among injection drug users (IDUs) occurs when the blood of an HIV-infected drug user is transferred to an uninfected IDU through the sharing of needles and syringes (drug injection equipment is also known as "works," "gimmicks," and "sets"). Needle sharing by IDUs is the leading cause of HIV transmission by blood, and the second leading mode of HIV transmission in the United States, after sexual transmission. CDC figures for 1995 showed that HIV transmission among IDUs accounted for 24% of reported AIDS cases in men that year nationwide and 38% among women. HIV can spread rapidly and efficiently through needle sharing. In New York City, HIV infection among IDUs went from less than 10% to more than 50% in five years in some groups studied. In Edinburgh, Scotland, the number of HIV-infected IDUs in one group went from zero to more than 40% in one year.

Because a vast majority of IDUs are heterosexual, they are also a leading factor in the spread of HIV to the heterosexual population and in the rapid increase in the numbers of women with HIV disease and AIDS and, hence, also in the numbers of newborns with HIV disease.

Two drug-injection practices in particular set the stage for HIV transmission during needle sharing: the initial drawing of blood into the barrel of the syringe to verify that the needle is inserted into a vein, and the practice of refilling the syringe repeatedly with blood following drug injection to rinse out any remaining drug.

Noninjection Drugs and HIV Transmission

The use of alcohol, crack cocaine, and other mind-altering drugs also increases the risk of acquiring or transmitting HIV infection. Mind-altering drugs affect judgment and increase the probability of unsafe behavior. Trading sex for crack or other drugs is a practice that usually involves unprotected sex. It is thought to be responsible for the significant increases in the incidence of syphilis and other STDs, as well as that of HIV infection. Because syphilis produces genital ulcers, an increase in syphilis incidence also means, for the people affected, a higher risk of acquiring HIV infection through sexual contact.

Transmission by Transfusion: Safety of the Blood Supply

There never has been—nor is there now—any risk at all of acquiring HIV through the process of *donating* blood. However, HIV can be transmitted by transfusion of whole blood, the cellular components of blood, plasma, and clotting factors derived from blood. In the early 1980s, virtually 100% of the people who received transfusions of HIV-contaminated blood became infected because of the high dose of virus that can be present in a single unit of blood. In all, an estimated 12,000 people became HIV infected by contaminated transfusions.

The self-disqualification as blood donors of individuals at high risk for HIV/AIDS, and the screening of all blood donations have, since 1985, virtually eliminated this mode of HIV transmission in the Western world.

In the United States, testing the blood supply for HIV began in early 1985. In early 1997, the risk of receiving a pint of blood infected with HIV was estimated to be about 1 in 700,000. Transfusion of infected blood, however, remains the third leading cause of HIV transmission in Africa and many other developing countries, after sexual transmission and mother-to-infant transmission.

Also prior to testing, many of the estimated 15,000 hemophiliacs in the United States became infected with HIV in the early years of the HIV epidemic after receiving contaminated clotting factors. Hemophilia is a disorder of the blood-clotting system that is corrected by administration of clotting factors. These are proteins derived from plasma that is obtained by pooling many units of donated blood. Prior to 1985, clotting factor preparation methods did not inactivate HIV. One unit of HIV-infected blood in the entire blood pool could infect all the clotting factor preparations derived from it.

As a result, in the early 1980s, between 80% and 90% of people with hemophilia A in the United States became infected with HIV, and so did between 35% and 45% of people with hemophilia B. (People with hemophilia B require less frequent infusions of clotting factors.)

The screening of all blood donations and the heat treatment of clotting factors during their preparation have virtually eliminated clotting factors as a source of HIV infection in the Western world.

Transmission from HIV-Positive Patients to Health-Care Workers

The transmission of HIV from an infected patient to an uninfected health-care worker is possible if the health-care worker accidentally cuts himself or herself during surgery or sticks himself or herself with a needle that contains infected blood from the patient. This kind of on-the-job exposure to HIV is known as "occupational exposure." It can also occur if a health-care worker has open wounds—even tiny ones—or skin abrasions that come in contact with an infected patient's blood or other virus-laden body fluids. Exposure to any infectious agent that involves a cut, abrasion, or break in the skin—including a break caused by a needle stick—is referred to as "percutaneous exposure."

Evidence indicates that the risk of acquiring HIV infection from percutaneous exposure is low. Several studies have estimated the risk of HIV infection from such exposure. A 1990 study[6] followed 2,200 health-care workers exposed to HIV following accidental needle sticks or other kinds of injuries. Of these, 8 workers later tested positive for HIV antibodies. This rate—8 infections per 2,200 exposure—yields a risk of 0.36 infection per 100 exposures. This falls into the range of 0.13 to 0.39 infection per 100 exposures found by other studies. By comparison, 12 to 17 infections occurred per 100 accidental needle sticks with needles that contained blood infected with hepatitis B virus.

Note that the risk of HIV transmission from accidental needle sticks is much lower than the risk of transmission from needle sharing by IDUs. The two types of exposures differ: An accidental needle stick is a one-time event and does not usually involve a deep or substantial injection. Exposure through needle sharing likely involves repeated injections of a larger dose of infectious material directly into a vein.

There is also a possible risk of transmission through exposure of the mucous membranes of a caregiver's eyes, nose, or mouth to a patient's HIV-infected blood or other body fluids. One study followed the outcome of 1,000 mucous membrane exposures and found no cases of HIV transmission.

Although the risk of acquiring HIV infection through percutaneous or mucous membrane exposure is slight, it is believed advisable that a person accidentally exposed to HIV should consider prompt treatment with a combination of antiretroviral drugs. Recent data strongly suggest that such treatment reduces the risk of infection.[7]

Transmission from HIV-Positive Health-Care Workers to Patients

In the United States, the only verified case of transmission from a health-care worker to patients involved a dentist who infected 6 of his patients. The mode of transmission in this unique case remains unknown. Testing of the dentist's 1,100 patients revealed 9 who were HIV infected. Infections in 3 of them proved to be unrelated to the dentist: Not only did all 3 have a history of recognized risk factors, but molecular analyses showed that the viral strains present in these 3 patients were only distantly genetically related to the viral strain present in the dentist. Viruses isolated from the remaining 6 patients, however, were closely related to the virus from the dentist.

Studies of more than 22,000 patients who were cared for by 63 HIV-positive physicians and dentists showed no other cases of HIV transmission to patients.

Perinatal Transmission

Perinatal transmission of HIV is thought to occur in 15% to 30% of births to HIV-positive women. The rate is lowest in developed countries and highest in developing countries. Worldwide, it is the second most common mode of HIV transmission after sexual transmission. Each year in the early 1990s, about 7,000 HIV-infected women in the United States gave birth to some 2,000 infected infants. Perinatal transmission may occur through a number of different pathways; it can happen before birth, during delivery, or during breast-feeding.

A seminal clinical trial concluded in 1994 found that azidothymidine (AZT) given orally to pregnant women for several weeks prior to delivery, intravenously during delivery, and orally to the newborns for six weeks could reduce perinatal transmission by two-thirds.[8] The study was a landmark because it was the first to show that a treatment for HIV could reduce the risk of virus transmission.

A strong correlation was later found between levels of free virus in the mother's blood (i.e., the mother's viral load) and perinatal transmission. A study found that high levels of free HIV in the mother's blood late in pregnancy or during delivery predicted risk of perinatal transmission.[9] The research also suggested that AZT helps prevent transmission by reducing the amount of free virus in the mother's blood prior to delivery. Other factors may also play a role, as some mothers with a low viral load did nevertheless transmit HIV to their infants. Some of these factors may be the following:

- The mother's immune status. A low CD4 count is also associated with an increased risk of perinatal transmission.
- Exposure of the infant's mucosal membranes to maternal blood during delivery.
- Prolonged period between the time the mother's water breaks and the time of delivery.
- Presence of ulcerations in the mother caused by sexually transmitted infections.
- Vaginal delivery. Some studies suggest that vaginal delivery increases the risk of transmission, but this has not been conclusively shown, and cesarean sections are not recommended as a means of reducing the risk of HIV transmission.
- Vitamin A deficiency. In Africa, vitamin A deficiency in pregnant women appears to increase the risk of perinatal transmission. However, it is not known yet whether supplements of vitamin A reduce this risk.

Breast-feeding

Breast milk can also transmit HIV, which is found in both the cells present and the liquid portion of the milk. The risk of transmission is believed to be highest during periods of high viral load in the mother, that is, during acute HIV infection and during advanced HIV disease, or AIDS.

In the United States and other developed countries that have safe alternatives to breast milk, breast-feeding by HIV-positive mothers is discouraged. In developing countries that lack safe and affordable alternatives to breast milk, breast-feeding by HIV-positive mothers is regarded as holding less risk of disease for the infant than the available alternatives, at least in environments with poor sanitation. (As the incidence of HIV infection increases in developing countries, the earlier recommendation that all HIV-positive mothers in these countries should breast-feed rather than use formula is being re-evaluated. The decision now often depends on local sanitary conditions.)

HOW HIV IS *NOT* TRANSMITTED

If HIV were spread by insects, like the plague or malaria; by casual contact, like influenza; by sneezing, like a cold; or by water, like cholera, the pattern of the AIDS epidemic would be far different from what it is. Either entire households would be affected, or individuals would be affected randomly, or the epidemic's spread would be determined by climate, altitude, quality of water supply, and other such environmental factors. This is not the case for the epidemic of HIV/AIDS. It is spread in specific ways: sexual contact, blood-to-blood contact, and from mother to infant. These modes of transmission were established early in the epidemic and continuing surveillance over a period of 15 years has revealed no additional routes of HIV transmission.

In addition, reviews of some 14 epidemiological studies that involved a total of 757 individuals sharing households with HIV-positive people found no cases of casual transmission.[10] These included households of infected hemophiliacs, households with infected foster children, households with HIV-contaminated transfusion recipients, and other households of people with HIV/AIDS.

Members of these households shared such things as combs, towels, bed linens, eating utensils, plates, and drinking glasses. They touched and kissed. None of the studies produced any evidence of HIV transmission when unprotected sexual contact or needle sharing did *not* occur. Thus, there *is no evidence* that HIV is transmitted by any of the following:

- Talking, shaking hands, or other casual contact
- Hugging or ordinary kissing (there is a remote risk that deep kissing—French kissing or tongue kissing—could lead to infection, especially if open sores are present on the lips, tongue, or mouth)
- Sharing kitchens, lunchrooms, dishes, or eating utensils
- Touching floors, walls, door knobs, or toilet seats; or sharing offices, restrooms, computers, telephones, or writing utensils
- Being bitten by mosquitoes, fleas, bed bugs, and other insects

If precautions are taken to avoid blood-to-blood contact, there is no evidence that HIV transmission occurs in a nonsexual, non-needle-sharing relationship with a person who is HIV positive.

▶ Endnotes

1. Centers for Disease Control and Prevention. *HIV/AIDS Surveillance Report* 1996;8(2):10.
2. *UNAIDS and WHO Fact Sheet: HIV/AIDS: The Global Epidemic.* Geneva, Switzerland: World Health Organization, December 1996. (World Health Organization document based on the *Final Report: The Status and Trends of the Global HIV/AIDS Pandemic,* Vancouver, July 5–6, 1996.)
3. Unpublished CDC AIDS surveillance data for 1985, provided by the National Center for HIV, STD, and TB Prevention, Bethesda, MD.
4. Centers for Disease Control and Prevention. *HIV/AIDS Surveillance Report* 1996;8(2):10.
5. Baba TW, et al. Infection and AIDS in adult macaques after nontraumatic oral exposure to cell-free SIV. *Science* 1996; 272: 1486–1489.
6. Gershon RRM, Vlahov D, Nelson KE. The risk of transmission of HIV-1 through non-percutaneous, non-sexual modes—a review. *AIDS* 1990;4:645–650.
7. Centers for Disease Control and Prevention. Case-control study of HIV seroconversion in health-care workers after percutaneous exposure to HIV-infected blood—France, United Kingdom, and United States, January 1988–August 1994. *Morbidity and Mortality Weekly Report* 1995;44:929–933.
8. Conner HM, et al. Reduction of maternal–infant transmission of human immunodeficiency virus type 1 with zidovudine treatment. *New England Journal of Medicine* 1994;331:1173–1180.
9. Dickover RE, et al. Identification of levels of maternal HIV-1 RNA associated with risk of perinatal transmission: effect of maternal zidovudine treatment on viral load. *Journal of the American Medical Association* 1996;275:599–605.
10. Gershon RRM, Vlahov D, Nelson KE. The risk of transmission of HIV-1 through non-percutaneous, non-sexual modes—a review. *AIDS* 1990;4:645–650.

Chapter
12

Testing and Prevention

Comprehensive HIV Prevention

UNAIDS

The steady growth of the AIDS epidemic stems not from the deficien-cies of available prevention strategies but rather from the world's fail-ure to use the highly effective tools at its disposal to slow the spread of HIV. Some 25 years after the epidemic was first recognized, most people at high risk of HIV infection have yet to be reached by HIV prevention, as many policy-makers refrain from implementing approaches that have been shown to work.

This chapter discusses the programmatic interventions and policy actions that are essen-tial to all strong national HIV prevention programmes. It specifically addresses the urgent pre-vention needs of women and young people, as well as the complex prevention opportunities and challenges presented by expanding access to treatment. Most importantly, it emphasizes the urgent need for comprehensive, robust national HIV prevention programmes to be scaled up, to cover sufficient numbers of people and target resources where they can be most effective.

▶ Intensifying HIV Prevention

If anything has been learnt from the past 25 years of the epidemic, it is that HIV prevention works. The early successes of Brazil, Thailand and Uganda in reversing their national AIDS epidemics through courageous political leadership and starting strong prevention efforts early have been well documented. More recent evidence suggests that prevention efforts are now also contributing to reductions in HIV prevalence in Cambodia and Zimbabwe, and in parts of Burkina Faso, Haiti, Kenya and the United Republic of Tanzania (UNAIDS, 2005a).

HIV prevention, like treatment, is for life. Instead of short-term or isolated prevention initia-tives, effective national programmes need to sustain essential programmatic and policy actions at a sufficient scale over the long term, adapting them as the epidemic evolves, responding to changes in infection patterns and social environments. In recognition of the inherent long-term nature of the HIV prevention enterprise, implementation and scaling up of available prevention strategies should be coupled with longer-term efforts to address human resource challenges and to develop new prevention technologies, including the ultimate prevention tool, a preventive vaccine.

Although much progress has been made, the global prevention response falls far short of the urgent, scaled-up effort needed to curb the epidemic's expansion. While funding for HIV programmes has increased in recent years, many countries are failing to direct financial resources towards activities that address the prevention needs of the populations at highest risk, opting instead to prioritize more general prevention efforts that are less cost effective and less likely to have an impact on the epidemic.

There are also disturbing signs that support for HIV prevention in some regions may be diminishing. In recent years, Thailand, for example, has reduced its HIV prevention budget by two thirds, even though injecting drug use is contributing to substantial new HIV infections. (UNDP/UNAIDS, 2004).

▶ Decisive Action Can—and Must—Make the Difference

The world's failure to make proven prevention methods available to those who need them represents a remarkable missed opportunity. Scaling up available prevention strategies in 125 low- and middle-income countries would avert an estimated 28 million new HIV infections between 2005 and 2015—more than half of those that are projected to occur during this period—and would save US$ 24 billion in associated treatment costs (Stover et al., 2006).

Countries also need to ensure that both prevention and treatment are scaled up in a balanced way, in order to capitalize fully on synergies between the two. Globally, it is estimated that a response focusing solely on treatment would result in only 9 million averted new HIV infections. In contrast, simultaneous scaling up of both prevention and treatment would avert 29 million new HIV infections by the end of 2020 (Salomon et al., 2005). Figures 12-1 and 12-2

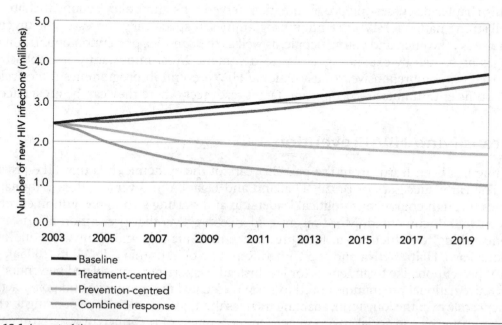

FIGURE 12-1 Impact of three scenarios on HIV infection in sub-Saharan Africa, 2003–2020
Source: Salomon JA et al. (2005). Integrating HIV prevention and treatment: from slogans to impact.

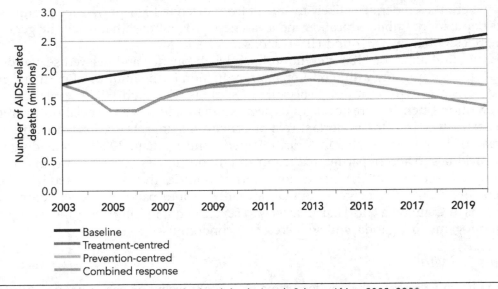

FIGURE 12-2 Impact of three scenarios on AIDS-related deaths in sub-Saharan Africa, 2003–2020
Source: Salomon JA et al. (2005). Integrating HIV prevention and treatment: from slogans to impact.

illustrate the benefits of scaling up prevention and treatment together (the combined response scenario), compared with concentrating on either prevention or treatment alone or with doing nothing (the baseline).

▶ Preventing Sexual Transmission of HIV

Unprotected vaginal intercourse accounts for the vast majority of HIV infections globally. Effective prevention of sexual transmission of HIV requires a combination of programmatic interventions and policy actions that promote safer behaviours, reduce biological and social vulnerability to transmission, encourage use of key prevention technologies, and promote social norms that favour risk reduction, as stated in the UNAIDS' policy position paper *Intensifying HIV Prevention* (see end of this chapter).

Safer Behaviours and Sexual Norms

Analysis of prevention interventions to change behaviour has consistently found that such programmes reduce the frequency of sexual risk behaviours (Crepaz et al., 2005; Elwy et al., 2002; Merson et al., 2000). Behavioural change programmes typically include basic information about the virus, personal risk assessment, counselling, building skills, such as negotiating condom use with sex partners, and access to condoms and other prevention technologies.

Behavioural change programmes targeting populations at especially high risk are among the most cost-effective prevention interventions available and represent a core component of any national HIV prevention programme. Although these are indispensable in all national responses, broader-based programmes are also essential in generalized epidemics or in settings where the epidemic is likely to spread from discrete high-prevalence groups into the broader population. Public education and awareness programmes that reach the general population are essential to any sound HIV response.

Behavioural aims for HIV prevention include: abstinence and delayed sexual debut for young people; monogamy within relationships; reduction in the number of partners; and correct and consistent condom use. Especially in settings with high HIV prevalence, effective HIV prevention often requires changes to deep-seated traditions and social norms regarding human sexuality. Given the important role of concurrent unprotected sexual partnerships in the spread of HIV in sub-Saharan Africa (Halperin and Epstein, 2004), persuading sexually active individuals to accept partner reduction and monogamy as valued norms may be critical to the long-term success of HIV prevention efforts. Countries that have lowered HIV incidence have benefited from the emergence of new sexual behaviour patterns—fewer commercial sex transactions in Cambodia and Thailand, delayed sexual debut in Zimbabwe, increasing emphasis on monogamy in Uganda, and an increase in condom use.

Condoms Still Vital

For sexually active people, the condom remains a vital prevention technology (UNFPA et al., 2004). Correct and consistent use of the male condom reduces the risk of sexual transmission of HIV by 80–90%—an efficacy rate that exceeds those reported for many of the world's standard vaccines (Halperin et al., 2004; Cohen and Farley, 2004). Observational studies, laboratory experiments and mathematical modelling indicate that female condoms also offer strong protection against HIV infection (Hoffman et al., 2004).

In addition to promoting condom access for especially vulnerable populations, prevention efforts should prioritize encouraging condom use for all sexually active adults, especially in countries with generalized epidemics. According to one global estimate, condoms supplied by the public sector were used in only 21% of unprotected sex acts involving non-regular partners in 2003 (USAID et al., 2004).

Many men harbour negative attitudes towards condoms, feeling that condom use reduces sexual pleasure or impedes sexual intimacy with regular partners. However, strong and sustained promotion of condoms helps overcome such resistance, significantly increasing condom use. For example, with the goal of normalizing condom use, this year the Brazilian Ministry of Health distributed 25 million condoms at parades, dances, parties and on the street during the annual carnival—just one component of the government's plan to distribute 1.5 billion condoms in 2006. In Singapore, following implementation in 1995 of energetic condom promotion for sex workers and their clients, consistent condom use increased from 45% before the intervention to more than 95% in 2002, and sex workers experienced significant declines in gonorrhoea incidence (Wong, Chan and Koh, 2004). In addition to condom social marketing, condoms should be also made available free of charge, as even extremely low prices for over-the-counter condoms can serve as a deterrent to use (Cohen and Farley, 2004).

Urgent Action: Increasing Knowledge of HIV Serostatus

Once diagnosed with HIV, and particularly if they receive proper counselling, most individuals take steps to avoid exposing others to the virus. Unfortunately, however, most people living with HIV are unaware of their serostatus.

Worldwide, only 12% of people who want to be tested are currently able to do so (UNAIDS et al., 2005c). In 2003, it was estimated that only 0.2% of adults in low- and middle-income countries received voluntary HIV counselling and testing services (USAID et al., 2004).

There are many reasons why people at risk of HIV infection fail to be tested: fear of discrimination, fear that the test result will be positive, lack of access to treatment or lack of access to testing services. According to ILO, fear of losing employment often discourages individuals from making use of available testing services. Workplaces with 'Know your status' campaigns administered jointly by managers and workers' representatives report improved uptake of testing, treatment and prevention services. For example, trade unions in Rwanda that maintain solidarity funds to

> ### THE PERSISTENT GAP IN CONDOM SUPPLY
>
> UNFPA, the largest public-sector purchaser of male condoms, estimates the global supply of public-sector condoms is less than 50% of that needed to ensure adequate condom coverage. The agency estimates that the gap between supply and actual need totals 8.3 billion condoms. While donor support for condom programmes increased by 16% between 2003 and 2004, to US$ 72 million, such funding was nearly US$ 20 million below amounts spent in 2001. To ensure a sufficient condom supply to halt the AIDS epidemic by 2015, the level of funding for condom procurement and distribution must increase threefold. In 2005, UNFPA launched the Global Programme to Enhance Reproductive Health Commodity Security. The five-year initiative seeks to catalyse national efforts to define, own and drive strategies to ensure access to all sexual and reproductive health technologies, including male and female condoms.

care for workers who test positive report that nearly all their members have been tested for HIV (UNAIDS/ILO/ICFTU, 2006).

Recognizing the urgency of increasing knowledge of HIV serostatus, in June 2004, UNAIDS and WHO recommended that traditional voluntary testing and counselling programmes be supplemented by enhanced diagnostic HIV testing and by the routine offer of HIV testing in clinics for sexually transmitted infections, in programme sites for the prevention of mother-to-child HIV transmission, and in clinical and community-based health-service settings in areas with high levels of HIV and access to antiretroviral drugs (UNAIDS and WHO, 2004).

In recommending a scaled-up approach to HIV testing, UNAIDS and WHO built on lessons learnt in Botswana, where the national government decreed in early 2004 that public and private health-care sites must offer HIV testing as a routine part of medical check-ups—a policy change that has led to more rapid uptake of testing (WHO, 2005a). For example, since up to half of all people living with HIV develop tuberculosis, clinics for tuberculosis represent an ideal venue for the promotion of HIV testing and linkage of HIV-positive individuals to HIV services. However, as this trend is taken up by health systems, care must be taken to ensure that the routine offer of testing does not lead to the imposition of a test.

In addition to a lack of testing locations, other obstacles need to be addressed including cost and convenience. A number of approaches have proven effective. Experience in the United Republic of Tanzania has shown that eliminating out-of-pocket costs associated with HIV testing services can significantly increase use of the services and their cost–effectiveness (Thielman et al., 2006). Another approach is to reduce the time that testing takes. According to a survey of adults in Malawi, 90% who wished to know their HIV serostatus preferred to learn their results the same day of the test (Degraft-Johnson et al., 2005). Such a desire can be met by rapid HIV tests, which provide results in about 20 minutes and eliminate the need for individuals to return days later for their results. While rapid HIV testing technologies are not unduly complex, they nevertheless require training of laboratory personnel. WHO and the United States' Centers for Disease Control and Prevention have developed a comprehensive five-day training module for rapid testing that is being rolled out in 2006.

Preventing Sexually Transmitted Infections

More than 340 million people contract a curable sexually transmitted infection each year, with women having greater vulnerability to infection than men (WHO, 2005b). As untreated sexually transmitted infections increase the risk of HIV transmission by several orders of magnitude (Fleming and Wasserheit, 1999), efforts to ensure the prompt diagnosis and treatment of sexually transmitted infections represent an essential programmatic component of a strong and comprehensive response to HIV (Dallabetta and Neilson, 2004). Increased cooperation between HIV prevention efforts and programmes to diagnose and treat other sexually transmitted infections has been identified as an important means of increasing the effectiveness of both.

While available treatments for sexually transmitted infections are among the most potent HIV prevention tools, more effective technologies are still needed. Hepatitis B is the only sexually transmitted infection for which a preventive vaccine is licensed, although emerging evidence suggests that a vaccine to prevent human papilloma virus infection may be imminent. Syphilis control continues to depend on therapies that have barely changed in 60 years, as newer antibiotics have not systematically been studied to assess their potential in treating syphilis and other sexually transmitted infections (Hook and Peeling, 2004). Two large-scale trials are currently under way to assess the HIV prevention efficacy of mass administration of acyclovir. If successful, this will provide a relatively inexpensive treatment for herpes simplex virus type 2 infection, a condition which increases the risk of HIV acquisition threefold (Freeman et al., 2005).

CIRCUMCISION: HOW EFFECTIVE IN HIV PREVENTION?

Although it has long been documented that circumcised males have lower infection rates than uncircumcised males, until recently no prospective study had specifically tested the efficacy of adult male circumcision in preventing the acquisition of HIV (Siegfried et al., 2005; Weiss et al., 2000). In 2005, researchers announced the results of a randomized controlled trial recruiting 3274 men aged 18 to 24 years in Orange Farm, South Africa, in an area where almost one in three adults are HIV-positive. The trial found that adult male circumcision reduced the men's risk of contracting HIV during sexual intercourse by over 60% during the 18-month study period. (Auvert et al., 2005.) Research suggests that among other possibilities, male circumcision may help to protect against HIV infection by removing cells in the inner foreskin that serve as entry points for the virus (Reynolds et al., 2004).

In July 2005, UNFPA, UNICEF, WHO and the UNAIDS Secretariat advised that the South Africa trial results should be confirmed before male circumcision is broadly promoted as a standard measure within comprehensive HIV prevention programmes (UNFPA et al., 2005). Two efficacy trials for adult male circumcision are underway in Kenya and Uganda, with results anticipated in 2007. The Kenyan trial of 2776 men uses the same circumcision method as the one tested in South Africa while the Uganda trial of 5000 men uses a different circumcision method. Both trials are designed to follow participants over a longer period to assess the duration of any observed benefit and to determine whether the intervention has an effect on overall levels of sexual risk behaviour. A third trial in Uganda is assessing the degree of protection that male circumcision may offer to female partners of HIV-positive men.

HIV Prevention in Emergency Situations

Displacement as a result of conflict can sometimes increase the affected population's HIV risk by reducing their access to HIV prevention services, disrupting social support networks, increasing exposure to sexual violence, encouraging sex in return for food, shelter or other necessities, or simply moving to a higher HIV prevalence location (UNAIDS and UNHCR, 2005). In Nepal, where a continuing violent conflict has displaced between 200 000 and 400 000 people, widespread population displacement may be accelerating the country's HIV epidemic. In particular, the conflict is severely curtailing the ability of nongovernmental organizations to provide HIV prevention services in such chaotic and dangerous circumstances (Singh et al., 2005).

UNAIDS and UNHCR recommend that refugee programming should include culturally and linguistically relevant community-based prevention interventions (UNHCR, 2005). In Uganda, where more than 220 000 refugees share health services with 135 000 people from surrounding communities, UNHCR works with the government to provide refugees with access to voluntary HIV testing and counselling, screening and treatment for sexually transmitted infections, and services to prevent mother-to-child HIV transmission. Recent evidence has documented an increase in condom use among refugees at the Kyaka II refugee settlement in Uganda.

Humanitarian relief efforts now routinely integrate HIV prevention into their work. UN agencies and nongovernmental organizations, for example, prioritized HIV prevention from the outset of the international response to the 2004 Asian tsunami.

HIV PREVENTION IN THE TRANSPORT SECTOR

HIV prevention efforts designed for specific occupational groups, often targeting the purchase of sex while on the road, have met with considerable success. For example, there is ample evidence that HIV prevention programmes aimed at truck drivers can reduce their frequency of unprotected sex. In Tamil Nadu, for example, research carried out after an HIV prevention programme for truck drivers found the percentage of drivers reporting that they had had commercial sex declined from 14% in 1996 to 2% in 2003. Moreover, the percentage of drivers whose last instance of commercial sex was unprotected fell from 45% to 9% in the same period (MAP, 2005).

Although long-haul truck drivers are more likely to engage in casual sex due to extended periods of time away from home, short-haul drivers have more access to communities and have been known to withhold goods and food in exchange for sex. This is particularly likely to happen when the goods being delivered are urgently needed, for instance in emergency situations. Opportunities for sexual exploitation and abuse and unprotected sex may increase in such situations and need to be addressed (WFP, 2006).

Programmes targeting truck drivers are most effective if carried out with the agreement of both employers and employees. In South Africa, an agreement between representatives of workers and employers has led to the establishment of a network of roadside clinics that provide general health services and HIV prevention interventions (ILO, 2005). In Malawi, the World Food Programme is in partnership with private companies, nongovernmental organizations and the government to provide HIV prevention information, condoms, treatment of sexually transmitted infections, voluntary HIV counselling and testing and referrals for HIV treatment to truck drivers and sex workers in two locations in the country.

▶ Preventing Mother-to-Child Transmission of HIV

Each day, 1800 children worldwide become infected with HIV—the vast majority of them newborns. More than 85% of children infected with HIV live in sub-Saharan Africa, although incidence of mother-to-child transmission of HIV is rapidly rising in Eastern Europe and Central Asia (UNICEF, 2005).

Effective prevention of mother-to-child HIV transmission involves a combination of strategies. These include primary HIV prevention for women (including integration of HIV prevention into reproductive and sexual health services), prevention of unintended pregnancies in HIV-positive women, access to comprehensive antenatal care, promotion of voluntary HIV testing and counselling for pregnant women and their partners in antenatal and community-based settings, antiretroviral therapy for mother and newborn and counselling on strategies to reduce the risk of HIV transmission via breastfeeding.

Although pilot projects are currently delivering HIV prevention services in antenatal settings, few countries have effectively scaled up such services. Globally, just less than 8% of pregnant women are currently offered services to prevent mother-to-child transmission of HIV. In sub-Saharan Africa, fewer than 6% of pregnant women in 2005 were offered services for the prevention of mother-to-child HIV transmission.

Timely administration of antiretroviral drugs to the HIV-diagnosed pregnant woman and her newborn significantly reduces the risk of mother-to-child HIV transmission. Combination regimens appear to be most effective but were until recently regarded as too costly for widespread use in low- and middle-income countries. In recent years, projects to prevent mother-to-child transmission in resource-limited settings have primarily focused on the provision of single-dose intrapartum and neonatal nevirapine, which cuts the risk of HIV transmission by more than 40% (Jackson et al., 2003). However, studies indicate that women who receive single-dose nevirapine to prevent transmission to their newborn may develop resistance to the drug, potentially compromising the effectiveness of future antiretroviral regimens (Johnson et al., 2005; Flys et al., 2005; Jourdain et al., 2004). While the benefits of single-dose nevirapine outweigh the risk of resistance in resource-limited settings, development of affordable regimens with superior resistance profiles represents an urgent global priority.

Prolonged breastfeeding by HIV-infected mothers significantly increases the risk of HIV transmission to the infant. Breastfeeding is preferable to artificial feeding in the first six months of life, regardless of the mother's HIV status, as replacement feeding poses a greater risk of death to the infant than breastfeeding from an HIV-infected mother in the first months (Ross and Labbok, 2004). HIV-infected mothers are advised to wean their infants early to avoid prolonged exposure of the infant and to avoid combining breastfeeding with replacement feeding, which appears to heighten the risk of transmission. The complex relationship between breastfeeding and HIV transmission risk to the newborn underscores the importance of extensive, culturally appropriate counselling on breastfeeding to new mothers who are living with HIV. Current research is focused on the potential of an extended course of nevirapine therapy to reduce the risk of HIV transmission through breastfeeding.

Because the women and households served by prevention of mother-to-child transmission services have multiple, often overwhelming needs, efforts to scale up such services require extensive investments in programmes that extend well beyond the delivery of counselling and short-course antiretroviral drugs in antenatal settings. Founded in 2002, the MTCT-Plus initiative administered by Columbia University's Mailman School of Public Health in the United States seeks to accelerate uptake of HIV prevention services by ensuring long-term access to antiretroviral drugs by women reached by prevention of mother-to-child transmission programmes. As of early 2006, the initiative was supporting 13 sites in 9 countries in Africa and Asia and providing HIV care and treatment to more than 8000 individuals.

In 2004, WFP issued formal guidance to the field on the integration of food and nutrition support into programmes for the prevention of mother-to-child transmission. In Rwanda, WFP provides food assistance from the 7th month of pregnancy until the baby is 12 months old. Such assistance not only contributes to the health of HIV-infected mothers and their newborns, but also helps reduce economic burdens associated with childbirth and HIV infection. (WFP, 2004.)

The Family Planning Association of Kenya provides an example of such integration in action. Working closely with the International Planned Parenthood Federation, the Family Planning Association of Kenya developed a model of services that offers comprehensive sexual and reproductive health care together with a wide range of services related to HIV including antiretroviral therapy for people living with HIV. The association's pioneering programme offers antiretroviral therapy in a sexual and reproductive health setting. All nine clinics of the association provide voluntary HIV counselling and testing; several offer prevention of mother-to-child HIV transmission as part of their maternal health services, and four of the nine are geared up to provide antiretroviral therapy. The provision of antiretroviral therapy is part of the BACKUP Initiative (Building Alliances—Creating Knowledge—Updating Partners in the fight against HIV/AIDS, tuberculosis and malaria) of the German development agency, Deutsche Gesellschaft für Technische Zusammenarbeit. Thus, the Family Planning Association of Kenya has demonstrated that the provision of antiretroviral therapy within sexual and reproductive health settings is both possible and practical. The strong network of community health volunteers attached to the clinics provides an excellent infrastructure for delivery of antiretroviral therapy and has good prospects of reaching the poor and marginalized with this life-saving therapy.

LINKING HIV RESPONSES WITH REPRODUCTIVE AND SEXUAL HEALTH SERVICES

There is an inherent association between HIV and sexual and reproductive health as many more than 75% of HIV infections are acquired through sexual transmission or through transmission during pregnancy, labour and delivery, or during breastfeeding. The presence of sexually transmitted infections other than HIV increases the risk of HIV transmission. Apart from these obvious direct associations, many of the same root causes affecting sexual and reproductive health status are also linked with the epidemic, such as gender inequality, poverty, stigma and discrimination, and marginalization of populations vulnerable to HIV (UNFPA, 2005).

Experience teaches that strengthening links between sexual and reproductive health and HIV programming can lead to important public health benefits. The commitment of the international community to intensify links between sexual and reproductive health and HIV at the policy and programme level is expressed in the June 2005 UNAIDS policy position paper *Intensifying HIV Prevention*. This reflects and builds upon two internationally agreed-upon policy statements: (i) the New York Call to Commitment: Linking HIV/AIDS and Sexual and Reproductive Health (UNFPA, 2004a); and (ii) The Glion Call to Action on Family Planning and HIV/AIDS in Women and Children (UNFPA, 2004b).

The New York Call to Commitment was issued in June 2004 by UNAIDS, UNFPA and Family Care International, at a high-level consultation that stressed the critical need to link HIV and sexual and reproductive health services. Noting that failure to link these systems has diminished the effectiveness of global efforts, the Glion Call to Action called for necessary resources to promote links between HIV and sexual and reproductive health, integration of links in national development plans and budgets, and a coordinated and coherent HIV response built on the principles of the "Three Ones."

▶ HIV Prevention for Women and Girls: A Global Priority

Extensive evidence demonstrates that HIV prevention initiatives that are specifically tailored to women's needs can reduce women's risk of HIV infection. Nevertheless, there are still far too few evidence-based prevention programmes that are designed for the particular needs of women and girls. These are sorely needed. For the most part, HIV prevention strategies have yet to grapple effectively with the gender dimensions of HIV prevention, treatment and impact mitigation. As well as being more physiologically vulnerable to sexual HIV transmission than men, women face a host of social, economic and legal disadvantages that severely limit their ability to protect themselves against HIV infection. In many countries, married women have little means of insisting on abstinence or that their husbands use a condom during sexual intercourse, even if they suspect he is having unprotected sex outside their marriage.

Effective HIV prevention for women has many components. These include easy access to HIV prevention services and commodities, intensified research efforts to develop new prevention methods that women can control, policy reforms to reduce women's vulnerability to HIV infection, and longer-term efforts to develop new gender norms and influence the behaviour and attitudes of men and boys. Sustained advocacy will be necessary for these to be realized, and with this in mind, the Global Coalition on Women and AIDS was launched by UNAIDS in 2004. The coalition aims to increase global awareness of the epidemic's growing burden on women and girls and to catalyse effective action to address the many sources of women's vulnerability to HIV infection. The coalition unites a broad array of stakeholders—including civil society groups, networks of women living with HIV, governments and UN agencies—to advocate for policies that address fundamental gender inequities and that promote women's empowerment.

Empowerment of Women and Gender Equality

Provision of clinical services and HIV prevention commodities are far from sufficient, however, to contain the epidemic among women and girls. In the long run, effective HIV prevention for women will require policy reforms that empower women and promote gender equality. Central to an effective prevention response for women is a strong commitment to universal education. Higher education levels for girls are associated with a higher age of marriage, reduced fertility, improved health-seeking behaviour, lower vulnerability to genital mutilation, and reduced risk of HIV and other sexually transmitted infections (Grown et al., 2005).

CHANGING THE ATTITUDES OF MEN AND BOYS

Forging new gender norms requires changing the attitudes and practices of men and boys. The International Planned Parenthood Federation currently has a number of projects around the world that aim to engage men in efforts to build healthier norms. For example, as a component of an initiative to build sexual and reproductive health capacity in Haiti, support from the foundation enabled the PROFAMIL (Association pour la Promotion de la Famille Haïtienne) project to help women and men negotiate sexual decision-making and to recognize that both partners should together decide whether to use a condom (IPPF, 2003a). With the aim of changing men's gender attitudes and to promote communication between men and women regarding condom use, the foundation sponsored a project in Kenya that included male-only clinics, motivational exercises to encourage male use of condoms, and various male-targeted information, education and communications approaches (IPPF, 2003b). In Brazil, it supports men's discussion groups that encourage men to reformulate certain beliefs about sexuality and the role of men in sexual and reproductive health.

Other policy actions that support HIV prevention for women and girls include legal reform to secure women's property and inheritance rights, implementation and enforcement of strong legal measures tackling violence against women, enhanced global and regional collaboration to fight human trafficking, and mainstreaming of gender issues into programmes and policies. Leaders in government, religion, business and the media should vocally lead efforts to promote equality and empowerment for women, and education sectors should prioritize initiatives to inculcate healthier gender norms among boys.

▶ Protecting Young People

UNAIDS estimates that people aged under 25 years account for half of all new HIV infections. Young people's risk of HIV infection is closely correlated with age of sexual debut (Pettifor et al., 2004). Accordingly, abstinence from sexual intercourse and delayed initiation of sexual behaviour are among the central aims of HIV prevention efforts for young people (Santelli et al., 2006). For the many young people who are sexually active, access to comprehensive prevention services, including prevention education and provision of condoms, represents an urgent global health necessity and a fundamental human right.

Young people who need HIV prevention services include both males and females, school students and young people who do not attend school, sexually inexperienced young people and those who are sexually active, and a substantial percentage (especially among girls) who are already married. No single prevention approach will meet the diverse needs of all young people who are vulnerable to HIV infection.

To be effective, HIV prevention services for young people should be widely accessible, evidence-based, grounded in human rights, age-specific and gender-responsive, and should help build life skills to enable young people to reduce their vulnerability. Such services should also involve young people living with HIV, and support balanced and comprehensive prevention strategies that promote abstinence, faithfulness, women's equality and empowerment, reduction in the number of partners, and consistent condom use (UNICEF, 2005). Young people themselves are often especially effective deliverers of HIV prevention interventions to their peers and thus have an important role to play in the development, implementation and evaluation of youth-oriented HIV prevention programmes.

Open discussion of sex is necessary to the provision of effective HIV prevention for young people. In some cultures, many young people, especially girls seeking to preserve their virginity, may engage in anal or oral sex in the belief that such behaviours do not constitute sex. Veiled or euphemistic discussion of sexuality may inadvertently permit such misconceptions to persist, potentially placing young people at risk of HIV infection.

School-Based HIV Prevention Programmes

Ensuring young people's access to school or other educational opportunities plays a critical role in HIV prevention efforts. Not only are higher levels of education associated with safer sexual behaviours and delayed sexual debut (UNICEF, 2005; Prata, Vahidnia and Fraser, 2005), but school attendance enables students to benefit from school-based sexuality education and HIV prevention programming. In a review of studies of school-based HIV prevention programmes in Africa, 10 of 11 studies found they were associated with significant improvements in young people's HIV-related knowledge, and all studies that assessed students' attitudes detected positive behavioural changes. The review found evidence that school-based programmes can contribute to delayed sexual initiation, a reduction in the number of sexual partners, and increases in condom use, although producing sustained behavioural change appears more difficult than increasing knowledge (Gallant and Maticka-Tyndale, 2004).

Contrary to common fears or stereotypes, extensive research has detected little evidence that sex education leads to an increase in sexual activity (Kirby et al., 2005; Cowan, 2002). In recent years, programmes that promote abstinence as the sole HIV prevention strategy for young people have attracted considerable attention from researchers, programme implementers, policy-makers, advocates and commentators. On the basis of extensive experience in low- and middle-income countries as well as in high-income countries, experts in adolescent health broadly agree that comprehensive HIV prevention programmes—which simultaneously promote condom use and delayed initiation of sex for those who are sexually active—represent the most effective approach to HIV prevention for young people. A formal position statement of the Society for Adolescent Medicine, released in January 2006, supports a "comprehensive approach to sexual risk reduction, including abstinence, as well as correct and consistent use of condoms and contraception among teens who choose to be sexually active" (Santelli et al., 2006).

However school-based HIV prevention programmes cannot reach young people who are not sent to school. Provision of in-school meals helps to bring vulnerable children to school and provides them with access to education including HIV education. WFP is working with governments, nongovernmental organizations and UN agencies to integrate HIV prevention education into its school feeding programmes, thereby serving a dual purpose of protecting young people.

Given the links between HIV infection and injecting drug use, HIV prevention programmes for young people should integrate strong, evidence-based drug prevention messages. Youth-oriented HIV prevention initiatives should also address the many other factors that increase the risk of HIV transmission, such as violence or sexual abuse. Moreover, programmes are needed to meet the HIV prevention needs of the millions of school-age children who do not attend school.

In 2005, in response to the urgent need for HIV prevention with and for young people, UNAIDS and UNICEF, with the support of UNFPA and UNESCO, initiated the *Unite for Children, Unite against AIDS* campaign, which seeks, among other things, to ensure achievement of the 2001 Declaration of Commitment's target of a 25% reduction in HIV prevalence among young people by 2010.

HIV Education Through the Mass Media

The mass media has an important role to play in promoting greater awareness and understanding of HIV and thus its prevention. A study of a youth-oriented media campaign in Zambia called the Helping Each Other Act Responsibly Together (HEART) campaign found that young people who saw the campaign

USING THEATRE TO PROMOTE HIV PREVENTION FOR YOUNG PEOPLE

In Burkina Faso, the International Building Workers Union supports a drama group that uses music, drama and poetry to educate communities about HIV. Called Yamwekre, which means 'prick your conscience,' the group has reached more than 10 000 people. Discussion sessions follow each performance. The group has particularly focused on reaching young people and their parents. Since good practice emphasizes the participation of children in designing the programmes that affect them, children from 30 schools have been asked to take part in a competition to choose the themes the theatre group should incorporate in its work.

were 60% more likely than those who had not to report being abstinent and more than twice as likely to have ever used a condom (Underwood et al., 2006). Similarly, a youth-oriented mass media and interpersonal communication campaign in Cameroon increased condom use during the last episode of sex with a regular partner by 32% (Meekers, Agha and Klein, 2005). To achieve successful results, reporters and editors must themselves be properly educated about HIV. Not doing so can have serious consequences, as was shown in three case studies in Guinea, Sudan and Uganda. In each case, inaccurate, misleading and stigmatizing media reports on HIV and refugees risked inflaming the local population and exposing refugees to discrimination (Lowicki-Zucca, Spiegel and Ciantia, 2005).

> **TELEVISION FOR CHILDREN TEACHES TOLERANCE**
>
> In South Africa, Takalani Sesame Street teaches children about HIV and AIDS. Started by the Public Broadcasting System in the United States in 1969, Sesame Street was introduced in South Africa in 1996, and in 2000 the country's own version was launched with the support of the United States Agency for International Development and South African Department of Education. In September 2002, Kami, a five-year-old girl puppet became part of the show. She is an orphan whose mother died of AIDS-related illness and her role is to humanize and destigmatize people living with HIV and encourage open discussion about issues such as coping with illness and loss.

Since the UN Secretary-General Kofi Annan convened a special meeting of media leaders in January 2004 to establish the Global Media AIDS Initiative, the media's engagement in the response has significantly increased at a global level. Meetings of regional- and national-level media leaders have been held in Moscow and New Delhi and in November 2004, 100 creative individuals from 35 media companies attended the first ever meeting to encourage greater integration of HIV prevention messages in entertainment programming. Transatlantic Partners Against AIDS and the Heroes Project have launched public education campaigns in the Russian Federation and India, respectively. At a meeting in Johannesburg, in October 2005, African broadcast media leaders adopted the Old Fort Declaration on HIV/AIDS, which called for a redoubling of regional media efforts including incorporating HIV and AIDS as an integral part of the strategic business plans of media companies.

▶ Linking Treatment Access to HIV Prevention

Today's global efforts towards universal treatment access for people living with HIV provide critical opportunities to strengthen and accelerate HIV prevention efforts. Strong evidence demonstrates that increased treatment access enhances awareness, reduces stigma, increases use of HIV testing services and promotes the mobilization of communities affected by HIV (Global HIV Prevention Working Group, 2004). Many people believe that antiretroviral drugs may reduce the per-contact likelihood that an HIV-infected individual will transmit the virus, although this hypothesis is not substantiated by data.

A complicated dynamic exists between HIV prevention and treatment. As treatment access expands in resource-limited countries, the health, longevity and quality of life for people with HIV will improve, potentially increasing opportunities for sexual transmission. At the same time, optimism about the treatment or misperceptions about the effects of antiretroviral drugs may also cause some people to increase their risk behaviour. Concern about this potential effect is not without foundation. In a study of 1168 HIV-positive women in the United States, initiation of antiretroviral therapy was associated with an increased likelihood of engaging in unprotected sex (Wilson et al., 2004). Among men who have sex with men in Sao Paolo, men who were optimistic about HIV treatment prospects were significantly more likely to engage in unprotected sex (da Silva et al., 2005).

HIV Prevention Services for HIV-Positive People

One strategy for maximizing the prevention benefits of greater treatment access is to increase prevention services for people living with HIV. While most people who test HIV-positive take careful steps to avoid exposing others to the virus, studies indicate that a minority of people with diagnosed HIV infection often have difficulty implementing and sustaining safer sexual practices (Denning and Campsmith, 2005). Relatively few studies have been undertaken to measure the effectiveness of behavioural interventions for people living with HIV, but emerging evidence indicates that such programmes are effective in reducing the likelihood that people with HIV will engage in sexual activity that might expose others to the virus (Crepaz et al., 2005). Integration of HIV prevention counselling in a home-based antiretroviral therapy programme in Uganda, combined with voluntary HIV counselling and testing for the partners of persons on antiretroviral therapy, resulted in a 70% drop in unprotected sex, including an 85% reduction in unprotected sex among married couples (Bunnell, 2006).

As a result of expanded treatment access, millions of people living with HIV are periodically visiting health-care delivery sites to monitor their treatment progress. This provides important opportunities for the delivery and reinforcement of HIV prevention for people living with HIV (Global HIV Prevention Working Group, 2004; CDC, 2003). A study of six HIV clinics in California, found that the delivery of brief HIV prevention counselling by medical providers reduced reported episodes of unprotected sex by 38% among HIV-infected patients seen at the clinic (Richardson et al., 2004).

▶ Safe Injections and Health-care Precautions

Although bloodborne exposure results in substantially fewer new HIV infections each year than does sexual intercourse, direct exposure of blood to HIV is the most efficient means of transmission. Effective HIV prevention measures exist for the major sources of bloodborne transmission—injecting drug use, injections in health-care settings and blood transfusion—although many countries are making inadequate use of these highly effective tools.

Unsafe injections in health-care settings account for an estimated 5% of new HIV infections worldwide, including 2.5% of new infections in sub-Saharan Africa (Hauri, Armstrong and Hutin, 2004). Although unsafe injections account for substantially fewer new HIV infections than does sexual intercourse (Schmid et al., 2004), an estimated 250 000 people contracted HIV through medical injections in 2003, underscoring the need for all national HIV prevention programmes to promote adherence to sound infection control practices in health-care settings, including prohibitions on the reuse of injection equipment. Relatively inexpensive auto-disable syringes help prevent HIV transmission in health-care settings by making reuse impossible and by eliminating the risk of inadvertent needle-stick injuries. International guidelines recommend use of auto-disable syringes as the equipment of choice for immunization initiatives (WHO et al., 1999).

While use of auto-disable syringes for routine immunization has significantly increased in recent years, 38% of low- and middle-income countries did not use such syringes in their national vaccine programmes in 2004 (WHO, 2005c). The Global Alliance for Vaccines and Immunization has significantly contributed to the implementation of safer injection practices worldwide, financing the purchase and delivery of nearly 1 billion auto-disable syringes between 2000 and 2005.

Preventing unsafe injections is only one component of a broader effort to ensure sound infection control practices in health and emergency settings, where workers may be exposed to blood or other body fluids. This risk can be significantly lowered through workers' adherence to universal precautions, which involve the routine use of gloves and other protective equipment to prevent occupational exposures, safe disposal of sharps, and timely administration of a four-week prophylactic course of antiretroviral drugs (CDC, 2001). Where workers have the potential to encounter blood or other body fluids in the course of their work, employers have an obligation to train these workers in infection control and to ensure ready access to protective equipment and post-exposure prophylaxis.

Blood Safety

While blood transfusions were an important source of HIV transmission in the epidemic's early stages, the incidence of blood-related HIV infection has declined over time as countries have implemented recommended strategies to improve the safety of the blood supply. Despite recent progress, ensuring the safety of the blood supply remains a particular challenge in times of emergency, when wars, civil strife, disasters or epidemics damage health infrastructure.

One important measure for public health systems to carry out is to reduce and eventually stop paying for blood and increase the use of voluntary donors, who are the least likely to transmit infectious agents such as HIV and hepatitis viruses. Only 40 countries in the world have achieved 100% voluntary blood donation. However, some countries have made substantial progress in this direction. In China, for example, the percentage of blood units obtained from voluntary donors increased from 22% to 94.5% between 1998 and 2005 (Ministry of Health China, 2006).

▶ Prevention Technologies

Although available prevention strategies are highly effective, they have important limitations. Existing tools for the prevention of sexual HIV transmission are not 100% efficacious, do not confer lifelong protection and typically depend on the individual's correct and consistent use during each instance of sex, as well as the individual's ability to negotiate condom use with his or her partner. The current array of prevention options is notably insufficient for women, who lack access to unobtrusive prevention methods under their control.

However, recent years have witnessed an acceleration of efforts to develop new prevention approaches. By early 2006, large-scale human trials had been initiated to assess the HIV prevention efficacy of microbicides, the female diaphragm and adult male circumcision, and research continues on vaccine development.

Supporting Research

Although progress on HIV vaccine research has been slow, the search for a vaccine remains one of the world's most urgent scientific priorities. A Phase III trial is under way in Thailand to assess the efficacy of a vaccine based on a canary-pox vector containing genetic components of HIV. Numerous other candidates are also in earlier stages of development, with clinical trials currently under way in Africa, Asia, Australia, Europe, South America and North America.

However, a host of complex scientific challenges has slowed progress on development of a vaccine. No perfect animal model exists for HIV, the correlates of immunity are unknown, the virus can be transmitted in multiple ways, and there is substantial viral variability around the world.

In an effort to overcome obstacles to accelerated vaccine development, diverse partners in 2003 launched the Global HIV/AIDS Vaccine Enterprise. This is a multi-stakeholder alliance of independent research organizations dedicated to greater strategic collaboration on HIV vaccine research. Following extensive deliberations by working groups focused on the key scientific and logistic barriers to swifter vaccine development, the enterprise published a strategic scientific plan in 2005 that is intended to guide the collaboration and resource allocations of key actors in the field (Global HIV/AIDS Vaccine Enterprise, 2005).

A founding member of the Global HIV/AIDS Vaccine Enterprise, the International AIDS Vaccine Initiative—which celebrates its tenth anniversary this year—has assembled research consortia to improve understanding of the mechanisms of action of live-attenuated vaccines and of the requirements for broadly neutralizing HIV antibodies. Since its creation, this initiative has advanced five vaccine candidates into human trials, and mobilized roughly US$ 300 million in new funding for HIV vaccine research.

Political support for HIV vaccine development has increased, as has available funding. In October 2005, 2000 African leaders, international scientists and vaccine stakeholders gathered in Yaoundé, Cameroon, to devise strategies concerning legislation and other policy responses to ensure regional preparedness for future vaccine trials. The Group of Eight lead-

---

KEEPING UP MOMENTUM ON MICROBICIDES

In light of the critical need for unobtrusive prevention technologies that women can control, increased global energy has been focused on research to develop topical microbicides that protect against HIV transmission during vaginal intercourse (Weber et al., 2005; Moore, 2005). Microbicides are gels, creams or other substances that can be inserted in the vagina to reduce the risk of HIV transmission. It is believed that microbicides might also potentially offer a measure of protection against transmission of HIV and other sexually transmitted microorganisms during rectal intercourse, although research and development for such a product is much less advanced than for vaginal microbicides. More than 60 candidate vaginal microbicides are under development, including 5 that are now being tested in large Phase III human trials in 10 countries.

Spending by the public and philanthropic sectors on microbicide research and development has more than doubled since 2000. On World AIDS Day in 2005, the governments of Denmark, Ireland, Sweden and the United Kingdom announced nearly US$ 30 million in new funding for the International Partnership for Microbicides, the result of sustained advocacy by the international partnership and other partners such as the Global Campaign for Microbicides and the Alliance for Microbicide Development.

ing industrialized countries reaffirmed their commitment to a robust vaccine research effort at their annual summit meeting in Gleneagles, in 2005.

Obstacles to Research and Development

The quickened pace of research on new HIV prevention approaches is merely one outcome of a new approach to global health, catalysed by strong and sustained activism and new sources of funding. However, HIV prevention clinical trials are often complex and expensive, requiring the enrolment and retention over several years of thousands of uninfected volunteers. Between 2004 and 2010, it is estimated that capacity for at least 96 000 volunteers in clinical trials will be needed to prevent delays in the development of potentially promising new HIV prevention tools.

Prevention research can often be highly controversial. For example, activist criticism regarding the fairness of planned multi-country research led to termination in 2005 of trials in Cambodia and Cameroon that were to test the use of the antiretroviral drug tenofovir in pre-exposure prevention. The experience with tenofovir highlights the need for researchers to engage a broad range of national and community stakeholders in the planning and conduct of prevention trials (UNAIDS, 2006; International AIDS Society, 2005). UNAIDS initiated a global consultation process in 2005 designed to inform the development of guidelines for durable partnerships between HIV prevention researchers and key stakeholders.

▶ A Sound Policy Environment

Implementing a strong national HIV prevention programme involves more than the selection of an appropriate mix of programmatic actions. It also requires a strong national policy framework that encourages safer behaviours, reduces vulnerability, maximizes the accessibility and effectiveness of HIV prevention services, promotes gender equality and women's empowerment, and reduces stigma and discrimination.

To mount a comprehensive, sustained HIV prevention effort with the appropriate coverage and intensity, financing for such efforts must significantly increase. UNAIDS and its research partners estimate that US$ 11.4 billion in financing for HIV prevention activities will be needed by 2008 to ensure that the world is on track to achieve the Millennium Development Goal of halting and beginning to reverse the global AIDS epidemic by 2015. Were the world to mount such a comprehensive, evidence-based response in all regions, HIV prevention would account for 52% of all HIV and AIDS spending worldwide in 2008 (UNAIDS, 2005c).

In 2005, with the aim of promoting universal access to HIV prevention, UNAIDS published a policy position paper, *Intensifying HIV Prevention,* which articulates basic principles and strategies that form the basis of strong national HIV prevention plans (UNAIDS, 2005a). For all countries, HIV prevention requires specific policy actions and programmatic actions, implemented with sufficient coverage, scale and intensity. These actions are detailed below. While national prevention programmes in all settings should incorporate each essential programmatic and policy action, the relative emphasis of specific HIV prevention measures may differ, based on the nature and severity of national and subnational HIV epidemics.

Essential Policy Actions for HIV Prevention

- Ensure that human rights are promoted, protected and respected and that measures are taken to eliminate stigma and discrimination.
- Build and maintain leadership from all sections of society, including governments, affected communities, nongovernmental organizations, faith-based organizations, the education sector, media, the private sector and trade unions.
- Involve people living with HIV in the design, implementation and evaluation of prevention strategies, addressing their distinct prevention needs.
- Address cultural norms and beliefs, recognizing both the key role they play in supporting prevention efforts and the potential they have to fuel HIV transmission.
- Promote gender equality and address gender norms and relations to reduce the vulnerability of women and girls to HIV infection, involving men and boys in this effort.
- Promote widespread knowledge and awareness of how HIV is transmitted and how infection can be averted.
- Promote the links between HIV prevention and sexual and reproductive health.
- Support the mobilization of community-based responses throughout the continuum of prevention, care and treatment.
- Promote programmes targeted at HIV prevention needs of key affected groups and populations.
- Mobilize and strengthen financial, human and institutional capacity across all sectors, particularly in health and education.
- Review and reform legal frameworks to remove barriers to effective, evidence-based HIV prevention, eliminate stigma and discrimination, and protect the rights of people living with HIV or vulnerable to or at risk of HIV infection.
- Ensure that sufficient investments are made in the research and development of, and advocacy for, new prevention technologies.

Essential Programmatic Actions for HIV Prevention

- Prevent the sexual transmission of HIV.
- Prevent mother-to-child transmission of HIV.
- Prevent the transmission of HIV through injecting drug use including harm reduction measures.
- Ensure the safety of the blood supply.
- Prevent HIV transmission in health-care settings.
- Promote greater access to voluntary HIV counselling and testing while promoting principles of confidentiality and consent.
- Integrate HIV prevention into AIDS treatment centres.
- Focus on HIV prevention among young people.
- Provide HIV-related information and education to enable individuals to protect themselves from infection.
- Confront and mitigate HIV-related stigma and discrimination.
- Prepare for access to and use of vaccines and microbicides.

New Approaches to HIV Prevention: Summary of Findings and Recommendations

Global HIV Prevention Working Group

▶ I. HIV Prevention Research: State of the Science

A wide range of promising HIV prevention approaches are in late-stage clinical trials:

- **Male circumcision:** Researchers have long observed that countries with higher rates of male circumcision have lower rates of HIV infection. In 2005, the first randomized efficacy trial of male circumcision for HIV prevention, conducted in South Africa, showed that circumcised men were 60 percent less likely than uncircumcised men to become infected with HIV from female partners.

  Three additional efficacy trials of male circumcision are underway in Kenya and Uganda to assess the applicability of the South African findings in other settings and populations, and to determine if male circumcision also reduces the risk of HIV transmission from men to their female partners. Results are expected in 2007.

- **Cervical barriers:** Researchers hypothesize that cervical barriers such as diaphragms, which are currently used for contraception, may help protect women from HIV and other sexually transmitted diseases. An efficacy trial of the diaphragm for HIV prevention is nearing completion in South Africa and Zimbabwe, and results are expected in 2007.

- **Pre-exposure prophylaxis with antiretrovirals:** Research in animals suggests that antiretroviral drugs used for HIV treatment may also be effective at preventing infection in HIV-uninfected adults, an approach called pre-exposure prophylaxis, or PREP. Efficacy trials of this approach are underway in Botswana, Peru, and Thailand. Results could be available as early as 2007 or 2008.

- **Herpes suppression:** Herpes, which infects up to 70 percent of people in some parts of sub-Saharan Africa, can triple the risk of HIV acquisition, as well as increase the risk of transmission to others. The inexpensive, off-patent drug acyclovir is approved for herpes suppression, and two trials are being conducted in Africa, Latin America,

327

and the U.S. to test the efficacy of suppressing herpes to lower HIV risk. Results are expected in 2007 and 2008.

- **Microbicides:** Microbicides are topical substances, such as gels or creams, that could be applied to the vagina or rectum to reduce HIV transmission. Five first-generation vaginal microbicide candidates are currently in late-stage clinical trials; results from some of these trials could be available by 2008. In addition, a number of second-generation microbicide candidates—which specifically target HIV or molecules of the cells it infects—are in earlier stages of research, and could complete clinical trials within 10 years.

- **HIV vaccines:** The best long-term hope for HIV prevention is a vaccine, although developing an effective vaccine has proven to be a highly complex scientific challenge. Most experts predict that it could be 10 years or more before an HIV vaccine candidate is shown to be effective. An effective vaccine will likely need to stimulate two types of immune response, although most of the vaccine candidates developed to date are designed to target only one arm of the immune system. Currently, 30 HIV vaccine candidates are in clinical trials, including two in advanced efficacy or proof-of-concept trials.

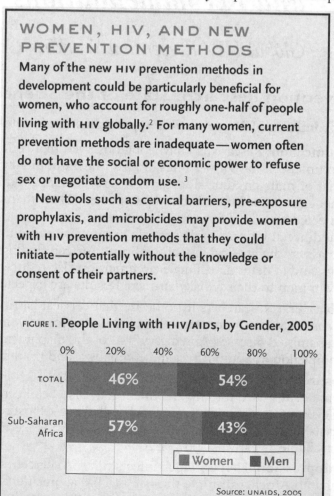

WOMEN, HIV, AND NEW PREVENTION METHODS

Many of the new HIV prevention methods in development could be particularly beneficial for women, who account for roughly one-half of people living with HIV globally.[2] For many women, current prevention methods are inadequate—women often do not have the social or economic power to refuse sex or negotiate condom use. [3]

New tools such as cervical barriers, pre-exposure prophylaxis, and microbicides may provide women with HIV prevention methods that they could initiate—potentially without the knowledge or consent of their partners.

FIGURE 1. **People Living with HIV/AIDS, by Gender, 2005**

	Women	Men
TOTAL	46%	54%
Sub-Saharan Africa	57%	43%

Source: UNAIDS, 2005

FIGURE 12-3 People Living with HIV/AIDs, by Gender, 2005
Source: UNAIDs, 2005

▶ 2. Accelerating HIV Prevention Research

As new HIV prevention approaches move forward into advanced stages of development, the world faces serious financial, logistical, and ethical challenges in completing ongoing prevention trials, and in mounting the additional large-scale trials that will be needed to fully test new prevention tools and strategies. Key challenges—and recommendations from the Global HIV Prevention Working Group—include:

- **Clinical trials capacity:** Current efficacy trials of new HIV prevention approaches will require a total of approximately 80,000 study participants. Even more participants will be needed to mount additional efficacy studies and to conduct confirmatory trials. Yet current global clinical trials capacity—including an adequate number of participants, properly equipped study sites, and trained research staff—falls far short of the need.

  Recommendations: Trial sponsors, national governments, and international donors should make significant new investments in global capacity for HIV prevention trials. Agencies should work together to inventory existing capacity, determine specific needs in key regions, and identify sites for scaling up capacity. Given limited capacity, trial sponsors should better coordinate decision-making about which prevention interventions to prioritize for large-scale trials, and share trial sites as necessary.

- **Ethical issues:** While current HIV prevention trials are being conducted according to internationally and locally accepted ethical standards, existing guidelines do not sufficiently address some key issues that have emerged in recent years. These include defining the standard set of existing prevention methods that should be provided to all trial participants; defining and ensuring fully informed consent; and determining how to facilitate HIV treatment access for participants who become HIV-infected during the course of a trial, or who are found to be HIV-infected at the initial screening for a trial.

  Recommendations: Key stakeholders in HIV prevention research—including trial sponsors, affected communities, and developing country governments—should work with UNAIDs and the World Health Organization (WHO) to convene a broadly inclusive panel of experts to develop updated ethical guidelines for conducting HIV prevention research. This guidance should be continually revised as HIV prevention research evolves.

- **Community engagement:** Community involvement and support are vital to successful clinical research. Yet some HIV prevention trials have been criticized for not properly reaching out to communities. In some cases, misinformation and lack of communication between researchers and communities have been factors in the cancellation of HIV prevention trials.

  Recommendations: Investigators and sponsors of HIV prevention trials should foster strong partnerships with the communities where trials are conducted—through Community Advisory Boards, regular communications to the broader community, and involvement of key local and national officials. Community input should inform key aspects of the clinical research process, including development of trial protocols, recruitment of participants, and ongoing trial oversight. International agencies such as UNAIDS and WHO should compile and publish best practices in community engagement.

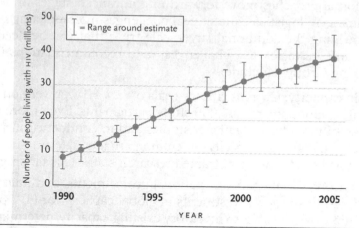

FIGURE 2. **Global HIV/AIDS Epidemic, 1990–2005**

FIGURE 12-4 Global HIV/AIDs Epidemic, 1990–2005
Source: UNAIDs, 2006

▶ 3. Preparing for Access

As soon as they are shown to be effective, new HIV prevention methods should be made accessible and affordable for people at risk. But the world is virtually unprepared to ensure rapid access. Key challenges and recommendations include:

- **Resources:** While there have been significant increases in global spending to fight the HIV/AIDs epidemic in recent years, there are still severe resource gaps. UNAIDs estimates that $11.4 billion will be needed annually for HIV prevention by 2008—two-and-a-half times current spending.[4] Ensuring timely, widespread access to new prevention methods will require significant additional resources. Many countries will need donor assistance to purchase new prevention tools such as pre-exposure prophylaxis, microbicides, and vaccines. New resources will also be needed to support provider training and community education programs, to ensure that new prevention methods are safely and properly implemented.

  Recommendations: The international community—including major donors such as the Global Fund to Fight AIDs, Tuberculosis, and Malaria, and the U.S. government's President's Emergency Plan for AIDs Relief—should commit to providing the resources necessary to ensure the roll-out of new HIV prevention tools as soon as they are shown to be effective. It is critical to begin estimating now the resources that will be needed to implement new prevention methods. It is also vital that these resources do not take funding away from current HIV prevention, treatment, and care programs.

- **Public health guidance:** As results become available from clinical trials, national and global decision-makers will need to carefully determine how to integrate new HIV prevention methods into health programs. In the case of new technologies such as microbicides and HIV vaccines, regulatory review and licensure will be required as well. Yet there are significant gaps in global capacity to provide timely public health guidance and regulatory review for new HIV prevention interventions.

Recommendations: Key stakeholders in HIV prevention—including national governments, donors, and international agencies such as UNAIDs and WHO—should establish systems to anticipate and provide needed guidance on the introduction of new prevention methods. Key issues include developing formal public health guidance on the proper use of new prevention approaches, and developing tools to help decision-makers in developing countries assess the relative cost and benefit of new prevention interventions. In addition, regulatory agencies in the U.S. and Europe should provide assistance to their counterparts in developing countries on evaluating new prevention methods.

- **Provider training:** Health care professionals and community health providers will require training in the safe and proper use of new HIV prevention methods. For example, in many developing countries, few health care providers have experience in circumcising adult males, and if the procedure is improperly performed it can result in serious injury or death. The problem of health worker training is compounded by the fact that many developing countries suffer acute shortages of qualified health care personnel in general.

Recommendations: International agencies such as UNAIDs and WHO should develop regional and country-level provider training programs to help promote the safe and proper use of new HIV prevention methods. Where possible, training in providing new HIV prevention methods should be integrated into ongoing health provider training programs, and traditional healers should be included in these programs.

- **Preventing "disinhibition":** It is essential that the introduction of new prevention methods does not lead people to become complacent about HIV risk behavior. Such behavioral disinhibition could cancel out the benefits of new HIV prevention methods, and lead to an inadvertent increase in HIV infections

Recommendations: Strong communications and public education campaigns, grounded in scientific evidence of effectiveness, should accompany the introduction of new prevention methods, to reinforce the importance of minimizing risk behavior and using new prevention methods in combination with existing tools and strategies. It is also critical to monitor and evaluate efforts to counter potential disinhibition on an ongoing basis to ensure they are effective.

▶ Expanding Access to Existing HIV Prevention Approaches

As research moves forward on new HIV prevention methods, it is also critical to expand access to existing prevention methods.

Fewer than one in five people at high risk for HIV currently have access to effective prevention (see Figure 12-5).[5] According to an analysis by UNAIDs and the World Health Organization, expanded access to proven prevention strategies could avert half of the 62 million new HIV infections projected to occur between 2005 and 2015.[6]

The following tools and strategies are proven to reduce the risk of HIV transmission:[7]

Preventing Sexual Transmission

- **Behavior change, including abstinence and condom use:** A number of scientific studies have documented the effectiveness of behavior change programs that encourage people to adopt safer sexual behaviors. These include remaining sexually abstinent or delaying initiation of sexual activity, decreasing the number of sexual partners, and using condoms consistently and correctly if sexually active.

- **HIV testing:** Encouraging HIV testing is critical for prevention—people who know their HIV status are more likely to protect themselves and others from infection.
- **Diagnosis and treatment of other STDs:** Infection with other sexually transmitted diseases (STDs) such as gonorrhea increases the risk of HIV transmission, and prompt diagnosis and treatment of STDs can help reduce HIV risk.

Preventing Blood Borne Transmission

- **Harm reduction for injection drug users:** Harm reduction programs that provide clean needles and syringes have been proven to be effective in reducing the risk of HIV transmission among injection drug users, without contributing to an increase in drug use.
- **Blood supply safety:** Routine screening of the blood supply can virtually eliminate the risk of HIV transmission through donated blood.
- **Infection control in health care:** Countries that require health workers to adopt "universal precautions" such as wearing gloves and masks have succeeded in making HIV transmission extremely rare in health care settings.

Preventing Mother-to-Child Transmission

- **Antiretroviral drugs:** The inexpensive antiretroviral drug nevirapine can reduce the risk that an HIV-infected pregnant woman will transmit HIV to her child by nearly 50 percent. Combinations of antiretrovirals can reduce the risk even further.
- **Breastfeeding alternatives:** The chance of an HIV-infected mother transmitting HIV to her newborn increases by up to half with prolonged breastfeeding, and HIV-infected mothers should have access to breastfeeding alternatives.
- **Caesarean delivery:** Caesarean delivery significantly reduces the risk of mother-to-child HIV transmission.

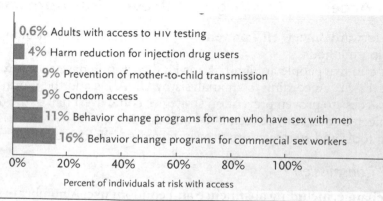

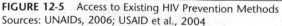

FIGURE 12-5 Access to Existing HIV Prevention Methods
Sources: UNAIDs, 2006; USAID et al., 2004

Supportive Policies

HIV prevention is most effective when it is supported by strong and visible political leadership, and by policies that address the root causes of vulnerability to HIV, including:

- **Anti-stigma measures** that prevent discrimination against people with HIV and vulnerable groups
- **Gender-equality initiatives,** including programs to enhance women's education and economic independence, and laws to combat sexual violence and trafficking
- **Involvement of communities and HIV-infected individuals** in educating people about HIV, and in developing, implementing, and evaluating prevention programs
- **Visible political leadership** that prioritizes a comprehensive response to the HIV/AIDs epidemic, including prevention, treatment, and care

▶ 1. HIV Prevention Research: State of the Science

A range of promising new HIV prevention approaches are currently under investigation. If shown to be effective, these new tools and strategies could help avert millions of new infections, and have a substantial impact on the course of the HIV/AIDs epidemic. They include:

- Male circumcision
- Cervical barriers
- Pre-exposure prophylaxis with antiretrovirals
- Herpes suppression
- Microbicides
- HIV vaccines

Some of these new prevention methods—including male circumcision, cervical barriers, pre-exposure prophylaxis with antiretrovirals, and herpes suppression—could potentially be shown to be effective within the next few years. While the successful development of prevention methods such as microbicides and vaccines is likely to take longer, important progress is being made on these fronts as well.

Many of these new HIV prevention methods could be particularly beneficial for women, who represent approximately one-half of HIV infections globally, and nearly 60 percent of people living with HIV in sub-Saharan Africa.[8] Physiologically, women are more vulnerable to HIV infection than men. In addition, many women have difficultly negotiating abstinence and condom use with male partners, especially in countries where women lack legal rights and are economically dependent on men.[9]

It is important to note that there is no "magic bullet" for HIV, and that none of these new HIV prevention methods is likely to be 100 percent effective. All would require the continued use of current prevention methods that have already been proven to be effective—including behavior change programs, condoms, HIV testing, and treatment of other sexually transmitted diseases.[10] As discussed in section 3 of this report, it is also essential to ensure that risk behavior does not increase with the introduction of new prevention methods.

This section describes the state of research into new prevention tools and strategies. Figure 12-6 summarizes current efficacy trials of new HIV prevention methods.

NEW HIV PREVENTION APPROACHES IN DEVELOPMENT

- **Male circumcision:** Observational studies have shown that countries with high rates of male circumcision—removal of the foreskin of the penis—have lower HIV infection rates.
- **Cervical barriers:** Cervical barriers, such as the diaphragm, cover the cervix, the site where most HIV infections in the female genital tract are believed to occur.
- **Pre-exposure prophylaxis with antiretrovirals:** Antiretroviral drugs, which improve the health of HIV-infected people, may also prevent HIV infection.
- **Herpes suppression:** Data suggest that infection with HSV-2, the primary cause of genital herpes, increases the risk of HIV acquisition and transmission. Suppressing herpes with the inexpensive, off-patent drug acyclovir may reduce HIV risk.
- **Microbicides:** Microbicides are topical substances applied to the vagina or rectum to potentially prevent HIV infection.
- **HIV vaccines:** Preventive vaccines enhance the body's immune defenses, enabling the immune system to fight off diseases that it cannot naturally control.

▶ Male Circumcision

Male circumcision—removal of the foreskin of the penis—may reduce the risk of HIV acquisition and transmission during sexual intercourse.

Theoretical Basis

Observational studies have long noted that, on average, countries with high rates of male circumcision have lower HIV infection rates.[11] Circumcision may reduce HIV risk because the mucosal surface of the foreskin of the penis contains Langerhans cells that are highly susceptible to HIV infection.[12] Circumcision may reduce HIV risk directly, or have an indirect effect by preventing other sexually transmitted diseases that facilitate HIV acquisition and transmission.

Status of Research

In 2005, French and South African researchers announced encouraging results from the first randomized clinical trial of the efficacy of male circumcision for HIV prevention. The investigators reported that men who were randomly assigned to receive circumcision had a 60 percent lower risk of subsequently acquiring HIV infection from female partners than men randomized to the control arm of the study, who were offered circumcision after the trial ended. The trial was conducted among 3,274 men in a community near Johannesburg, South Africa, and the findings have generated hope that circumcision could be an important new HIV prevention strategy.[13]

Three efficacy trials of male circumcision are underway in Kenya and Uganda, and UNAIDs and other international health agencies have emphasized the importance of waiting for these results before recommending widespread adoption of male circumcision for HIV prevention.[14] The trials in Kenya and Uganda involve more than 8,000 men, and are likely to offer important insights regarding the applicability of male circumcision in different settings. For example, the Uganda trials involve a broader age range (15–49) than the South Africa and Kenya

Prevention Method	Trial Sites and Participants	Primary Sponsors and Funders
Male Circumcision	Kenya—2,500 men	University of Illinois, U.S. National Institutes of Health (NIH)
	Uganda—5,000 men	Johns Hopkins University, NIH
	Uganda—1,361 men and 7,000 women	Columbia University, Gates Foundation
Cervical Barriers Female diaphragms	South Africa and Zimbabwe—5,045 women	University of California at San Francisco, Gates Foundation
Pre-Exposure Prophylaxis with Antiretrovirals		
Tenofovir	Thailand—1,600 injection drug users	U.S. Centers for Disease Control and Prevention (CDC)
Tenofovir plus emtricitabine	Botswana—1,200 men and women	CDC
	Peru—1,400 men who have sex with men	NIH
Herpes Suppression	Peru, South Africa, Zambia, Zimbabwe, and U.S.—3,277 men and women	University of Washington, NIH
	Botswana, Kenya, Rwanda, South Africa, Tanzania, Uganda, and Zambia—3,000 male-female couples in which one partner is infected with HIV and HSV-2	University of Washington, Gates Foundation
Microbicides		
C31G (Savvy)	Nigeria—2,142 women	Family Health International (FHI), U.S. Agency for International Development (USAID)
Carbopol 974p (BufferGel)	Malawi, South Africa, Tanzania, Zambia, Zimbabwe, and U.S.—3,220 women	NIH
Cellulose sulfate	Nigeria—2,160 women	FHI, USAID
	Benin, Burkina Faso, India, South Africa, and Uganda—2,574 women	CONRAD, Gates Foundation, USAID
Naphthalene sulfonate (PRO2000)	Same as Carbopol trial (see above)	NIH
	South Africa, Tanzania, Uganda, Zambia, and Zimbabwe—10,000 women	U.K. Medical Research Council, U.K. Department for International Development
PC-515 (Carraguard)	South Africa—6,299 women	Population Council, Gates Foundation, USAID
HIV Vaccines		
gag, pol, nef in adenovirus type 5 (MrkAd5)	Australia, Brazil, Canada, Dominican Republic, Haiti, Jamaica, Peru, and U.S.—3,000 men and women	Merck & Co., NIH
env, gag, pol in canarypox + gp120 (ALVAC + AIDsVAX)	Thailand—16,000 men and women	Thailand Ministry of Public Health, NIH, U.S. Military HIV Research Program

FIGURE 12-6 Current Efficacy Trials of New HIV Prevention Methods

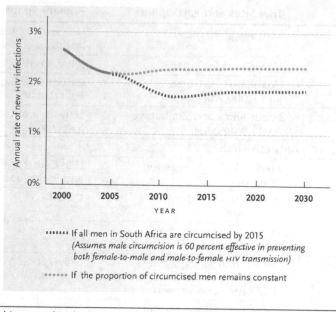

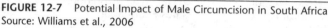

FIGURE 12-7   Potential Impact of Male Circumcision in South Africa
Source: Williams et al., 2006

---

trials (18–24), and use a different circumcision procedure (sleeve circumcision versus the forceps-guided procedure used in South Africa and Kenya). Results from these trials are expected in 2007.

In addition to studying the efficacy of male circumcision for preventing female-to-male HIV transmission, one of the trials in Uganda is following 7,000 women—including approximately 4,000 female partners of male participants in the circumcision trials—to determine if circumcising men also reduces the risk of HIV transmission from men to women, as suggested by observational data.[15] The findings among women in the Uganda trial could have important public health significance, because most HIV infections in women are the result of male-to-female transmission of the virus.

Potential Prevention Impact

Used in combination with other HIV prevention methods, male circumcision could have a substantial impact on reducing HIV acquisition and transmission. One modeling study predicts that widespread implementation of male circumcision could avert 2 million new HIV infections over the next 10 years in sub-Saharan Africa, and a further 3.7 million new infections over the 10 years after that (see Figure 12-7 for South Africa projections).[16] Circumcision is also potentially important as a prevention option because it is a one-time intervention that could offer life-long benefit. Research indicates that circumcision would be acceptable to men in Africa: a study of adult males circumcised in Kenya found that 99 percent were satisfied with the procedure, as were their female partners.[17]

When performed by a trained practitioner, male circumcision is a safe procedure (typically defined as resulting in surgical complications in fewer than 2 percent of cases), and analgesia effectively mitigates pain. However, as noted in section 3 of this report, concerns have been raised about the safety of circumcision procedures performed by medical practitioners or traditional healers who have not been properly trained, underscoring the importance of coupling future introduction of male circumcision for HIV prevention with strong training and quality assurance initiatives.

▶ Cervical Barriers

Cervical barriers such as the diaphragm and cervical caps are currently used with spermicides as contraceptives. Made of latex or silicone, they are inserted into the vagina to cover the cervix and serve as a barrier against sperm.

Theoretical Basis

Research suggests that most HIV infections in the female genital tract occur in the cervix and endocervix.[18] Cervical barriers such as diaphragms cover the cervix, and by doing so may significantly reduce women's risk of becoming infected with HIV. In addition, cervical barriers may prevent HIV by preventing infection with other sexually transmitted diseases that facilitate HIV transmission.

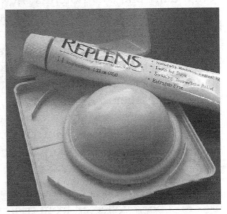
Diaphragm and lubricant gel

Status of Research

A clinical trial in South Africa and Zimbabwe is testing the efficacy of the latex diaphragm used with a non-contraceptive lubricant gel for preventing male-to-female HIV transmission. The trial involves 5,045 women and is comparing use of the diaphragm plus condoms with use of condoms alone. Results are expected in 2007.

Potential Prevention Impact

If proven to be effective for HIV prevention, cervical barriers such as diaphragms would have a number of distinct advantages. Diaphragms are inexpensive, reusable, and already approved and available for pregnancy prevention. In addition, diaphragms can be inserted in advance of sexual activity, left in place up to 24 hours, and potentially used without the knowledge of the woman's sexual partner. Studies in Zimbabwe suggest that the diaphragm is accepted among women at risk for HIV,[19] and women and their male partners prefer the diaphragm to other female-initiated prevention methods such as the female condom.[20]

Cervical barriers such as diaphragms could also potentially be used to deliver microbicides for HIV prevention (see discussion of microbicides on page 341).

▶ Pre-Exposure Prophylaxis with Antiretrovirals

Antiretroviral drugs, which improve the health of HIV-infected people, may also prevent HIV infection.

Theoretical Basis

Antiretroviral drugs, which have improved the health and prolonged the lives of people infected with HIV, are currently also used to prevent some forms of HIV transmission. Timely administration of antiretrovirals reduces the risk of HIV transmission from HIV-infected mothers to their newborns,[21] and to health care workers with occupational percutaneous exposure to HIV (i.e., by needle stick), if administered shortly after exposure.[22] It is hypothesized that daily pre-exposure administration of antiretrovirals to HIV-uninfected individuals may prevent HIV infection by disabling or interfering with HIV within the initial period after an individual is exposed to it.

Status of Research

In recent years, researchers have begun studying the antiretroviral drug tenofovir, taken as a once-daily pill, as a potential new method to prevent HIV infection in high-risk individuals, an approach known as pre-exposure prophylaxis, or PREP. Tenofovir is approved for the treatment of HIV infection; it is especially long-lasting in the body, unusually slow to cause HIV to develop resistance, and rarely causes serious side effects.[23] In monkey studies, tenofovir has shown promise in preventing infection with HIV-like viruses,[24] although other animal studies have suggested that tenofovir's effectiveness may decrease over time.[25]

Researchers are also beginning to test a combination pill containing tenofovir plus emtricitabine.[26] A monkey study with the combination regimen showed that it provided strong protection against HIV-like infection.[27]

Over the past few years, a number of clinical trials have been initiated to evaluate the safety and efficacy of pre-exposure prophylaxis with antiretrovirals for HIV prevention:

- *Safety:* Data on the safety of administering tenofovir to HIV-uninfected people has been collected from trials involving more than 900 women in Ghana, Cameroon, and Nigeria. An additional safety trial is ongoing among men in the United States.
- *Efficacy:* Clinical trials to assess the efficacy of daily administration of tenofovir, or tenofovir plus emtricitabine, for HIV prevention are being conducted in three countries—Botswana, Peru and Thailand. The trials will enroll approximately 4,200 participants from a number of groups at high risk for HIV, including injection drug users, men who have sex with men, and high-risk women. The first results on the efficacy of pre-exposure prophylaxis for HIV prevention could be available by 2007 or 2008.

Research is in earlier stages for the potential prevention application of other antiretroviral agents, including new classes of drugs that are also being developed as potential HIV treatments.

Potential Prevention Impact

If shown to be effective, pre-exposure prophylaxis with antiretrovirals could be an important new prevention method for people at high risk for HIV infection. A modeling study sponsored by AIDs Partnership California concluded that providing PREP to high-risk groups such as men who have sex with men, injection drug users, and high-risk women could quickly reduce the rate of new HIV infections, depending on the level of PREP's efficacy, and the percentage of people at risk who received the intervention.[28]

While PREP is likely to be more expensive than other new HIV prevention methods under investigation, if found to be highly efficacious, studies suggest it could nonetheless be a cost-

RESEARCH TO IMPROVE EXISTING PREVENTION METHODS

In addition to efforts to develop new HIV prevention methods, researchers are exploring ways to improve the prevention impact of existing approaches:

- **Next-generation female condoms:** The FC® female condom was developed in the 1990s by the Female Health Company and provides an alternative to male condoms for the prevention HIV and other sexually transmitted diseases.[33] However, the product, which is made of polyurethane, has not been widely used because of its relatively high cost. The Female Health Company is developing a new female condom made of synthetic latex (nitrile polymer), which is expected to be considerably less expensive. Other organizations, including the Program for Appropriate Technology in Health, are also working on other models of female condoms. The World Health Organization (WHO) is currently reviewing data on the new female condom to determine its suitability for use in HIV prevention. The redesign of the female condom could also facilitate its use for HIV prevention during anal sex, for both heterosexual couples and men who have sex with men.[34]

- **Treatment of drug addiction:** Methadone is currently used to treat addiction to opiate drugs such as heroin, and has been shown to reduce the risk of HIV transmission through injection drug use. Although roughly three-quarters of people who initiate methadone maintenance therapy respond well, the intervention does not suit all patients with opioid dependence.[35] Researchers are testing buprenorphine in China and Thailand as an alternative to methadone for treating heroin addiction and reducing HIV risk. The U.S. Food and Drug Administration has already approved buprenorphine for treatment of heroin addiction when administered by a physician, and buprenorphine is also prescribed in several European countries. WHO has added both methadone and buprenorphine to its List of Essential Medicines.

- **Improved mother-to-child prevention strategies:** Researchers are studying ways to improve the effectiveness of current strategies for preventing mother-to-child transmission. For example, a clinical trial in Africa will assess an extended regimen of the antiretroviral drug nevirapine to reduce the risk of HIV transmission to newborns during breastfeeding. Other clinical trials will test a range of antiretrovirals for mother-to-child prevention. At the same time, an important shortcoming of mother-to-child prevention programs is the fact that they reach fewer than 10 percent of women who could potentially benefit from them.[36] WHO has identified research into the barriers to providing access to existing mother-to-child prevention programs as a top priority.

- **Improved behavior change strategies:** Researchers are studying ways to strengthen behavior change interventions that encourage people at high risk for HIV infection to reduce risk behavior. For example, a clinical trial in Thailand and the United States will test a peer-based HIV prevention program for injection drug users. In the trial, injection drug users will be given a four-week training course to learn skills for educating other drug users about ways to reduce the risk of HIV acquisition and transmission.

- **New "prevention for positives" strategies:** Because so few people in developing countries are aware of their HIV status,[37] prevention programs have often relied on general messages that implicitly assume that all individuals are HIV-uninfected—an approach that may be limiting the effectiveness of HIV prevention efforts. Although a positive HIV test result typically prompts HIV-infected people to avoid transmitting HIV to others,[38] evidence in developed countries indicates that a notable share of people with HIV infection have difficulty implementing and sustaining safer behavior.[39] In recent years, WHO, the International Planned Parenthood Federation, and the U.S. Centers for Disease Control and Prevention, among others, have begun examining behavior change strategies tailored specifically for people living with HIV.[40]

- **Antiretroviral therapy to reduce the risk of HIV transmission:** Antiretroviral therapy reduces viral load in HIV-infected individuals, and studies have shown that lower viral load is strongly associated with lower transmission risk.[41] On this basis, it has been hypothesized that appropriate

(continued)

therapeutic administration of antiretrovirals may reduce the infectiousness of people with HIV and their likelihood of transmitting the virus to others. Currently, 1,700 HIV-discordant couples are being enrolled in a six-country, seven-year clinical trial to assess whether administering combinations of antiretrovirals to HIV-infected individuals reduces the risk of HIV transmission. The trial is also assessing whether the prevention impact of antiretroviral therapy can be enhanced by administering antiretrovirals to HIV-infected people earlier than would currently be medically indicated.

- **Improving the safety of health care injections:** Unsafe injections and blood-draws in health care settings account for an estimated 5 percent of new infections worldwide.[42] In 1999, WHO, UNICEF, and the United Nations Population Fund issued a joint statement identifying the inexpensive "auto-disable" syringe as the "equipment of choice" for routine and mass immunization.[43] However, as of 2004, 38 percent of developing countries did not use auto-disable syringes in their immunization programs.[44] In addition to ensuring universal adoption of auto-disable syringes, research efforts in both public and private sectors continue to focus on other methods to improve injection safety.

effective prevention method for high-risk groups, when used in combination with other prevention methods.[29]

One potential concern regarding pre-exposure prophylaxis is resistance. Any resistance developed to antiretrovirals such as tenofovir when used for prevention could limit the usefulness of the drugs for later HIV treatment. Several of the ongoing or planned trials are examining this important question.

▶ Herpes Suppression

Data suggest that infection with herpes simplex virus type 2 (HSV-2), the primary cause of genital herpes, increases the risk of HIV acquisition and transmission. Suppressing HSV-2 with the inexpensive, off-patent drug acyclovir may reduce HIV risk.

Theoretical Basis

An HIV-uninfected individual is up to three times more likely to contract HIV infection during sexual intercourse if he or she is infected with HSV-2.[30] In addition, because HSV-2 appears to accelerate HIV replication and shedding, HIV-infected individuals may be more likely to transmit HIV if they are also infected with HSV-2.[31]

Researchers aim to determine whether the drug acyclovir, which suppresses HSV-2, can help reduce the risk of HIV transmission.* Acyclovir is safe and well tolerated, and slow to cause HSV-2 to develop resistance in both HIV-infected and HIV-uninfected people.[32]

---

*It is important to note that even if herpes suppression is not proved efficacious for HIV prevention, expanded access to acyclovir treatment could significantly decrease the global burden of herpes.

Status of Research

Two clinical trials are evaluating the efficacy of suppressing HSV-2 with acyclovir as an HIV prevention strategy. The first trial involves 3,227 men and women who are infected with HSV-2 but uninfected with HIV in Africa, Latin America, and the United States; this study will help determine whether HSV-2 suppression decreases the risk of HIV acquisition. The second trial involves 3,000 HIV-discordant couples in Africa in which one partner is infected with both HIV and HSV-2 and the other is not HIV-infected. This study will help determine whether HSV-2 suppression decreases the likelihood that people infected with HIV will transmit it to others. Results are expected in 2007 for the trial among HIV-uninfected people, and in 2008 for the trial among HIV-discordant couples.

Potential Prevention Impact

If proven to be effective and used in combination with other prevention methods, suppression of HSV-2 with acyclovir could significantly strengthen efforts to reduce sexual HIV transmission. In some parts of southern Africa, up to 70 percent of adults are infected with HSV-2,[45] and a recent four-city study in Africa linked HSV-2 with more than one-third of all new HIV infections over a 15-year period (see Figure 12-8).[46]

From a cost perspective, acyclovir is an attractive prevention option. Because its patent has expired, the drug is inexpensive and already available in many developing countries.

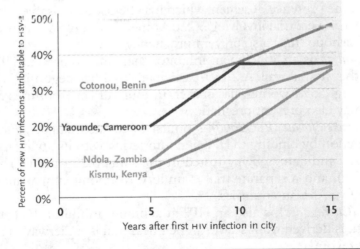

FIGURE 12-8   Four-City Study: Herpes Infection Fuels HIV Spread
Source: Freeman et al., 2005

▶ Microbicides

Microbicides are topical substances designed to be applied to the vagina or rectum to prevent HIV infection. Some vaginal microbicides may also prevent pregnancy.

Theoretical Basis

Microbicide candidates currently in research and development are designed to operate in a variety of ways to prevent HIV infection. These include:

- Disabling HIV
- Providing a barrier between HIV in semen and vaginal or rectal tissue
- Interfering with the process by which HIV enters cells and establishes infection
- Strengthening the body's natural defenses against HIV[47]

Status of Research

As of mid-2006, the microbicide research pipeline included 28 candidate products.[48] Microbicide candidates can be divided into two groups, first- and second-generation candidates.

First-generation microbicide candidates: Five microbicide candidates—all formulated as clear, colorless gels— are furthest along in development and are being tested in large-scale clinical trials for efficacy:

- *C31G (Savvy)* is a surfactant compound designed to disable HIV by breaking down its outer membrane. The product is being tested in a clinical trial involving 2,142 women in Nigeria. C31G may also protect against pregnancy.
- *Carbopol 974p (BufferGel)* is a buffering compound designed to function as a barrier between HIV in semen and vaginal tissue. It is also designed to maintain the vagina's acidity in the presence of semen, which may help kill or disable HIV. Carbopol is being tested in a clinical trial involving 3,220 women in five African countries and the United States. Carbopol may also prevent pregnancy.
- *Cellulose sulfate* is an attachment inhibitor that aims to prevent HIV from attaching to cells in the vaginal wall. A 2,160-participant trial has begun in Nigeria, and a second trial among 2,574 women has started in four African countries and India. Cellulose sulfate may also prevent pregnancy.
- *Naphthalene sulfonate (PRO2000)* is similar to cellulose sulfate, and is designed to prevent infection by binding to HIV and interfering with its ability to attach to and enter cells. The candidate is being tested in the same 3,220-participant trial as Carbopol (see above), and a separate trial is underway among approximately 10,000 participants in five African countries.
- *PC-515 (Carraguard)* is also an HIV attachment inhibitor. Its active ingredient, carrageenan, is derived from seaweed. A clinical trial is underway in South Africa involving 6,299 women.

The first results from efficacy trials of first-generation microbicide candidates could potentially be available in 2008.

Second-Generation Microbicide Candidates

While the microbicide candidates above are in late-stage trials and could potentially be shown to be effective within the next five years, there is growing interest in second-generation microbicide approaches that are approximately 10 years away from completing testing. Second-generation microbicide candidates specifically target HIV or molecules of the cells it infects, and some of these microbicide approaches involve using existing or new classes of antiretroviral compounds as microbicides.[49]

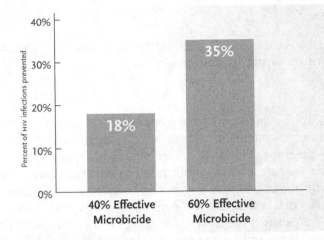

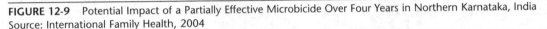

FIGURE 12-9 Potential Impact of a Partially Effective Microbicide Over Four Years in Northern Karnataka, India
Source: International Family Health, 2004

Researchers are also investigating new ways of formulating microbicides, such as using them in vaginal rings or cervical barriers.[50] In addition, although most development efforts have concentrated on vaginal microbicides, a number of early research projects are advancing the development of rectal microbicides, which could reduce the risk of HIV transmission during anal sex.[51]

Potential Prevention Impact

A modeling study from the London School of Hygiene and Tropical Medicine estimated that a 60 percent effective microbicide could avert 2.5 million new HIV infections in low- and middle-income countries over three years.[52] A separate modeling project concluded that a microbicide that is 60 percent effective against HIV and other STDs could prevent more than one-third of new HIV infections that are projected to occur over four years in a district in northern Karnataka, India, where infection is migrating from high-risk groups to the broader population (see Figure 12-9).[53]

Other studies have predicted that even a microbicide with a relatively low effectiveness rate could prevent 9 percent of new infections over four years in a high-prevalence neighborhood of Johannesburg, South Africa, and nearly 40 percent of new infections projected in a lower-prevalence setting in Benin.[54]

Like many of the other new HIV prevention methods in development, microbicides would be female-initiated, and may be able to be used by women without requiring the cooperation of male partners. Developers of potential microbicides have conducted extensive research into the acceptability of their products, and evidence to date indicates that women and men in both developing and developed countries are interested in using microbicides. Further research is needed to identify the specific product characteristics that would be most acceptable to women and men.[55]

▶ HIV Vaccines

Preventive vaccines enhance the body's immune defenses, enabling the immune system to fight off diseases that it cannot naturally control.

Theoretical Basis

The ultimate goal for an HIV vaccine is to prevent HIV infection. Scientists have identified rare individuals whose immune systems appear to have a natural ability to resist HIV infection, a finding that provides clues for the design of an effective vaccine.

However, an HIV vaccine that does not prevent infection but, in the event of infection, suppresses the amount of virus circulating in the body could also have a substantial impact. Such a vaccine would work much like antiretroviral drugs that lower viral load in order to keep people with HIV healthy, except that a vaccine would stimulate the immune system to do this, rather than requiring daily doses of medicine. An HIV vaccine that lowered viral load may also reduce HIV transmission.

FUNDING FOR HIV PREVENTION RESEARCH

Only a small percentage of total global spending on biomedical research and development focuses on HIV/AIDs and other diseases that primarily affect developing countries.[63] Funding for research on new HIV prevention methods is inadequate.

The best available information on funding for HIV prevention research is for microbicide and vaccine development (see Figure 12-10):[64]

- **Microbicide funding:** The HIV Vaccines and Microbicides Resource Tracking Group estimates that a total of $142 million was invested worldwide in microbicide development in 2004. The public sector was the main source of this funding, accounting for 87 percent of total funding. The United States provided nearly three-quarters of public sector funding—largely through the National Institutes of Health and the U.S. Agency for International Development. European governments and the European Commission provided roughly one-quarter of public sector funding in 2004.
- **HIV vaccine funding:** In 2004, an estimated total of $682 million was spent on HIV vaccine development, of which 88 percent was public sector funding. U.S. government agencies provided a significant share (86 percent) of this funding.

Although current levels of funding for microbicide and vaccine development represent substantial increases over previous years—public sector investments in both microbicide and HIV vaccine development doubled between 2000 and 2004—far more resources are needed. The International Partnership for Microbicides (IPM) has called for an additional $280 million to be invested in microbicide development annually, and the Global HIV Vaccine Enterprise has urged an additional $500 million annually to fully fund HIV vaccine development.[65]

Experience thus far underscores the critical need for increased financing for prevention research. In some cases, large-scale efficacy trials for new prevention approaches have proven to be significantly more expensive than originally anticipated. As this report describes in section 2, large prevention trials require substantial outlays for pre-trial epidemiological and behavioral studies, involve time-consuming efforts to enroll sufficient participants, and require close monitoring by well-trained clinical and non-clinical staff. The emergence of effective new prevention methods that may need to be included as part of the standard package of prevention interventions offered to all trial participants could further increase the cost of future prevention trials by requiring the enrollment of significantly larger numbers of trial participants.

Increasing Private Sector Investments

Private industry has generally been reluctant to invest in new health products intended for primary use in developing countries because of the concern that these products are unlikely to obtain a return on investment. While public and philanthropic financing has a played a vital role in advancing research on new prevention methods, it cannot replace the unique contributions of the private sector. Expertise regarding development and licensure of new health products resides largely with the private sector—failing to capitalize on the essential know-how of private industry will inevitably slow efforts to develop new methods to prevent HIV transmission.[66]

A number of public policy measures have been proposed to encourage greater private sector engagement in research and development for HIV/AIDs and other diseases that primarily affect developing countries. These include:

- **Direct financing:** The public and philanthropic sectors can provide direct financing to private companies to conduct research. In exchange, the companies agree to make any resulting products available at affordable prices in low-income countries. This approach is being pursued by a number of public-private partnerships, such as IPM and the International AIDs Vaccine Initiative.

	2000	2001	2002	2003	2004
Microbicides					
Public sector	36	62	81	90	124
Philanthropic sector	29	3	25	17	18
Total microbicides	**65**	**65**	**106**	**107**	**142**
HIV Vaccines					
Public sector	307	359	436	532	602
Philanthropic sector	20	7	112	15	12
Private sector*					68
Total HIV vaccines	**327**	**366**	**548**	**547**	**682**
		US$ MILLIONS			

*Private sector spending figures available only for HIV vaccines in 2004

Source: HIV Vaccines and Microbicides Resource Tracking Group, 2005

FIGURE 12-10 Spending on Microbicide and HIV Vaccine Development, 2000–2004

- **Patent extensions:** The Project Bioshield II legislation introduced in 2005 in the U.S. Congress proposed that companies that successfully develop new HIV prevention tools could extend the patent on any other product in their portfolio.
- **Predictable markets:** Governments and donors could make legally binding agreements to pay a specific price for a specific quantity of a product, should it be successfully developed.[67] For example, the G-8 is exploring "advance purchase commitments" to help spur companies to develop new tools to fight major global health problems such as malaria.

These approaches are designed to generate greater private sector investment in biomedical research by reducing uncertainties in the market for new health technologies in developing countries. Other nonfinancial reforms—such as improved demand forecasting, strong expressions of political commitment by developing country leaders to put new technologies to use, and measures to strengthen health service delivery systems—are discussed in section 3 of this report.

Status of Research

Developing an effective HIV vaccine has proven to be a highly complex scientific challenge, and most research is at an early stage.[56] To date, traditional vaccine designs have not worked for HIV, in part because the virus is able to evade the immune system by rapidly mutating. Some experimental vaccines have been shown to protect monkeys from HIV-like viruses, although the results have not yet been replicated in humans.[57]

The one HIV vaccine candidate to complete the full course of clinical trials was found to be ineffective.[58] More than 30 other HIV vaccine candidates are currently in clinical trials, including two vaccine candidates in advanced efficacy or proof-of-concept trials (see Figure 12-6 on page 335).[59]

Most experts predict that it will be 10 years or more before an HIV vaccine is shown to be effective. A major challenge facing researchers is that it is likely that an effective vaccine will need to stimulate the immune system's two main arms, called humoral immunity (broadly neutralizing antibodies) and cellular immunity. Most HIV vaccine candidates currently being tested are designed only to stimulate cellular immunity, and research is in the very early stages to identify vaccine candidates capable of stimulating broadly neutralizing antibodies.[60]

Recently, a number of leading HIV vaccine research agencies and funders formed a cooperative alliance to accelerate progress in developing an HIV vaccine. The Global HIV Vaccine Enterprise seeks to overcome the major scientific challenges to developing an HIV vaccine by bringing new collaboration, strategic focus, and resources to the field.[61]

Potential Prevention Impact

A preventive vaccine is the best long-term hope to control the global HIV epidemic. Vaccines have been successfully developed for other serious viral diseases—including polio and hepatitis B—and have been critical to controlling these diseases.

For HIV, a number of modeling studies suggest that even a partially effective vaccine could have a substantial impact on the course of the epidemic, although—like other prevention approaches—it would need to used in combination with other proven methods. For example, a modeling study by the World Bank found that a 50 percent efficacious HIV vaccine could reduce HIV infection rates by up to 60 percent in developing countries, provided that it was delivered to a majority of adults at risk.[62]

▶ 2. Accelerating HIV Prevention Research

The proper design and conduct of clinical trials is essential to the development of any new health tool or strategy.[68]

Clinical trials can be complicated and expensive. This is especially true for HIV prevention trials, which often require thousands of trial participants, who must be followed for up to several years in order to reliably detect whether the prevention method being studied is effective in reducing HIV transmission. Because it is critical to test new health tools and strategies under the conditions in which they will ultimately be used, many HIV prevention trials are conducted in developing countries where the need is most acute. This can increase their complexity, since clinical trials infrastructure in many developing countries often needs to be established in order to conduct a trial.

As a result of the expanding pipeline of new prevention methods and the increasing complexity of trials, substantial additional clinical trials capacity will be needed to prevent delays in testing new prevention methods. New ways of doing business are also needed to prioritize testing of the prevention methods that offer the greatest public health promise, and to promote collaboration among researchers to ensure the optimal use of scarce trial resources.

This section examines the following issues related to accelerating the pace of HIV prevention research, and ensuring that HIV prevention trials are conducted properly:

- Creating substantial additional clinical trials capacity that can be readily adapted for testing a range of new prevention methods, and identifying populations to participate in trials
- Resolving critical issues pertaining to the ethical conduct of HIV prevention trials
- Engaging affected communities as key partners in prevention research

---

ACCELERATING HIV PREVENTION RESEARCH—KEY RECOMMENDATIONS

- **Clinical trials capacity:** To avoid delays in testing promising new HIV prevention methods, leading trial sponsors, governments, and international donors should make significant new investments in increasing global capacity for HIV prevention trials. There is also a need to strengthen regulatory capacity to review trial protocols.
- **Trial design:** Researchers should develop improved models for accurately estimating the number of participants needed for HIV prevention trials, and create innovative trial designs that could reduce the number of participants needed to obtain valid results.
- **Coordination among trial sponsors:** Trial sponsors and international agencies should develop clear criteria to prioritize prevention methods for clinical trials. Sponsors should share data and information, and ensure that study sites can be adapted as needed and appropriate to test different prevention interventions.
- **Ethical issues:** Trial sponsors and international agencies should convene a broadly inclusive panel of experts to develop formal guidance on ethical issues in HIV prevention research that have recently emerged and are not addressed by existing guidance.
- **Community engagement:** Investigators and sponsors of HIV prevention trials should ensure meaningful involvement of local communities in trial design and conduct.

▶ Clinical Trials Capacity

Global capacity to conduct HIV prevention clinical trials falls far short of what will be needed to expedite the development and testing of promising new prevention approaches over the coming years. Unless immediate steps are taken to increase the number of sites prepared to conduct HIV prevention trials, the world could soon face a situation where there is a pipeline of promising new prevention methods ready for trials, but inadequate capacity to test them.

Developing Additional Clinical Trial Sites

As research on new HIV prevention methods advances, the need for additional sites to conduct clinical trials will increase sharply. For example, in addition to the five microbicide candidates currently in large-scale clinical trials, a number of other candidates are in earlier stages of trials, and still more candidates are undergoing pre-clinical investigation. Key issues include:

- **Recruitment and retention of potential participants:** Fully testing just one new HIV prevention method for safety and effectiveness typically requires thousands of trial participants. Current efficacy trials of new HIV prevention approaches will require a total of approximately 80,000 participants, with most of this capacity needed in developing countries.

- **Confirmatory and bridging trials:** Although a number of large-scale trials of new HIV prevention methods are underway, and some are already fully enrolled, these trials are unlikely to be the definitive word on the effectiveness of these tools and strategies. New health interventions typically must be tested in multiple large-scale trials, to confirm the results and ensure they are accurate and broadly applicable.[69] For example, in a review of 39 heavily cited randomized clinical trials, nine of the trials were contradicted by subsequent trials, underscoring the importance of confirming early results.[70] In addition, for entirely new technologies such as microbicides and HIV vaccines, it is probable that the first candidate products to be found efficacious will have shortcomings, and it is likely there will need to be an iterative process of refinement and improvement, which will require substantial trials capacity. Furthermore, "bridging" trials are sometimes needed to determine the applicability of new health interventions in settings or populations that differ markedly from those in which the original trial was conducted.

- **Infrastructure and training:** To develop new trial sites in developing countries, trial sponsors, national governments, and donors must invest substantial additional resources in building physical infrastructure and training staff. In a multi-center trial, for example, the failure of a single trial site to adhere to international standards for good clinical practice may undermine the ability to draw definitive conclusions from the trial.

- **Basic health services:** Preparing a trial site also requires ensuring that there is sufficient capacity to provide basic health services in the community to support the trial, such as HIV testing and counseling, access to condoms and other supplies, and referrals to medical care when needed. These resources are vital to the successful conduct of any prevention trial, yet they are lacking in many developing countries.

- **Regulatory capacity:** Regulatory authorities play an important role in the approval and oversight of clinical trials. Greater regulatory capacity, particularly in developing countries, is needed to ensure that HIV prevention trial protocols are thoroughly and efficiently reviewed before the trials begin. (See section 3 of this report for a full discussion of regulatory capacity issues.)

Recommendations

- **New investments in trials capacity:** Leading sponsors of HIV prevention research, national governments, and international donors should make significant new investments in increasing global capacity for HIV prevention trials. Agencies should inventory existing capacity, identify specific needs in key regions, and prioritize sites for scaling up capacity. Increased resources should also be directed toward increasing regulatory capacity, particularly in developing countries, to help expedite review and approval of prevention trials. It is important, however, that scarce resources are not diverted from other health care needs, since many countries already face acute shortages of doctors and nurses.

- **Collaboration on HIV prevention research:** Leading sponsors of HIV prevention research—including bilateral donors, public sector biomedical research agencies, and leading foundations—should undertake joint planning and information-sharing to expedite developing new clinical trial sites for HIV prevention research. It is also critical for sponsors of prevention trials to collaborate with sponsors of HIV treatment studies, to identify opportunities for clinical trials capacity to be shared and used to optimal benefit across prevention and treatment research.
- **Confirmatory trials:** To ensure as little delay as possible in bringing new prevention tools to people in need, leading sponsors of HIV prevention research should plan—at the outset of a clinical trial—for confirmatory or bridging trials that may be needed after the original trial is completed.

Cohort Development

Clinical trials determine if a new HIV prevention method is effective by comparing the rate of new HIV infections among individuals who receive the intervention with the rate of new infections among a control group of individuals who do not receive the intervention. In order to yield valid results, the population being studied must be similar to the population that would benefit most from the intervention under study.[71]

As part of the process of mounting a major prevention trial, researchers undertake epidemiological studies to identify populations with appropriate behavioral and demographic characteristics to be enrolled in the trial—so-called "cohorts"—including those with high rates of HIV infection. However, in some cohorts currently enrolled in prevention trials, there have been much lower rates of infection during the trials than researchers had expected based on pre-trial estimates. For example, in one site studying pre-exposure use of tenofovir, HIV incidence was found to be one-third as high as pre-trial studies estimated it would be.[72] This difference could stem from a variety of factors, including the positive impact of the other prevention services that are routinely provided to trial participants. Nonetheless, such a difference is critical, since it may require enrolling significantly more participants to yield statistically significant results.

Key issues in identifying appropriate cohorts for HIV prevention trials include:

- **Accurately estimating HIV incidence:** An accurate estimate of HIV incidence—that is, the rate of new HIV infections in the study population—is needed to enable researchers to project with accuracy the number of participants that will be needed for a given trial. While obtaining information on HIV prevalence—the proportion of people currently infected in a particular population—can be relatively straightforward, it is much more difficult to obtain a valid estimate of incidence, and to discern the characteristics of those who are more likely than others to become infected. In addition, the likely impact of other prevention services provided to trial participants must be taken into account when estimating needed trial size.
- **Challenges in enrolling and retaining participants:** In some trials, enrollment of trial participants has taken significantly longer than anticipated, and drop-out rates can be high. In some prevention trials that have enrolled large numbers of women of childbearing age, substantial numbers of participants have become pregnant and were

required—temporarily or permanently—to drop out of the study. A large number of drop-outs can compromise the ability of a trial to arrive at valid conclusions.

Recommendations

- **Enhancing models for estimating trial size:** Principal investigators from past and ongoing prevention trials should collaborate with leading sponsors of prevention research, the World Health Organization (WHO), the U.S. Centers for Disease Control and Prevention (CDC), and other agencies to develop improved models for accurately estimating HIV incidence in trial populations and the number of participants that should be enrolled. Researchers should take into account the likelihood of participant drop-outs due to pregnancy and other factors. Until improved models are developed to estimate needed trial size, investigators should overestimate the number of participants needed, in order to increase the likelihood that the trial will have sufficient statistical power.
- **New trial designs:** Researchers should develop new trial designs that shorten the time and participants required to identify effective interventions, as well as develop new methods of increasing retention of trial participants. In addition, to minimize the number of pregnant women who must discontinue or suspend participation in HIV prevention trials, more research is needed to assess the safety of new prevention methods during pregnancy, and to identify ways that pregnant women may be able to be safely retained in trials.

Prioritizing Among Multiple Candidates

At present, clinical trials capacity is typically developed by individual trial sponsors or investigators in order to test a specific product that they are researching, without considering how that capacity might be used by other sponsors or investigators. As a result, limited trials capacity may not be used strategically to test the most promising products first. In addition, trials

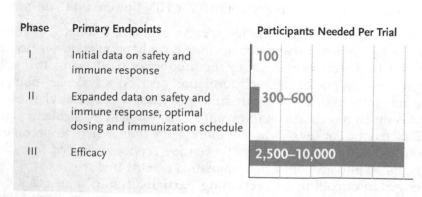

FIGURE 12-11 Phases of HIV Vaccine Clinical Trials
Source: Klausner et al., 2003

may miss opportunities to undertake complementary behavioral studies or other research that might advance knowledge in the field as a whole.

In some cases, a better-financed sponsor may advance its own product through clinical trials even when other sponsors' products appear more promising. In other cases, a product may be pushed forward simply because it is the first to be available for testing, even though more promising candidates are in earlier stages of development. This approach can waste resources, as well as erode general confidence in the field if disappointing trial results are reported. For example, in the case of microbicide and HIV vaccine development, while the mounting of large-scale trials should be viewed as significant progress for the field, questions have also been raised regarding whether the microbicide and vaccine candidates that have proceeded to advanced trials are sufficiently different from each other to warrant testing each among large numbers of participants.

Recommendations

- **Prioritizing prevention candidates:** Key stakeholders should develop clear criteria and mechanisms for prioritizing among multiple prevention methods for large-scale clinical trials. For example, researchers could agree to use comparable tests for assessing potential new HIV prevention methods, openly share information, and agree to common benchmarks at each stage of the research process for determining whether a new prevention method is sufficiently promising to warrant further development. Some efforts are already underway to increase coordination among trial sponsors—including a working group of donors that support microbicide clinical trials, and the Global HIV Vaccine Enterprise—and these efforts should be strengthened and expanded.[73]
- **Flexible trial sites:** Where feasible, trial sites should be capable of being adapted for testing a range of different new prevention methods, including those developed by different sponsors and investigators, and prevention trial sites should be shared with HIV treatment research programs as appropriate. In awarding grants for prevention research, the major funders of such research should make such funding contingent on researchers' agreement to create flexible research sites that may be used for the most appropriate and promising research, regardless of sponsor.

▶ Ethical Conduct of Prevention Trials

All clinical trials must adhere to ethical standards that are recognized both internationally and in the local community in which the trial occurs.[74] While the HIV prevention trials that have been conducted to date have adhered to these standards, new issues have arisen that are not addressed by existing ethical guidance, and that must be resolved in order to ensure the proper design and rapid conduct of trials. In particular, clarity is needed on the following issues:

- Provision of appropriate prevention counseling and interventions to trial participants
- Provision of antiretroviral treatment to individuals who become HIV-infected while participating in the trial, or who test positive for HIV infection while being screened for trial participation
- The best process for ensuring that trial participants give informed consent and remain properly informed throughout the duration of the trial

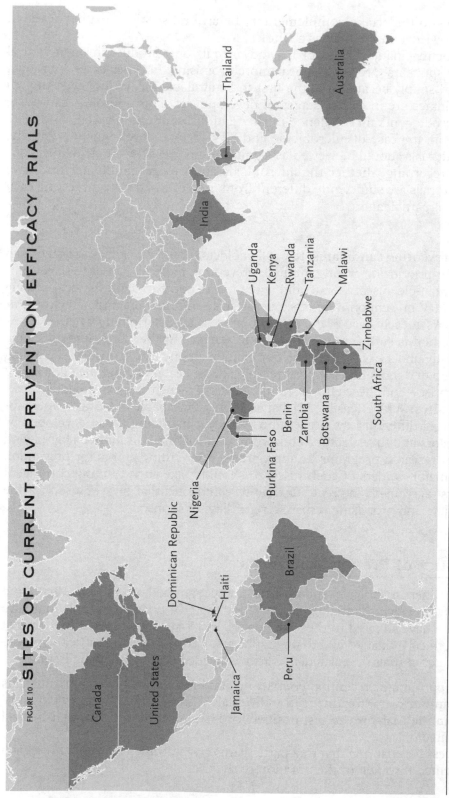

FIGURE 12-12 Sites of Current HIV Prevention Efficacy Trials

Prevention Standards for Trial Participants

Researchers are obligated to minimize potential harms to research participants, and trials are not permitted to withhold proven HIV prevention interventions from trial participants. Recently, this obligation has raised a number of issues that need to be addressed:

- **Range of prevention services provided:** There is not yet consensus on the range of existing prevention methods that should be provided to participants in trials of new HIV prevention approaches. For example, several governments prohibit the provision of sterile injection equipment, a proven strategy for the prevention of HIV transmission among injection drug users.[75]
- **Quality assurance:** Although the basic principles of HIV prevention counseling are well established, the delivery of such counseling can vary widely in quality. For example, interactive, client-centered counseling appears to be more effective than didactic approaches.
- **Future changes in prevention standards:** As new HIV prevention methods are successfully developed, the obligations of trial sponsors may evolve. For example, if male circumcision is confirmed as an effective strategy for HIV prevention, it may need to be incorporated in the package of prevention interventions provided to trial participants or their partners. Because the addition of new prevention tools and strategies is likely to decrease the rate of new HIV infections in the study population, the number of participants in prevention trials may need to increase.

Recommendations

- **Guidance on prevention standards:** Trial sponsors and international agencies should convene a standing committee to provide timely guidance on the list of prevention interventions that have been proven in scientific studies to be effective in reducing the risk of HIV transmission, and should be provided to participants in prevention trials. Such a committee may be able to be linked to existing efforts, such as groups established as part of UNAIDs's Intensifying Prevention effort.[76]
- **Access to comprehensive prevention services:** Trial sponsors should ensure access for trial participants to all proven prevention services, given the local context, including, as appropriate, evidence-based prevention interventions for participants who are injection drug users. Funding from international donors—such as the Global Fund to Fight AIDs, Tuberculosis, and Malaria, and the U.S. government's President's Emergency Plan for AIDs Relief (PEPFAR)—should be used to support access to comprehensive prevention for clinical trial participants.
- **Monitoring:** Trial sponsors should work with communities and others to establish mechanisms to monitor and document the ongoing provision of prevention services.

Access to Treatment

In recent years, extensive debate has focused on the obligation of sponsors of HIV prevention trials to provide antiretrovirals and other HIV treatments to trial participants who contract HIV during a trial. Generally speaking, the initial debate over whether to provide antiretrovirals to trial participants who become infected has given way to discussions over how best to deliver the medications.[77]*

*It is important to note that people who become HIV-infected during the course of a prevention trial do not become infected from the investigational tool or strategy.

A consensus is emerging that antiretroviral provision is an indispensable part of the agreement between trial sponsors and trial participants. In exchange for the inconvenience and potential risks of participating in clinical research, many believe that participants have the reasonable expectation of receiving antiretroviral therapy if they become infected with HIV during the trial. In addition, many in the field view antiretroviral provision to trial participants as an obligation that is owed to the communities in which trials are conducted. Dramatic reductions in the price of antiretrovirals in developing countries, combined with the demonstrated feasibility of administering antiretrovirals in low-income countries, have also influenced the debates on the obligations to trial participants.

Ethical guidance for HIV vaccine trials released in 2000 by UNAIDs called for the provision of "care and treatment for HIV/AIDs and its complications" to participants who become HIV-infected during the trial, although the recommendations did not specify at that time the nature or duration of such an obligation.[78] In 2005, the International AIDs Society convened a meeting of stakeholders involved in pre-exposure tenofovir research to explore key issues associated with these trials, including access to antiretrovirals for trial participants who become infected.[79]

In recognition of the evolving discussion on this issue, UNAIDs is in the process of developing updated guidance on antiretroviral access and other issues associated with HIV prevention research. In addition, a number of trial sponsors have made arrangements with national HIV treatment programs to refer trial participants who become HIV-infected during the trial (see the discussion of treatment for HIV vaccine trial participants later in this section).

Key issues currently being debated and discussed regarding provision of antiretroviral treatment to participants in HIV prevention trials include:

- **Duration of obligation:** It must be assumed that antiretroviral therapy, once initiated, is likely to be needed for life. Yet no consensus currently exists on the appropriate timeframe for ensuring treatment for trial participants who become HIV-infected. It should be noted that participants who become HIV infected during a trial are unlikely to need antiretroviral treatment until five to 10 years after they become infected, complicating the practical implications of providing treatment to these trial participants.

- **Scope of obligation:** There is a lack of consensus about whether trial sponsors are obliged to ensure access to antiretrovirals for individuals who are screened for participation in a prevention trial but are found to be ineligible because they are HIV-infected. Current standard practice is to refer would-be participants who are excluded due to prior HIV infection to existing sources of care and support, although questions have been raised about whether it is ethical to conduct prevention trials where there are severe gaps in local capacity to provide HIV treatment and care. At the same time, others, especially those from settings in which treatment is not available or imminent, have urged that researchers not avoid their communities merely because antiretrovirals are not widely available.

- **Financial responsibility:** There is no clear agreement as to who should be responsible for covering the long-term costs associated with treatment of trial participants who become HIV-infected, especially in countries where treatment services are limited or do not exist. Funding is also needed for scaling up treatment services in the trial communities generally. If trial sponsors were to assume the financial costs and complexity associated with treatment provision, this would significantly increase the costs of prevention research. Some have proposed that an independent fund be established to cover costs of providing antiretrovirals and other care and treatment to individuals who become HIV-infected during trial participation, or who are found to be HIV-infected during a trial's screening stage.[80]

- **Community access:** In addition to arranging treatment access for trial participants, some have argued that the larger communities that host prevention trials should be prioritized for roll-out of broad-based treatment access.

Recommendations

- **Guidance on antiretroviral access:** Trial sponsors and international agencies such as UNAIDs and WHO should convene a broadly inclusive panel of experts—including clinical trial investigators, developing country health ministries, trial sponsors, private industry, ethicists, affected communities, and people living with HIV—to develop guidance on key principles for the provision of antiretroviral therapy to individuals who become HIV-infected while participating in an HIV prevention trial, or who are found to be ineligible for the trial during the screening stage. This would include guidance on scope and duration of obligation, and financial responsibility.
- **Community access:** Where feasible and appropriate, communities that host prevention trials should be prioritized for introduction of antiretroviral treatment access. Provision of treatment to communities that host trials should be supported by international donors such as the Global Fund and PEPFAR.

Informed Consent

Informed consent requires (1) disclosure of critical information to potential trial participants, (2) comprehension by the potential participant of this information, and (3) the informed individual's voluntary choice to participate in the trial.[81] Although a participant's informed consent is typically obtained in writing on a consent form, informed consent should be viewed as an ongoing, interactive process that permits individuals to obtain and understand the information they need to make an informed decision.

In developing countries, where literacy rates are low and there may be little community experience with clinical trials, a major challenge is to ensure that participants understand basic facts about the trial before consenting to participate. Key issues include:

- **Presentation of information:** It has not been fully determined what amount of information should be provided, and in what manner, to ensure that consent is truly informed. For example, some prevention studies have incorporated visual images or group exercises into the informed consent process as a strategy to communicate risks, benefits, and other details regarding trial participation. However, there are no international standards for how information should be presented in order to obtain informed consent.
- **Verifying comprehension:** Ideally, researchers should be able to verify the individual's comprehension of critical information about the trial prior to enrollment, and throughout the trial. To date, most HIV prevention trials have included some strategy to measure comprehension, although optimal strategies to make such measurements remain unclear.

HIV VACCINE RESEARCH AS A POTENTIAL MODEL FOR TREATMENT ACCESS

HIV vaccine trial sponsors have discussed for some time the ethical issues of providing antiretroviral treatment to participants who become infected with HIV during HIV vaccine clinical trials. In recent years, both the U.S. government-sponsored HIV Vaccine Trial Network (HVTN) and the International AIDs Vaccine Initiative (IAVI) have established policy guidance regarding the provision of treatment to volunteers who become infected with HIV while participating in their trials. This guidance provides a potential model for trials of other HIV prevention methods.

IAVI works with local partners to ensure the provision of long-term treatment and care, and in some cases, the partners assume responsibility for the costs of any needed care. If IAVI's partners are unable to do this, the organization commits to providing antiretroviral treatment for participants who become infected during a trial, for a period of five years after the start of treatment is clinically indicated.[82] Similarly, HVTN has pledged to provide "long-term" treatment to trial participants, although it has not specified a time-period for its treatment commitment.[83]

Both IAVI and HVTN have developed plans for ensuring access to treatment. IAVI has established an escrow account to pay for treatment needs in its trials, and HVTN has set up a foundation to fund treatment provision in its trials (HVTN is prohibited by U.S. law from providing treatment that is not the specific focus of research).

IAVI and HVTN acknowledge that providing treatment over the longer term will require establishing partnerships with governments, nongovernmental agencies, and communities. In a 2003 commentary in *The Lancet*, members of HVTN noted that while researchers cannot "reverse the global inequities" in HIV care they "can work with communities to develop, implement, and assess high-quality treatment models for participants in research programs, and encourage the development of sustainable community access to good HIV-1 care."[84]

Recommendations

- **Guidance on informed consent:** Trial sponsors and international agencies should consult a broadly inclusive panel of experts—including clinical trial investigators, developing country health ministries, private industry, ethicists, and affected communities—to develop guidance on key principles for informed consent in HIV prevention trials.
- **Assessment of comprehension:** All prevention trials should incorporate mechanisms for assessing trial participants' comprehension of information disclosed for purposes of obtaining informed consent. In addition to the participant's informed consent upon enrollment, assessments of comprehension and, as needed, re-education should occur periodically throughout the trial to ensure that understanding of key aspects of the trial does not diminish over time.
- **Community participation:** The Institutional Review Boards that oversee HIV prevention trials, as well as Community Advisory Boards, should include representatives of the communities from which trial participants are drawn, and people living with HIV. These community representatives can provide input into the substantive content of the information that should be disclosed to potential trial participants, interactive mechanisms for communicating key information, and strategies to maximize and monitor trial participants' comprehension. Trial sponsors should also undertake efforts to assist the communities from which participants will be drawn in understanding the basic nature of clinical research—including the purpose, benefits, and limitations of clinical research.

- **Best practices:** UNAIDs and WHO should work with trial investigators and sponsors to identify, define, and publish best practices with respect to informed consent in HIV prevention research.

▶ Engaging Communities in Prevention Research

The communities in which prevention trials occur should be empowered to function as genuine partners with researchers and other stakeholders in conducting research that is vital to the fight against AIDs. Communities that host clinical trials must be educated about the research that is being conducted and be involved in all aspects of trial design and implementation. Moreover, community support is often vital to researchers' ability to enroll eligible individuals as trial participants, to successfully complete trials, and to eventually support roll-out of successful tools and strategies.

In recent years, community concerns about plans for large-scale studies of tenofovir for the prevention of HIV transmission were a major factor in the closing of two of the trials.[85] Although the concerns expressed about the tenofovir trials have varied, a common theme has focused on the degree to which researchers effectively engaged the communities in which trials would take place.[86]

In 2005, UNAIDs held a series of consultations on creating effective partnerships between HIV prevention researchers and civil society, which acknowledged there is a need "to define new approaches to collaboration that will facilitate critically important research while at the same time being responsible and accountable to community needs and priorities."[87] Key issues include:

- **Identification of "community":** Efforts to engage affected communities require researchers to define the community and determine who speaks on its behalf. In all instances, trial sponsors should forge strong relationships with national and district-level political and public health leaders. In addition, a May 2005 expert consultation convened by the International AIDs Society concluded that "community" includes "potential participants, domestic and international activists, non-governmental organizations, and human rights organizations."[88]
- **Nature and timing of community engagement:** Community engagement should extend beyond education and outreach to include the meaningful involvement of community representatives in Institutional Review Boards and/or Community Advisory Boards. Community involvement should begin well before trial recruitment begins. Community representatives can have invaluable input regarding trial recruitment, informed consent, prevention counseling, and community relations.
- **Optimal strategies for engaging the community:** UNAIDs is in the process of developing guidelines on forging strong partnerships between affected communities and HIV prevention researchers. Potential strategies include retaining qualified staff to conduct community outreach, forging formal linkages with respected NGOs and community groups, and integrating community participation into Institutional Review Boards, Community Advisory Boards, and other institutions.

Recommendations

- **Strong community partnerships:** Sponsors of HIV prevention trials should build strong and genuine partnerships with the communities from which trial participants are drawn. Early community input should inform development of trial protocols, community education, and ongoing trial oversight.

- **Building research literacy:** Sponsors of HIV prevention trials should implement strong education programs to increase community awareness and understanding of the goals, nature, and purpose of planned research. This should also include reporting back to the community after the research has been completed.
- **Guidance:** International agencies such as UNAIDs and WHO should widely disseminate formal guidance on best practices for engaging communities.

▶ 3. Preparing for Access

Given the global health imperative of curbing the AIDs epidemic, it is vital that the world rapidly introduce new HIV prevention methods after they prove effective in trials, and avoid the historic delays in making life-saving health interventions available to those who need them in poor countries. For example, for new vaccines for other infectious diseases, 15 years or more have typically passed after licensure to achieve even modest coverage in low- and middle-income countries.[89] There is considerable cause for concern in the case of new HIV prevention methods, since the global community has not yet succeeded in ensuring meaningful access to current interventions for HIV/AIDs, including both prevention and treatment services.[90]

While introduction of new HIV prevention methods poses significant challenges, particularly in developing countries, there are feasible strategies to address the obstacles. It is too late, though, to wait until after a new prevention method has been shown to be effective to take the steps needed to expedite introduction and uptake. To accelerate the implementation of new prevention methods, development of sufficient manufacturing capacity will likely need to begin years in advance, systems to purchase and deliver the intervention must be put in place, public health guidance must be developed, and national regulatory expertise may need to be strengthened. In many cases, extensive operations research will be needed to identify the best strategies and tactics for addressing these implementation challenges. In short, the world must act now to ensure that future prevention breakthroughs will be accessible to those who need them.

Even if they are accessible, new HIV prevention methods will only have an impact on reducing the number of new infections if they are used by people at risk, and in combination with existing prevention tools. Introduction of new prevention methods must be accompanied by communications campaigns to encourage adoption of new approaches, and by educational initiatives to ensure that these prevention methods are used safely and properly.

It is also vital that strong, evidence-based education campaigns are undertaken to avoid complacency about risk behavior that could result from a mistaken belief that new interventions are 100 percent effective. If risk behavior increases, modeling studies suggest this could undermine rather than strengthen HIV prevention efforts, and actually result in a growth of new HIV infections. Efforts to introduce new tools must be accompanied by strong public health steps to reinforce the importance of current prevention methods, and ongoing monitoring and evaluation to ensure that these public health steps are in fact effective.

PREPARING FOR ACCESS—KEY RECOMMENDATIONS

- **Public health recommendations and regulatory capacity:** To avoid delays in rolling out new HIV prevention methods after they are shown to be effective in clinical trials, international agencies should maintain a standing committee to anticipate and provide needed guidance on new HIV prevention methods, and regulatory agencies in the United States and Europe should provide assistance to their counterparts in developing countries in evaluating new prevention methods.
- **Provider training:** The World Health Organization and others should develop provider training programs to promote the safe and proper use of new HIV prevention methods.
- **Preventing "disinhibition":** Because no new HIV prevention method will be 100 percent effective, strong, evidence-based communications and public education campaigns will need to accompany the introduction of new prevention methods, to prevent an inadvertent increase in risk behavior. It is essential that efforts to prevent behavioral "disinhibition" are monitored on an ongoing basis to ensure they are effective.
- **Resources for implementation:** Ensuring the rapid deployment of new prevention methods will require significant new resources, both to purchase new tools and to support programs such as the development of public health guidance, provider training, and community education. National governments and donors should commit to providing the resources necessary for the rapid roll-out of new HIV prevention methods, as part of a comprehensive response to the global

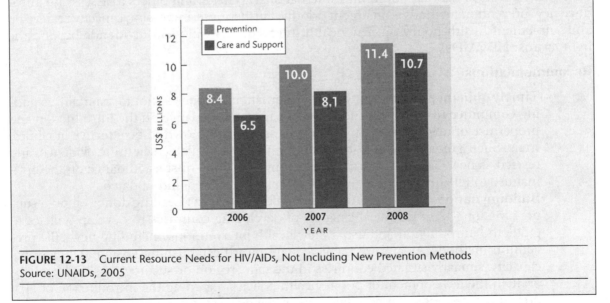

FIGURE 12-13 Current Resource Needs for HIV/AIDs, Not Including New Prevention Methods
Source: UNAIDs, 2005

This section covers the following issues that are critical for expediting the introduction of new HIV prevention methods:

- Providing sound and timely public health recommendations regarding adoption of new prevention methods
- Developing public and provider education strategies to guide the safe and proper introduction of new prevention methods and prevent inadvertent increases in risk behavior
- Ensuring adequate resources and capacity to expedite introduction of new prevention methods
- Establishing strong, sustainable systems for monitoring and evaluation

► Public Health Guidance

The availability of new HIV prevention methods could raise important policy questions. National decision-makers, as well as donors and international NGOs, will need to determine whether, and how, to integrate new HIV prevention methods into their health programs. In addition, public health guidelines must be developed to guide the safe and proper use of new prevention methods.

Guidance on use of new health tools is currently provided on an ad hoc basis. For example, in the case of initial efficacy results on male circumcision, informal discussions among key global health stakeholders resulted in consensus that additional studies should be completed before circumcision as an HIV prevention method could be recommended. In other instances, where consensus has been less clear, UNAIDs and the World Health Organization (WHO) have convened experts to advise on the proper public health approach to difficult questions. In some cases, these consultations have led to the development of formal public health guidance for use by national health ministries and other key stakeholders.[91]

To be effective, guidance on emerging prevention methods must be timely so that donors, national policy-makers, and program implementers can move swiftly to take advantage of new prevention approaches. Guidance must also be grounded in rigorous scientific evidence. Because several new prevention methods could be shown to be effective in the coming years, strengthening the capacity of national authorities, international agencies, and others to assess and introduce new prevention methods is an urgent priority. Furthermore, increasing capacity to develop and implement health policy on new health interventions will yield dividends beyond the fight against HIV/AIDs.

Recommendations

- **Timely guidance on emerging tools:** International agencies should maintain a standing committee to anticipate and assess the need for guidance on the introduction and proper use of new prevention approaches as they are shown to be effective in clinical trials. Such guidance should be based on the best available scientific evidence, and revised as new data and information become available—just as guidance on the optimal use of HIV treatment regimens is regularly reviewed and updated.
- **Building national and regional policymaking capacity:** Leading donors should support the long-term technical capacity of developing countries to develop policies to guide the introduction and use of new health interventions, including new HIV prevention methods. As an intermediate step toward establishing sustainable national capacity, similarly situated countries in the same region or sub-region should collaborate in the development of public health policies regarding the introduction of HIV prevention methods that could emerge in the next several years.
- **Donor support for operations research:** In many cases, operations research will be needed to identify the best strategies and tactics for rolling out new prevention methods. International donors—such as the Global Fund to Fight AIDs, Tuberculosis, and Malaria, and the U.S. government's President's Emergency Plan for AIDs Relief—should commit funding specifically to support this operations research, and to assist countries in applying for such funding.

▶ Regulatory Capacity

To be eligible for use in a country, some new health technologies require the approval of the national regulatory authority. Technically sophisticated new HIV prevention methods—such as HIV vaccines, microbicides, and pre-exposure antiretroviral prophylaxis—will almost certainly require official licensure before they can be introduced in countries. Although WHO publishes a list of essential medications and pre-qualifies drugs and vaccines that meet accepted standards of quality, safety, and efficacy, the organization does not undertake a comprehensive regulatory review of new health products. Therefore, unless national regulators are prepared for the potentially complex issues that some new HIV prevention technologies are likely to present, significant delays could result in the introduction of new prevention methods. Key issues include:

- **Building national regulatory capacity:** Regulatory systems for drugs, vaccines, and medical devices are weak in most developing countries, potentially delaying the introduction and uptake of new health technologies. Historically, relatively few new health products have been designed for initial introduction in developing countries, and investment in strong regulatory infrastructure has not been viewed as a major priority in developing countries. To facilitate the rapid introduction of new products in countries where they are most needed, substantially greater national regulatory capacity must be built.[92]
- **Capitalizing on regulatory capacity in high-income countries:** Applicable laws, policies, and practices have historically barred regulatory authorities in high-income countries from undertaking regulatory review on behalf of another country or for products not intended to be used in the regulatory authority's home country. In recent years, however, a growing number of global health experts have advocated mechanisms to use the regulatory capacity in high-income countries to buttress regulatory systems in developing countries.
- **Unanswered scientific questions:** In the case of certain new HIV prevention technologies, such as microbicides and vaccines, there are unanswered scientific questions about what criteria should be used to make a decision regarding licensure—this applies to industrialized countries as well as developing countries.

Recommendations

- **Capacity building:** Leading donors should support sustained efforts to increase national regulatory capacity in developing countries. For new prevention technologies such as microbicides and vaccines, for which clear regulatory criteria for safety and efficacy do not exist, donors should also provide support to international agencies to convene appropriate regulatory experts to develop guidance for regulatory review.
- **Regulatory collaboration:** At the request of one or more developing countries, the U.S. Food and Drug Administration (FDA), European Medicines Evaluation Agency (EMEA), and other leading regulatory bodies should be prepared to undertake a regulatory review and analysis of a complete regulatory submission regarding new health interventions intended for primary use in developing countries, including new

HIV prevention methods. Upon completion of the review or analysis, the regulatory body would provide the requesting party with a summary of findings, with ultimate licensure decisions remaining the province of national regulatory authorities in countries where the new tool or strategy will be used. FDA, EMEA, and other leading regulatory bodies should set aside sufficient budget to support such regulatory reviews. It should be noted that under a new initiative by EMEA, European regulators will, at the request of a developing country, review and analyze regulatory submissions for new health products that are designed for primary or exclusive use in developing countries. Under this new policy, licensure of any new product ultimately remains the province of individual national regulatory authorities.[93]

- **Regional collaboration:** Regional collaboration among national regulators could strengthen the ability of developing countries to expedite the review and approval of promising new HIV prevention methods. By pooling regulatory expertise, regions could capitalize on available capacity to accelerate the introduction of new products. Supported by donors, regulatory bodies in different regions should develop strategic plans for timely, collaborative review and information-sharing regarding new HIV prevention methods that are candidates for licensure.

- **Harmonization:** International efforts to harmonize regulatory requirements for new health interventions should be broadened to include national regulatory authorities from developing countries. Although national regulatory agencies in North America, Europe, and Japan have worked under the umbrella of the International Conference on Harmonization of Technical Requirements for Registration of Pharmaceuticals for Human Use to reduce the duplication and expense associated with regulatory approval in multiple countries, this process has yet to address regulatory processes in developing countries.[94]

▶ Public and Provider Education

Effective communication and education strategies are vital to the introduction of new HIV prevention tools and strategies. Individuals will not adopt a new prevention method if they are not aware of it, and sustained marketing efforts may be needed to promote uptake of some new methods. In addition, training may be required—for providers as well as consumers—to ensure that new prevention methods are used properly. Most importantly, strong, proactive communication and education strategies will be essential to ensure that the introduction of new prevention methods does not inadvertently lead to overall increases in sexual risk behavior.

Community Education and Marketing

Proof in clinical trials that a new prevention method, such as male circumcision, is safe and effective will not automatically result in its widespread adoption by consumers or providers. And if individuals who adopt a new prevention method use it improperly, this could diminish its effectiveness in reducing the risk of HIV transmission.

For example, studies indicate that education and experience using condoms significantly reduce the likelihood of condom failure.[95] As new HIV prevention methods emerge, community education initiatives will be needed to raise awareness of the new method and to encourage its adoption and proper use. Social marketing approaches to community education have proven to be highly effective in increasing consumer adoption of new health products.[96]

Acceptability studies can inform efforts to ensure broad and correct adoption of new prevention methods. Developers of candidate microbicides, for example, have performed extensive research on the acceptability of the products among sexually active women and their male partners.[97] In the case of male circumcision, surveys and anecdotal data indicate widespread demand for circumcision in some parts of Africa,[98] although there is a need for further research, given strong cultural norms and practices surrounding circumcision in many countries. And in Zimbabwe, researchers conducted a female diaphragm acceptability study,[99] and are continuing to assess acceptability by the community and providers while they test the diaphragm's effectiveness for HIV prevention.

Recommendations

- **Acceptability studies:** Sponsors of efficacy trials of new HIV prevention methods should undertake studies to assess the acceptability of the method to consumers and, when appropriate, to their sexual partners. These studies should also assess acceptability among providers.
- **Financing:** Additional donor financing for new prevention methods should include funding for community education initiatives and social marketing campaigns to identify and implement strategies to encourage adoption and proper use of new prevention methods.

BEHAVIORAL DISINHIBITION—LESSONS FROM TREATMENT ACCESS

As new HIV prevention methods are introduced, it is critical to ensure that risk behavior does not increase as a result of complacency about HIV. Researchers have modeled the impact of even small increases in risk behavior as the result of expanded treatment access, which could also have a "disinhibiting" effect on risk behavior.

For example, in India, projections by the World Bank estimate that even small decreases in condom use as a result of expanded access to treatment could actually result in a loss of millions of life-years. However, if treatment access is accompanied by strong prevention campaigns, and condom use remains stable or increases, expanded access to treatment and prevention together could save millions of life-years.

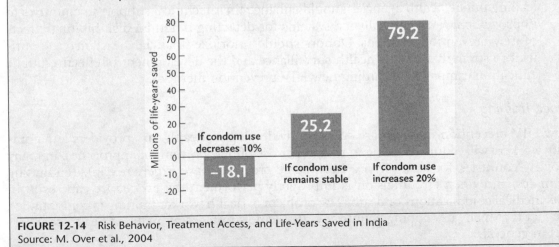

FIGURE 12-14 Risk Behavior, Treatment Access, and Life-Years Saved in India
Source: M. Over et al., 2004

Preventing Behavioral "Disinhibition"

It is critical that the introduction of new HIV prevention methods does not inadvertently lead people to become complacent about risk behavior.[100] If the introduction of a new prevention method is accompanied by an overall increase in risk behaviors, the protective benefits of the new method, as well as of other prevention measures, may be canceled out. In the most extreme case, a "disinhibiting" effect of a new prevention method could result in an actual increase in the number of new HIV infections. The need to address potential disinhibition as a result of prevention advances is especially important for the classes of prevention methods currently under development, as all would offer only partial protection against infection. Key issues include:

- **Community education:** Integration of new prevention methods into national AIDs programs should be accompanied by strong, sustained campaigns to educate affected communities regarding the benefits and limitations of the new methods. These campaigns must be grounded in rigorous scientific evidence of effectiveness. Both donors and national authorities should understand that the costs of introducing new prevention methods include substantial investments in education to avoid disinhibition.
- **Monitoring of behavioral changes:** To inform public health measures to prevent disinhibition, behavioral surveillance will be needed to assess the effect, if any, of new HIV prevention approaches on risk behavior decision-making. Currently, behavioral surveillance systems are extremely weak in many developing countries.

Recommendations

- **Education campaigns:** It is essential that the introduction of new prevention methods be accompanied by strong, sustained, well-financed public education campaigns that warn against disinhibition, emphasize the benefits and limitations of new prevention methods, and encourage use of the full range of proven prevention measures, including sexual abstinence, partner reduction, and condoms. The development of these campaigns should be informed by social science research to identify the most effective education strategies.
- **Technical support:** WHO, the Centers for Disease Control and Prevention, and other leading public health agencies should enhance their technical support to countries to improve behavioral surveillance systems for detecting potential disinhibiting effects of new prevention methods. Donors should prioritize financial assistance to countries to strengthen public health surveillance and the development of effective public education campaigns regarding new HIV prevention methods.

Provider Training

As new HIV prevention methods are successfully developed, health care providers and community workers will require training in the proper use of new prevention approaches. In many developing countries, for example, few health care providers have experience in circumcising adult males, and when circumcision is improperly performed, the procedure can result in serious medical complications or death. The problem of health worker training is compounded by the fact that many developing countries suffer acute shortages of qualified health care personnel in general.

Recommendation

- **Training:** With targeted financial support from donors, WHO should develop regional and country-level training measures to promote proper use of new HIV prevention methods. In some cases it may be advisable to implement accreditation and supervision programs, although such efforts would need to account for the fact that in many countries, traditional healers and religious leaders play a critical role in providing and advising on health care.

▶ Supply and Delivery

Substantial financial investments will be needed to build the long-term capacity essential for ensuring the adequate supply and swift delivery of new HIV prevention methods in developing countries.

Procurement and Supply Management

Some new HIV prevention methods will present significant procurement and supply management challenges for the developing countries most seriously affected by HIV. In the case of technically sophisticated prevention methods—such as HIV vaccines, microbicides, and antiretrovirals for prophylaxis—the cost of the new prevention methods will likely substantially exceed most countries' ability to purchase them. In countries where annual per capita health spending is especially constrained, even inexpensive prevention options will compete with other national priorities for budget allocations. In addition, recent experience in the introduction of antiretrovirals for the treatment of HIV underscores the potential for logistical issues to impede introduction of life-saving health interventions, as countries have found that roll-out of HIV treatment requires the capacity to forecast demand and manage supplies on a large scale.[101]

In addition to the need for increased and sustained political commitment to provide resources to purchase and deliver new prevention methods, key issues include:

- **Estimating demand:** Ensuring sufficient supply and, if necessary, manufacturing capacity for new HIV prevention methods requires accurate demand forecasting. Future demand for new HIV prevention methods will depend on a variety of variables, including existence of a means to purchase the product, accessible delivery systems, and consumer acceptance, among other factors. Demand is not static and can be influenced by external factors, such as donor assistance and social marketing.
- **Country-level systems for procurement and supply management:** Limited or nonexistent national capacity to manage the purchase, delivery, and inventory of health commodities has limited countries' ability to rapidly expand access to antiretroviral therapy in recent years. Similar impediments could slow uptake for new prevention methods, although experience gained through the global push for universal HIV/AIDs treatment access is rapidly helping countries build capacity and expertise that will assist in expediting introduction of new prevention methods.

Recommendations

- **Political commitment to provide resources:** Both developed country donors and developing country leaders should honor the commitments made at the United Nations General Assembly Special Session on HIV/AIDs[102] to support the rapid introduction of new methods for the prevention of HIV transmission. In addition, further action is needed on measures currently being examined to increase resources for international health and development, including advance purchase mechanisms for new prevention methods,[103] use of securities markets to generate funds for health and development initiatives (e.g., the International Finance Facility for Immunization),[104] and implementation of a tax on air travel.[105]
- **Pricing agreements:** With the close cooperation of developing countries and multilateral institutions, leading donors should implement, monitor, and refine new mechanisms to purchase new prevention commodities at favorable prices for developing countries.
- **Capacity building:** Countries should receive targeted support to build the capacity to develop timely analyses of future demand for emerging HIV prevention methods such as microbicides and to implement sound purchase, delivery, and supply management systems for new prevention methods.

Manufacturing Capacity

For technologies such as HIV vaccines and microbicides, several years can be required to build sufficient production capacity, and manufacturers may need to make decisions regarding initial manufacturing capacity in advance of initial regulatory licensure—that is, before large-scale efficacy trials have been completed.[106] Even for less complicated technologies, it is often challenging to gauge future demand and to calibrate manufacturing capacity to meet anticipated demand. Key issues include:

- **Creating and sustaining sufficient manufacturing capacity:** Even for relatively simple technologies, construction of manufacturing capacity to meet global demand involves substantial financial outlays and adherence to regulatory requirements. In many cases, owners of new prevention technologies are small biotech companies, academic centers, or not-for-profit organizations that have limited access to capital.

Recommendation

- **Innovative mechanisms for ensuring sufficient manufacturing capacity:** Leading donors, multilateral organizations, and developing countries should collaborate in the development of strategies to ensure timely and sufficient manufacturing capacity to meet global demand for a wide variety of new HIV prevention methods.

▶ Monitoring and Evaluation

A key role of regulatory agencies in developed countries is to monitor health interventions after they are approved for use. Such monitoring helps to document the impact of new tools and strategies, detect side effects not identified in clinical trials, and refine public health guidelines for optimal use of health interventions. In the case of side effects, for example, use of improper circumcision techniques by untrained practitioners can result in severe infections, permanent disability, and even death, underscoring the need for strong quality assurance mechanisms.

At the same time, documentation of the public health impact of new interventions will help generate momentum for investment in even better tools and strategies for the future.

Recommendation

- **Quality assurance:** Additional donor financing for new HIV prevention methods should include sufficient support for the implementation and maintenance of strong national monitoring, evaluation, and quality assurance programs. These programs should include components that monitor for potential disinhibiting effects of new HIV prevention methods.

▶ References

1. UNAIDS, *Report on the Global AIDS Epidemic,* 2006.

2. UNAIDS, *AIDS Epidemic Update,* 2005.

3. UNAIDS, *Women and HIV/AIDS: Confronting the Crisis,* 2004.

4. UNAIDS, *Resource Needs for an Expanded Response to AIDS in Low- and Middle-Income Countries,* 2005.

5. USAID et al., *Coverage of Selected Services for HIV/AIDS Prevention, Care, and Support in Low- and Middle-Income Countries in 2003,* 2004. See also Global HIV Prevention Working Group, *Access to HIV Prevention: Closing the Gap,* 2003.

6. J. Stover et al., The global impact of scaling up HIV/AIDS prevention programs in low- and middle-income countries, *Science;* published online February 2, 2006.

7. For a review of the effectiveness of current HIV prevention methods, see Global HIV Prevention Working Group, *Global Mobilization for HIV Prevention: A Blueprint for Action,* 2002 (and studies cited therein). See also J. Auerbach et al., Overview of effective and promising interventions to prevent HIV infection, in D. Ross et al. (eds.), *Preventing HIV/AIDS in Young People: A Systematic Review of the Evidence From Developing Countries,* 2006.

8. *Ibid.,* UNAIDS, *Epidemic Update,* 2005.

9. *Ibid.,* UNAIDS, *Women and AIDS,* 2004.

10. *Ibid.,* Global HIV Prevention Working Group, *Blueprint for Action,* 2002 (and studies cited therein).

11. H. Weiss et al., Male circumcision and risk of HIV infection in sub-Saharan Africa: a systematic review and meta-analysis, *AIDS* 2000;14:2361–70.

12. S. Reynolds et al., Male circumcision and risk of HIV-1 and other sexually transmitted infections in India, *Lancet* 2004;363:1039–40.

13. B. Auvert et al., Randomized, controlled intervention trial of male circumcision for reduction of HIV infection risk: the ANRS 1265 trial, *PLoS Med* 2005;2:e298.

14. UNAIDS, *Statement on South African Trial Findings Regarding Male Circumcision and HIV,* July 26, 2005.

15. R. Gray et al., Male circumcision and the risks of female HIV and STI acquisition in Rakai, Uganda, abstract presented at 13th Conference on Retroviruses and Opportunistic Infections, 2006.

16. B. Williams et al., The potential impact of male circumcision on HIV in sub-Saharan Africa, *PLoS Med* 2006;3:e262.

17. J. Krieger et al., Adult male circumcision: results of a standardized procedure in Kisumu District, Kenya, *BJU Int* 2005;96:1109–13.

18. T. Moench et al., Preventing disease by protecting the cervix: the unexplored promise of internal vaginal barrier devices, *AIDS* 2001;15:1595–1602.

19. A. van der Straten et al., Predictors of diaphragm use as a potential sexually transmitted disease/HIV prevention method in Zimbabwe, *STD* 2005;32:64–71.

20. J. Buck et al., Barrier method preference and perceptions among Zimbabwean women and their partners, *AIDS Behav* 2005;9:415–22.

21. L. Guay et al., Intrapartum and neonatal single-dose nevirapine compared with zidovudine for prevention of mother-to-child transmission of HIV-1 in Kampala, Uganda: HIVNET 012 randomized trial, *Lancet* 1999;354:795–802. See also Institute of Medicine, *Review of the HIVNET 012 Perinatal HIV Prevention Study,* 2005.

22. D. Cardo et al., A case-control study of HIV seroconversion in health care workers after percutaneous exposure, *New Eng J Med* 1997;337:1485–90.

23. For an overview of tenofovir's drug profile, see J. Gallant & S. Deresinski, Tenofovir disoproxil fumarate, *Clin Infect Dis* 2003;37:944–50.

24. C. Tsai et al., Prevention of SIV infection in macaques by (R)-9-(2-phosphonyl-methoxypropyl)adenine, *Science* 1995;270:1197–9.

25. S. Subbarao et al., Chemoprophylaxis with oral tenofovir disoproxil fumarate (TDF) delays but does not prevent infection in rhesus macaques given repeated rectal challenges of SHIV, abstract presented at 12th Conference on Retroviruses and Opportunistic Infections, 2005.

26. For an overview of emtricitabine's drug profile, see S. Michael et al., Efficacy and safety of emtricitabine vs. stavudine in combination therapy in antiretroviral-naive patients: a randomized trial, *JAMA* 2004;292:180–190.

27. W. Heneine et al., Prevention of rectal SHIV transmission in macaques by tenofovir/FTC combination, abstract presented at 13th Conference on Retroviruses and Opportunistic Infections, 2006.

28. G. Szekeres et al., *Anticipating the Efficacy of HIV Pre-Exposure Prophylaxis (PREP) and the Needs of At-Risk Californians,* 2004.

29. *Ibid.*

30. E. Freeman et al., Herpes simplex virus 2 infection increases HIV acquisition in men and women: systematic review and meta-analysis of longitudinal studies, *AIDS* 2006;20:78–83.

31. N. Nagot et al., Effect of HSV-2 suppressive therapy on HIV-1 genital shedding and plasma viral load: a proof-of-concept randomized double-blind placebo controlled trial (ANRS 1285 trial), abstract presented at 13th Conference on Retroviruses and Opportunistic Infections, 2006.

32. M. Reyes et al., Acyclovir-resistant genital herpes among persons attending sexually transmitted disease and human immunodeficiency virus clinics, *Arch Intern Med* 2003;163:76–80.

33. J. Trussell et al., Comparative contraceptive efficacy of the female condom and other barrier methods, *Fam Plan Perspect* 1994;26:66–72.

34. M. Gross et al., Use of Reality female condoms for anal sex by U.S. men who have sex with men, *Am J Pub Health* 1999;89:1739–41.

35. WHO, *Substitution Maintenance Therapy in the Management of Opioid Dependence and HIV Prevention*, 2004.

36. *Ibid.*, UNAIDS, *Global Report*, 2006.

37. *Ibid.*

38. Voluntary HIV-1 Counseling and Testing Efficacy Study Group, Efficacy of voluntary HIV-1 counseling and testing in individuals and couples in Kenya, Tanzania, and Trinidad: a randomized trial, *Lancet* 2000;356:103–12.

39. N. Crepaz & G. Marks, Toward an understanding of sexual risk behavior in people living with HIV: a review of social, psychological, and medical findings, *AIDS* 2002;16:135–49.

40. CDC, Incorporating HIV prevention into the medical care of persons living with HIV, *MMWR* 2003;52:1–24.

41. T. Quinn et al., Viral load and heterosexual transmission of human immunodeficiency virus type 1, *N Eng J Med* 2000;342:921–9.

42. A. Hauri et al., The global burden of disease attributable to contaminated injections given in health care settings, *Int J STD AIDS* 2004;15:7–16.

43. WHO, *Statement on the Use of Auto-Disable Syringes in Immunization Services*, 1999.

44. WHO, *The Safety of Immunization Practices Improves Over Last Five Years, but Challenges Remain*, news release, November 11, 2005.

45. W. Hogrefe et al., Detection of herpes simplex virus type 2-specific immunoglobulin G antibodies in African sera by using recombinant gG2, Western Blotting, and gG2 inhibition, *J Clin Microbiol* 2002;40:3635–40.

46. E. Freeman et al., The impact of HSV-2 on new HIV infections increases over time: the changing role of sexually transmitted infections in sub-Saharan African HIV epidemics, abstract presented at 16th Biennial Meeting of the International Society for Sexually Transmitted Diseases Research, 2005.

47. For an overview of potential microbicide approaches, see J. Weber et al., The development of vaginal microbicides for the prevention of HIV transmission, *PLoS Med* 2005;2:e142. See also J. Moore, Topical microbicides become topical, *New Eng J Med* 2005;352:298–300.

48. For up-to-date information on microbicide candidates in development, see the websites of the Global Campaign for Microbicides (www.global-campaign.org), and the Alliance for Microbicide Development (www.microbicide.org).

49. For example, R. Veazey et al., Protection of macaques from vaginal SHIV challenge by vaginally delivered inhibitors of virus-cell fusion, *Nature* 2005;438:99–102.

50. For example, K. Barnhart et al., BufferGel with diaphragm found to be an effective contraceptive in two phase II/III trials, abstract presented at Microbicides 2006 conference, 2006.

51. For an overview of rectal microbicide research, see International Rectal Microbicide Working Group, *Rectal Microbicides: Investment and Advocacy*, 2006 (and studies cited therein).

52. Public Health Working Group, Microbicides Initiative, *The Public Health Benefits of Microbicides in Lower-Income Countries: Model Projections*, 2002.

53. International Family Health et al., *The Potential Impact of Microbicides in Bagalkot District, Karnataka, India: Model Projections and Implications for Product Promotion,* 2004.

54. International Family Health et al., *A Comparison of the Potential Impact of Microbicides in Two Contrasting African Settings, Johannesburg, South Africa, and Cotonou, Benin,* 2004.

55. See J. Mantel et al., Microbicide acceptability research: current approaches and future directions, *Soc Sci Med* 2005;60:319–30.

56. For a comprehensive review of the state of HIV vaccine research, see Coordinating Committee of the Global HIV Vaccine Enterprise, The Global HIV Vaccine Enterprise Scientific Strategic Plan, *PLoS Med* 2005;2:e25. See also International AIDS Vaccine Initiative, *AIDS Vaccine Blueprint 2006: Actions to Strengthen Global Research and Development,* 2006. In addition, see AIDS Vaccine Advocacy Coalition, *AIDS Vaccines: The Next Frontiers,* 2006.

57. For example, J. Shiver et al., Replication-incompetent adenoviral vaccine vector elicits effective anti-immunodeficiency-virus immunity, *Nature* 2002;415:331–5.

58. D. Follmann, An independent analysis of the effect of race in VAX004, abstract presented at 11th Conference on Retroviruses and Opportunistic Infections, 2004.

59. Databases of HIV vaccine candidates in clinical trials are maintained by the International AIDS Vaccine Initiative (www.iavi.org) and the HIV Vaccine Trials Network's Pipeline Project (chi.ucsf.edu/vaccine).

60. G. Pantaleo & R. Koup, Correlates of immune protection in HIV-1 infection: what we know, what we don't know, what we should know, *Nat Med* 2004;10:806–10.

61. *Ibid.,* Global HIV Vaccine Enterprise, Scientific Strategic Plan, 2005. See also R. Klausner et al., The need for a global HIV vaccine enterprise, *Science* 2003;300:2036–9.

62. World Bank, *The Epidemiological Impact of an HIV/AIDS Vaccine in Developing Countries,* 2002.

63. Global Forum for Health Research, *Monitoring Financial Flows for Health Research,* 2004.

64. HIV Vaccines and Microbicides Resource Tracking Group, *Tracking Funding for Microbicide Research and Development: Estimates of Annual Investments,* 2005. HIV Vaccines and Microbicides Resource Tracking Group, *Tracking Funding for Preventive HIV Vaccine Research and Development: Estimates of Annual Investments and Expenditures,* 2005. See also www.hivresourcetracking.org.

65. *Ibid.*

66. A. Batson, The problems and promise of vaccine markets in developing countries, *Health Affairs* 2005;24:690–3. See also M. Pauly, Improving vaccine supply and development: who needs what? *Health Affairs* 2005;24:680–9.

67. Center for Global Development, *Making Markets for Vaccines: Ideas to Action,* 2005.

68. For an overview of issues concerning clinical trial design and conduct, see S. Chow & J. Liu, *Design and Analysis of Clinical Trials: Concepts and Methodologies, 2nd Edition,* 2003.

69. In the case of community-based sexually transmitted disease control as an HIV prevention strategy, initial trial results indicating a high level of effectiveness were followed by results from other studies that failed to detect a significant benefit. For a discussion, see P. Hitchcock & L. Fransen, Preventing HIV infection: lessons from Mwanza and Rakai, *Lancet* 1999;353:513–5.

70. J. Ioannidis, Contradicted and initially stronger effects in highly cited clinical research, *JAMA* 2005;294:218–28.

71. S. Buchbinder, HIV vaccine efficacy trials: lessons learned and future directions, abstract presented at 11th Conference on Retroviruses and Opportunistic Infections, 2004.

72. Family Health International & Cellegy Pharmaceuticals, *Joint Statement on Savvy Phase III Trial in Ghana to Test the Effectiveness of Savvy Gel in Preventing HIV,* November 8, 2005.

73. *Ibid.,* Global HIV Vaccine Enterprise, Scientific Strategic Plan, 2005.

74. For an overview of ethical standards for clinical trials, see R. Levine, *Ethics and Regulation of Clinical Research, 2nd Edition,* 1988.

75. For a review of the evidence on the effectiveness of prevention strategies for injection drug users, see S. Hurley et al., Effectiveness of needle exchange programs for prevention of HIV infection, *Lancet* 1997;349:1797–800. See also A. Wodak & A. Cooney, Do needle syringe programs reduce HIV infection among injecting drug users? A comprehensive review of the international evidence, *Sub Use & Misuse* 2006;41:777–813.

76. UNAIDS, *Intensifying HIV Prevention,* 2005.

77. WHO, Treating people with intercurrent infection in HIV prevention trials: report from a WHO/UNAIDS consultation, *AIDS* 2004;18:W1–12. See also A. Forbes, Moving toward assured access to treatment in microbicide trials, *PLoS Med* 2006;3:e153.

78. UNAIDS, *Ethical Considerations in HIV Preventive Vaccine Research,* 2000.

79. International AIDS Society, *Building Collaboration to Advance HIV Prevention: Global Consultation on Tenofovir Pre-Exposure Prophylaxis Research,* 2005.

80. J. Ananworanich et al., Creation of a drug fund for post-clinical trial access to antiretrovirals, *Lancet* 2004;364:101–2.

81. For an overview of issues related to informed consent, see C. McGrory et al., *Informed Consent in HIV Prevention Trials: Report of an International Workshop,* 2006.

82. S. Berkley, Thorny issues in the ethics of AIDS vaccine trials, *Lancet* 2003;362:992.

83. D. Fitzgerald et al., Provision of treatment in HIV-1 vaccine trials in developing countries, *Lancet* 2003;362:993–4.

84. *Ibid.*

85. K. Page-Shafer et al., HIV prevention research in a resource-limited setting: the experience of planning a trial in Cambodia, *Lancet* 2005;366:1499–503.

86. E. Mills et al., Designing research in vulnerable populations: lessons from HIV prevention trials that stopped early, *BMJ* 2005;331:1403–6.

87. UNAIDS, Creating effective partnerships for HIV prevention trials: report of a UNAIDS consultation, *AIDS* 2006;20:W1–11.

88. *Ibid.,* International AIDS Society, *Consultation on Tenofovir,* 2005.

89. J. Clemens & L. Jodar, Introducing new vaccines into developing countries: obstacles, opportunities and complexities, *Nat Med* 2005;11:S12–5. See also J. Andrus & J. Fitzsimmons, Introduction of new and underutilized vaccines: sustaining access, disease control, and infrastructure development, *PLoS Med* 2005;2:e286.

90. *Ibid.,* USAID et al., *Coverage of Selected Services for HIV,* 2004. See also WHO, *Progress on Global Access to HIV Antiretroviral Therapy: An Update on "3 by 5,"* 2006.

91. For example, UNFPA et al., *New Data on the Prevention of Mother-to-Child Transmission of HIV and Their Policy Implications: Technical Consultation,* 2001.

92. For a discussion of issues involved in strengthening the national regulatory capacity of developing countries, see WHO, *Aide-Memoire: Strengthening National Regulatory Authorities,* 2003.

93. Article 58 of European Commission regulation 726/2004 allows the EMEA's Committee for Medicinal Products for Human Use to provide opinions on products intended for markets outside of the European Union.

94. For information on ICH, see www.ich.org.

95. U.S. National Institute of Allergy and Infectious Diseases, *Scientific Evidence on Condom Effectiveness for Sexually Transmitted Disease Prevention,* 2001.

96. For example, UNAIDS, *Condom Social Marketing: Selected Case Studies,* 2000.

97. *Ibid.,* J. Mantel et al., Microbicide acceptability research, 2005.

98. *Ibid.,* J. Krieger et al., Adult male circumcision, 2005.

99. *Ibid.,* J. Buck et al., Barrier method preference, 2005.

100. For a discussion of disinhibition in the context of the potential future introduction of tenofovir pre-exposure prophylaxis, see AIDS Vaccine Advocacy Coalition, *Will a Pill a Day Prevent HIV?: Anticipating the Results of the Tenofovir PREP Trials,* 2005. For a discussion of disinhibition in the context of expanded access to HIV treatment, see M. Over et al., *HIV/AIDS Treatment and Prevention in India: Modeling the Costs and Consequences,* 2004.

101. *Ibid.,* WHO, *Progress on Global Access to Antiretroviral Therapy,* 2006.

102. United Nations, *Declaration of Commitment on HIV/AIDS, United Nations General Assembly Special Session on HIV/AIDS,* 2001 (see paragraph 70).

103. *Ibid.,* Center for Global Development, *Making Markets for Vaccines,* 2005.

104. See www.iffim.com.

105. Reuters, *13 Countries Join Forces on Air Ticket Tax for Poor,* March 1, 2006.

106. International AIDS Vaccine Initiative, *Speeding the Manufacture of an HIV Vaccine: Policy Issues and Options,* 2005.

Unfinished Business—Expanding HIV Testing in Developing Countries

Kevin M. De Cock, M.D., D.T.M.H., Rebecca Bunnell, Sc.D., and Jonathan Mermin, M.D., M.P.H.

When the Group of Eight (G8) major industrial countries (France, the United States, Britain, Germany, Japan, Italy, Canada, and Russia) made a commitment in July 2005 to work toward universal access by 2010 to the prevention and treatment of human immunodeficiency virus (HIV) infection and AIDS, the move brought to light an HIV testing emergency: knowledge of serologic status is required for the appropriate targeting of services and interventions. The World Health Organization and the Joint United Nations Program on HIV/ AIDS recently published revised guidelines for HIV testing,[1] but field experience in Africa indicates that testing must be greatly expanded. It seems clear that to maximize benefit, a public health approach to HIV testing and treatment—including case finding and testing of partners—should become the norm.

Meeting the targets for antiretroviral treatment that had been set for the end of 2005 would have required testing as many as 180 million persons worldwide annually,[2] far exceeding the current rates.[3] Current guidelines recommend offering testing to persons with symptoms and signs that are potentially attributable to HIV infection or AIDS.[1] However, since advanced immunodeficiency can be clinically silent, it would be more effective to offer testing to all patients attending health care facilities in locations with a high prevalence of HIV infection. Botswana, with a prevalence of more than 35 percent among people 15 to 49 years of age, has initiated such routine testing at clinics and hospitals nationwide. Kenya is increasing routine testing of pregnant women, hospitalized patients, and patients with tuberculosis; with an "opt-out" approach, less than 20 percent have chosen not to be tested. With routine testing of inpatients in selected hospitals in Uganda, 95 percent of inpatients agreed to be tested, and the prevalence of HIV was discovered to exceed 50 percent.

Current guidelines restrict the use of routine testing to settings in which antiretroviral therapy is available.[1] We believe that the recommendations should support routine testing wherever basic HIV care and prevention are available. Such a change would improve efforts at prevention, allow infected persons to receive care such as cotrimoxazole prophylaxis, and normalize HIV testing. Prophylaxis against opportunistic infections is within the reach of even the poorest countries, and the identification of those who will need it benefits the entire public health system. In the United States, it is cost-effective to provide routine testing and counseling to all patients in hospitals with a prevalence of HIV of more than 1 percent, a practice recommended by the Centers for Disease Control and Prevention (CDC); in Africa, the prevalence among hospitalized patients is often greater than 50 percent.

Providing testing to family members of infected persons is critical; 50 percent of the spouses of infected African adults are also infected.[3] The testing of partners is the first step toward providing care for those who are infected—and protecting those who are not. Knowledge of HIV status is associated with reductions in high-risk behavior; and providing preventive services, including condoms to HIV-discordant couples, decreases the risk of transmission by 80 percent.[4] The children of infected women have an increased likelihood of infection, and pediatric HIV infection may indicate the presence of infection in other family members. The identification and treatment to HIV-infected mothers are important for their children, since their risk of death is at least doubled if their mother dies.

The prevalence of HIV infection among adolescents, especially young women, is high in much of Africa. Counseling and testing among young people is an important preventive strategy, although it may be ethically and legally challenging. Although premarital HIV testing is not cost-effective where prevalence is low, it is an important preventive practice in regions with generalized epidemics. Careful guidance is required, however, to determine how to implement such testing without coercion and how to limit the negative social consequences of a premarital diagnosis of HIV infection, especially for young women.

Approximately 2.3 million children worldwide are living with HIV infection, and children account for 18 percent of AIDS-related deaths. Signs of HIV disease are often nonspecific, and more than half of infected African children die before two years of age. Antiretroviral therapy, therefore, must be started early, and universal HIV testing in pediatric clinical settings—an issue omitted from recent guidelines[1]—will be required. Pediatric testing is complex: the possible presence of passively transferred maternal antibody limits diagnostic confidence until 18 months of age, and venipuncture is difficult. Moreover, exposure to HIV may continue during breast-feeding. Algorithms for testing children of various ages should be evaluated and endorsed by international public health authorities. For younger children, the algorithms could include rapid testing, with positive results verified by a central laboratory—a system being examined in Uganda and Kenya.

Since the denial of an HIV test may restrict an infected person's access to life-prolonging therapy, health care systems must determine whose role it is to grant permission for the testing of children, including orphans with no official guardians. In some countries, pediatric testing has been avoided for fear that HIV-infected children might be abandoned or neglected by families or caregivers, but this has not, to our knowledge, been documented. Guidance is also required with regard to the appropriate timing and methods of disclosing to children their HIV status.

In Africa, AIDS-related mortality is high among the providers of essential services—not only health care workers, but also teachers, police, and the military—so that stability, security, and economic development are all threatened. We recommend routine testing for HIV for persons in key occupations, with guarantees of confidentiality, protection against discrimination, free treatment for infected persons, and postexposure prophylaxis as appropriate.

The equitable expansion of HIV testing requires innovative approaches to reaching people in remote settings. New methods, such as finger-stick or salivary testing, are being used, and services are being provided in innovative ways, including testing of entire families in health care facilities and homes. Testing and counseling services have been delivered at community and religious institutions, youth centers, and military barracks. The shortage of health care professionals in Africa will have to be addressed in part by the training of community and lay workers to provide testing and counseling, treatment support, and other services.

Successful HIV-testing programs provide respectful and convenient service, confidentiality, accurate testing, full information, and effective referral. Rapid test algorithms involving the use of different tests in combination have a validity similar to that of standard approaches,[5] do not require laboratory facilities or confirmation by Western blot assay, and can be performed by trained lay personnel. Performing rapid tests on fingerstick specimens in front of clients increases confidence in the results and prevents clerical errors. Tests may be performed sequentially or in parallel, with a third test used as a "tie breaker" for discrepant results. A subgroup of specimens may be sent to a laboratory for quality assurance.

Vigorous treatment and prevention programs limit the devastation wrought by AIDS, motivating a reassessment of attitudes toward HIV testing. The initial experience in Africa shows that the benefits outweigh the risks. According to Rose Apondi, a researcher at CDC–Uganda who studied HIV-infected persons in rural Uganda, home-based HIV testing and three months of antiretroviral therapy were associated with exclusively positive social experiences, such as community and partner support, in 79 percent of cases and with exclusively negative ones, such as stigma, in less than 1 percent.

HIV epidemics have also emerged in countries such as China, India, and Russia, where they are concentrated among injection-drug users, sex workers and their clients, and paid blood donors. Ensuring the appropriate distribution of services will require sentinel surveillance, followed by HIV testing targeted according to local epidemiologic trends. These countries have an opportunity that was not afforded to countries in Africa: before their epidemics become generalized, they may develop integrated strategies linking surveillance, prevention, HIV testing, antiretroviral therapy, and other care.

The increased resources available for combating HIV and AIDS, the strong emphasis on treatment, and the commitment of the G8 to universal access necessitate a massive expansion of HIV testing. The ideal that all citizens of high-prevalence countries should know their serologic status and should be tested repeatedly over the course of their lives should become explicit targets of preventive efforts. Increased rates of testing will, of course, generate other challenges, such as the provision of preventive services for HIV-infected persons, the disclosure of serologic status, and the notification of partners—all areas in which we must define the best practices for a new era.

▶ Notes

The opinions and statements in this Perspective are those of the authors and do not represent the official policy, endorsement, or views of the CDC, the U.S. Public Health Service, or the U.S. Department of Health and Human Services. Dr. De Cock is the director of CDC–Kenya; Dr. Bunnell is the associate director for science at CDC–Uganda; and Dr. Mermin is the director of CDC–Uganda. The other participants in the Kenya–Uganda HIV Testing Group were Elizabeth Marum, Ph.D., Barbara Marston, M.D., Dorothy Mbori-Ngacha, M.B., Ch.B., M.Med.,and Laurence Marum, M.D., M.P.H., in Kenya, and Donna Kabatesi, M.B., Ch.B., M.P.H., in Uganda.

1. UNAIDS/WHO policy statement on HIV testing. Geneva: Joint United Nations Programme on HIV/AIDS, June 2004.

2. The right to know: new approaches to HIV testing and counseling. Geneva: World Health Organization, 2003.

3. Central Bureau of Statistics (CBS) [Kenya], Ministry of Health (MOH) [Kenya], ORC Macro. Kenya demographic and health survey 2003. Calverton, Md.: ORC Macro, July 2004:227–8.

4. Weller S, Davis K. Condom effectiveness in reducing heterosexual HIV transmission. Cochrane Database Syst Rev 2001;3: CD003255.

5. Downing RG, Otten RA, Marum E, et al. Optimizing the delivery of HIV counseling and testing services: the Uganda experience using rapid HIV antibody test algorithms. J Acquir Immune Defic Syndr Hum Retrovirol 1998;18:384–8.

The Search for Effective HIV Vaccines

Howard Markel, M.D., Ph.D.

In February 2003, after more than a decade of work, a team of scientists representing the biotechnology company VaxGen announced the results of the first phase 3 trial to test the efficacy of a vaccine against the human immunodeficiency virus (HIV). Despite the highest of hopes, their product, AIDSVax—which contains a synthetic monomeric glycoprotein based on glycoprotein 120 (GP120), the CD4-binding site on the outer coat, or envelope, of the virus— did not prevent HIV infection in the study cohort as a whole. It was a frustrating setback for HIV-vaccine research, a field that has endured a Sisyphean onslaught of disappointments. But if the virus that causes AIDS is persistent, the vaccine researchers are no less so. Indeed, on July 14, 2005, the National Institute of Allergy and Infectious Diseases (NIAID) announced a grant of more than $300 million for a new Center for HIV/AIDS Vaccine Immunology. The center aims to address key immunology roadblocks to HIV-vaccine development and to design, develop, and test novel vaccine candidates.

As of this writing, two phase 2 trials that are testing therapeutic HIV vaccines are under way—these vaccines are designed not to prevent infection but, rather, by stimulating T lymphocytes that can identify and kill HIVinfected cells, to prevent or limit viral replication and delay disease progression. Although experts have not given up the ultimate goal of a preventive vaccine, they are hopeful that a therapeutic vaccine will, at least, help stem the devastating tide of disease, disability, and death from AIDS.

Because the AIDS epidemic has occurred at a time when medical science is progressing at a rapid clip, unrealistic expectations or promises about its conquest have played a supporting role in this drama since the epidemic's earliest days. Historians have pinpointed April 23, 1984, as the moment of the most wildly optimistic prediction about an AIDS vaccine. At a press conference in Washington, D.C., at which the identification of the virus we now call HIV was announced, Margaret Heckler, the Secretary of Health and Human Services, proclaimed that a preventive vaccine would be ready for testing within two years.

Several scientists seated in the packed auditorium "blanched visibly" at Heckler's declaration.[1] Their reaction was understandable. After all, it had taken 105 years to develop a vaccine for typhoid after the discovery of its microbiologic cause; the *Haemophilus influenzae* vaccine took 92 years; pertussis vaccine, 89 years; polio vaccine, 47 years; measles vaccine, 42 years; and hepatitis B vaccine, 16 years.

And so, after a mere 21 years, we continue to struggle to contain the pandemic of our age. This year, 34 candidate HIV vaccines are in the early phases of human clinical trials in 19 countries. But, as in 1984, a safe and effective preventive vaccine remains elusive.

Some delay can justly be blamed on inadequate funding. According to Mitchell Warren, executive director of the AIDS Vaccine Advocacy Coalition, in New York, "Last year, about $680 million, primarily from the public sector but in smaller amounts from the private sector and philanthropy, went toward the development of AIDS vaccines—less than 1 percent of the total global spending on health-product research and development."

During the past century especially, the major pharmaceutical companies have led the way in developing most vaccines. Yet when it comes to HIV, many of these companies have been slow to participate, in part because there is so much uncertainty about which approach is most promising (see diagram) and in part because the return on the massive investment required is likely to be small, especially as compared with the profits generated by blockbuster drugs such as statins or antidepressants.

"A substantial proportion of the entire investment in AIDS vaccines comes from the National Institutes of Health," notes Dr. Anthony Fauci, the director of NIAID. "We need to overcome the scientific barriers to the point that leads industry to say we can afford to get involved. But . . . at the end of the day, we—and academe—must partner with industry. The government or universities do not manufacture vaccines, the pharmaceutical companies do."

But even if we could vanquish the economic challenges, as well as the myriad cultural, social, and ethical problems that attend the development of any vaccine, there remains one Himalayan obstacle: the remarkable pathogenic power of HIV itself. Even now, scientists do not know the correlates of immune protection—the specific types of immune responses that an effective HIV vaccine must stimulate in order to prevent infection.

Typically, successful immune responses against viral infections include humoral and cellular components. The humoral reaction yields virus-neutralizing antibodies that prevent viral particles from infecting new cells. The cellular response mobilizes specific CD8+ cytotoxic T lymphocytes that target and kill cells that express viral antigens. Thus, an optimal HIV vaccine would elicit both types of responses.

Unfortunately, HIV has a large menu of mechanisms that enable it to undermine immune responses. "HIV is astounding," says Fauci. "Of the 60-million-plus people who have been infected with it, there's not a single documented case of someone who has ultimately cleared the infection from his or her body. The initial infection wipes out specific immune responses, the virus permanently integrates into the host cell's chromosome and establishes what appears to be a permanent reservoir of infected cells, and . . . the antigens that induce broadly reactive neutralizing antibodies do not appear to present themselves in a way that allows the host to elicit a protective immune response."

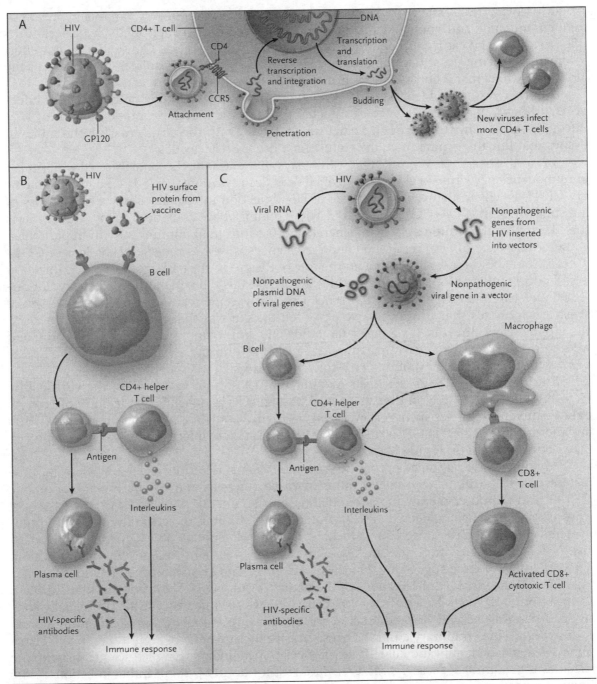

FIGURE 12-15 Approaches to HIV-Vaccine Development
The mechanism of normal HIV infection is shown (Panel A), along with mechanisms of three types of potential vaccines: a subunit vaccine containing a synthetic protein from the CD4-binding site on the envelope of the virus (Panel B), a naked DNA vaccine, and a recombinant vaccine with a bacterial or viral vector (Panel C).

Moreover, the plasticity of the virus affords a steady stream of new variants by means of frequent mutation and, sometimes, recombination. Three major groups of HIV have been identified to date, and these have been divided into nine subtypes or clades. Consequently, any effort to create a vaccine must use the broadest possible range of HIV isolates from around the globe and will demand constant surveillance of the virus in ensuing years.

Another vexing problem has to do with an evolving understanding of the routes of infection. Although many people become infected through the bloodstream, 90 percent of HIV infections are contracted through sexual transmission, with the virus crossing the mucosal tissues that line the genital tract, the rectum, and other body cavities.

In April, researchers reported that within days after macaques become infected with simian immunodeficiency virus—a close relative of HIV—it destroys more than 50 percent of the memory CD4+ T cells in their guts.[2,3] Studies of HIV infection in humans show a similar loss of intestinal memory CD4+CCR5+ T cells.[4,5] These findings have convinced many AIDS experts that the mucosal immune system in general, and the intestinal immune system in particular, is the primary site of viral replication and persistence, as well as the site of the loss of CD4+ T cells. Some now argue that, although the role of the gut in the pathogenesis of the infection is still poorly understood, vaccine strategies that target this type of immunity may revolutionize HIV research and therapy. Dr. Lawrence Corey, a vaccine researcher at the University of Washington, notes that "until now, we never felt the gut was that much different from, say, the bloodstream. But it is. It's a major target for HIV in the first two weeks of infection, and we never see patients that early, making the concept of utilizing a therapeutic vaccine to stabilize or preserve immunity among HIV-infected persons . . . difficult."

During the mid-1980s, scientists identified GP120 on the envelope of the virus as the CD4-binding site, the region that attaches to human cells and facilitates the entry of HIV. As a result, much energy was spent on developing a vaccine based on genetically engineered GP120 and the larger glycoprotein GP160 to prevent the acquisition of infection. This was the approach taken by VaxGen in designing its vaccine.

Although AIDSVax failed to provide protection against infection, its failure held some critical lessons: the structure of the HIV outer envelope differs from the structure of monomeric GP120, and the outer membrane of circulating HIV strains hides its epitopes in a variety of ways that genetically engineered GP120 proteins do not mimic successfully. The viral glycoproteins appear to have a protective shield, consisting of variable loop sequences and extensive *N*-linked glycosylation, that makes them relatively resistant to antibody neutralization. There is little evidence suggesting that these difficulties can be surmounted anytime soon.

One of the sentinel observations of the natural history of HIV infection is that although some amount of T-cell depletion occurs in everyone who is infected, the virus is usually controlled for at least several years before it begins multiplying so rapidly that the immune system is destroyed. This temporary control corresponds to the presence of high numbers of T lymphocytes that can identify and kill HIV-infected cells. Such findings have led scientists to explore vaccines that stimulate these T cells, even though they do not prevent initial infection, in the hope of preventing or limiting viral replication and delaying disease progression.

A number of such vaccines are now being tested. Some are live-vector vaccines containing a bacterium or virus that has been modified so that it does not cause disease but can transport a gene or genes into the body that will make one or more HIV proteins and confer some immunity. For example, a canarypox-vector vaccine containing HIV genes for both internal and envelope HIV proteins is being tested in a phase 3 trial in Thailand, but preliminary data on its immunogenicity are not encouraging.

Another vaccine, now in the early stages of a "proof of concept," or phase 2B trial, contains replication-defective adenovirus type 5 that transmits the HIV genes *gag, pol,* and *nef* (which code for internal HIV proteins and may stimulate cellular immunity); this vaccine looks far more promising. The trial, a collaboration between Merck and the NIAID-funded HIV Vaccine Trials Network, is being conducted under the direction of Dr. Corey. So far, only about 250 people have been enrolled in the United States, Peru, Brazil, and the Caribbean, but the target is 3000 volunteers.

A different and propitious candidate, which is being developed at NIAID's Vaccine Research Center and is currently in a phase 2 trial, entails a combination approach: first, a vaccine is administered that uses naked DNA to prime an immune response to both internal HIV proteins and external HIV proteins; then, a booster shot involving an inactivated adenovirus vector is administered, which stimulates specific antibody responses to HIV envelope proteins and internal proteins. The hope is that this prime-boost strategy will be far more potent than the single adenovirus-vector or canarypox-vector vaccine and that it will address some of the challenges posed by the diversity of envelope proteins found among the various HIV isolates throughout the world.

When asked whether changing the focus from prevention to therapy turns the concept of vaccination upside down, Dr. Gary Nabel, the director of the Vaccine Research Center, explains that what we are really doing is testing immune concepts. "I am an empiricist," says Nabel. "I will look for any kind of protection we can get. In the end, we are searching to identify the critical immune parameters that will predict success in protecting against infection or disease. We need to define both variables."

"These cellular-immunity-producing vaccines are primarily blunting mechanisms to dampen the progression of infection," said Fauci, "but if they do work, we will be scrambling to produce one in combination with a vaccine that would induce neutralizing antibodies to protect against infection. This should be seen as a first step rather than an end point. No one is relying on these vaccines alone."

But a comprehensive vaccine has yet to be found. Dr. James Curran, the dean of Emory University's School of Public Health in Atlanta, was the director of AIDS research at the Centers for Disease Control in 1984 when he heard Margaret Heckler make her vaccine prediction. He recalls that afternoon well, and even today, despite our inability to predict with any certainty when we will have a vaccine, Curran counsels optimistic patience.

"Secretary Heckler was actually responding to a reporter's question," he said, "and I think her answer was a natural response that still occurs in an era of rapid scientific progress. Everyone understands we need a vaccine, and I think people back then were caught up with the enthusiasm of our initial successes. We now know that it is considerably more complicated."

► Notes

Dr. Markel is a professor of the history of medicine and a professor of pediatrics and communicable diseases at the University of Michigan Medical School, Ann Arbor, where he directs the Center for the History of Medicine.

1. Shilts R. And the band played on: politics, people, and the AIDS epidemic. New York: St. Martin's Press, 1987:451.

2. Mattapallil JJ, Douek DC, Hill B, Nishimura Y, Martin M, Roederer M. Massive infection and loss of memory CD4+ T cells in multiple tissues during acute SIV infection. Nature 2005;434:1093–7.

3. Li Q, Duan L, Estes JD, et al. Peak SIV replication in resting memory CD4+ T cells depletes gut lamina propria CD4+ T cells. Nature 2005;434:1148–52.

4. Mehandru S, Poles MA, Tenner-Racz K, et–al. Primary HIV-1 infection is associated with preferential depletion of CD4+ T lymphocytes from effector sites in the gastrointestinal tract. J Exp Med 2004;200:761–70.

5. Brenchley JM, Schacker TW, Ruff LE, et al. CD4+ T cell depletion during all stages of HIV disease occurs predominantly in the gastrointestinal tract. J Exp Med 2004; 200:749–59.

Chapter 13

Treatment

Treatment of HIV Disease

Darrell Ward

Antiretroviral drugs—drugs specifically targeted to HIV—are the primary treatment for HIV disease. This chapter describes the antiretroviral drugs that are currently available, explains why resistance to them can develop, and provides a summary of the scientific principles that underlie their use. It concludes with strategies under development. (Note: Optimal antiretroviral therapy varies with the individual, the stage of disease, and other factors. In addition, the field of antiretroviral therapy continues to evolve. For these reasons, specific HIV-treatment regimens are not presented in this book. For information on antiretroviral regimens call the HIV/AIDS Treatment Information Service or visit their Web site, or see the latest issue of AmFAR's *AIDS/HIV Treatment Directory*.

In the past few years, potent new drugs have been developed to manage HIV infection, numerous advances have been made in the understanding of HIV and how it causes disease, and tests became available to measure the amount of HIV in the blood (i.e., viral load). This progress has redefined how HIV infection is treated and managed. The new drugs, for example, are combined in treatment regimens that as a group are known as "highly active anti-retroviral therapy" (HAART), which in many people suppresses the reproduction (i.e., replication) of HIV to levels undetectable in blood by currently available tests and allows the body to at least partially replenish the number of CD4 lymphocytes in the blood. Physicians experienced in HIV disease also now have a much better idea of when antiretroviral therapy should begin (largely because of viral-load testing) and what drug combinations to use in particular patients.

The success of HAART has allowed many people with advanced HIV disease to return to an active life. It has also led some researchers to believe that a cure for the disease, at least at some stages, may be possible one day. At the same time, however, a great deal of uncertainty remains about HAART regimens. Researchers do not yet know how quickly HIV will develop resistance to combination therapy, or how well the human body will tolerate its long-term use. The development of cross-resistance—which occurs when viral resistance to one drug also results in resistance to other drugs of the same class—is also a concern. Scientists are also uncertain about how effectively the CD4 cells that arise during the use of HAART can fight infections. These questions are under investigation.

The cost of anti-HIV drugs also presents problems for many people who need them. A course of treatment for a single antiretroviral drug approved by the Food and Drug Administration (FDA) can range from $2,000 to $7,000 annually, and HAART regimens typically require taking three drugs simultaneously. Help with the cost of HIV treatment is available through private insurance, state Medicaid programs, and the Ryan White CARE Act, a federal assistance plan (provided under Title II of the AIDS Drugs Assistance Program [ADAP]). Individuals should ask their physician, social worker, or local AIDS service organization about the financial assistance programs for which they may qualify.

▶ Antiretroviral Therapies

Currently approved antiretroviral drugs work by inhibiting the action of one or the other of two viral enzymes that are essential for HIV replication, reverse transcriptase (RT) and protease. Consequently, antiretroviral drugs are known as "reverse transcriptase inhibitors" (RTIs) and "protease inhibitors." Note that the use and side effects of all anti-HIV drugs should be discussed with an experienced physician before the drugs are taken.

Reverse Transcriptase Inhibitors

RTIs work by blocking the viral enzyme RT. This enzyme is used by HIV to construct a DNA copy of its RNA genome shortly after the virus enters a host cell. RTIs are classified as either nucleoside analogues or nonnucleoside analogues.

Nucleoside Analogues

The nucleoside analogue RTIs (Table 13.1) work by mimicking nucleosides, molecules found in the cell that are needed for assembly of DNA strands. Nucleosides are modified versions of the so-called bases that form the cross pieces in the DNA double helix. The bases, named adenine, cytosine, guanine, and thymine, are first converted to nucleosides before they can be incorporated into DNA. A nucleoside is produced when a base is chemically linked to a sugar molecule; a nucleotide is produced when a phosphate group is linked to a nucleoside.

When RT is assembling a viral DNA strand in a newly infected cell, it hijacks nucleotides made by the cell for the cell's own needs. When an HIV-infected person takes a nucleoside analogue RTI such as AZT, cells take up the drug and add a phosphate group to the molecules of AZT, thereby converting them to their nucleotide form. RT will then add AZT to the growing strand of viral DNA in place of the normal thymine nucleotide. Once this happens, however, AZT blocks any further assembly of the viral DNA, thereby putting an early stop to that virus's replication cycle.

A molecule with a structure that resembles that of another molecule is known as an "analogue." Because all RTI drugs work by masquerading as nucleosides, they are known as nucleoside analogue RTIs. Nucleoside RTIs are the oldest class of anti-HIV drugs, and more are in development (as are drugs that work as nucleotide analogues). Nucleoside RTIs in current use include the following:

- Abacavir (also known as 1592-U89) is an analogue of the nucleoside guanosine that is in phase III testing as of this writing.
- Didanosine (ddI) is an analogue of the nucleoside adenosine. It was the second drug to be approved for the treatment of HIV infection.

TABLE 13.1 Nucleoside Analogue Reverse Transcriptase Inhibitors*#

| Generic Name | Brand Name | Manufacturer | Development Stage | |
			Adults	Children
abacavir	Ziagen	Glaxo-Wellcome	In clinical trials	
didanosine (ddI)	Videx	Bristol-Myers Squibb	Approved	Approved
lamivudine (3TC)	Epivir	Glaxo-Wellcome	Approved	Approved
stavudine (d4T)	Zerit	Bristol-Myers Squibb	Approved	Approved
zalcitabine (ddC)	Hivid	Hoffman-LaRoche	Approved	
zidovudine (ZDV) (also known as AZT or azidothymidine)†	Retrovir	Glaxo-Wellcome	Approved	Approved
zidovudine & lamivudine	Combivir	Glaxo-Wellcome	Approved	

*FDA-approved drugs have at least three names: a generic name, a brand name, and a chemical name. The generic name is the name used when referring to the drug during clinical trials, in medical-research papers, and usually in the media; generic names are not capitalized. Brand names are given to a drug by its manufacturer for marketing purposes; brand names are registered and the initial letter is always capitalized. The chemical name of a drug is derived from its chemical structure. The chemical name for AZT, for example, is 3′-azido-3′-deoxythymidine (chemical names are not included in the tables in this chapter). In addition, during a drug's testing phase, pharmaceutical company may initially refer to it using a combination of letters and numbers.

†As of May 1997, AZT was the only antiretroviral drug approved for pregnant women.

- Lamivudine (3TC) is an analogue of the nucleoside cytidine. The FDA announced the accelerated approval of 3TC in November 1995 for use in combination with AZT. It is noteworthy that 3TC has also been found to suppress the hepatitis B virus.
- Stavudine (d4T) is an analogue of thymidine. d4T was approved by the FDA in June 1994 for patients who were intolerant of zidovudine and didanosine, or whose disease was advancing while taking these treatments.
- Zalcitabine (ddC) is an analogue of the nucleoside cytidine.
- Zidovudine (ZDV), also known as azidothymidine, or AZT, is an analogue of the nucleoside thymidine. AZT was first synthesized as a potential anticancer agent in 1963. In 1986, during a phase II clinical trial, it became the first drug to show benefit to people with HIV disease by reducing the incidence of opportunistic disease or prolonging their lives. This finding greatly stimulated research to discover and test agents with similar or possibly better antiretroviral properties.

Nonnucleoside RTIs

Nonnucleoside RTIs (NNRTIs) (Table 13.2) work by binding to RT and stopping its action. NNRTIs are very specific for inhibiting HIV-1; they have no activity against HIV-2, a closely related retrovirus that also causes AIDS. Viral resistance (see below) to NNRTIs develops quickly, but the process is slowed when the drugs are used in combination with a nucleoside analogue RTI. One NNRTI, nevirapine, is also able to cross the blood-brain barrier. Clinical trials using NNRTIs are under way. Two of these drugs, nevirapine and delavirdine, have been approved by the FDA.

Protease Inhibitors

Late in its replication, HIV produces an enzyme called protease (sometimes called proteinase). Its job is to cleave a large viral "polyprotein" as HIV buds from cells. If this large protein is not

TABLE 13.2 Nonnucleoside Reverse Transcriptase Inhibitors#

Generic Name	Brand Name	Manufacturer	Development Stage	
			Adults	Children
delavirdine (DLV)	Rescriptor	Pharmacia & Upjohn	Approved	
efavirenz	Sustiva	DuPont-Merck	In clinical trials	
nevirapine (NVP)	Viramune	Boehringer Ingelheim	Approved	

TABLE 13.3 Protease Inhibitors#

Generic Name	Brand Name	Manufacturer	Development Stage	
			Adults	Children
indinavir	Crixivan	Merck	Approved	
nelfinavir	Viracept	Agouron Pharm.	Approved	Approved
ritonavir	Norvir	Abbott Laboratories	Approved	Approved
saquinavir	Fortovase and Invirase*	Hoffman-LaRoche	Approved	

*Invirase is the original hard-gel formulation of saquinavir, which is more poorly absorbed by the body than the newer Fortovase, which is a soft-gel preparation.

#Warning: Some of the antiretroviral drugs listed in Tables 13.1, 13.2, and 13.3 have similar names. As a result, pharmacies have been known to make serious mistakes when filling prescriptions, such as confusing ritonavir (a protease inhibitor) with Retrovir (a nucleoside analogue RTI), or Viramune (a nonnucleoside RTI) with Viracept (a protease inhibitor).

cleaved, the virus cannot assemble properly and only "defective" noninfectious virus particles are produced. Protease inhibitors (Table 13.3) work by blocking that essential cleavage reaction.

As a group, protease inhibitors are tolerated relatively well. However, they are metabolized in the liver by a group of cellular enzymes known as the "P450 enzyme system." These enzymes metabolize many other drugs as well. When a protease inhibitor is used in combination with such drugs, this can affect how quickly drugs (as well as the protease inhibitor itself) are cleared from the body, thereby possibly increasing their toxicity. Protease inhibitors also may not cross the blood-brain barrier in amounts sufficient to affect HIV-infected cells located in the brain. In addition, these drugs must be taken at specific times relative to meals; that is, some must be taken on a full stomach and others on an empty stomach.

A possible side-effect of protease-inhibitor use in combination therapy reported in a substantial fraction of patients—from 7% to over 60%—is the development of abnormal fat deposits in the abdomen (so-called "protease belly") and on the shoulders at the base of the neck ("buffalo hump"). This is accompanied by wasting of the face, arms, and legs (a condition known as "lipodystrophy"), along with elevations of certain lipids in the blood, particularly triglycerides. The cause of these deposits and blood abnormalities is presently unknown.

Although similar changes have occurred in HIV-positive individuals who were not taking any anti-HIV medications, it appears to be worsened or initiated by the use of protease inhibitors, and it can occur as early as four weeks after use of a protease inhibitor begins. All currently approved protease inhibitors have been associated with this condition, but the combination of ritonavir plus saquinavir may have the highest incidence. Its clinical significance is unknown. Further study of large numbers of patients for longer periods is needed before any change in antiretroviral therapy or use of lipid-lowering drugs can be recommended.

Which protease inhibitor to use in a drug regimen depends on many factors, including the individual patient's medical profile and lifestyle. While research has established sound principles of HIV treatment (presented below), all anti-HIV drugs have advantages and disadvantages, and there is still no standard way of combining and using them. The treatment of HIV disease remains in flux, and the use of HAART is still under study. For this reason, an individual seeking treatment for HIV disease is best advised to rely on a physician experienced in this disease.

Drug Resistance and Antiretroviral Therapy

When AZT alone is used to treat HIV disease (that is, as monotherapy), it typically produces an increase in CD4 counts of 30 to 50 cells per mm^3, and it decreases the viral load by 60% to 70%. But after a few months, the viral load begins to increase again and the CD4 counts drop. A similar course is seen when many other antiretroviral drugs are used alone. The rebound in viral load and the renewed drop in CD4 cells occur because HIV quickly becomes resistant to single drugs.

It is generally believed that HIV develops drug resistance so effectively largely because of the high rate at which genetic mutations occur during its replication. These gene mutations occur because RT is prone to making errors when it copies HIV's RNA genes into DNA. Thus, when an HIV particle enters a cell and produces a provirus, it is the provirus that contains the gene mutations introduced by RT. When that provirus begins producing new virions, those virions will have genetic characteristics that are different from those of the virion that originally infected the cell (some proviruses end up with so many mutations that they cannot produce viable HIV particles at all).

This tendency of RT to make inexact copies of the virus's original RNA genes results in great genetic diversity among the HIV particles infecting an individual. Thus, a person with HIV is soon infected with many genetically different populations of virions. Some of these populations consist of HIV particles that have relatively unmodified (or "wild-type") genes. These virions are sensitive to antiretroviral drugs and therefore cannot replicate in their presence. Other populations, however, consist of small numbers of HIV particles that, by chance, have mutations that make them resistant to one or more antiretroviral drugs. The growth of these mutated HIV particles is not slowed in the presence of these drugs. In fact, they then have a selective advantage over the wild-type HIV particles: The "drug-adapted" virions can infect cells and replicate, even as the wild-type virions are prevented from doing so, as long as the patient continues to be treated with those drugs to which the mutated virions are resistant. Some of these virion populations will have mutations that make them resistant to AZT, some will have mutations that make them resistant to ddl, others will be resistant to the nonnucleoside inhibitor nevirapine. Still others might have mutations that confer resistance to the protease inhibitors ritonavir or saquinavir. Quite possibly, virus populations might arise that are resistant to multiple drugs.[1]

Occasionally, chance produces mutations in HIV that confer resistance to one drug and reverse resistance to another drug. Take for example virions that have the most common mutation that confers resistance to AZT. If those mutant virions replicate and produce progeny virions that also have the most common mutation for resistance to ddl, this second mutation makes the virions again highly vulnerable to AZT.

The number of genetic mutations needed to make a virus resistant to any one drug can be very small. For example, a single mutation that causes a change of one amino acid in the structure of HIV's RT enzyme can produce a virus that is 1,000 times more resistant to the drug 3TC. It would take a dose of 3TC that is a thousand times stronger to block the replication of that mutated virus, a dose that would also be deadly to the individual.[2]

Compliance, Drug Resistance, and Antiretroviral Therapy

Compliance—the taking of drugs according to prescribed directions—plays an important role in preventing or slowing the development of drug resistance. Compliance is important for the effective use of all medications, but it is critical for antiretroviral regimens that are designed to suppress HIV. Skipping doses or reducing a drug's dosage even briefly allows the level of drug in the body to drop, giving HIV an opportunity to replicate and develop genetic mutations that confer drug resistance. In the worst case, resistance to one drug can result in cross-resistance to all the drugs in the same class. Should this happen for protease inhibitors, it would make all protease inhibitors, the most effective weapons against HIV currently available, ineffective thereafter for that individual.

Therefore, it is of the utmost importance to comply with the requirements of HAART so as to suppress viral replication as completely as possible, to prevent or forestall the development of drug resistance.

Sometimes, side effects or other problems might prevent patients from taking full doses of all their antiretroviral drugs. In such cases, it is better to either stop taking all these drugs altogether for a time, or to try a different combination of drugs, than to reduce the dosage.[3] In the absence of any drugs, all virus populations replicate and compete with each other, although the wild-type virions replicate most effectively. The presence of any antiretroviral drug at low levels, however, favors the replication of the mutated drug-adapted, or drug-resistant, virions that then become the most numerous HIV particles in the body.

▶ Principles of Antiretroviral Therapy for HIV

In 1997, the Office of AIDS Research of the National Institutes of Health (NIH) convened a panel of experts to assess the advances in basic research on HIV, treatment research, and testing in order to translate them into information useful to physicians and people with HIV. The result was the "Report of the NIH Panel to Define Principles of Therapy of HIV Infection."[4] The report presents 11 principles that guide current antiretroviral therapy. They are summarized here as follows:

> 1. HIV infection is always harmful, and true long-term survival without signifiant loss of immune function is unusual; continuous HIV replication damages the immune system and leads to AIDS.

About 5% of people infected with HIV have survived for more than 10 or 12 years without treatment and with no signs of HIV disease. Presently, however, there is no way to identify at the time of diagnosis individuals who may be long-term slow progressors or nonprogressors. For this reason, all persons with HIV infection must be considered at risk for progressive disease.

The goal of HIV therapy is to prevent disease progression: that is, maintain immune function in a state as close to normal as possible, preserve quality of life, and prolong survival by effectively suppressing HIV replication. These goals can be accomplished only by initiating therapy, whenever possible, before significant damage has occurred to the immune system.

> 2. Regular, periodic viral-load tests and CD4 lymphocyte counts are necessary to determine when to initiate or modify antiretroviral therapy and to assess the risk of disease progression.

Levels of HIV in the blood—viral load—are measured using HIV genome tests and indicate the rate of HIV replicaton and suggest the rate of CD4 lymphocyte destruction; CD4 lymphocyte counts indicate the extent of HIV-induced immune damage already present.

Viral load first rises, then falls during the first six months after initial infection. After about six to nine months, it stabilizes and reaches a baseline level, or "set point." In many people with HIV infection, the baseline remains fairly constant from several months to several years, although it tends to rise over time. An increase in the baseline viral load is a predictor of disease progression. Two baseline measurements should be made one to two weeks apart by the same laboratory using the same assay to ensure that a true baseline viral load is obtained. Other important points about testing include the following:

- In individuals newly diagnosed with HIV, viral-load measurements should be performed during a period of clinical stability. Thereafter, testing should be done every three to four months to monitor risk of disease progression and to help determine when to initiate therapy.
- Measurements of viral load within six months after initial infection do not accurately predict the risk of disease progression because the level of HIV is probably still unstable.
- If the individual is experiencing symptoms of acute infection at the time of diagnosis, viral-load testing can be used to establish an HIV diagnosis even if the HIV antibody test result is negative or indeterminate.
- Viral-load testing should also be done before and after starting anti-retroviral therapy as described under "When Therapy Is Initiated" under Principle 3.
- CD4 lymphocyte counts should be made at the time of diagnosis and generally every three to six months thereafter. CD4 cell counts are subject to significant variability, so treatment decisions must be based on trends in CD4 numbers over time, not on any one count.
- Prior to making treatment decisions, both viral load and CD4 cell counts should be determined at least on two occasions by the same laboratory using the same assay to ensure that the measurements are accurate.
- A threefold or greater (i.e., 0.5-log or more) change in viral load is considered significant; a drop of 30% or more in CD4 lymphocyte count from baseline is considered significant, as is a 3% or greater drop from baseline when CD4 lymphocytes are monitored as a percentage of total lymphocytes (this figure is used by some physicians instead of absolute numbers of CD4 lymphocytes).

> 3. The time to initiate anti-HIV therapy should be based on risk of disease progression and degree of immune deficiency, and these vary with individual patients.

All individuals with symptomatic HIV disease (i.e., thrush, wasting, unexplained fever, or AIDS) should be offered antiretroviral therapy. Determining when to initiate therapy in individuals who are asymptomatic or in the acute stage of HIV infection is more complicated (for acute infection, see "Considerations for Initiating Antiretroviral Therapy during Acute Infection").

SOME OF THE BENEFITS AND RISKS OF EARLY ANTIRETROVIRAL THERAPY IN ASYMPTOMATIC DISEASE

Potential Benefits

- Control of viral replication and mutation, and reduction of viral load.
- Prevention of progressive immune deficiency.
- Potential preservation of a normal immune system.
- Delay in progression to AIDS and perhaps prolongation of life.
- Decrease of the risk that resistant HIV will emerge.
- Lessening of the risk of drug toxicity.

Potential Risks

- Reduced quality of life due to possible drug side effects.
- Earlier development of drug resistance.
- Limitations on future choices of antiretroviral agents.
- Risk of dissemination of drug-resistant HIV in the community.
- Long-term toxicity and treatment benefit of certain anti-HIV drugs are both still unpredictable.

There is no known threshold of HIV replication below which disease progression will not eventually occur. In theory, beginning antiretroviral therapy *before* the onset of disease progression as indicated by falling CD4 counts and rising viral load should have the greatest and most long-lasting effect on preserving health. But the benefits of initiating therapy in asymptomatic individuals must be weighed against the disadvantages (see "Some of the Benefits and Risks of Early Antiretroviral Therapy in Asymptomatic Disease").

In general, asymptomatic individuals with CD4 lymphocyte counts below 500 cells per mm^3 and viral loads greater than 10,000 by bDNA testing or 20,000 by RT-PCR testing should be offered therapy. The strength of the recommendation, however, should be based on an individual's readiness for treatment, and on the relative risk of disease progression. Disease progression, in turn, is based on *rates* of change in viral load and CD4 lymphocyte counts. (No data are available yet on the degree of benefit in starting antiretroviral therapy in individuals with CD4 counts above 500 cells per mm^3 and viral loads lower than those mentioned above; for pregnant women.)

When Therapy Is Initiated

When the decision is made to initiate therapy in an asymptomatic person, the goal should be maximum suppression of HIV replication, preferably to undetectable levels (see Principle 4). Viral load and CD4 T-cell counts should be determined immediately before therapy begins and again four weeks later. After four weeks, the individual should experience a significant drop (tenfold or 1 log) in viral load; if such a drop is not seen, the physician should check for patient adherence to the treatment regimen or poor drug absorption. Viral-load testing should be repeated to verify the lack of response. At that point, the physician may recommend changing the treatment regimen. Viral load tends to reach a low (ideally, below the level of detection) within approximately eight weeks of HAART, although this can take up to 16 weeks in individuals with high initial viral loads.

The continued effectiveness of the treatment regimen should be monitored by viral-load testing every three to four months. By six months, the regimen should have reduced viral load to undetectable levels. If viral load remains detectable after six months, the viral-load test should be repeated to rule out the possibility of a temporary increase (this can happen, for example, when an immunization or concurrent infection activates the immune system, either of which can trigger a temporary increase in HIV replication and viral load). If the repeat viral-load test also shows a detectable viral load, a change in therapy should be considered (see "Considerations for Changing a Failing Antiretroviral Therapy").

When Therapy Is Postponed

When therapy is postponed in an asymptomatic person infected with HIV, viral-load measurements and CD4 counts should be performed (as described under Principle 2) at the time of diagnosis and then every three to four months thereafter. Note that these intervals can be flexible to meet the circumstances of individual cases.

> 4. The goal of therapy is to suppress HIV replication below levels detectable by viral-load tests.

The emergence of drug-resistant forms of HIV is the major reason why antiretroviral therapy fails. The development of drug resistance can be delayed, and perhaps even prevented, through the use of combinations of antiretroviral drugs, the only regimens that can suppress HIV replication below levels detectable by current viral-load tests. As described earlier, suppressing HIV replication slows or suppresses the accumulation of viral mutations that give rise to drug-resistant virions. Furthermore, the extent and duration of viral suppression also predict the degree to which an individual will clinically benefit from antiretroviral treatment.

Suppression of HIV replication to undetectable levels does not mean that the infection has been eradicated or that virus replication has been stopped altogether. Virus replication may continue in certain tissues such as the lymph nodes or the central nervous system, and suppression may be temporary. For these reasons, viral-load monitoring should continue as described above.

If suppression of HIV replication to undetectable levels cannot be achieved, the goal of therapy should be to suppress viral replication as much as possible for as long as possible.

> 5. The antiretroviral drugs used in combination therapy must be carefully chosen and given simultaneously.

Effective suppression of HIV replication by combination therapy is not due simply to the number of drugs used; it also depends on which drugs are used. Careful drug selection is also important because the decision will affect the therapeutic options available to the individual in the future. The rational selection of drugs for combination antiretroviral therapy is based on the following:

- The combination should not include antiretroviral drugs previously taken by the individual, or drugs that are cross-resistant with drugs previously taken by the individual.
- The drugs should work together to show additive or synergistic activity against HIV.
- None of the drugs should interfere with the anti-HIV activity of any of the other drugs in the combination.

- When possible, it is best if the drugs used in a combination work together to delay the development of viral mutations that lead to drug resistance. That is, certain antiretroviral drugs when used in combination make it more difficult for viral resistance to develop. For example, there is evidence that it is difficult for HIV to simultaneously develop a certain mutation that leads to resistance to 3TC and mutations that lead to resistance to AZT. This phenomenon is known as molecular antagonism.
- When possible, it is best to choose a drug combination that leaves as many future therapeutic options as possible, in case the regimen should fail (although it is most important to use a combination of drugs that a person can tolerate and that drives his or her viral load to undetectable levels).

Effective Regimens

Presently, the most effective combinations for suppressing HIV replication in individuals who have not previously taken antiretroviral therapy (i.e., antiretroviral "naive" persons) incorporate two nucleoside analogue RTIs plus a potent protease inhibitor. The use of two nucleoside analogue RTIs and an NNRTI is also reported to be effective in antiretroviral naive persons, but this combination needs further study and is not recommended at this time as a first-line therapy. This regimen is also less effective in persons previously treated with nucleoside analogue RTIs.

Antiretroviral drugs such as lamivudine (3TC) or the NNRTIs, which may be potent but to which HIV readily develops high-level resistance, should not be used in regimens that are expected to produce incomplete suppression of HIV replication (i.e., HIV levels in the blood are reduced, but remain detectable) because resistance is likely to develop quickly against them.

Use of Monotherapy

The NIH panel noted that no currently available single antiretroviral drug used by itself (i.e., as monotherapy)—not even the most potent protease inhibitor—can provide significant, long-lasting suppression of HIV replication. This is because drug resistance inevitably develops to any single drug. Even worse, cross-resistance may develop. For these reasons, monotherapy is not recommended for the treatment of HIV infection, with one exception: the temporary use of AZT by pregnant women to prevent perinatal HIV transmission.

Use of Two-Drug Combinations

Some physicians and HIV-infected individuals may consider using a two-drug combination, but they should recognize that no combination of two currently available nucleoside analogue RTIs has been shown to provide long-lasting suppression of HIV replication. An inability to profoundly suppress replication allows drug-resistant forms of HIV to develop. These may be cross-resistant to related drugs, thereby severely limiting future treatment options. The same is true of combinations consisting of one nucleoside analogue RTI and one NNRTI, or of two protease inhibitors. The latter combination has resulted in durable suppression of HIV replication in pilot studies, but this regimen needs further testing (a danger here is that if cross-resistance develops between protease inhibitors, it would eliminate this whole class of extremely potent antiretroviral drugs from future treatment options).

> 6. Each antiretroviral drug in a combination therapy regimen should always be used according to optimum schedules and dosages.

As stated above, maximum suppression of HIV replication is the best approach to prevent development of drug-resistant variants of HIV. Ideally, the drugs used in combination therapy should be started within one or two days of each other; they should not be added in stages, as this may lead to temporary incomplete viral suppression during which the accumulation of viral mutations that lead to drug resistance may occur. Giving reduced doses or administering fewer than all the drugs of a combination at the same time should therefore be avoided. It is essential for physicians to educate and counsel patients about the goals and rationale for their HAART treatment, even if this means a short delay in initiating it.

Adherence to a Regimen Is Crucial to Its Success

Current combination therapy regimens require that individuals take multiple medications at specific times of day, and at specific intervals relative to meals. Deviating from prescribed intervals, or using one or all of the drugs only intermittently, greatly increases the risk for developing drug-resistant strains of HIV and failure of the treatment (as described earlier under "Compliance, Drug Resistance, and Antiretroviral Therapy"). For this reason, there should be an active collaboration between patient and physician once therapy is started. This should include a review of the drug-dosing intervals, the possibility of taking several medications at the same time, the relationship of drug dosing to meals and snacks, and concerns about the cost of therapy.[5]

Individuals who are homeless or who for other reasons have unstable living conditions or limited social-support mechanisms may find it particularly difficult to adhere to a combination therapy regimen. The NIH panel recommended that health-care providers work with HIV-infected individuals to assess their readiness and ability to commit to a HAART regimen. This assessment should be made on an individual basis; health-care workers should not assume that any specific group of people as a whole is unable to adhere to a particular regimen. No individual should be automatically excluded from consideration for antiretroviral therapy simply because he or she simply appears to exhibit characteristics judged by some to be predictable of noncompliance.

On the other hand, concern for the public health requires that if a patient does not respond to HAART because of a documented history of noncompliance with treatment requirements, and is not practicing safer sex, that individual's antiretroviral treatment may be discontinued. Under such circumstances, HAART is useless to the patient and may in fact lead to drug-resistant HIV mutants that are likely to be transmitted to his or her sexual partners.

---

7. Any change in antiretroviral therapy reduces future therapeutic options.

Any decision to change a therapeutic regimen is likely to limit an individual's future treatment options. It is therefore important not to abandon any regimen prematurely. During antiretroviral therapy, increases in viral load and in the rate at which they occur (which suggest higher HIV replication rates) indicate the urgency with which therapy should be altered.

A change in treatment regimen should be considered for any individual whose viral load steadily increases from an undetectable to a detectable level. A change in treatment is also usually considered for individuals who show evidence of drug toxicity or intolerance (sometimes these manifestations are temporary, and therapy may be safely continued along with patient counseling and continued evaluation).

To avoid making an unnecessary change in therapy, it is important, whenever possible, to determine why viral load is increasing. An individual may not adhere closely to his or her regimen because of a lack of understanding about the need for strict compliance. Such problems can be corrected. Also, a recent vaccination or concurrent infection could have stimulated immune responses that produce a temporary increase in HIV replication. Thus, clinicians should always perform two viral-load tests on separate occasions before changing therapy to rule out a transient increase in HIV replication.

Biological factors can also be responsible for rising viral loads. These include the emergence of drug-resistant variants of HIV, decreased absorption of antiretroviral drugs, and a change in the body's ability to metabolize the drugs. For more information, see "Considerations for Changing a Failing Antiretroviral Therapy."

8. Women should receive optimal antiretroviral therapy even when pregnant.

The preceding principles concerning the use and initiation of HAART therapy apply equally to men and women, both adult and adolescent. In general, the NIH panel recommended that the use of antiretroviral drugs and the initiation of treatment follow the same guidelines in pregnant HIV-infected women as in other adults. Thus, a pregnant woman's clinical condition, viral load, and CD4 lymphocyte counts should guide treatment decisions.

But the use of antiretroviral therapy in pregnant HIV-infected women also raises unique concerns. Two important considerations are the use of antiretroviral drugs to preserve the health of the mother, and the possible effect of these drugs in reducing the risk of HIV transmission to her child.

Use of Antiretroviral Drugs to Preserve the Health of the Mother

Determining whether to initiate HAART becomes more difficult if a woman is in the first trimester—weeks 1 to 14—of pregnancy (particularly the first 8 weeks). During this time, the embryo is most vulnerable to birth defects caused by chemicals in the body. Furthermore, no long-term studies have examined the safety of antiretroviral drug combinations during pregnancy. Therefore, pregnant women should discuss the potential advantages and hazards of such treatment with their physicians. Considerations include the stage of pregnancy; a woman's general state of health, viral load, and CD4 counts; and what is and is not known about the potential effects of antiretroviral drugs on the fetus.

The NIH panel advised that physicians consider delaying antiretroviral therapy until after 14 weeks of pregnancy (and particularly until after the first 8 weeks) when feasible.

Women who are already on a HAART regimen when pregnancy occurs should continue the therapy. However, if pregnancy is anticipated or diagnosed early in the first trimester (during the first 8–14 weeks), some women may choose to discontinue therapy until the end of the first trimester. It is not known if such a temporary discontinuation of therapy is harmful, although an increase in viral load should be expected and could increase the risk of disease progression in the mother and HIV transmission to the fetus. If therapy is temporarily stopped, all drugs should be discontinued simultaneously; when therapy is resumed, all drugs should be reintroduced simultaneously.

The antiretroviral regimen used for a pregnant woman should suppress HIV replication to undetectable levels; incomplete suppression increases the risk that drug-resistant forms of HIV will emerge, which will limit the woman's future treatment options. It may also limit the ability of the same drugs to decrease the risk of perinatal transmission.

Use of Antiretroviral Drugs to Reduce the Risk of Perinatal HIV Transmission

Transmission of HIV from mother to infant (perinatal transmission) can occur at all levels of viral load, although a high viral load is associated with a higher probability of transmission. AZT therapy effectively reduces perinatal HIV transmission regardless of the maternal viral load. Therefore, the use of AZT alone or in combination with other antiretroviral drugs should be offered to all HIV-infected pregnant women, regardless of viral load.

> 9. The principles of antiretroviral therapy presented above apply to both HIV-infected children and adults, although the treatment of HIV-infected children involves unique pharmacological, virological, and immunological considerations.

The data available on HIV infection in children support the principles of antiretroviral therapy as outlined for adults. Therefore, HIV-infected children should also be treated with combination antiretroviral therapy with the goal of long-term suppression of HIV replication to undetectable levels. Unfortunately, not all of the antiretroviral drugs used for HAART in adults are available in formulations (such as palatable liquid formulations) for infants and young children. In addition, studies on the action of many antiretroviral drugs in children have not been completed. Drugs for which this information is unavailable may produce undesirable side effects in children and should therefore be used only as part of a controlled clinical trial.

> 10. Persons with acute HIV infection may also benefit from combination antiretroviral therapy and suppression of virus replication to undetectable levels.

Theoretically, people in the acute stage of HIV infection should also benefit from combination therapy and suppression of virus replication to undetectable levels. Such therapy may curb the high levels of HIV replication that otherwise occur during acute infection, reduce HIV-related damage to the immune system, and produce a lower baseline (or set-point) level of HIV replication during asymptomatic disease. Such effects would help preserve the function of the immune system and possibly improve the subsequent clinical course of the infection. It has also been suggested that the best opportunity to eradicate HIV infection may arise, in the future, during acute infection.

These benefits, however, are all theoretical. Preliminary data from small-scale studies support these predictions, but they have not yet been formally demonstrated to be valid. Therefore, the benefits of antiviral treatment during acute infection must be weighed against the risks; see "Considerations for Initiating Antiretroviral Therapy during Acute Infection."

> 11. All HIV-infected persons, including those with viral loads below detectable levels, should be considered infectious and should avoid sexual and drug-use behaviors associated with the transmission or acquisition of HIV and other infectious pathogens.

It is not yet known whether HIV-infected individuals who are on therapy and have undetectable viral loads can transmit HIV infection to others through unsafe sex or needle sharing. For this reason, all HIV-infected individuals should continue to practice safer sex. Similarly, any HIV-infected person who injects drugs, whether illicit or medically prescribed, should not share injection equipment with others and use a sterile, disposable needle and syringe for each injection.

Restored CD4 Lymphocyte Counts and Prophylaxis

Suppression of HIV replication to undetectable levels is often accompanied by increases in CD4 lymphocyte counts, often to levels above 200 cells per mm³. Current research indicates that these new immune cells are unable to provide adequate protection against at least certain opportunistic infections. It is therefore important to continue the use of prophylactic therapy, even if CD4 counts return to levels above 200 cells per mm³.

▶ Considerations for Initiating Antiretroviral Therapy during Acute Infection

The acute phase of HIV infection produces no noticeable symptoms in about half of the people infected, and of those who do experience symptoms, only about 20% to 30% consult a physician because of them (the clinical symptoms of acute infection often resemble those of the "flu" or other common illnesses).

But many experts recommend antiretroviral therapy for individuals with laboratory evidence of acute HIV infection, including those in whom infection has been documented to have occurred within the previous six months (individuals who believe themselves recently infected but for whom the time of infection cannot be documented should be considered to be in the asymptomatic phase of infection).[6] The goal of therapy is suppression of viral load to undetectable levels; the DHHS guidelines note that any regimen that is not expected to achieve maximal suppression of viral replication is not appropriate for the treatment of acute HIV infection.

The use of antiretroviral therapy during acute infection, however, is based almost entirely on theoretical considerations—evidence of actual clinical benefit based on information from clinical trials is presently very limited. The theoretical rationale for the early use of HAART is based on four points:

- It should suppress the burst of viral replication that occurs during acute infection and decrease the number of virus particles dispersed throughout the body.
- It should decrease the severity of acute disease.
- It should decrease the initial baseline (or set-point) level of HIV, which is widely believed to affect disease progression.
- It should slow the rate of viral mutation by suppressing viral replication.

These potential benefits must be weighed against risks that are similar to those of HAART for individuals with asymptomatic disease and include the following:

- Drug toxicity and compliance with regimen of treatment might adversely affect the individual's quality of life.
- Should therapy fail to completely suppress viral replication, drug resistance may develop and limit future treatment options.
- Antiviral therapy may need to be continued indefinitely.
- It might blunt the development of an effective immune response. Triple-drug therapy taken within a few weeks following HIV infection may delay development of anti-HIV antibodies from months to more than a year, and it often prevents a CTL response. This occurs because the early use of HAART reduces the viral load to such low levels that not enough viral antigen is produced to provoke an immune response. Because

of this, many scientists want to test the hypothesis that injections of recombinant HIV proteins should be combined with HAART when the latter is used soon after HIV infection.

To help define the optimal approach to the treatment of acute infection, the NIH panel recommended that newly diagnosed patients should be encouraged to enroll in clinical trials that study this question. If enrolling in a clinical trial is not feasible or desired, the panel recommended that combination antiretroviral therapy be given, with the goal of suppressing HIV replication to undetectable levels. Therapy should continue indefinitely until clinical trials provide data to establish its appropriate duration.

If Therapy Is Initiated

If the decision is made to initiate antiretroviral therapy, viral load and CD4 counts should be determined as described already (at initiation of therapy, after four weeks,[7] and every three to four months thereafter). How long therapy should be continued is a matter of opinion. Many experts would continue to treat with antiretroviral therapy indefinitely because viremia is known to recur or increase when therapy is discontinued; others might be tempted to treat for a year, then discontinue therapy and evaluate the individual using CD4 cell counts and viral-load testing. In reality, the optimal treatment strategy in terms of what drugs to use and for how long is not yet known, although clinical trials are under way to help answer these questions.

▶ Considerations for Initiating Antiretroviral Therapy during Late-Stage HIV Disease

Some people are first diagnosed with HIV infection only after advanced disease has developed (i.e., those diagnosed with any condition meeting the 1993 CDC definition of AIDS). HAART can slow disease progression and prolong life even in individuals with late-stage HIV disease (e.g., CD4 lymphocyte counts below 50 cells per mm^3). For this reason, and after possible complications are taken into consideration, all individuals with advanced HIV disease should be treated with antiretroviral drug combinations regardless of their viral load. If the decision is made to initiate HAART, the goal should again be to suppress the viral load to undetectable levels.

A number of factors complicate the use of antiretroviral therapy in individuals who are acutely ill, however. They include drug toxicity, drug interactions, and the ability of the individual to adhere to the therapeutic regimen.

The possibility of drug interactions is particularly a problem in persons being treated with multiple drugs, and it can influence the choice of drugs to be used in combination. For example, protease inhibitors affect the metabolism of the drug rifampin, which is sometimes given for active tuberculosis. At the same time, rifampin lowers the blood level of protease inhibitors, which can reduce their therapeutic effectiveness.

Medical complications of advanced disease also influence the use of combination antiretroviral therapy. Wasting and anorexia can prevent individuals from following the dietary requirements necessary for effective absorption of protease inhibitors. Protease inhibitors may also not be an option for individuals with HIV-related liver dysfunction. Because of the broad possibilities for detrimental drug interactions, individuals taking antiretroviral therapy should always discuss with their physician any new drugs they may consider taking, including over-the-counter and "alternative" medications.

▶ Considerations When Interrupting Antiretroviral Therapy

Reasons for interrupting HAART may include intolerable side effects, drug interactions, the first trimester of pregnancy, and the unavailability of the drugs. If one antiretroviral drug must be discontinued, all other antiretroviral drugs that are part of the combination therapy being taken should be discontinued simultaneously, rather than continuing the use of only one or two of them. Discontinuing all drugs at once has the theoretical advantage of minimizing the emergence of drug-resistant viral strains (as described earlier in this chapter).

▶ Considerations for Changing a Failing Antiretroviral Therapy

The decision to change a failing regimen involves taking many complex factors into account. They include such things as the results of a physical examination and of clinical tests; remaining treatment options; viral load (measured on two separate occasions); the trend in CD4 counts; the stage of disease; and the individual's potential ability to tolerate a new regimen in terms of side effects, drug interactions, and dietary requirements.

The physician must distinguish between the need to change therapy due to drug failure versus drug toxicity. In the case of drug toxicity, the drug or drugs thought to be responsible for the toxicity should be replaced by alternatives of equal potency and from the same class as the agent being discontinued.

When a regimen is changed because of drug failure, the new regimen should incorporate drugs not previously taken by the individual. With triple-drug combinations, at least two, and preferably all three, agents should be changed to reduce the risk of drug resistance; changing only a single drug, even if it is a very potent one, is likely to result in viral resistance to the new drug.

In addition, the drugs chosen for a new regimen should not be cross-resistant to previously used antiretroviral drugs or induce similar patterns of viral mutations that are associated with resistance.[8] Specific criteria that should prompt considering a change in combination antiretroviral therapy include the following:

- A less than tenfold (1.0-log) reduction in the viral load by four weeks following initiation of HAART.
- Failure of the viral load to reach an undetectable level within four to six months of initiating HAART. (Although consideration should be given here to the viral load at the start of therapy. For example, an individual with 1 million virions per ml of plasma who then stabilizes after six months of therapy with a viral load that is detectable but below 10,000 virions per ml may not need an immediate change of therapy.)
- Repeated detection of virus in plasma after it has been initially suppressed to undetectable levels. This occurrence suggests the development of drug resistance.
- A threefold (i.e., 0.5-log) or greater increase in viral load from its stable low, as determined by repeated testing (to eliminate the possibility of a temporary increase in viral

load due to simultaneous infection from another pathogen or vaccination, or to a spurious measurement due to the testing methodology).

- Persistently declining CD4 lymphocyte counts, as measured on at least two separate occasions.
- Clinical deterioration. A new AIDS-defining illness that develops after the initiation of HAART may or may not suggest a failure of that therapy. A poor antiviral response (e.g., a less than tenfold drop in viral load) does suggest such a failure. But if the individual was already severely immunocompromised when treatment began, and therapy produced a good antiviral response, the new opportunistic infection may reflect severely impaired immunity and not a failure of antiviral therapy.

Clearly, obtaining the expert advice of a physician very knowledgeable in the treatment of HIV disease—by referral or consultation, if necessary—is essential when considering a change in therapy. That expertise is also essential to those who require a change in antiretroviral therapy but who have exhausted their options among the currently approved drugs. These individuals should be referred for possible inclusion in an appropriate clinical trial.

▶ Antiretroviral Compounds Under Development

Research is under way to develop new, safer, and more effective RTIs and protease inhibitors, but other types of drugs and treatment strategies are also under investigation. The following compounds have shown activity against HIV in cell and animal studies and are in clinical trials. In most cases, there is little or no information as yet on their effectiveness, toxicity, or side effects in humans. For additional information on the treatments described below, as well as on new RTIs, protease inhibitors, and others, see the AmFAR *AIDS/HIV Treatment Directory* (which also lists the sites at which testing is being done).

Integrase Inhibitors

Integrase is the third HIV enzyme necessary for the replication of HIV (along with RT and protease). After RT produces a DNA copy of HIV's RNA genome, the viral DNA travels to the cell nucleus where it is inserted into a chromosome of the host cell. The insertion of the viral DNA into the host DNA is accomplished (catalyzed) by the viral enzyme integrase. Zintevir (AR-177) is an experimental integrase inhibitor that is in early clinical testing.

CI-1012, a Zinc Finger Inhibitor

Zinc fingers are structures present in some protein molecules that resemble narrow outpouchings (or "fingers"). These outpouchings enable these proteins to bind with DNA or RNA. HIV's nucleocapsid protein, which encapsulates HIV RNA inside the virion, is a protein that has zinc fingers. It is thought that the zinc fingers help stabilize HIV RNA when viral RT copies the viral RNA into DNA early in replication, and that they are also important during the assembly of new virions prior to budding. CI-1012 is a compound that disrupts zinc fingers of the nucleocapsid protein, probably by ejecting their zinc atoms. In this way, CI-1012 could block viral replication by interfering with both reverse transcription and virus assembly.

Hydroxyurea

Hydroxyurea is an oral anticancer drug used in the treatment of inoperable ovarian cancer and some leukemias. There is also laboratory evidence that hydroxyurea inhibits viral RT from copying viral RNA into DNA. In anti-HIV clinical testing, hydroxyurea has been used in combination therapy with a nucleoside analogue—AZT, ddl, or d4T.

Pentafuside

Pentafuside, or T-20, is a small, 36 amino acids long, peptide. It is derived from the HIV-1 gp41 protein. Pentafuside blocks the fusion of HIV with the cell membrane. This peptide has shown anti-HIV activity in the small number of patients who have received it, but human testing has been limited because presently there is no oral formulation of pentafuside, and it must be given intravenously.

Immune-Based Therapy

Immune-based therapies attempt to strengthen the immune system's response to HIV infection or to restore immune function. A number of immune-based strategies are undergoing testing in clinical trials, but to date none have been shown to be of clinical benefit. Immune-based therapies undergoing testing are described below.

Cytokines

Cytokines are compounds naturally produced by cells to regulate the activity and behavior of other cells. The following three cytokines are being tested for their ability to stimulate immune activity against HIV.

Interleukin-12

Interleukin (IL)-12 has a variety of effects on immune cells. One effect is to stimulate the activity of a subgroup of helper T cells known as helper T cells type 1, or TH1 cells. TH1 cells are important in activating the cell-mediated immune response, specifically cytotoxic T cells, which are believed to be important in fighting HIV.

Interleukin-2

IL-2 stimulates the proliferation of T lymphocytes and natural killer cells, as well as the proliferation of B lymphocytes and the production of antibodies by plasma cells. Several clinical trials have shown that IL-2 given along with combination antiretroviral therapy increases CD4 counts rather dramatically in some patients whose initial CD4 counts are over 200. It is not known how effective these new cells will be in fighting infections, and a larger controlled trial needs to be performed to determine IL-2's clinical benefit. IL-2 increases HIV replication because it activates the replication of T cells; it is therefore important to stress that IL-2 must be taken only by people who are receiving highly effective antiretroviral therapy, otherwise T-cell activation alone would stimulate HIV replication and increase viral load.

Interleukin-10

IL-10 has a number of effects on a variety of immune-system cells. For example, it promotes B-cell proliferation and antibody production. It also suppresses cell-mediated immunity, which is thought to be a major defense mechanism against HIV. However, at low doses it appears to have anti-HIV properties, although the mechanism of this effect is unclear.

Gene Transfer Therapy

Gene transfer therapy, or gene therapy, uses gene-splicing techniques (i.e., genetic engineering) to place one or more new or altered genes into cells. The new genes may be intended to replace faulty ones, augment the action of normal genes, or inactivate disease-causing genes. Foreign genes are delivered into target cells (which have been removed from the body) using a harmless virus such as an adenovirus or a mouse retrovirus. If all goes well, the genetically modified cells are returned to the body and the foreign gene(s) begins producing the desired protein. Other means of delivering foreign genes into cells include injecting, or "bombarding," genes directly into cells or encapsulating them in laboratory-produced, microscopic spheres of fat known as "liposomes," which cells take up.

Two major forms of anti-HIV gene therapy are known as "immunotherapeutics" and "intracellular immunization."

- *Immunotherapeutics* is an approach that uses cells that are genetically engineered to overproduce HIV antigens to stimulate antibody and cellular immune responses to HIV. One method that has undergone phase I testing in humans uses connective-tissue cells known as "fibroblasts." Fibroblasts are removed from an HIV-infected person and two HIV genes, *env* and *rev,* are transferred into them. The cells are then returned to the body, where they are intended to produce the viral envelope (Env) and Rev proteins and so stimulate stronger immune responses to HIV.
- *Intracellular immunization* encompasses one of three possibilities: Introducing an "antisense" gene that produces mRNAs that can bind to viral RNA and DNA and inactivate them; introducing genes that code for mutated HIV proteins that interfere with the function of normal HIV proteins; or introducing genes that code for anti-HIV antibodies, which can bind to and inactivate HIV proteins within the cell.

A third strategy, which may or may not use genetically engineered lymphocytes, is adoptive T-cell transfer. This involves removing T lymphocytes from HIV-infected patients, selecting those with anti-HIV activity, growing them to large numbers, and returning them to the patient.

Therapeutic Vaccines

Therapeutic vaccines—as opposed to protective vaccines—are designed to stimulate a more effective immune response to HIV in people who are already HIV infected. Most therapeutic vaccines tested have used the gp120 or gp160 envelope proteins produced by recombinant DNA technology. Using genetic engineering techniques, viral genes coding for these proteins were introduced into bacteria or other kinds of cells. These cells were then grown in large numbers and produced the viral recombinant proteins in large quantities for use as experimental vaccines.

An example of a therapeutic vaccine is the HIV-Immunogen vaccine, which uses whole inactivated HIV particles. During early testing, this vaccine was given to HIV-positive individuals with CD4 counts higher than 600 cells per mm^3, and it produced significant increases in p24 antibody levels relative to the control group. Whether this can delay disease progression is being tested in two phase III trials. Enthusiasm for therapeutic vaccines, however, has waned over recent years because of disappointing results so far, particularly in the ability of such vaccines to stimulate cell-mediated immunity, believed to be important to an effective immune response to HIV. Nevertheless, trials are ongoing.

▶ Buyers' Clubs

Unfortunately, even antiretroviral combinations that benefit many people do not work well for everyone. Some people experience side effects so severe that they are forced to discontinue using antiretroviral drugs. Others are able to tolerate them, but their viral load does not fall. This leaves these individuals with no effective anti-HIV treatment. Many of them, as well as others who are HIV positive, then often turn to buyers' clubs for drugs and other agents that might either slow the progression of their disease or alleviate its symptoms.

Through buyers' clubs, people can obtain some drugs that are approved in other countries but are either not, or not as yet, approved by the FDA for use in the United States. They may also obtain agents that are unproven and sometimes illegal. Some buyers' clubs, for example, specialize in medicinal marijuana, which may help treat AIDS wasting syndrome, appetite loss, nausea, and pain. Some clubs also provide alternative or complementary treatments, Chinese herbs, and nutritional and other supplements.

People who are considering the use of unapproved, experimental, untested, or alternative treatments should first carefully investigate any agent before using it. They should learn how effective the agent is purported to be, how it is administered, what its potential side effects are, whether it is toxic at certain levels, and whether it is thought to interact with other drugs.

Anyone preparing to use a buyers' club should be sure to ask questions to learn if the club is reputable. The characteristics of a reputable buyers' club include the following:

- It is not-for-profit.
- It refrains from giving medical advice.
- It provides unbiased information.
- It minimizes the cost of its services and provides services to some who cannot afford them.
- It does its best to ensure that its products are truthfully labeled and free of contaminants.
- Its products meet the highest possible standards of purity and potency. Some buyers' clubs, for example, send samples to testing laboratories to check for purity. Nonetheless, buyers' clubs have limited control over the quality of their products.
- Also, ask if the club provides mail-order service, accepts major credit cards, or has an annual membership fee.

▶ Conclusions

In research on antiretroviral therapy, as in all areas of HIV/AIDS research, much has been accomplished and much remains to be done. Combination antiretroviral therapies are now extending and improving the quality of the lives of many who take them, but formidable problems remain.

The treatment and care of people with HIV has become extremely complex. The success of HAART depends on a thorough understanding by physicians of how HIV causes disease and of how to optimally use the greater number of drugs now available to treat it. Physicians must also be willing to effectively educate their patients regarding the use of antiretroviral drugs: New and potent drugs are of little help to a person with HIV if the drugs are not used correctly, and this is the responsibility of both the physician and the patient. If the drugs are used incorrectly, this can reduce the effectiveness of other anti-HIV drugs that may be needed in the future.

Drug resistance remains a major problem. The best hope for people who have failed several drugs is new drugs that attack novel targets in HIV or the same target in novel ways. In addition, the side effects of anti-HIV drugs taken over the long term are only beginning to emerge. Much more basic and clinical research remains to be done.

Individuals who respond well to HAART also experience an increase in CD4 lymphocyte counts. This has raised a new and vexing problem: Although the immune system in these individuals seems to have at least partially restored itself in terms of numbers of CD4 lymphocytes, the new cells appear unable to marshal effective immune responses. Thus, even people responding well to antiretroviral therapy must continue taking prophylaxis, at least for the time being, for protection from opportunistic infections. Overcoming this hurdle and fully restoring immune-system functions is a major challenge. If HIV/AIDS is to become a controllable chronic infection with which people can live without constant fears, research on immune reconstitution is essential.

The cumulative costs of HAART and prophylaxis for opportunistic infections, as well as both medical and laboratory monitoring, confront a growing number of people living with HIV disease, the federal and state governments, and community-based service organizations with difficult decisions related to the allocation of resources. Economic and socio-political issues indeed also limit the potential effectiveness of the new therapies.[9]

The use of costly, high-tech, antiretroviral regimens is a major problem globally: they will predictably remain largely unavailable to HIV-infected people in developing countries who make up 90% of people with HIV/AIDS worldwide. Even in the United States, a significant number of people cannot access, tolerate, or comply with the rigors of combination antiretroviral therapy; others do not respond to it.

The inescapable conclusion is that the epidemic of HIV/AIDS is far from over. Only through continued basic and clinical biomedical research dedicated to achieving a more complete knowledge of HIV; to finding ways of reconstituting immune-system functions damaged by HIV; and to understanding the correlates of anti-HIV immunity, which is necessary for the development of a protective HIV vaccine, can the epidemic come under control.

▶ Endnotes

1. Note that drug resistance is never a matter of the HIV somehow "knowing" what drugs are present and deliberately adapting to them. The presence or absence of antiretroviral drugs only creates a set of conditions for the growth of HIV in the body. Because of the range of viral genetic variants present, some virions can survive and replicate in the presence of one or more given drugs and others cannot, just as the genetic makeup of some flies or mosquitoes allows them to survive an insecticide treatment while others are killed by it.

2. Genetic mutation is not the only way HIV acquires drug resistance. It can also happen when two genetically different HIV particles infect the same cell. Under these conditions, each virion can assemble part of its DNA strand using RNA from the other virion as well as from its own. The DNA strands and proviruses that will result will be mixtures of the genes from the two genetic variants. This type of genetic shuffling is known as "genetic recombination," and it can produce new and different populations of virus.

3. It is important to avoid unnecessary interruption of HAART, even when a drop in viral load is not seen. A recent study has shown that continuing to take a triple combination despite a persistently detectable viral load and documented resistance may still, by an unclear mechanism, preserve some T-cell function. See Kaufmann D, et al. CD4-cell count in HIV-1-infected individuals remaining viraemic with highly active antiretroviral therapy (HAART). *Lancet* 1998;351:723–24.

4. Centers for Disease Control and Prevention. Report of the NIH panel to define principles of therapy of HIV infection and guidelines for the use of antiretrovial agents in HIV-infected adults and adolescents. *MWWR* 1998;47(RR-5):1–83.

5. Cost is a major reason why some people do not take a medication as prescribed. Because of the risk of developing drug-resistant strains of HIV, it is a serious mistake to skip doses of antiretroviral therapy to make a prescription last longer or as a way of saving money. If the cost of a medication causes anxiety, by all means the problem should be discussed with one's physician or an AIDS service organization that can provide advice on possible financial assistance.

6. The NIH treatment guidelines recommend that with one exception, no individual be treated for HIV infection until the infection is documented by an ELISA and an accepted confirmatory test such as Western blot. The one exception is the treatment of individuals for postexposure prophylaxis.

7. Some experts believe testing at four weeks is not helpful in evaluating the response to therapy in acute infection because viral levels are typically decreasing at this time even in the absence of therapy.

8. Although assays are commercially available for determining the viral mutations in HIV that are associated with drug resistance, these methods have not yet been field tested to demonstrate their clinical usefulness, and they have not been approved by the FDA. Therefore, they are not recommended at present by the Department of Health and Human Services (DHHS) for routine use.

9. Several studies have shown that HAART therapy is cost effective as compared to the annual cost of treating a person with AIDS. In addition, a person responding to combination antiretroviral therapy can be a productive, taxpaying citizen.

▶ Suggested Readings and Resources for Part 3

HIV: Structure and Life Cycle
http://www.avert.org/wwhiv.htm

The Origin of HIV and the First Cases of AIDS
http://www.avert.org/wwhiv.htm

Introduction to HIV Types, Groups and Subtypes
http://www.avert.org/wwhiv.htm

The different stages of HIV infection
http://www.avert.org/wwhiv.htm

HIV-Related Opportunistic Infections (2007)
http://www.avert.org/hivtreatment.htm

HIV and TB (2007)
http://www.avert.org/hivtreatment.htm

CDC Fact Sheet: HIV Transmission
http://www.cdc.gov/hiv/resources/factsheets/transmission.htm

San Francisco AIDS Foundation
http://www.sfaf.org/aids101/transmission.html

You can get AIDS from. . . .
http://www.avert.org/howcan.htm

Women's Health Information Center: Pregnancy and HIV
http://womenshealth.gov/hiv/livingwith/pregnant.cfm

Mother to Child Transmission
http://www.cdc.gov/nchstp/od/gap/pa_pmtct.htm

HIV/AIDS and Pregnancy (2007)
http://www.avert.org/trans.htm

Preventing Mother to Child Transmission Worldwide
http://www.avert.org/hivprevention.htm

Preventing Mother-to-Child Transmission of HIV (2007)
http://www.avert.org/hivprevention.htm

Topical Microbicides: Preventing STIs 2003 NIAID
http://www.niaid.nih.gov/publications/topical_microbicides.pdf

AIDS Vaccines and Microbicides (2007)
http://www.avert.org/hivprevention.htm

AIDS Info September 2006
http://www.cdc.gov/mmwr/preview/mmwrhtml/rr5514a1.htm

Circumcision and HIV (2006)
http://www.avert.org/hivprevention.htm

HIV and Infant Feeding (2007)
http://www.avert.org/hivprevention.htm

Wainberg M. A. (2005) Generic HIV Drugs: Enlightened Policy for Global Health; New England Journal of Medicine; 352:8:747–750.
   http://content.nejm.org/cgi/reprint/352/8/747.pdf

UNAIDS 2006 Report on the Global AIDS Epidemic:
Chapter 7: Treatment and Care
   http://www.unaids.org/en/HIV_data/2006GlobalReport/default.asp

Kim et al (2005). Scaling Up Treatment: Why We Can't Wait. The New England Journal of Medicine. 353:22:2392–2393.
   http://content.nejm.org/cgi/content/full/353/22/2392

Steinbrook (2006). Message from Toronto: Deliver AIDS Treatment and Prevention. The New England Journal of Medicine; 355:11:1081–1084.
   http://content.nejm.org/cgi/content/full/355/11/1081

▶ Part 3

Critical Thinking

1. Discuss the challenges of developing a vaccine for HIV.
2. Why is it difficult to get people to test for HIV/AIDS?
3. Is it important to know how a person acquires HIV/AIDS? Why or why not?

Discussion Questions

1. List and describe three opportunistic infections associated with HIV/AIDS.
2. How is HIV transmitted?
3. What is the origin of HIV?
4. What are the different biological characteristics of HIV?
5. What are the different types of testing for HIV?
6. What are some prevention measures for HIV?

PART FOUR

Global Issues

Chapter
14

Social Conditions and HIV/AIDS

Women, Inequality and the Burden of HIV

*Bisola O. Ojikutu, M.D., M.P.H.,
and Valerie E. Stone, M.D., M.P.H.*

Driving through KwaZulu-Natal, South Africa, one is struck by the lush farmland and beautiful coast. Beyond this panorama, however, lie rural communities such as Umbumbulu, with its unemployment rate of 60 percent and rampant violence, where 40 percent of women seeking prenatal care are positive for the human immunodeficiency virus (HIV).[1]

Thandi Dlamini (not her real name) grew up in a crowded four-room house in Umbumbulu with 13 family members. As the youngest girl, she was charged with cooking, cleaning, and caring for her elders. At 19 years of age, she met her first boyfriend. From the perspective of Thandi and other women in her community, he was quite a catch—he was older, unmarried, and financially stable. She dreamed that one day he would offer to pay her *lobola* (bride price) and she would have her own home. Several months after meeting, he and Thandi had sexual intercourse. Thandi says this was her first sexual encounter.

Nine months later, she gave birth to a daughter, Zama. The baby had many episodes of bloody diarrhea and uncontrollable vomiting. By six months of age, Zama was clearly failing to thrive, and Thandi consented to have her tested for HIV. When the young mother returned to the hospital for the results, she was given three tragic pieces of information: she had given her daughter HIV, no treatment was available, and Zama would not live long.

Ichilo. Disgrace. *Amahloni.* Shame. This is how Thandi describes her feelings after leaving the hospital. She didn't really know what HIV was, except that it caused people to speak in hushed tones. It took months for Thandi to tell her boyfriend. Soon after hearing the news, he disappeared. Shortly after that, Zama died.

Around the same time, 9000 miles away in Denver, a 32-year-old black woman was sharing Thandi's fate. In 1991, Donna Williams (not her real name) went to her doctor because of fatigue and consented to an HIV test. Weeks later, two women from the Denver Public Health Department arrived at her apartment. They informed her that she was HIV-positive and that her only option was to go to a specialty clinic at the public hospital. When she overcame her

413

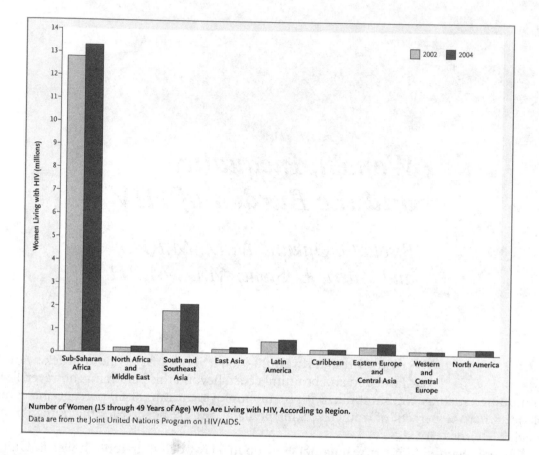

Number of Women (15 through 49 Years of Age) Who Are Living with HIV, According to Region.
Data are from the Joint United Nations Program on HIV/AIDS.

initial shock and went to the clinic, she was confronted by a sea of faces unlike her own—almost all men, many appearing near death. Terrified, she fled. A year passed before she obtained care for HIV.

Like Thandi, Donna grew up in a crowded home where she was the primary caregiver at a young age. Her mother had a series of abusive boyfriends, and in an effort to escape, Donna married an older man when she was 17 years old. During their first year of marriage, he was a good provider. Then his addiction to heroin surfaced and quickly destroyed their lives. For the next five years, he was in and out of prison, leaving his wife with their four children, unstably employed and transiently housed. After finally leaving her husband in 1987, Donna discovered that he was dying of AIDS. At the time, she was not sick and was struggling to survive as a single mother, so she did not get tested for HIV until 1991.

The differences between these two women are relatively few: native language, ethnic background, and land of birth. The list of similarities is substantially longer. Both are mothers and caregivers and both are poverty-stricken, transiently employed, and struggling to obtain basic daily requirements such as adequate housing. Both have had limited access to health care. Both have been dependent on men at some point in their lives for financial security. And all these similarities have contributed to their deadliest bond: HIV infection.

The legion of women with HIV infection now numbers in the millions (see graph). According to the World Health Organization, 19.2 million women were living with HIV or AIDS by the end of 2003.[1] An alarming increase in the number of women infected has been noted on almost every continent. The region that has been hit the hardest is sub-Saharan Africa, where 57 percent of infected persons are women. In the United States, HIV infection has begun to spread disproportionately among women of certain racial and ethnic groups. About 80 percent of all women living with HIV or AIDS in this country are members of minority groups—66 percent are black, and 14 percent are Hispanic.[2] Globally, most women have acquired HIV through heterosexual intercourse.

Biology provides a partial explanation for women's increased risk of becoming infected with HIV. It is well established that during unprotected sex, HIV is transmitted more efficiently from male to female than from female to male. The mucosal lining of the vagina provides a more permeable membrane than does the penile shaft, and microlesions in the vaginal mucosa caused by other sexually transmitted infections permit increased viral penetration.[3]

However, the spread of HIV among women has sociopolitical as well as biologic roots: it arises from the inequity between the sexes, societies' class structures, and the inaccessibility of health care. In many societies, educational and employment opportunities for women are limited. Throughout the world, women are placed in subservient positions and lack the freedom to ask questions or to demand the use of condoms. In most societies, if a woman chooses to remain single, she is choosing a life limited by poverty and instability.

Inequality between the sexes is not unique to the non-Western world. In the United States, sex-based income inequity has fueled disproportionate rates of poverty among women, and women's options are limited as a result. Poor women, regardless of their nationality, share a fear of losing a male partner if it also means the loss of financial security. Thandi articulated it best when, in a discussion of sexual relationships with men, she noted that for many women, "it's either that or nothing." When " nothing" means not being able to afford food or shelter for themselves or their children, there really is no choice.

Both these women's stories demonstrate that HIV is one small piece of a larger puzzle. As these pieces multiply and shift, health care needs are often low on the priority list. Donna is thankful that none of her children have HIV, but she has had to help each one through tumultuous circumstances. Currently, she is supporting her daughter through recovery from drug addiction. At 46,she has custody of her 5-year-oldgranddaughter. She is unemployed and recently had to move back to a subsidized housing project because of her limited income. Through all these difficulties, her adherence to her regimen of highly active antiretroviral therapy has been sporadic. Consequently, she has been hospitalized four times for pneumonia in the past two years.

After Zama's death, Thandi gave birth to a second daughter—who is also HIV-positive. Luckily, through the support of a benefactor, this child has access to the same medications that would be used to treat her in the United States. Thandi's life revolves around ensuring that her daughter takes her medications and stays well. Her greatest concern is that she and her daughter will never have financial security. She is training to become an HIV counselor because she would like to help other women obtain and benefit from HIV treatment, but she has no income and is therefore still dependent on a boyfriend for support.

The lives of these and many other women with HIV infection are mired in adverse circumstances. HIV adds to the overwhelming burden that they must bear. Here in the United States, there are disparities between the sexes in the care received for HIV infection[4]—partly because of the complexity of these women's lives, but also because they are frequently uninsured or underinsured and because they are often forced to seek care in systems that are not structured to meet their needs. For example, many HIV clinics have inflexible and inconvenient hours, long waiting times, and few staff members from the same racial or ethnic groups as the patients.

As antiretroviral medications become more widely available in the developing world, a major challenge will be finding ways not simply to dole out medications but also to simultaneously address the broader context. In both Thandi's world and Donna's, cultural, economic, and social structures must be changed to allow women more viable life options. Throughout the world, physicians can assist in this process by advocating a multidisciplinary approach to treatment and prevention that would address women's life circumstances along with their medical needs. Only when such change has been effected will HIV-infected women be able to obtain and benefit optimally from appropriate treatment, and only then will uninfected women be able to protect themselves from HIV infection and secure their own well-being.

▶ Notes

Dr. Ojikutu is a fellow in infectious diseases at the Massachusetts General Hospital and Brigham and Women's Hospital, Boston; and Dr. Stone is an associate professor in the Division of AIDS, Harvard Medical School, and the Department of Medicine, Massachusetts General Hospital, Boston.

1. 2004 Report on the global AIDS epidemic: 4th global report. Geneva: Joint United Nations Programme on HIV/AIDS (UNAIDS), 2004:22–58.

2. HIV/AIDS surveillance report. Vol. 15. Atlanta: Centers for Disease Control and Prevention, 2004:18–9.

3. Padian NS, Shiboski SC, Glass SO, Vittinhoff E. Heterosexual transmission of human immunodeficiency virus (HIV) in northern California: results from a ten-year study. Am J Epidemiol 1997;146:350–7.

4. Shapiro MF, Morton SC, McCaffrey DF, et al. Variations in the care of HIV-infected adults in the United States: results from the HIV Cost and Services Utilization Study. JAMA 1999;281: 2305–15.

Understanding and Addressing AIDS-Related Stigma: From Anthropological Theory to Clinical Practice in Haiti

Arachu Castro, Ph.D, M.P.H.,
and Paul Farmer, M.D., Ph.D.

For the past several years, diverse and often confused concepts of stigma have been invoked in discussions on AIDS. Many have argued compellingly that AIDS-related stigma acts as a barrier to voluntary counseling and testing. Less compelling are observations regarding the source of stigma or its role in decreasing interest in HIV care.

We reviewed these claims as well as literature from anthropology, sociology, and public health. Preliminary data from research in rural Haiti suggest that the introduction of quality HIV care can lead to a rapid reduction in stigma, with resulting increased uptake of testing. Rather than stigma, logistic and economic barriers determine who will access such services. Implications for scale-up of integrated AIDS prevention and care are explored. (*Am J Public Health.* 2005;95:53–59. doi: 10.2105/AJPH.2003.028563)

Most of those involved in the movement to slow the spread of AIDS and to improve the quality of life of those living with HIV view stigma and discrimination as human rights violations requiring redress. Both organizations and individuals have taken various actions to address stigma; however, these actions often have not been grounded in a broad biosocial understanding of stigma and AIDS-related discrimination. The Joint United Nations Programme on HIV/AIDS (UNAIDS) often refers to the need to fight stigma in order to combat HIV/AIDS,[1] but the definition of stigma remains unclear. Stigma undoubtedly poses several challenges, but the mechanisms by which it is at the heart of the AIDS pandemic need to be explored. Stigma and discrimination are part of complex systems of beliefs about illness and disease that are often grounded in social inequalities. Indeed, stigma is often just the tip of the iceberg; because it is visible and generally accepted in public health discourse without further qualification, the term has frequently served as a means of giving short shrift to powerful social inequalities (for example, in Valdiserri[2]) that are much harder to identify and conceptualize.

In addition, the tendency to use "rapid" methodologies has generated a wealth of information regarding people's knowledge and attitudes about AIDS-related stigma in different situations, but this information is often "desocialized"—decontextualized from larger social processes that are both historically rooted and linked to persons and processes that are not visible to the survey researcher. Such desocialized and disparate approaches have hindered the advancement of a theoretically sound understanding of AIDS-related stigma and have slowed effective actions to counter stigma.

Similar confusion surrounds debate over stigma as a barrier to introducing antiretrovirals to poor countries or to making voluntary HIV tests accessible. Again, such comments are insufficiently grounded in broader social analyses. The AIDS literature is rife with surveys that offer completely discrepant views on how stigma is related to events and processes as varied as sexual comportment, care-seeking behavior, and adherence to antibiotic regimens.[3-5] Without reference to any particular experience in delivering AIDS care in the world's poorest nations, 1 recent review claimed that

> in many countries hardest hit by HIV, the stigma of this disease is at least as powerful, if not more so, than in wealthy nations. Although the prospect of access to treatment may encourage individuals to determine their HIV status, the linkage of treatment to directly observed HIV therapy may paradoxically lower the use of counseling and testing services due to confidentiality concerns.[6(p1385)]

Elsewhere, we have termed those assertions "immodest claims of causality,"[7] since they are advanced authoritatively but may be readily countered by contrary claims.

Our concern in this review is to question the understanding of AIDS-related stigma and to assess its relationships to integrated HIV prevention and care. That AIDS-related stigma exists and needs redress is not debated. But where is the evidence that stigma stands as a ranking obstacle to treatment in poor countries when less than 5% of people with advanced AIDS in these countries have access to highly active antiretroviral therapy (HAART)?[8] Instead, some recent studies conducted in Botswana,[9] Senegal,[10] and Côte d'Ivoire[11] showed that the cost of medications borne by patients is the main stated reason for lack of adherence to therapy.

Still, "stigma" has become, in the popular press, one more argument used to walk a slow walk to fight the pandemic. A study conducted in Zambia claims that "despite increasing access to prevention of mother-to-child transmission initiatives, including antiretroviral drugs, the perceived disincentives of HIV testing, particularly for women, largely outweigh the potential gains from available treatments."[12(p347)] A closer look at the study shows that the use of antiretrovirals was limited to the prevention of mother-to-child transmission of HIV and did not include HAART to treat women (or any other adults) outside of pregnancy. What conclusions might be reached if proper therapy and a more equitable distribution of that therapy were introduced? A study conducted in Kenya showed that lack of access to drugs is the main factor compromising medical residents' ability to provide care to AIDS patients.[13]

On a more hopeful note, the evaluation of a mother-to-child transmission program in the Dominican Republic suggested that implementation of effective therapy for mothers has helped diminish the stigmatization of patients, in part because health professionals focused on pregnant women as potential conduits of antiretrovirals destined to prevent transmission to unborn children.[14] An AIDS program in rural Haiti also reported a sharp decline in AIDS-related stigma since the introduction of HAART.[15]

▶ Theoretical Framework

Our theoretical framework for the understanding of AIDS-related stigma has been developed over a decade of ethnographic research in rural Haiti. Our interpretations of the relevant literature are informed by more recent experience providing clinical services in rural Haiti.[15] Although the first references to the association between stigma and health in the social science literature date back to the 1880s,[16] sociologist Erving Goffman, beginning with his work in psychiatric hospitals in the late 1950s, developed what has become the benchmark social theory of the association between stigma and disease.[17,18] Goffman defined stigma as the identification that a social group creates of a person (or group of people) based on some physical, behavioral, or social trait perceived as being divergent from group norms. This socially constructed identification lays the groundwork for subsequent disqualification of membership from a group in which that person was originally included. Although Goffman emphasized the importance of analyzing stigma in terms of relationships rather than individual traits or attributes,[18] many subsequent interpretations of stigma have focused on individual attributes and are divorced from broader social processes, especially from relations of power.

Key anthropological and sociological contributions to our understanding of AIDS have introduced new components to Goffman's definition of stigma and offer the promise of novel conceptual frameworks.[19–22] Others have used a similar approach to understanding stigma associated with diseases such as hookworm, tuberculosis, cancer, polio, and sexually transmitted infections and the association of these diseases with racist ideology in the United States[23,24] or with cholera-related stigma in Venezuela.[25] Further contributions of anthropological work to the understanding of AIDS stigma have been obtained through research conducted in Zambia,[26] South Africa,[27] the Philippines,[28] Haiti,[29] and Puerto Rico and the United States.[30]

The field of social psychology has clarified the cognitive processes that lead to labeling and stereotyping. However, most psychological research focuses more on individualistic perceptions and attitudes than on the broader social context in which such perceptions are grounded. Most of these studies discuss the implications of these beliefs—in terms of misunderstandings, misinformation, and negative attitudes—as far as efforts to change the perceptions of the stigmatizers are concerned. Examples from Jamaica[31] and Mexico[32] are illustrative. Such approaches seek to improve HIV/AIDS education and to enhance sensitivity and empathy training or tolerance through personal contact with people living with HIV.[4,33–35] However, these laudable efforts have placed little emphasis on the larger economic and political processes in which stigma is grounded.

More recently, some anthropologists[20,36–39] have challenged approaches that emphasize cognitivist explanations of stigma rather than the structural violence that generates the social inequalities in which stigma is invariably rooted. According to Parker and Aggleton, the desocialization of stigma is not

> drawn directly from Goffman, who, on the contrary, was very much concerned with issues of social change. . . . Yet the fact that Goffman's framework has been appropriated in much research on stigma (whether in relation to HIV/AIDS or other issues), as though

stigma were a static attitude rather than a constantly changing (and often resisted) social process has seriously limited the ways in which stigmatization and discrimination have been approached in relation to HIV and AIDS.[20(p14)]

These authors proposed that stigma be analyzed within frameworks drawing on concepts of power, dominance, hegemony, and oppression.[40,41] They further proposed interventions that have deeper social, political, and economic roots, because "stigma is deployed by concrete and identifiable social actors seeking to legitimize their own dominant status within existing structures of social inequality."[20(p18)] This resocialized view of stigma defines discrimination, one of the consequences of stigma, as "when, in the absence of objective justification, a distinction is made against a person that results in that person's being treated unfairly and unjustly on the basis of belonging or being perceived to belong, to a particular group."[42] Other anthropologists have been scrupulous in ensuring that their interpretations of stigma are informed by the lived experience of those who suffer from it.[22,29,43-47]

A useful definition of AIDS-related stigma comes from the field of sociology:

In our conceptualization, stigma exists when the following interrelated components converge. In the first component, people distinguish and label human differences. In the second, dominant cultural beliefs link labeled persons to undesirable characteristics—to negative stereotypes. In the third, labeled persons are placed in distinct categories so as to accomplish some degree of separation of "us" from "them." In the fourth, labeled persons experience status loss and discrimination that lead to unequal outcomes. Finally, stigmatization is entirely contingent on access to social, economic, and political power that allows the identification of differentness, the construction of stereotypes, the separation of labeled persons into distinct categories, and the full execution of disapproval, rejection, exclusion, and discrimination.[48(p367)]

These authors noted that stigma is a "persistent predicament" and sought to understand "why the negative consequences of stigma are so difficult to eradicate."[48,49(p379)] The fundamental causes of stigma need to be addressed, they argued, by targeting multiple mechanisms to bring about change. Yet these authors limited the depth of required transformations to changing "deeply held attitudes and beliefs of powerful groups" and confining "the power of such groups to make their cognitions the dominant ones."[48(p381)] In acknowledging the centrality of social, economic, and political power differentials—emphasizing that cognitive processes are necessary but not sufficient causes for the production of stigma—they concluded that a better understanding of stigma requires an understanding of how these power differentials, along with issues of constraint and resistance, exert their impact on stigma.[48]

We propose *structural violence* as a conceptual framework for understanding AIDS-related stigma. Every society is shaped by large-scale social forces that together define structural violence. These forces include racism, sexism, political violence, poverty, and other social inequalities that are rooted in historical and economic processes that sculpt the distribution and outcome of HIV/AIDS. Structural violence predisposes the human body to pathogenic vulnerability by shaping risk of infection and also rate of disease progression.[7,50-53] Structural violence also determines who has access to counseling, diagnostics, and effective therapy for HIV disease. Finally, structural violence determines, in large part, who suffers from AIDS-related stigma and discrimination.

In societies marked by profound racism, it is expected that people of color with AIDS will be more stigmatized than in societies where racism is more attenuated. Similarly, gender inequality determines the extent to which sexism will mark the course of HIV disease. In highly sexist settings, the disclosure of HIV infection is more likely to provoke stigma and threat of domestic violence than in environments where women enjoy gender equity. Class often trumps both racism and sexism. The poor almost invariably experience violations of their social and economic rights. We can therefore conclude that poverty, already representing an almost universal stigma, will be the primary reason that poor people living with HIV suffer from greater AIDS-related stigma. Racism, sexism, and poverty exacerbate one another, especially where political violence and social inequalities are added to the equation. Together, social forces determine not only risk of HIV infection but also risk of AIDS-related stigma.

To improve our understanding of AIDS-related stigma, it is necessary to focus on a series of variables readily discernible across different societies; these include the experience of people living with HIV, public perceptions of AIDS, local experiences of stigma and discrimination and their influence in care-seeking activities, varied degrees of stigma over the course of HIV disease, impact of stigma on quality of life, and structural sources of stigma and discrimination (B. J. Good, written communication, May 2003). The understanding of these experiences and the analysis of these processes permit a better understanding of how different strategies, ranging from legal recourse to the introduction of HAART, can alter the course of AIDS-related stigma.

▶ Results

Public health experts prescribing health policies for poor countries believe that stigma, the high cost of treatment, the lack of infrastructure, and poor patient adherence to treatment constitute insurmountable barriers to effective AIDS control. From our experience providing health and social services in rural Haiti, this is not the case.[15,52,54,55] Haiti is by far the most impoverished country in Latin America and, not coincidentally, the hemisphere's most HIV-affected country, with an adult prevalence of around 5.6%.[56] To illustrate how structural violence is embodied and generates stigma, we explored the history of one of our patients in rural Haiti. Because the "texture" of dire affliction is better felt in the gritty details of biography, and since any example begs the question of its relevance, we argue that the story of our patient is anything but anecdotal. In the eyes of the epidemiologist as well as the political analyst, Samuel has suffered in exemplary fashion.

In 2001, Samuel Morin was dying of AIDS. Until then, Samuel, 40 years old, had farmed a small plot of land and had a tiny shop—which sold everything from matches to soap—in a town in central Haiti. He considered himself poor but was able to send his 4 children to school. Samuel was an active member of his church and sometimes used his meager earnings to help neighboring families in crisis, providing food if their crops failed, or helping with school fees. He also supported his sister and her 3 children after his brother-in-law died of AIDS.

When Samuel became ill in the mid-1990s, his wife had to assume all responsibility for the farming, although he could still sit and mind the shop. But after a while, Samuel recalled, "the disease transformed me. I looked like a stick." He continued to lose weight and then developed visible skin infections and thrush; he had difficulty swallowing food and began to cough. It was at this time, he felt, that people stopped coming to his shop. His children had to leave school because they were needed to help in the fields and because Samuel and his wife could no longer afford the school fees. Eventually, the shop failed completely. His wife left him and returned to her parents' home in Port-au-Prince.

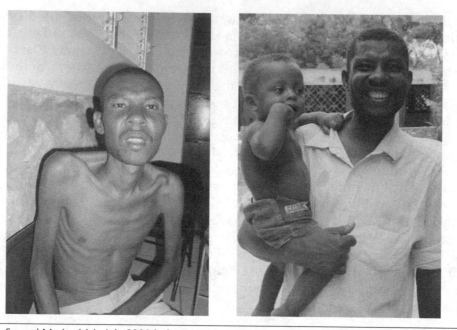

FIGURE 14-1   Samuel Morin, (a) in July 2001 before receiving HAART and (b) 1 year later, after a year of therapy. Photographs courtesy of Jen Singler and Laura Tarter.

In July 2001, when Samuel weighed only 80 pounds (Figure 14-1a), he decided to use his last 10 Haitian dollars to pay for a truck ride to the Clinique Bon Sauveur in Cange, a 6-hour walk from his home. Since then, Samuel has been receiving HAART under the supervision of an *accompagnateur* (community health worker), free of charge. In almost 3 years of therapy, Samuel stated, he has not missed a dose; he has responded clinically—he has gained 30 pounds, has normal skin color, and feels "great"—and has an undetectable viral load (Figure 14-1b shows Samuel a year after initiation of therapy). Moreover, his family has returned to him, his children are back in school, and he has reopened his shop. He also volunteers with the local Partners In Health team in HIV-prevention efforts. Of his recovery, Samuel said, "I was a walking skeleton before I began therapy. I was afraid to go out of my house and no one would buy things from my shop. But now I am fine again. My wife has returned to me and now my children are not ashamed to be seen with me. I can work again."

In reflecting on Samuel's experience, it is possible to argue that AIDS treatment can spark a "virtuous social cycle." Access to comprehensive AIDS care[57] saved Samuel's life; returning to work and securing school fees for his children has allowed him to surmount some of the miserable conditions faced by the majority of Haitians. It is also possible to discern direct links between access to care and stigma. There are the links mentioned by Samuel: proper HIV care can transform a disfiguring and consumptive disease into a manageable condition that is invisible to one's consociates. Integrating people living with HIV into the workforce of a community health program—around 5% of our current staff are persons living with HIV—permits them to receive comprehensive care, send their children to school, and earn steady wages. Further, the demonstrably favorable response of Samuel and others to HAART has sparked interest in voluntary counseling and testing. Together, these processes have contributed to lessening the impact of the AIDS stigma.

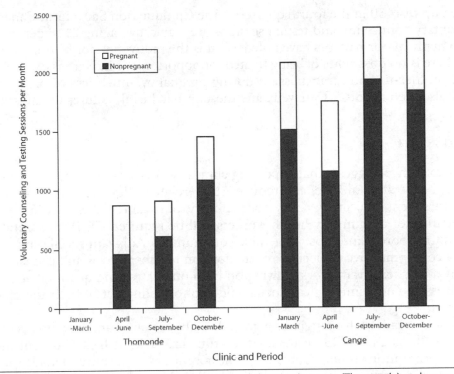

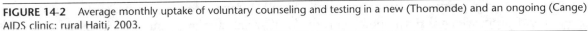

FIGURE 14-2   Average monthly uptake of voluntary counseling and testing in a new (Thomonde) and an ongoing (Cange) AIDS clinic: rural Haiti, 2003.

Years ago, before the advent of effective therapy for AIDS, anthropologists noted that the introduction of such therapy may alter profoundly the social interpretations of the disease.[43,58] Other social scientists have shown that stigma is aggravated by an undefined etiology and the lack of an effective treatment.[59] AIDS has afforded ample possibilities to study the social construction of stigma. Exposure to a new disease, as occurred with AIDS in Haiti in the 1980s, generates new cultural models of the etiology and expected course of disease.[29,60,61] These models change with time because diseases have a social course—that is, pathology is embedded in social experience.[42,60] The social experience of AIDS is affected profoundly by the advent of effective therapy.

The Haiti project already demonstrates that individuals who can access effective care are the most likely to get an HIV test,[15] which supports social theories on the social course of illness. The introduction of antiretrovirals has had a profound and positive impact on the demand for voluntary counseling and testing. It is possible to chart the rise in demand for testing and counseling in rural Haiti by following laboratory registers and daily reports. Since 1998, when we introduced the first free and comprehensive AIDS program in rural Haiti at the Clinique Bon Sauveur,[15] demand for such services has more than quintupled.

Samuel Morin was diagnosed and treated initially in Cange. But looking at his hometown of Thomonde, where community-based AIDS care was introduced only in 2003, is instructive. Figure 14-2 shows how rapidly voluntary counseling and testing may increase when comprehensive prevention and care are introduced. In Thomonde, voluntary counseling and testing sessions per month have skyrocketed from 0 to an average of 869 in the second quarter and up to 1450 in the fourth quarter; at the Clinique Bon Sauveur in Cange, the number of voluntary counseling and testing sessions are stable, averaging 2118 per month.

As so many of our patients have noted, what is the motivation for learning one's serostatus when there is no possibility of being treated for opportunistic infections or of access to prevention of mother-to-child transmission during pregnancy, much less of being treated with antiretrovirals when needed? Can we blame these public health failures on stigma alone?

▶ Discussion

The Haiti experience suggests that improving clinical services can raise the quality of prevention efforts, boost staff morale, and reduce AIDS-related stigma. As 1 of the first donor-supported treatment projects in a very poor country, our team's experience suggests that the full participation of community health workers will be required if HIV prevention and care are to reach the poorest and most vulnerable communities. Adjuvant social services must also be part of a comprehensive project, as must attention to tuberculosis and primary health care needs. Only a biosocial framework drawing on both qualitative and quantitative methods can hope to assess the epidemiological, social, and economic impact of both the epidemic and responses to it.

The last 2 decades have taught us a great deal about failure and how it is best measured; new HIV infections and AIDS deaths are the grim yardsticks. A lack of decent medical care and effective prevention strategies (including the absence of a vaccine and inadequate women-controlled barrier methods) frustrates public health efforts. However, a broad range of other events and processes are markers for failure: AIDS-related stigma and discrimination, unsafe blood transfusions, unattended childbirths, unclean water, and a lack of social services for HIV-affected individuals and families would figure high on this list of indirect markers.

And there's the analytic rub: we don't know how best to analyze such a diverse set of inextricably related problems. What evaluative framework might guide us as we attempt to measure phenomena as varied as HIV incidence and AIDS-related stigma and discrimination? How might we assess the impact of new projects? How do we address poverty and gender inequality in AIDS prevention and care, if they are so manifestly related to HIV transmission and outcomes? The best framework for analysis and evaluation would need to be robustly biosocial, since the phenomena it attempts to describe are nothing if not both biological and social. The framework would draw on conventional epidemiology, certainly, but also on complementary resocializing disciplines in which patients' voices and experiences are heard and documented. Anthropology and sociology are among these disciplines, as is the sociology of science. Unfortunately, ethnographic inquiry and community health worker reports are not often regarded, within public health, as reliable sources of information.

Could this evaluative framework be anything other than biosocial? It must not only assess the impact of stigma on morbidity and mortality but also address questions of stigma and equity; it must offer a resocialized understanding of how inequalities come to take their toll through disparities of risk for infection, radically different courses of disease, and disparities of access to proven therapies. Some of the indicators that we suggest be used include the number of patients with access to effective care, serosurveys in sentinel populations (e.g., prenatal clinics), HIV prevention checklists (sex education, condom distribution), number of person-hours of prevention through information and education campaigns, number of sites offering pre-

TABLE 14.1   Assessing the Impact of a Comprehensive AIDS Program: Possible Data Points

Indicators	Sources of Information Needed to Evaluate Indicators
Impact on patient outcomes	Patient charts, weight, activities of daily living
Impact on burden of disease	Prenatal screening
Response to local calls for equity	Community forums, focus groups
Reduced mortality	Chart review, community health workers' reports
Reduced rates of hospitalization	Daily reports, chart review
Reduced stigma	Ethnographic inquiry, case histories
Improved staff morale	Staff meetings, ethnographic study
Increased demand for voluntary	Laboratory registers, daily reports
counseling and testing	External Ministry of Health evaluation
Meeting public health goals	

vention of mother-to-child transmission of HIV, number of community health workers supervising therapy, reinforcement of public health infrastructures, creation of coalitions to expand and "harmonize" prevention and care services, transparent reporting of expenditures, and avoidance of drug stock depletions. We need, now, a novel synthesis of complementary methodologies, both quantitative and qualitative. We need to value the input of community groups, including community health workers and others who deliver services directly to those in greatest need.

The transformation of AIDS from an inevitably fatal disease to a chronic and manageable one has decreased stigma dramatically in Haiti, as Samuel's story shows. Our own experience in Haiti suggests that it is clear that the impact of a "low-tech" HIV prevention-and-care project could be measured without importing a new and costly "evaluation infrastructure." Table 14.1 lists some indirect indices of positive impact and the potential sources of data that might be made available in even the poorest communities. The most daunting challenges for which scale-up projects must be prepared are those having to do with the poverty of patients.

AIDS, stigma, and blame have been intertwined since the start of the epidemic. One of the characteristics of AIDS stigma is that, from the onset, this disease has been associated with lifestyles that society attributes, with little evidence, to being shaped by "voluntary acts." In America and Europe, where in the 1980s the epidemic ravaged groups of homosexuals and heroin addicts, there was very little solidarity with infected people because they were blamed for having "opted" for sexual practices or for addiction and reproached by society as immoral. The stigma that already existed toward these groups was amplified by AIDS.[62] This type of social discrimination was extended to poor countries where cases of HIV infection began to be diagnosed[29] and to other groups of vulnerable people, including poor women.

Some of these prejudices were reflected within universities, international organizations, foundations, bilateral organizations, governments, financing institutions, and pharmaceutical companies—institutions key to effective responses to the pandemic. A general hostility to people living with HIV is suggested by the fact that, until recently, AIDS prevention, not treatment, was the leitmotiv of international AIDS work; treatment was the privilege of those able to pay for it. These are powerful fora, and their position set the agenda for both funding and action. Freire might say that such positions are "sectarized": "Sectarization . . . transforms reality into something false that, thus, cannot be transformed."[63(p30)] By ignoring or giving short shrift to visible evidence of structural violence in the transmission of HIV and in the stigma that it generates, these "fora of knowledge" may perpetuate, sometimes by inaction, both stigma and discrimination.

Since the 1980s, blaming the victim has been a powerful current in the social experience of AIDS. Victim blaming helps to explain the lack of solidarity in providing appropriate care to people living with HIV; discrimination in the arenas of housing, employment, and education has been documented in the Caribbean[64-68] and in other parts of the world. The only people not often blamed for their own misfortune are those deemed infected by mechanisms considered unrelated to "personal choices in lifestyles." These exceptions include health professionals who, by occupational accident, are exposed to HIV-infected blood and hemophiliacs and other recipients of blood products infected by medical and political negligence, as occurred in France in 1985.[69] Additionally, children who contract HIV in utero or during birth or breastfeeding are also often exempt from blame (as noted in Puerto Rico[70]). These same children may face, as they grow older, discrimination when attending school (as in Mexico[71]). Even women infected through rape are often blamed for the violence of which they are victims.[53]

Exemptions from blame may be reflected at the national level within systems of social security or of private insurance that cover antiretroviral therapy for exempted groups but not for others. In the international arena, the division of people living with HIV into "blameworthy" and "blameless" categories reinforces the lack of will on the part of rich countries to finance AIDS treatment in poor countries. The funding gap, which reflects social inequalities between and among countries, is itself a reflection and source of structural violence contributing to AIDS-related stigma. Stigma and human-rights violations deriving from it are often the only visible part of deep-rooted social inequality. Addressing the root causes of stigma will require addressing structural violence, including the symbolic violence perpetuated by shallow theories about AIDS-related stigma. These theories may lead to inaction. To assess AIDS-related stigma and declare it a cause rather than both cause and consequence of inequality will probably weaken efforts to address AIDS among those with heightened risk of HIV because of poverty, racism, and gender inequality.

▶ About the Authors

The authors are with the Program in Infectious Disease and Social Change, Department of Social Medicine, Harvard Medical School; Partners In Health; and the Division of Social Medicine and Health Inequalities, Department of Medicine, Brigham and Women's Hospital, Boston, Mass.

Requests for reprints should be sent to Arachu Castro, PhD, MPH, Program in Infectious Disease and Social Change, Department of Social Medicine, Harvard Medical School, 641 Huntington Ave, Boston, MA 02115 (e-mail: arachu_castro@hms.harvard.edu).

This article was accepted March 13, 2004.

▶ Contributors

Both authors conceptualized the article, interpreted findings, and wrote the article.

▶ Acknowledgments

We acknowledge the Wilbur Marvin Fund of the David Rockefeller Center for Latin American Studies at Harvard University for the award of a 2003 Faculty Grant to the authors to work on the project "HIV/AIDS in the Caribbean: The Impact of Effective Therapy on Stigma." The scale-up of AIDS care in central Haiti has been made possible by the Global Fund to Fight AIDS, Tuberculosis and Malaria.

We are grateful to Yasmin Khawja, Haun Saussy, Joan Paluzzi, Alice Yang, and Rob Stavert for their contributions. We are most indebted to the Haitian clinical team, led by Dr Fernet Léandre, for its efforts to implement integrated AIDS prevention and care under very difficult circumstances.

▶ Human Participant Protection

No protocol approval was needed for this study.

▶ References

1. Piot P. From planning to implementation: success against AIDS in the region. Opening speech at: 2nd Latin American Forum on HIV/AIDS and STIs; April 8, 2003; Havana, Cuba.

2. Valdiserri RO. HIV/AIDS stigma: an impediment to public health. *Am J Public Health.* 2002;92: 341–342.

3. Fortenberry JD, McFarlane M, Bleakley A, et al. Relationships of stigma and shame to gonorrhea and HIV screening. *Am J Public Health.* 2002;92:378–381.

4. Herek GM, Capitanio JP, Widaman KF. HIV-related stigma and knowledge in the United States: prevalence and trends, 1991–1999. *Am J Public Health.* 2002;92:371–377.

5. Egger M, Pauw J, Lopatatzidis A, et al. Promotion of condom use in a high-risk setting in Nicaragua: a randomised controlled trial. *Lancet.* 2000;355: 2101–2105.

6. Liechty C, Bangsberg D. Doubts about DOT: antiretroviral therapy for resource-poor countries. *AIDS.* 2003;17:1383–1387.

7. Farmer P. *Infections and Inequalities: The Modern Plagues.* Berkeley: University of California Press; 1999.

8. *Scaling Up Antiretroviral Therapy in Resource-Limited Settings.* Geneva, Switzerland: World Health Organization; 2002.

9. Weiser S, Wolfe W, Bangsberg D, et al. Barriers to antiretroviral adherence for patients living with HIV infection and AIDS in Botswana. *J Acquir Immune Defic Syndr.* 2003;34(3):281–288.

10. Lanièce I, Ciss M, Desclaux A, et al. Adherence to HAART and its principal determinants in a cohort of Senegalese adults. *AIDS.* 2003;17(suppl 3): S103–S108.

11. Delaunay K, Vidal L, Msellati P, Moatti J-P. La mise sous traitement antirétroviral dans l'Initiative: l'explicite et l'implicite d'un processus de sélection. In: Msellati P, Vidal L, Moatti J-P, eds. *L'accès aux traitements du VIH/sida en Côte d'Ivoire. Aspects économiques, sociaux et comportementaux.* Paris, France: Agence Nationale de Recherches sur le Sida; 2001:87–113.

12. Bond V, Chase E, Aggleton P. Stigma, HIV/AIDS and prevention of mother-to-child transmission in Zambia. *Eval Program Plann.* 2002;25:347–356.

13. Raviola G, Machoki MI, Mwaikambo E, Good MJD. HIV, disease plague, demoralization and "burnout": resident experience of the medical profession in Nairobi, Kenya. *Cult Med Psychiatry.* 2002;26: 55–86.

14. Cáceres Ureña FI, Duarte I, Moya EA, Pérez-Then E, Hasbún MJ, Tapia M. *Análisis de la situación y la respuesta al VIH/SIDA en República Dominicana.* Santo Domingo, Dominican Republic: Instituto de Estudios de Población y Desarrollos (IEPD) and Asociación Dominicana Pro-Bienestar de la Familia (PROFAMILIA); 1998.

15. Farmer P, Léandre F, Mukherjee J, et al. Community-based approaches to HIV treatment in resource-poor settings. *Lancet.* 2001;358:404–409.

16. Tuke DH. The Cagots. *J Anthropol Instit Great Britain Ireland.* 1880;9:376–385.

17. Goffman E. *Asylums: Essays on the Social Situation of Mental Patients and Other Inmates.* Garden City, NY: Anchor Books; 1961.

18. Goffman E. *Stigma: Notes on the Management of Spoiled Identity.* Garden City, NY: Anchor Books; 1963.

19. Weiss MG, Ramakrishna J. Stigma interventions and research for international health. Paper presented at: Stigma and Global Health: Developing a Research Agenda; September 5–7, 2001; Bethesda, Md.

20. Parker R, Aggleton P. HIV and AIDS-related stigma and discrimination: a conceptual framework and implications for action. *Soc Sci Med.* 2003;57:13–24.

21. Das V. Stigma, contagion, defect: issues in the anthropology of public health. Paper presented at: Stigma and Global Health: Developing a Research Agenda; September 5–7, 2001; Bethesda, Md.

22. Alonzo AA, Reynolds NR. Stigma, HIV and AIDS: an exploration and elaboration of a stigma trajectory. *Soc Sci Med.* 1995;41(3):303–315.

23. Wailoo K. Stigma, race, and disease in 20th century America: an historical overview. Paper presented at: Stigma and Global Health: Developing a Research Agenda; September 5–7, 2001; Bethesda, Md.

24. Brandt A. *No Magic Bullet: A Social History of Venereal Disease in the United States Since 1880.* Oxford, England: Oxford University Press; 1985.

25. Briggs C, Mantini-Briggs C. *Stories in the Time of Cholera: Racial Profiling During a Medical Nightmare.* Berkeley: University of California Press; 2003.

26. Gausset Q. AIDS and cultural practices in Africa: the case of the Tonga (Zambia). *Soc Sci Med.* 2001; 52(4):509–518.

27. Wojcicki JM, Malala J. Condom use, power and HIV/AIDS risk: sex-workers bargain for survival in Hillbrow/Joubert Park/Berea, Johannesburg. *Soc Sci Med.* 2001;53(1):99–121.

28. Simbulan NP, Aguilar AS, Flanigan T, Cu-Uvin S. High-risk behaviors and the prevalence of sexually transmitted diseases among women prisoners at the women state penitentiary in Metro Manila. *Soc Sci Med.* 2001;52(4):599–618.

29. Farmer P. *AIDS and Accusation: Haiti and the Geography of Blame.* Berkeley: University of California Press; 1992.

30. Finlinson HA, Robles RR, Colón HM, et al. Puerto Rican drug users experiences of physical and sexual abuse: comparisons based on sexual identities. *J Sex Res.* 2003;40(3):277–285.

31. Hue LE. Children's [*sic*] involvement in HIV/AIDS support initiatives help reduce stigma and discrimination. Paper presented at: 14th International AIDS Conference; July 7, 2002; Barcelona, Spain.

32. McCauley A, Stewart H, Baker S, et al. HIV prevention programs can reduce stigma among students. Paper presented at: 14th International AIDS Conference; July 9, 2002; Barcelona, Spain.

33. Devine PG, Plant EA, Harrison K. The problem of "us" versus "them" and AIDS stigma. *Am Behav Sci.* 1999;42(7):1208–1224.

34. Herek GM. Illness, stigma, and AIDS. In: Costa P, Vanden GR, eds. *Psychological Aspects of Serious Illness.* Washington, DC: American Psychological Association; 1990:103–150.

35. Pryor JB, Reeder GD, Landau S. A social-psychological analysis of HIV-related stigma. *Am Behav Sci.* 1999;42(7):1189–1207.

36. Parker R, Camargo KR Jr. Pobreza e HIV/AIDS: aspectos antropológicos e sociológicos. *Cad Saúde Pública.* 2000;16(suppl 1):89–102.

37. Farmer P. Introducing ARVs in resource-poor settings. Plenary lecture. Paper presented at: 14th International AIDS Conference; July 10, 2002; Barcelona, Spain.

38. Castro A. Determinantes socio-políticos de la infección por VIH: violencia estructural y culpabilización de la víctima. Conferencia plenaria [Socio-political determinants of HIV: structural violence and the blaming of the victim. Plenary lecture]. Paper presented at: 2nd Latin American Forum on HIV/AIDS and STIs; April 10, 2003; Havana, Cuba.

39. Abadía-Barrero C. *"I Have AIDS but I Am Happy": Children's Subjectivities, AIDS, and Social Responses in Brazil.* Boston, Mass: Harvard School of Dental Medicine; 2002.

40. Foucault M. *Histoire de la sexualité [The History of Sexuality].* Paris, France: Gallimard; 1976.

41. Bourdieu P. *La distinction: Critique sociale du jugement [Distinction: A Social Critique of the Judgment of Taste].* Paris, France: Minuit; 1979.

42. Maluwa M, Aggleton P, Parker R. HIV- and AIDS-related stigma, discrimination, and human rights. *Health Hum Rights.* 2002;6(1):1–18.

43. Kleinman A, Wang W-Z, Li S-C, et al. The social course of epilepsy: chronic illness as social experience in interior China. *Soc Sci Med.* 1995;40(10): 1319–1330.

44. Good BJ, Good M-JDV. In the subjunctive mode: epilepsy narratives in Turkey. *Soc Sci Med.* 1994;38(6): 835–842.

45. Kleinman A, Kleinman J. Suffering and its professional transformation. *Cult Med Psychiatry.* 1991;15(3): 275–301.

46. Farmer P, Kleinman A. AIDS as human suffering. *Dædalus.* 1989;118(2):135–160.

47. Whittaker AM. Living with HIV: resistance by positive people. *Med Anthropol Q.* 1992;6(4): 385–390.

48. Link B, Phelan J. Conceptualizing stigma. *Annu Rev Sociol.* 2001;27:363–385.

49. Link BG, Phelan J. On stigma and its public health implications. Paper presented at: Stigma and Global Health: Developing a Research Agenda; September 5–7, 2001; Bethesda, Md.

50. Castro A, Farmer P. Anthropologie de la violence: la culpabilisation des victimes. *Notre Librairie: Revue des Littératures du Sud.* 2002;148:102–108.

51. Farmer P. *Pathologies of Power: Health, Human Rights, and the New War on the Poor.* Berkeley: University of California Press; 2003.

52. Castro A, Farmer P. El sida y la violencia estructural: la culpabilización de la víctima. *Cuadernos de Antropología Social.* 2003;17:31–49.

53. Farmer P, Connors M, Simmons J, eds. *Women, Poverty, and AIDS: Sex, Drugs, and Structural Violence.* Monroe, Me: Common Courage Press; 1996.

54. Farmer P, Castro A. Un pilote en Haïti: de l'efficacité de la distribution d'antiviraux dans des pays pauvres, et des objections qui lui sont faites. *Vacarme.* 2002;19:17–22.

55. Castro A, Farmer P. Infectious disease in Haiti: HIV/AIDS, tuberculosis, and social inequalities. *EMBO Rep.* 2003;4(6 suppl):S20–S23.

56. *Report on the HIV/AIDS Epidemic.* Geneva, Switzerland: UNAIDS; 2004.

57. Castro A, Farmer P, Kim JY, et al., eds. *Scaling Up Health Systems to Respond to the Challenge of HIV/AIDS in Latin America and the Caribbean.* Washington, DC: Pan American Health Organization; 2003.

58. Lévi-Strauss C. *Anthropologie structurale* [*Structural Anthropology*]. Paris, France: Plon; 1958.

59. Sontag S. *Illness as Metaphor.* New York, NY: Farrar, Straus and Giroux; 1978.

60. Farmer P. Sending sickness: sorcery, politics, and changing concepts of AIDS in rural Haiti. *Med Anthropol Q.* 1990;4(1):6–27.

61. Farmer P. AIDS-talk and the constitution of cultural models. *Soc Sci Med.* 1994;38(6):801–809.

62. Altman D. *AIDS in the Mind of America.* Garden City, NY: Doubleday; 1986.

63. Freire P. *Pedagogóa del oprimido* [*The Pedagogy of the Oppressed*]. Madrid, Spain: Siglo XXI; 1970.

64. Bacchus R. Legal and ethical dimensions of HIV/ AIDS. In: Howe G, Cobley A, eds. *The Caribbean AIDS Epidemic.* Kingston, Jamaica: University of the West Indies Press; 2000:151–185.

65. Walrond ER. Regional policies in relation to the HIV/AIDS epidemic in the Commonwealth Caribbean. In: Howe G, Cobley A, eds. *The Caribbean AIDS Epidemic.* Kingston, Jamaica: University of the West Indies Press; 2000:57–70.

66. Trotman L. HIV/AIDS in the workplace: the workers' perspective. In: Howe G, Cobley A, eds. *The Caribbean AIDS Epidemic.* Kingston, Jamaica: University of the West Indies Press; 2000:139–150.

67. Francis CR. The psychological dynamics of the AIDS epidemic in the Caribbean. In: Howe G, Cobley A, eds. *The Caribbean AIDS Epidemic.* Kingston, Jamaica: University of the West Indies Press; 2000:186–201.

68. Royes H. *A Cultural Approach to HIV/AIDS Prevention and Care: Jamaica's Experience.* Kingston, Jamaica: UNESCO, Cultural Policies for Development Unit; 1999. Studies and Reports, Special Series 8.

69. Sultan Y. Épidémiologie de l'infection par le virus LAV/HTLVIII chez les hémophiles polytransfusés en France. Résultats d'une enquête menée par 28 centres d'hémophiles. *Nouv Rev Fr Hematol.* 1986;28(5): 327–329.

70. Susser I, Kreniske J. Community organizing around HIV prevention in rural Puerto Rico. In: Bond GC, Kreniske J, Susser I, Vincent J, eds. *AIDS in Africa and the Caribbean.* Boulder, Colo: Westview Press; 1997:51–64.

71. Aggleton P, Parker R, Maluwa M. *Stigma, Discrimination and HIV/AIDS in Latin America and the Caribbean.* Washington, DC: Inter-American Development Bank; February 2003.

"I Have an Evil Child at My House": Stigma and HIV/AIDS Management in a South African Community

Catherine Campbell, Ph.D., Carol Ann Foulis, M.A., Sbongile Maimane, and Zweni Sibiya

We examined the social roots of stigma by means of a case study of HIV/AIDS management among young people in a South African community (drawing from interviews, focus groups, and fieldworker diaries). We highlight the web of representations that sustain stigma, the economic and political contexts within which these representations are constructed, and the way in which they flourish in the institutional contexts of HIV/AIDS interventions.

Stigma serves as an effective form of "social psychological policing" by punishing those who have breached unequal power relations of gender, generation, and ethnicity. We outline an agenda for participatory programs that promote critical thinking about stigma's social roots to stand alongside education and, where possible, legislation as an integral part of antistigma efforts. (*Am J Public Health*. 2005;95:808–815. doi:10.2105/AJPH.2003.037499)

Stigmatization of people living with AIDS is a key obstacle to HIV prevention and AIDS care. It is now generally accepted that efforts to reduce stigma should be an integrated part of all HIV/AIDS programming.[1] However, discussions of the form such efforts should take remain in their infancy. Here we discuss the social roots of stigma in the interest of contributing to debates about appropriate stigma reduction interventions, drawing on a case study of HIV/AIDS management among young people in South Africa.

The existing HIV/AIDS literature points to 3 antistigma strategies. The first is information-based awareness programs designed to reduce ignorance about people with AIDS. However, while ignorance often plays a key role in perpetuating stigma, providing people with factual information about the contagiousness of illnesses does not lead to widespread stigma reduction.[2] The second strategy is institution of legal safeguards making discrimination against people with AIDS a punishable offense. Antidiscrimination legislation has the potential to reduce the explicit and public stigmatization of such individuals.[3] However, manifestations of stigma are often too subtle to be immediately apparent, rooted within individual psyches, families, and communities and beyond the reach of the legal system. Thus, while education and legal safeguards may arguably be necessary conditions for fighting stigma, they are certainly not sufficient ones.

The third strategy—which we believe should go hand in hand with the first 2—involves participation of local community members in antistigma efforts. Our interest in this strategy informs the discussion provided here. Although community participation is repeatedly advocated, there is a lack of clarity regarding precisely *what* community members should participate in and *how* this participation should take place. Much work remains to be done in providing specific direction to calls for participatory initiatives, lest they result in nothing more than programs in which participants are encouraged to tell one another that stigma is a bad thing and that they should not contribute to it. Such didactic approaches are less likely to succeed than initiatives promoting debate and dialogue within a group of people, especially in marginalized communities where social obstacles may undermine attitude or behavior change. It is through such dialogue that a group may develop critical understandings of the social roots of health-damaging attitudes or behaviors, enhancing their awareness of the obstacles to change they will have to overcome and, ideally, leading to collective action to challenge such obstacles.[4]

What are the social roots of stigma? The theoretical literature emphasizes that stigma results not only from fear of physical contagion but also from fear of "symbolic contagion," a threat to both the health and well-being of individuals and to the well-being and legitimacy of the status quo. Whereas the form and content of stigma will vary from one context to another, various forms of stigma are united by the way in which they serve to support systems of social inequality and social difference and to reinforce the interests of powerful social actors seeking to legitimize their dominant status.[3] We examine the form taken by stigma in 1 small local community in the interest of understanding some of the ways in which stigmatization of people with AIDS is situated within other patterns of material and symbolic social exclusion. We conclude by discussing the implications of our findings for participatory strategies that challenge stigma.

▶ Conceptual Framework

Psychodynamic thinkers speak of the existence among humans of a universal unconscious fear of collapse and chaos.[5] People may cope by projecting their worst fears onto identifiable outgroups. This process of stigmatization or "othering" is thought to serve an "identity-protective" function by producing feelings of comfort and security and a sense of personal invulnerability to threats and dangers that might otherwise appear overwhelming.

Stigmatization is also argued to serve a "system-justifying" function.[6] The content of the psychological processes associated with "othering" may often reflect wider social interests. A study of representations of AIDS in Zambia highlighted how the stigmatization of women as vectors of AIDS, with men depicted as the "innocent parties," is part and parcel of a more general devaluing of women.[7] In another context, people with AIDS have been described as the symbolic markers of all that threatens to undermine American society and economic success.[8] In a country where economic success is built on traditional values of self-discipline, self-control, and prosperity, HIV/AIDS (stereotypically associated with promiscuous sex, drug abuse, and poverty) can be seen as standing for everything that threatens the middle American way of life. HIV/AIDS is an "epidemic of signification" at the same time as it is a biomedical epidemic, and stigmatization of people with AIDS has been an important vehicle for affirming the status quo.[9]

The widespread stigmatization of sex in South Africa and President Mbeki's well-publicized refusal to acknowledge the extent of the AIDS problem have been linked to the president's project of postapartheid nation building and to his conception of the type of citizen best equipped to carry forward his vision of an "African Renaissance." The president makes a strong distinction between South Africa's wretched past and a bright new postapartheid future. AIDS, and its association with promiscuous and diseased sexuality, threatens to blur this distinction. Public discourses and silences around sexuality are embedded in "a wider matrix of moral anxiety, social instability and political contestation" characterizing the current historical moment in South Africa, where people battle with "the complexities and vulnerabilities of the drive to produce a newly democratic unified nation."[10]

More broadly, Africanist historians have found that policing of sexuality, stigmatization, and social inequalities are linked. They have shown how the teachings of the church (particularly Victorian sexuality as mediated by Christian missionaries) were combined with the construction and reconstruction of so-called "traditional African culture" to place limits on the sexuality of African women, preserving the patriarchal social relations that continue to dominate in South Africa, despite challenges and resistances.[11,12]

▶ Methodology

We draw on a case study of a youth HIV prevention program run by an international body, the Christian Youth Alliance (CYA), in the South African community of Ekuthuleni, a periurban area near Durban in KwaZulu-Natal province. (Both the name of the community and that of the youth organization have been changed in line with the ethical principles of anonymity and confidentiality.) Sixteen percent of all KwaZulu-Natal adults aged 15 to 49 years are HIV positive,[13] as are 36% of women attending antenatal clinics.[14] Heterosexual sex is the most common mode of transmission, and levels of HIV among young people are particularly high.[4] Ekuthuleni is home to 20000 people, some living in formal housing with road access and services, but many living in makeshift shacks with minimal access to water and electricity. Unemployment and poverty are rife. Although many residents are HIV positive or suffering from AIDS, levels of disclosure are minimal. Nearly all of our research informants reported that they were not aware of anyone in the community who they were sure was HIV positive.

Funded by overseas donors, the CYA has established a nongovernmental organization in Ekuthuleni that promotes peer education among young people, both in and out of school, in the context of an integrated approach, including support groups and individual counseling for people with AIDS. We examined how local community contexts facilitated or hindered the success of CYA's peer education program. An open-ended topic guide focused on informants' views of the South African political context; local community life; the causes of HIV transmission, the impact of AIDS on their community; the role of their particular peer group in contributing to HIV/AIDS management; and their views on peer education, participation, and partnerships as strategies for HIV prevention.

This case study took the form of 3-hour interviews conducted in 2003 with 44 people, 11 focus groups involving a total of 55 people, and fieldworker diaries. Informants included young people and peer educators both in and out of school, teachers, a school principal, community health workers, community leaders (traditional leaders, the local ward councillor, youth leaders, and members of the local development committee), CYA staff, a traditional healer, clinic nurses, parents, people with AIDS, church ministers, a government official, and representatives of a multinational company that employs local people.

Thematic content analyses were used in analyzing interviews.[15] Stigma emerged as a central topic, and the goal of the preliminary data analysis was to identify the forms taken by stigma and its effects on the CYA's work. A more detailed secondary analysis sought to identify the material, symbolic, and organizational contexts associated with stigmatization of people with AIDS.

► Findings

Forms of Stigma and Effects on the Christian Youth Alliance's Work

We found that stigma was rife. One anecdote after another referred to the vicious stigmatization of HIV-positive individuals of all ages. As reported by a youth worker: "Children are not comfortable to disclose [their HIV status] to their parents. Their mothers gossip, saying 'I have an evil child at my house who has contracted this disease.' " Family members sometimes hid away sick relatives, depriving them of health care or support. According to a community health worker, "Neighbors will tell me there is a sick person in the bedroom at the back of the house. But when I arrive the family denies having such a person. The families themselves prevent anyone from helping them."

Families sometimes disowned dead relatives, refusing to collect their bodies from the mortuary, for example. Amidst stories of rejection and prejudice, there were a few stories of care and compassion among family members. However, even in such families it was not uncommon for both the dying person and his or her family members never to refer to the fact that the person had AIDS, even when everyone was fully aware of the situation. One woman reported that, even after her sister's death, no one in the family had ever strayed from the "official story" that she had died of tuberculosis, despite everyone secretly being aware that she had died as a result of AIDS-related illnesses.

People with AIDS who did disclose to family members often did so in indirect ways. One man stated that his brother, 2 weeks before his death, wrote the family a letter disclosing his status rather than telling them face to face. When the man told mourners at the funeral that his brother had died of AIDS, several friends and relatives berated him for "spoiling his brother's name."

Stigmatization by one's family members, at the very time one most needs their support, is often cited as the most hurtful and damaging form of stigma and the form that has the most negative effects on the HIV prevention struggle.[1] As one parent commented,

> We mothers and grannies play a key role in allowing HIV/AIDS to continue. Our refusal to disclose keeps the disease underground, and feeds into people denying the humanity of [people with AIDS] and their sense that they are no different to animals, with nothing to live for.

This stigmatization also served as a strong deterrent to young people seeking HIV/AIDS-related counseling.

One CYA worker reported that "there is fear of this place. Youth are scared to be seen entering our office that is known to be providing AIDS counseling. And the people who do come here are not from Ekuthuleni."

Other CYA workers reported that young people feared their parents would see them attending HIV prevention meetings and punish them. Many informants spoke of the way in which churches and schools also actively undermined HIV prevention efforts. According to a CYA worker,

> When we ask to talk about HIV in the churches they say we are encouraging the youth to sin. We recently called youth to attend a meeting on life skills [and had] a very poor turnout. Later we were told by youth that the minister said if they attended the workshop they would be demoted in the church.

Another CYA worker said "we sometimes use 'loveLife' brochures in schools, which have some sexual pictures in them. At one school the principal told us never to come again, that we were promoting pornography."

Symbolic Contexts of Stigma

What are the contexts that sustain the types of rejection and isolation of people with AIDS just outlined? We highlight 3 different aspects of context: the symbolic context (mapping out the wider field of social representations within which stigma is located); the economic, political, and local community contexts within which these representations are constructed; and the organizational context of efforts to address HIV/AIDS in Ekuthuleni.

Virtually every informant reported that stigma originated in the association between HIV/AIDS and sex. For example: "People know HIV/AIDS is here, but they won't talk about it because they believe if you have got AIDS you have got it through sex." Stigmatization of people with AIDS is supported by an associative network of symbolic links (sometimes logical and sometimes arbitrary) between such individuals and other negatively valued groups or attributes (in the very different context of the United States, a study of stigma highlighted the associative links between people with AIDS and homosexuality, death, drug use, and ethnic minorities).[16] In the following, we examine the web of representations within which stigma is located.

Many adults showed a strong unwillingness to acknowledge that their children were sexually active. When asked whether her son had ever told her he had girlfriends, one mother responded,

> Wow! Wow! He could never tell me that. Wow! There is no need for him to talk about that here. . . . I don't believe a parent must talk to their children about their love life. This is how I grew up. It wouldn't be right for me to know my children have relationships.

Such contexts exclude the possibility of parents providing a supportive environment for the promotion of safer sexual behavior by young people.

Some of the more frank adults in our sample wryly commented that this posturing by their peers was unconvincing, given that sexual activity among young people had been common for many years. According to one mother who was in her early 50s,

> In my time I could sleep with 7 men and only be infected with [a sexually transmitted disease]. I would go to the hospital or traditional healer and be cured in no time. The only difference now is that HIV has no cure. Nothing has changed in sexual behavior.

Denial of young people's sexual desire and relationships was particularly strong in the case of girls. Mothers refused to discuss sex in any way that resonated with their daughters' personal experiences of desires and relationships. They would darkly and indirectly allude to a link between sex, shame, and danger rather than accepting that their daughters were sexually active and teaching them how to protect themselves from sexually transmitted diseases and pregnancy.

According to one adolescent girl,

> Mother says that when you sleep with a boy you get a baby, he dumps you, and it's only afterwards that you regret that you ever slept with him. She says if you are a girl you must protect yourself against boys who will destroy your life.

Such denial of young girls' sexuality is related to what has been referred to as the wider "demonization of women" that the epidemic has provoked in sub-Saharan Africa.[17] In our interviews, many informants spoke of the way in which the weakness of women had fueled the epidemic. One of the church ministers stated, "The key to respect and good behavior is in the hands of women. A person who has the right to say no to sexual advances is a woman." Within such contexts, young women often had a particular investment in hiding their sexual activities. This made them less likely to seek out information about sexual health and to seek out or carry condoms. They often depicted sex as something that "just happened" to them, as something they did not expect and therefore did not prepare for.[18]

However, behind this public discourse is a thriving and dynamic world of young people's sexuality, away from the oversight of adults. In this world, many girls want and enjoy sex as often and as much as boys and adults. This counterstereotype emerged repeatedly in our interviews, and, not surprisingly, it was boys rather than girls who spoke of it. For example, according to one of the male youth informants: "Girls don't like trains that are not moving." Another stated: "Some girls say they don't want sex, but after an hour of kissing they always change their minds."

Another factor that supported stigmatization of HIV/AIDS was the link made by many between sex, sin, and immorality. The church was the main contributor of symbolic ammunition sustaining this link. According to one of the senior nurses, "If people reduce their sins God will cure their diseases. . . . It is the devil that overpowers people [when they engage in wrongful sex]."

Similarly, in the words of a parent, "The Bible says the end of the world will come when we are struck down by incurable diseases. The Kingdom of God will come to destroy all the evil that is prevailing in this world. I always tell myself that AIDS shows us this time has come."

Part of the link between sex and sin that was widely lamented in the interviews was the sin of disrespect by young people for their elders.[19] According to one of the health volunteers: "God is angry with us. We have sinned so much, and we are living in bad times. This younger generation does not listen when they are told, they have no respect. He is punishing us for this."

Informants in all age groups spoke of young people as a "menace" needing to be controlled and disciplined. Aside from young people's engagement in sexual activity, informants frequently referred to their involvement in crime and drugs as further evidence of youthful bad behavior, proposing strong discipline as the solution. Informants frequently linked alleged "youth disrespect" with the political freedoms characterizing postapartheid society, stating that so-called "children's rights" contradicted the traditional culture. An out-of-school youth informant reported,

> Government policies on children's rights make it difficult for parents to discipline their children. What used to be called punishment is now called abuse, and a social worker can be called in. These "rights" contradict our traditional culture. . . . It is wrong that the threat of social workers should be allowed to disrupt the smooth running of the household.

Several informants spoke approvingly of the link between harsh discipline of young people and the so-called "African culture." The view of young people as "mad, bad, and deviant" was underpinned by parents' lack of confidence in their ability to control their offspring in general or, in particular, to talk to them about sex.

A number of informants spoke, sometimes in a self-denigrating way, of HIV/AIDS as a problem facing Black Africans. According to one father,

> The cause of the problem of HIV in this country is that we Black people don't behave ourselves. We have many girlfriends, that is what spreads AIDS all over. I have never heard that Whites, Indians or 'coloreds' [people of mixed race] have AIDS, yet AIDS infects many Black people.

The conceptual rationale underlying these informants' linking of HIV/AIDS with specific ethnic groups varied. Some informants referred to the spread of HIV/AIDS as the White regime's last gasp attempt to undermine Black opposition. A teacher spoke of members of the apartheid regime injecting Black political prisoners with the virus and then releasing them back into the community to infect others. Informants also spoke of the spread of HIV/AIDS as resulting from postapartheid White envy, with Whites infecting Blacks to "reduce the Black vote." Several people spoke of Whites spreading HIV/AIDS through the lubricant contained in condoms. One influential local leader spoke of how he had boiled a condom in water and taken the water to a medical laboratory for HIV testing. The water tested positive, he said.

What are the contexts within which this web of representations is constructed and sustained? We focus on this topic in the 2 sections to follow.

Economic, Political, and Local Community Contexts

General context of poverty and political disempowerment. Life in Ekuthuleni is characterized by high levels of poverty and political marginalization.[20] Many young people have little tertiary education, few skills, and poor job prospects. Some families are refugees from political violence in the surrounding areas and have suffered traumatic experiences. Many unemployed young men from poor families engage in crime, and informants spoke of drug abuse among young people as a serious problem.

Furthermore, young people have virtually no political representation and play no decisionmaking role in the local political or community development structures, and there were many stories of petty adult elites squashing young people's attempts to develop local initiatives.

Youth representation on school councils was described as ineffectual by both students and teachers. Against this background, it was not surprising that many of the informants spoke of low morale among young people and a prevailing sense of apathy in regard to asserting their needs and rights.

Poor intergenerational communication. Informants reported that many young people have little support and guidance from their parents and that intergenerational communication is poor. Many young people spoke of their parents' failure to educate them about sex. According to one out-of-school youth: "Our parents have been shy to tell us the truth, they tell us children come from aeroplanes. This is a big mistake. They should have told us the truth. I got pregnant and I didn't know what had happened to me until my child was born."

Many parents refused to consider talking to their children about sex. A father of 10 told us that discussing condoms with his sons "would constitute pornography and only encourage them to have sex." A mother of 9 repeatedly insisted that it would be inappropriate to acknowledge that her children were sexually active outside of wedlock. Yet, 2 of her unmarried daughters (who lived with her) had their own children, and she herself had nursed a third unmarried daughter for the 18 months preceding her death from AIDS. Moreover, she spoke openly about the cause of her daughter's death.

Some women did speak of how important it was for mothers to be open with their children about sexual health. However, at different stages of their interviews, it became clear that they had not succeeded in doing so themselves. One who spoke at length about the importance of promoting intergenerational communication about sex later reported that she did not know whether her daughter had started menstruating and did not know how to broach the topic. Our sample did include parents who were more successful, however. One 41-year-old father of 5 praised the AIDS training his son was receiving at school. He also believed that young people received better guidance if their parents sat down and talked with them as opposed to disciplining them strongly. However, such parents appeared to be in the minority.

Community networks. Much has been written about the roles of "civic engagement" and local solidarity as key assets in poor communities.[21] It is frequently argued that health promotional projects have the greatest chance of succeeding in united communities with dense local networks.[4,22] There are strongly supportive relationships and support systems among Ekuthuleni residents, including women's groups, prayer groups, gardening collectives formed to cultivate food for the sick and the unemployed, community health volunteers sharing their own meager incomes and food with destitute patients, and savings clubs run by housewives and pensioners.

These groups are a key element in the social fabric and economic survival of the local people. Yet, while they provide effective social support in a range of ways, these networks do not serve as potential resources for HIV prevention efforts among young people. Rather, they are usually adult dominated, and they tend to have a narrow focus. Furthermore, to date there has been no effective community leadership to take up the challenge of mobilizing these small, dispersed, and fragmented networks in the pursuit of other goals (such as initiatives to reduce stigma).

The solidarity that does exist in Ekuthuleni is mostly that among micro-networks of older women united by their commitment to "respectability." According to social identity theory,[23] human beings have a fundamental need for positive self-esteem and often seek to achieve this need through making favorable comparisons between themselves and others. Two types of "social competition" form the basis of these comparisons: objective competition (competition for material resources such as money) and subjective competition (competition for symbolic resources such as respect or recognition). Sex and alcohol use constitute 2 key ways in which a person's respectability might be compromised.[24,25]

In the context of poverty and disempowerment, many people lack access to the conventional social advantages of a highly materialistic society (e.g., expensive clothing and cars) and thus to those objective resources that might boost their self-esteem. Symbolic resources—such as respectability—come to constitute valuable currency in individuals' efforts to enhance their self-esteem. In the case of many Ekuthuleni residents, openly expressed stigmatization of people with AIDS has become a way of asserting claims to respectability.

AIDS-Related Institutional Contexts

Many of the informants commented regretfully on the shortcomings of government services aimed at HIV prevention and AIDS care. Lack of national government leadership and services went hand in hand with a lack of local leadership and inadequate or nonexistent local services. According to a health worker,

> I don't see the government having any care for [people with AIDS]. Here there is no proper hospital treatment, people can't afford medication for opportunistic infections, there are delays in grants . . . until patients are dead—the money arrives too late to help them eat and get tablets to survive—so far I haven't heard of 1 who was still alive when the grant [government grant for people in the later stages of AIDS] came through.

Both the school principal and the clinic director expressed bewilderment in the face of frequent media publicity highlighting the availability of government funds for HIV/AIDS management, stating that such resources had never materialized at schools or clinics of which they were aware. Informants also remarked on the poor networking between local health professionals involved in caring for people with AIDS (another symptom of the failure of local leadership and local coordination of networks and services). In the words of a community health worker,

> There are so many people that need us. This is a frustrating job. When we complain or make suggestions, we don't get any response from the hospital. The lines of communication are very poor. Social work referrals are even worse. Sometimes I have to hide from my patients in the street because the response from the social workers has been so slow I no longer know what to say to them.

The lack of adequate government leadership, resources, and infrastructure went hand in hand with lack of action in Ekuthuleni schools. The school principal who participated in the present study, who was head of the local school in which the CYA had instituted its most extensive peer educator program, repeatedly referred in glowing terms to the positive contribution the CYA was making to young people in the local community and how the school found its support invaluable, because there was so little aid from the government.

The principal also insisted that despite his compassion for affected pupils, he did not have the resources or time to take any action in relation to AIDS (while informally estimating that up to 50% of his pupils might be HIV positive). He stated that the school could not address a problem of this magnitude without counseling and welfare backup: "If the 14 schools in this area were to take up this problem we would need a clinic, a psychologist, and a social worker to back us up." This seems like a reasonable requirement given that such an effort would involve more than 7000 pupils, many infected or affected by AIDS.

Lack of resources was often identified as a cause of loss of hope among people with AIDS. A support worker reported that "we visit people with AIDS in their homes and offer emotional support through counseling. But you find people expecting more from us because they are sick and don't have anything to eat. How can you motivate people to live positively if they are hungry?"

The CYA's work is further complicated by the dual leadership system that prevails in Ekuthuleni, with hereditary traditional chiefs existing side by side with municipal councillors elected according to political party affiliations (in this case, the African National Congress). According to CYA workers, the councillors tended to have a relatively progressive attitude toward women and sexuality that appealed to many young people. Traditional leaders tended to be more conservative, highly critical of sexually active young people, and supportive of the "policing" of young people's sexuality, particularly that of young women, through practices such as virginity testing.[26,27]

CYA employees stated that they had to take care not to offend either of these constituencies, usually through working with different sets of leaders on different occasions. For example, they might work with traditional leaders in setting up HIV/AIDS events on the more traditional Heritage Day, and they might work with councillors in setting up other types of HIV/AIDS activities on holidays such as June 16, which celebrates South Africa's history of radical political protest.

▶ Discussion

In unequal societies, social dynamics are often inherently conservative, and a series of multi-level symbolic, material, and institutional dynamics are in place that ensure that inequalities are perpetuated even in the face of challenges or resistance.[28,29] Foucault's work highlights the way in which power hierarchies are policed not only by *overt* systems of power and government (inherent in laws and police forces, for example) but also by *covert* systems of power: the internal "psychological policing" through which people at all levels of the social hierarchy are socialized to voluntarily behave in ways that support the status quo.[30] Integrating our Ekuthuleni findings with this theoretical frame, we argue that stigmatization is 1 form of covert psychological policing whereby those who breach power relations of gender, generation, or ethnicity are disciplined and punished. Stigmatization of people with AIDS serves as a mechanism for highlighting the literally fatal consequences that face young people or women who step out of line, for example.

High levels of HIV/AIDS among youth expose the previously hidden ways in which many young people in general, and young women in particular, have resisted adult attempts to control their sexuality (with such control playing a key role in the perpetuation of male and adult authority). They have done so through their active participation in a thriving sexual subculture.[10] In many ways, this subculture is a positive element in Ekuthuleni, part of young persons' assertion of energy and creativity in a community where they tend to be marginalized at best and denigrated at worst. Some of the excitement and mystique of this world comes from the fact that many aspects of young people's sexual relations take place away from the eyes of adults and are shrouded in secrecy. Yet, the secret nature of young people's participation in this world—secret not only from adults but often, in the case of girls, from each other—places it beyond the reach of the best-intentioned (and almost always adult-orchestrated) HIV prevention efforts.

The nature of this world also places it out of the reach of adults, such as parents. Many parents are particularly ill placed to contribute to the fight against HIV because of their (often well-founded) fear that their children are more worldly wise than they are in regard to much of the new way of life in South Africa. Their refusal or downright unwillingness to talk about AIDS is part and parcel of their attempt to maintain what they believe is their "traditional" or "cultural" right to dominance over young people.

Many authors have pointed to the important role the church has played in sanctioning and sustaining unequal relationships between men and women and between adults and young people, postulating a strong link between the moral order of the church and the sexuality of its members. The very public nature of the HIV/AIDS epidemic brings the church face to face with the dramatic contradictions between (1) its teachings that sex should take place only within the context of a faithful marriage and (2) the epidemic's very public and assertive evidence of the church's failure to reinforce these teachings. By implication, the existence of the HIV/AIDS epidemic highlights the loss of the church's moral authority. One of the strategies now being used by representatives of many churches to regain this lost moral authority is that of vigorously linking sexual transgressions and AIDS with sin, immorality, and, sometimes, even the end of the world.

In a similar way, the existence of the epidemic—drawing attention to the sexual activity of large numbers of people who are not located within monogamous marriages—highlights the lack of influence of traditional chiefs and the traditional leadership system over the sexuality of many women and young people. Supporters of traditional systems of authority seek to reassert this influence by reinstating old-fashioned practices such as virginity testing, rewarding girls who pass this test with "goods" ranging from enhanced social status to virginity certificates. In short, stigmatization of people with AIDS is part and parcel of a conservative reassertion of power relations of gender and generation and a public reinforcement of social institutions whose moral authority rested on their ability to control the sexuality of women and young people (or to at least be seen as controlling this sexuality at the level of rhetoric, if not at the level of reality, in the pre-AIDS days when it was easier for sexual "transgressors" to be discreet about their activities).

Stigmatization also serves as 1 aspect of a vicious reassertion of the racial and economic marginalization of many Black South Africans. At the symbolic level, the close link that several of our informants made between HIV/AIDS and Black African people both draws on and feeds back into negative stereotypes of Black people that have a long history in South Africa. At the material and political levels, stigmatization of people with AIDS dramatically undermines the likelihood that they or their families will stand up openly and challenge inadequate levels of social recognition and support in a society that often fails to acknowledge even their existence, let alone their needs and rights.

Much has been written about the way in which AIDS undermines the economic well-being of both sufferers and their families.[31,32] In the absence of appropriate medical and welfare treatment and support, people with AIDS and their families become trapped in a downward economic spiral that has extremely negative consequences for individual families and communities and threatens to undermine many of the development gains of recent years; examples are the negative effects of AIDS on life expectancies, which had previously been rising, and on the material well-being and morale of communities.[33]

▶ Implications for Intervention

Although the strategies of education and legislation are vital elements in the fight against stigma, they will not be adequate on their own. Communities need to be mobilized to engage in critical thinking about the wider webs of representation and practice that feed into stigmatization of people with AIDS. Arguments that provision of free and accessible medical treatment to people with AIDS will contribute to the end of stigma are increasingly common.[34] We have no doubt that a key facet of the fear and denial surrounding HIV/AIDS in many of the poorer countries where the disease flourishes is linked to its currently incurable status in the case of those who do not have access to drugs. However, we believe that even after treatment is available and HIV/AIDS is no longer fatal, the link between HIV/AIDS and "bad behavior" (i.e., sexual behavior) will still exist in ways that associate the disease with shame and embarrassment. In the absence of initiatives to tackle root social causes, the potential impact of treatment on stigma will be reduced.

Paulo Freire argued that marginalized groups are most likely to improve their circumstances in projects that simultaneously work to challenge the social conditions that contribute to their exclusion.[35,36] Writing in the context of HIV/AIDS among more confident and articulate groups residing in wealthier countries (e.g., gay men in San Francisco and Australia), researchers have pointed to the positive role of collective action by members of stigmatized groups.[5] These groups have often organized themselves in a strong and assertive way to improve their access to health services and challenge those who seek to discriminate against them.

In South Africa, the Treatment Action Campaign (TAC) has opened up the exciting possibility of collective action by people with AIDS, engaging in many high-profile actions highlighting the ways in which people's lives are blighted by various forms of interpersonal stigma and institutional discrimination.[37] CYA workers in Ekuthuleni were aware of the existence of the TAC and had invited individual TAC speakers to address local meetings on different occasions. However, much work remains to be done to extend the reach of this high-profile organization in South Africa and to mobilize collective action by people in the marginalized communities (such as Ekuthuleni) within which many of the country's people with AIDS reside.

Furthermore, the necessary support must be in place if people are to be expected to disclose their HIV status even to 1 close friend or family member, let alone stand on public platforms asserting their rights and needs. Freire would contend that a key stage in doing the necessary groundwork would be development of critical thinking about the social roots of the problem of stigma and about the social obstacles standing in the way of its solution.

We agree with Freire and argue that an important first step toward mobilizing people with AIDS would involve initiatives that work toward facilitating the participation of local community groups in critical thinking programs. Such programs would aim to expose, confront, and resist the webs of signification and practice that sustain stigma and undermine the confidence of communities and individuals who might otherwise challenge it. Our case study suggests that, in contexts such as Ekuthuleni, programs could include critical thinking about the marginalization of young people and women, denial of young people's sexuality, and, more particularly, denial of the sexual activities of women. Programs might also seek to generate critical thinking about the ways in which social institutions such as the church, the family, and the traditional leadership system do or do not contribute to these forms of marginalization and denial, which are so undermining of effective HIV prevention and the humane treatment and care of people with AIDS.

Such critical thinking might also seek to challenge the fictional notion that young people of the current generation are necessarily more sexually active than those of earlier generations. It might seek as well to deconstruct and challenge the distinction between "good" and "bad" behavior and, particularly, the invariable association of sex outside faithful marriage with "bad" behavior. Finally, it might highlight the possibility that sexual activity need not "destroy" a young woman's life if she is discreet and protects her sexual health.

Our case study highlights the gap between rhetoric and reality in terms of the way in which people often seek to give the impression that they or other family members are sexually inactive or HIV/AIDS free when, behind this curtain of social desirability, the truth might be very different. It also highlights the way in which the conventions of what constitutes social desirability may often both feed on and perpetuate unequal power relations between young and old, men and women, Black and White, and rich and poor. Community participation has a key role to play in promoting forms of critical consciousness that both expose and challenge the unequal social relations drawn on and sustained by stigma. As such, it should stand alongside education and legislation as a powerful weapon against stigma.

▶ About the Authors

Catherine Campbell is with the Department of Social Psychology, London School of Economics and Political Science, London, England, and the Centre for HIV/AIDS Networking, University of KwaZulu Natal, KwaZulu-Natal, South Africa. At the time of this study, Carol Ann Foulis was with the Centre for HIV/AIDS Networking, University of KwaZulu-Natal. Sbongile Maimane and Zweni Sibiya are with the Centre for HIV/AIDS Networking, University of KwaZulu-Natal.

Requests for reprints should be sent to Catherine Campbell, PhD, Social Psychology, London School of Economics, Houghton Street, London WC2A 2AE, England (email: c.campbell@lse.ac.uk).

This article was accepted July 27, 2004.

▶ Contributors

C. Campbell conceptualized and designed the study, analyzed the data, and wrote the article. C. A. Foulis established and maintained the partnership between the researchers and the study community and managed the data collection. S. Maimane and Z. Sibiya conducted the field-work and kept detailed fieldworker diaries. All of the authors engaged in discussions of every aspect of the research.

▶ Acknowledgments

We are grateful to Mpume Nzama and colleagues at the Christian Youth Alliance and to Eleanor Preston-Whyte and Debbie Heustice from the Centre for HIV/AIDS Networking for enabling this research. We also wish to thank the Atlantic Philanthropies and the Carnegie Corporation of New York, whose grants made this study possible.

Note. The views expressed in this article are those of the authors alone and do not necessarily reflect the views of the Christian Youth Alliance, the Centre for HIV/AIDS Networking, or the funding agencies.

References

1. *Stigma and AIDS in Africa: Setting an Operational Research Agenda.* Dar es Salaam, Tanzania: Joint United Nations Programme on HIV/AIDS; 2001.

2. Hayes R, Vaughan C. Stigma directed toward chronic illness is resistant to change through education and exposure. *Psychol Rep.* 2002;90:1161–1173.

3. Parker R, Aggleton P. HIV and AIDS-related stigma and discrimination: a conceptual framework and implications for action. *Soc Sci Med.* 2003;57:13–24.

4. Campbell C. *Letting Them Die: Why HIV/AIDS Prevention Programmes Fail.* Bloomington, Ind: Indiana University Press; 2003.

5. Joffe H. *Risk and the Other.* Cambridge, England: Cambridge University Press; 1999.

6. Jost J, Banaji M. The role of stereotyping in system-justification and the production of false consciousness. *Br J Soc Psychol.* 1994;33:1–27.

7. Joffe H, Begetta N. Social representations of AIDS among Zambian adolescents. *J Health Psychol.* 2003;8: 616–631.

8. Crawford R. The boundaries of the self and the unhealthy other: reflections on health, culture and AIDS. *Soc Sci Med.* 1994;38:1347–1365.

9. Treichler P. AIDS, homophobia and biomedical discourse. In: Crimp D, ed. *AIDS: Cultural Analysis/Cultural Activism.* Cambridge, Mass: MIT Press; 1988: 164–182.

10. Posel D. "Getting the nation talking about sex": reflections on the politics of sexuality and "nation-building" in post-apartheid South Africa. *Afr Aff.* In press.

11. Gaitskell D. "Wailing for purity": purity unions, African mothers and adolescent daughters, 1912–1940. In: Marks S, Rathbone R, eds. *Industrialisation and Social Change in South Africa: African Class Formation, Culture and Consciousness, 1870–1930.* Harlow, England: Longman; 1982:338–357.

12. Marks S. Patriotism, patriarchy and purity: Natal and the politics of Zulu ethnic consciousness. In: Vail L, ed. *The Creation of Tribalism in Southern Africa.* Berkeley, Calif: University of California Press; 1989: 226–247.

13. Shisana O. *Nelson Mandela/HSRC Study of HIV/AIDS: South African National HIV Prevalence, Behavioral Risks and Mass Media.* Cape Town, South Africa: Human Sciences Research Council; 2002.

14. South African Department of Health. Summary report: National HIV and syphilis antenatal seroprevalence survey in South Africa, 2002. Available at: http://www.doh.gov.za/aids/index.html. Accessed December 1, 2002.

15. Flick U. *An Introduction to Qualitative Research.* 2nd ed. London, England: Sage Publications; 2002.

16. Pryor J, Reeder G. Collective and individual representations of HIV/AIDS stigma. In: Pryor J, Reeder G, eds. *The Social Psychology of HIV Infection.* London, England: Lawrence Erlbaum Associates; 1993: 263–286.

17. Leclerc-Madlala S. On the virgin cleansing myth: gendered bodies, AIDS and ethnomedicine. *Afr J AIDS Res.* 2002;1:87–95.

18. MacPhail C, Campbell C. 'I think condoms are good but, aai, I hate those things': condom use among adolescents and young people in a southern African township. *Soc Sci Med.* 2001;52:1613–1627.

19. Campbell C. Intergenerational conflict in township families: transforming notions of "respect" and changing power relations. *S Afr J Gerontol.* 1994;3:150–159.

20. Campbell C, Foulis CA, Maimane S, Sibiya Z. *Supporting Youth: Broadening the Approach to HIV/AIDS Prevention Programmes.* Durban, South Africa: Centre for HIV/AIDS Networking; 2004.

21. Moser C. The asset vulnerability framework: reassessing urban poverty reduction strategies. *World Dev.* 1998;26:1–19.

22. Baum F. Social capital: is it good for your health? Issues for a public health agenda [editorial]. *J Epidemiol Community Health.* 1999;53:195–196.

23. Hogg M, Abrams D. *Social Identifications.* Oxford, England: Blackwell; 1988.

24. Campbell C. The social identity of township youth (part 1): an extension of social identity theory. *S Afr J Psychol.* 1995;25:150–159.

25. Campbell C. The social identity of township youth (part 2): social identity theory and gender. *S Afr J Psychol.* 1995;25:160–167.

26. Scorgie F. Virginity testing and the politics of sexual responsibility: implications for AIDS intervention. *Afr Stud.* 2002;61:55–75.

27. Geisler G. "Women are women *or* how to please your husband": initiation ceremonies and the politics of "tradition" in southern Africa. In: Goddard V, ed. *Gender, Agency and Change: Anthropological Perspectives.* London, England: Routledge; 2000:203–229.

28. Bourdieu P. The forms of capital. In: Richardson J, ed. *Handbook of Theory and Research for the Sociology of Education.* New York, NY: Greenwood Press; 1986: 241–248.

29. Bourdieu P. *Distinction: A Social Critique of the Judgement of Taste.* Cambridge, England: Cambridge University Press; 1984.

30. Rose N. *Governing the Soul: The Shaping of the Private Self.* New York, NY: Routledge; 1991.

31. Barnett T, Whiteside A. *AIDS in the 21st Century: Disease and Globalisation.* New York, NY: Palgrave Macmillan; 2002.

32. Nattrass N. *The Moral Economy of AIDS in South Africa.* Cambridge, England: Cambridge University Press; 2004.

33. Nnko S, Chiduo B, Wilson F, Msuya W, Mwaluko G. Tanzania: AIDS care—learning from experience. *Rev Afr Political Economy.* 2000;86:547–557.

34. Cameron E. Speech to the Second Annual Conference of People Living with AIDS, Durban, South Africa, 10 March 2000. Available at: http://www.tac.org.za. Accessed September 20, 2003.

35. Freire P. *The Pedagogy of the Oppressed.* London, England: Penguin Books; 1993.

36. Freire P. *Education for Critical Consciousness.* New York, NY: Continuum; 1993.

37. Treatment Action Campaign. About TAC. Available at: http://www.tac.org.za. Accessed September 20, 2003.

Culture, Poverty and HIV Transmission
The Case of Rural Haiti

Paul Farmer

Violent deaths are natural deaths here. He died of his environment.
DR. MAGIOT, IN GRAHAM GREENE'S *The Comedians, 1966*

The preceding chapter describes some of the important work regarding HIV transmission that has been conducted in urban Haiti over the course of the past fifteen years. Haiti, however, a country of well over seven million inhabitants, is generally considered to be a substantially rural nation,[1] and it is significant that few studies of HIV transmission have been conducted in rural parts of the country. As the ties that link rural and urban Haiti are economically and affectively strong, an understanding of the urban epidemic is a necessary prologue to an investigation of HIV transmission in rural areas, the subject of this chapter.

Early reports by Pape and Johnson, based on small studies conducted in 1986–87, noted that the seroprevalence rate for HIV averaged 3 percent "in rural areas."[2] The seroprevalence in 97 mothers of children hospitalized with dehydration was 3 percent; of 245 unscreened rural blood donors, 4 percent had antibodies to HIV. In an area even more distant from urban centers, only 1 percent of 191 adults who came for immunizations were seropositive. Unfortunately, we know little about the individuals bled for these studies. Just how rural were they? What was the nature of their ties to Port-au-Prince and other high-prevalence cities? How did the seropositive individuals come to be at risk for HIV? How did they differ from seronegative controls? How rapidly was HIV making inroads into the rural population? What, in short, are the dynamics of HIV transmission in rural Haiti?

To understand the rural Haitian AIDS epidemic, we must move beyond the concept of "risk groups" to consider the interplay between human agency and the powerful forces that constrain it, focusing especially on those activities that promote or retard the spread of HIV. In Haiti, the most powerful of these forces have been inequality, deepening poverty, and political dislocations, which have together conspired to hasten the spread of HIV. This chapter details research on HIV transmission in a rural area of Haiti—and also recounts some of the ways such large-scale social forces become manifest in the lives of particular individuals.

▶ AIDS in a Haitian Village

The setting for the research described here is the Péligre basin of Haiti's Central Plateau, home to several hundred thousand mostly rural people. Although all parts of Haiti are poor, the Péligre basin region and its villages may be especially so.

Before 1956, the village of Kay was situated in a deep and fertile valley in this area, near the banks of the Rivière Artibonite. For generations, the villagers farmed the broad and gently sloping banks of the river, selling rice, bananas, millet, corn, and sugarcane in regional markets. Harvests were, by all reports, bountiful; life then is now recalled as idyllic. With the construction of Haiti's largest hydroelectric dam in 1956, however, thousands of families living in this region were flooded out. The displaced persons were largely peasant farmers, and they received little or no compensation for their lost land.

The hilltop village of Do Kay was founded by refugees from the rising water. The flooding of the valley forced most villagers up into the hills on either side of the new reservoir. Kay became divided into "Do" (those who settled on the stony backs of the hills) and "Ba" (those who remained down near the new waterline). By all standard measures, both parts of Kay are now very poor; its older inhabitants often blame their poverty on the massive buttress dam a few miles away and note bitterly that it brought them neither electricity nor water.

Though initially a dusty squatter settlement of fewer than two hundred persons, Do Kay has grown rapidly in the past decade and now counts about two thousand inhabitants. In spite of the hostile conditions, most families continue to rely to some extent on small-scale agriculture. But many villagers are involved in a series of development projects designed to improve the health of the area's inhabitants. Since 1984, for example, a series of outreach initiatives have complemented the work of our growing team of clinicians, based in Do Kay at the Clinique Bon Sauveur. The most significant efforts were undertaken under the aegis of Proje Veye Sante, the "health surveillance project." Proje Veye Sante, conducted in large part by village-based community health workers from about thirty nearby communities, provides preventive and primary care to close to fifty thousand rural people.

Through Proje Veye Sante, AIDS surveillance began well before the epidemic was manifest in the region. It is thus possible to date the index, or first, case of AIDS to 1986, when a young schoolteacher, Manno Surpris, fell ill with recurrent superficial fungal infections, chronic diarrhea, and pulmonary tuberculosis. Seropositive for HIV, he died a year later.[3]

Although Manno Surpris was from another part of the Central Plateau, it was not long before we began to diagnose the syndrome among natives of Do Kay. The sections that follow offer brief case histories of the first three villagers known to have died of AIDS. None had a history of transfusion with blood or blood products; none had a history of homosexual contact or other "risk factors" as designated by the CDC. They did, however, share two important, if poorly understood, risk factors: poverty and inequality.

Anita

Anita Joseph was born in approximately 1966 to a family that had lost its land to the Péligre dam. One of six children, she briefly attended school until her mother, weakened by the malnutrition then rampant in the Kay area, died of tuberculosis. Anita was then thirteen. Her father became depressed and abusive, and she resolved to run away: "I'd had it with his yelling. . . . When I saw how poor I was, and how hungry, and saw that it would never get any better, I had to go to the city. Back then I was so skinny—I was saving my life, I thought, by getting out of here."

Anita left for Port-au-Prince with less than $3 and no clear plan of action. She worked briefly as a *restavèk*, or live-in maid, for $10 a month but lost this position when her employer was herself fired from a factory job.

Cast into the street, Anita eventually found a relative who took her in. The kinswoman, who lived in a notorious slum north of the capital, introduced her to Vincent, a young man who worked unloading luggage at the airport. Anita was not yet fifteen when she entered her first and only sexual union. "What could I do, really?" she sighed as she recounted the story much later. "He had a good job. My aunt thought I should go with him."

Vincent, who had at least one other sexual partner at the time, became ill less than two years after they began sharing a room. The young man, whom Anita cared for throughout his illness, died after repeated infections, including tuberculosis. Not long after his death, Anita herself fell ill with tuberculosis.

Upon returning to Do Kay in 1987, she quickly responded to anti-tuberculous therapy. When she relapsed some months later, we performed an HIV test, which revealed the true cause of her immunosuppression. Following a slow but ineluctable decline, Anita died in February 1988.

Dieudonné

Dieudonné Gracia, born in Do Kay in 1963, was also the child of two "water refugees." One of seven children, he attended primary school in his home village and, briefly, secondary school in a nearby town. It was there, at the age of nineteen, that he had his first sexual contact. Dieudonné remarked that his girlfriend had had "two, maybe three partners" before they met; he was sure that one of her partners had been a truck driver from a city in central Haiti.

When a series of setbacks further immiserated his family, Dieudonné was forced to drop out of secondary school and also to drop his relationship with the young woman. He returned to Do Kay to work with his father, a carpenter. In 1983, however, the young man decided to "try my luck in Port-au-Prince." Through a friend from Do Kay, Dieudonné found a position as a domestic for a well-to-do family in a suburb of the capital.

While in the city, Dieudonné's sexual experience broadened considerably. He had five partners in little more than two years, all of them close to his own age. Asked about the brevity of these liaisons, Dieudonné favored an economic explanation: "A couple of them let go of me because they saw that I couldn't do anything for them. They saw that I couldn't give them anything for any children."

In 1985, Dieudonné became ill and was dismissed from his job in Port-au-Prince. He returned to Do Kay and began seeing his former lover again. She soon became pregnant and moved to Do Kay as the young man's *plase*, a term designating a partner in a more or less stable conjugal union.[4]

During this interlude, Dieudonné was seen at the Do Kay clinic for a number of problems that suggested immunodeficiency: herpes zoster and genital herpes, recurrent diarrhea, and weight loss. In the months following the birth of their baby, the young mother fell ill with a febrile illness, thought by her physician to be malaria, and quickly succumbed. Less than a year later, Dieudonné, much reduced by chronic diarrhea, was diagnosed with tuberculosis. Although he initially responded to antituberculous agents, Dieudonné died of AIDS in October 1988.

Acéphie

Acéphie Joseph was born in 1965 on a small knoll protruding into the reservoir that had drowned her parents' land. Acéphie attended primary school somewhat irregularly; by the age of nineteen, she had not yet graduated and decided that it was time to help generate income for her family, which was sinking deeper and deeper into poverty. Hunger was a near-daily occurrence for the Joseph family; the times were as bad as those right after the flooding of the valley. Acéphie began to help her mother, a market woman, by carrying produce to a local market on Friday mornings.

It was there that she met a soldier, formerly stationed in Port-au-Prince, who began to make overtures to the striking young woman from Do Kay. Although the soldier had a wife and children and was known to have more than one regular partner, Acéphie did not spurn him. "What would you have me do? I could tell that the old people were uncomfortable, worried—but they didn't say no. They didn't tell me to stay away from him. I wish they had, but how could they have known? . . . I looked around and saw how poor we all were, how the old people were finished. . . . It was a way out, that's how I saw it."

Within a short time, the soldier fell ill and was diagnosed in the Do Kay clinic with AIDS. A few months after he and Acéphie parted, he was dead.

Shaken, Acéphie went to a nearby town and began a course in what she euphemistically termed a "cooking school," which prepared poor girls for work as servants. In 1987, twenty-two years old, Acéphie went to Port-au-Prince, where she found a $30-per-month job as a housekeeper for a middle-class Haitian woman who worked for the U.S. embassy. She began to see a man, also from the Kay region, who chauffeured a small bus between the Central Plateau and Port-au-Prince.

Acéphie worked in the city until late in 1989, when she discovered that she was pregnant. This displeased both her partner and her employer. Sans job and sans boyfriend, Acéphie returned to Do Kay in her third trimester.

Following the birth of her daughter, Acéphie was sapped by repeated opportunistic infections, each one caught in time by the staff of the clinic in Do Kay. Throughout 1991, however, she continued to lose weight; by January 1992, she weighed less than ninety pounds, and her intermittent fevers did not respond to broad-spectrum antibiotics.

Acéphie died in April 1992. Her daughter, the first "AIDS orphan" in Do Kay, is now in the care of Acéphie's mother. The child is also infected. A few months after Acéphie's death, her father hanged himself.

Sadly, however, this is not simply the story of Acéphie and her family. The soldier's wife, who is much thinner than last year, has already had a case of herpes zoster. Two of her children are also HIV-positive. This woman, who is well known to the clinic staff, is no longer a widow; once again, she is the partner of a military man. Her late husband had at least two other partners, both of them poor peasant women, in the Central Plateau. One is HIV-positive and has two sickly children. The father of Acéphie's child, apparently in good health, is still plying the roads from Mirebalais to Port-au-Prince. His serostatus is unknown.

Individual Experience in Context

When compared to age-matched North Americans with AIDS, Anita, Dieudonné, and Acéphie have sparse sexual histories: Anita had only one partner; Dieudonné had six; Acéphie had two. Although a case-control study by Pape and Johnson suggested that HIV-infected urban men, at least, had larger numbers of partners than our patients did,[5] research conducted in Anita's neighborhood in Port-au-Prince suggests that her case is not as unique as it would seem:

> The high seropositivity rate (8%) found in pregnant women 14 to 19 years of age suggests that women [in Cité Soleil] appear to acquire HIV infection soon after becoming sexually active. Moreover, this age group is the only one in which a higher seropositivity rate is not associated with a greater number of sexual partners. Women with only one sexual partner in the year prior to pregnancy actually have a slightly higher prevalence rate (although not significantly so) than the others. This suggests that they were infected by their first and only partner.[6]

The stories of Anita, Dieudonné, and Acéphie are ones that reveal the push-and-pull forces of contemporary Haiti. In all three cases, the declining fortunes of the rural poor pushed young adults to try their chances in the city. Once there, all three became entangled in unions that the women, at least, characterized as attempts to emerge from poverty. Each worked as a domestic, but none managed to fulfill the expectation of saving and sending home desperately needed cash. What they brought home, instead, was AIDS.

How representative are these case histories? Over the past several years, the medical staff of the Clinique Bon Sauveur has diagnosed dozens more cases of AIDS and other forms of HIV infection in women who arrive at the clinic with a broad range of complaints. In fact, the majority of our patients have been women—a pattern rarely described in the AIDS literature. With surprisingly few exceptions, those so diagnosed shared a number of risk factors, as our modest case-control study suggests.

We conducted this study by interviewing the first twenty-five women we diagnosed with symptomatic HIV infection who were residents of Do Kay or its two neighboring villages. Their responses to questions posed during a series of open-ended interviews were compared with those of twenty-five age-matched, seronegative controls. In both groups, ages ranged from 16 to 44, with a mean age of about 27 years. Table 14.2 presents our findings.

None of these fifty women had a history of prostitution, and none had used illicit drugs. Only two, both members of the control group, had received blood transfusions. None of the women in either group had had more than five sexual partners in the course of their lives; in fact, seven of the afflicted women had had only one. Although women in the study group had

TABLE 14.2 Case-Control Study of AIDS in Rural Haitian Women

Patient Characteristics	Patients with AIDS (N = 25)	Control Group (N = 25)
Average number of sexual partners	2.7	2.4
Sexual partner of a truck driver	12	2
Sexual partner of a soldier	9	0
Sexual partner of a peasant only	0	23
Ever lived in Port-au-Prince	20	4
Worked as a servant	18	1
Average number of years of formal schooling	4.5	4.0
Ever received a blood transfusion	0	2
Ever used illicit drugs	0	0
Ever received more than ten intramuscular injections	17	19

on average more sexual partners than the controls, the difference is not striking. Similarly, we found no clear difference between the two groups in the number of intramuscular injections they had received or their years of education.

The chief risk factors in this small cohort seem to involve not number of partners but rather the professions of these partners. Fully nineteen of the women with HIV disease had histories of sexual contact with soldiers or truck drivers. Three of these women reported having only two sexual partners: one a soldier, one a truck driver. Of the women diagnosed with AIDS, none had a history of sexual contact exclusively with peasants (although one had as sole partner a construction worker from Do Kay). Among the control group, only two women had a regular partner who was a truck driver; none reported contact with soldiers, and most had had sexual relations only with peasants from the region. Histories of extended residence in Port-au-Prince and work as a domestic were also strongly associated with a diagnosis of HIV disease.

How can we make sense of these surprising results? In the socio-graphically "flat" region around the dam—after all, most area residents share a single socioeconomic status, poverty—conjugal unions with non-peasants (salaried soldiers and truck drivers who are paid on a daily basis) reflect women's quest for some measure of economic security. In the setting of a worsening economic crisis, the gap between the hungry peasant class and the relatively well-off soldiers and truck drivers became the salient local inequality. In this manner, truck drivers and soldiers have served as a "bridge" from the city to the rural population, just as North American tourists seemed to have served as a bridge to the urban Haitian population.

But just as North Americans are no longer important in the transmission of HIV in Haiti, truck drivers and soldiers will soon no longer be necessary components of the rural epidemic. Once introduced into a sexually active population, HIV will work its way to those with no history of residence in the city, no history of contact with soldiers or truck drivers no history of work as a domestic. But these risk factors—all of which reflect a desperate attempt to escape rural poverty—are emblematic of the lot of the rural Haitian poor, and perhaps especially of poor women.

HIV in a Haitian Village

Extended residence in Port-au-Prince, work as a servant, and sexual contact with nonpeasants—although these risk factors were far different from those described for North Americans with AIDS, they characterized the majority of our male and female patients afflicted with AIDS. The majority of the residents of the area served by Proje Veye Sante shared none of these attributes, however. Did this suggest that few would prove to be infected with HIV? Although a good deal of ethnographic research into the nature of AIDS had already been conducted in the region, no research had addressed the question of HIV prevalence among asymptomatic adults.

Troubled by this lacuna, the staff of the clinic and of Proje Veye Sante established the Groupe d'étude du SIDA dans la Classe Paysanne.[7] GESCAP has a mandate to research the mechanisms by which poverty puts young adults, and especially young women, at risk of HIV infection.[8] With community approval, GESCAP is attempting to illuminate case histories with serologic surveys, an expanded case-control study, and cluster studies (such as those that revealed how a single HIV-positive soldier came to infect at least eleven natives of the region, one of whom was Acéphie).

After considerable discussion, the members of GESCAP decided to undertake a study of all asymptomatic adults living in Do Kay. The study was to include all members of the community who might plausibly be sexually active (fifteen years and older) and who were free of any suggestion of immunodeficiency; patients with active tuberculosis were excluded from this study. Anyone who was the regular sexual partner of a person with known HIV infection was also excluded.

Of the first one hundred villagers enrolling in the program, ninety-nine were seronegative for HIV.[9] The one young woman with HIV infection, Alourdes, had a history of extended residence in Port-au-Prince and also in 1985 of regular sexual contact with a salaried employee of the national electric company. This man, who had several sexual partners during his tenure in central Haiti, was rumored to have died of AIDS. In 1986, Alourdes had been the partner of a young man from her home village, a construction worker. He later developed tuberculosis, initially attributed to respiratory contact with his wife, who had pulmonary tuberculosis. Both were later found to be infected with HIV; neither had ever had sexual contact outside the Do Kay area. The discovery of HIV infection in Alourdes, who was known to have risk factors as defined in the case-control study, helped to identify the routes of exposure of the couple who had HIV-related tuberculosis.

Such discrete studies do not, however, fully define the nature of the large-scale social forces at work. The discussion in the following sections summarizes the factors that seem to be most significant in the ultimate rate of progression of HIV in rural Haiti. Perhaps an examination of these forces can serve to inform understandings of the dynamics of HIV transmission in other parts of Latin America and also in areas of Asia and Africa where prevalence rates in rural regions are currently low. It is a cautionary tale that argues for aggressive preventive measures.

> If a disaster is to be prevented in rural Haiti, vigorous and effective prevention campaigns must be initiated at once. And although such efforts must begin, the prospects of stopping the steady march of HIV are slim. AIDS is far more likely to join a host of other sexually transmitted diseases—including gonorrhea, syphilis, genital herpes, chlamydia, hepatitis B, lymphogranuloma venereum, and even cervical cancer—that have already become entrenched among the poor.[10]

Only massive and coordinated efforts may yet avert the ongoing disaster that has befallen urban Haiti, Puerto Rico, inner-city North America, Thailand, Brazil, and many nations in sub-Saharan Africa.

▶ The Dynamics of HIV Transmission in Rural Haiti

Wherever HIV infection is a sexually transmitted disease, social forces necessarily determine its distribution. Cultural, political, and economic factors, while each inevitably important, cannot be of equal significance in all settings. In rural Haiti, we can identify a number of differentially weighted, synergistic forces that promote HIV transmission.

Population Pressures

Haiti, which covers 27,700 square kilometers, is one of the most crowded societies in the hemisphere. In 1980, only 8,000 square kilometers were under cultivation, giving an effective population density of 626 persons per square kilometer. Unfortunately, Haiti's topsoil is now prey, to runaway forces that further compound the overcrowding: "The land suffers from defor-estation, soil erosion and exhaustion; the country is periodically ravaged by hurricanes which cause enormous damage."[11] As the land becomes increasingly exhausted, more and more peasants abandon agriculture for the lure of wage-labor in cities and towns.

Indeed, one of the most striking recent demographic changes has been the rapid growth of Port-au-Prince. More than 20 percent of the Haitian population now lives in the capital, a city of over 1.5 million. Although this concentration is not impressive by Caribbean standards (more than 30 percent of Puerto Ricans live in San Juan), the rate of growth in Port-au-Prince has been striking: "The urban population was 12.2% of the total in 1950, 20.4% in 1971 and an estimated 27.5% in 1980."[12] Haitian demographers estimate that by the year 2000 urban dwellers will constitute 37 percent of the total population.

As is the case with so many Third World countries, internal migration has played the most significant role in the growth of the capital, Locher estimates that "between 1950 and 1971 rural-urban migration accounted for 59% of Haitian urban growth, while natural population increase accounted for only 8%."[13] Neptune-Anglade has observed that the growth of Port-au-Prince is substantially the result of a "feminine rural exodus," leaving the city approximately 60 percent female.[14] Younger women of rural origin—women like Anita and Acéphie—are most commonly employed as servants.[15] Migrants of both sexes maintain strong ties with their regions of origin. In these respects, the three index cases of AIDS from Do Kay are illustrative of the trends documented by demographers and others who speak of Port-au-Prince as "a city of peasants."

Economic Pressures

Rural Haiti, always poor, has become palpably poorer in recent decades. A per capita annual income of $315 in 1983 masked the fact that income hovered around $100 in the countryside; in the late 1990s the average annual per capita income is down to around $175.[16] Accompanying the population growth and a loss of arable land to erosion and alkalinization has been an inevitable growth in landlessness. All of these factors have inevitably had a devastating effect on agricultural production. For example, Girault typifies the decade preceding 1984 as marked chiefly "by the slow-down of agricultural production and by a decrease in productivity."[17]

This decline has been further compounded by striking rural-urban disparities in every imaginable type of goods and service. In 1984, Girault was able to complain that "Port-au-Prince with 17–18% of the national population consumes as much as 30% of all the food produced in the country and a larger share of imported food."[18] Government statistics reveal that the "Port-au-Prince agglomeration" consumed 93 percent of all electricity produced in the country in 1979. As Trouillot notes, the city "houses 20% of the national population, but consumes 80% of all State expenditures."[19]

In short, current economic conditions push people out of the country-side and into the city or, often enough, out of the country altogether. The Haitian people have long since left behind a peasant standard of living (which did not necessarily mean an exceptionally low one). Whereas Haiti was once a nation with an extremely high percentage of landholders, late-twentieth-century Haiti is increasingly a country of unemployed and landless paupers. When the Population Crisis Committee published its "international index of human suffering" in 1992, based on a variety of measures of human welfare, Haiti had the dubious distinction of heading the list of all countries in this hemisphere. Of the 141 countries studied, only three were deemed to have living conditions worse than those in Haiti—and all three of these countries were at the time being consumed by civil war.[20]

Patterns of Sexual Union

In the numerous studies of conjugal unions in rural Haiti, most have underlined the classic division between couples who are *marye* (joined by civil or religious marriage) and those who are *plase* (joined in a conjugal union that incurs significant and enduring obligations to both partners). *Plasaj* (from French, *plaçage*) has generally been the most common form of conjugal union in rural Haiti, outnumbering marriages by two or three to one.

Early studies usually considered *plasaj* to be polygamous, with one man having more than one *plase* partner. This is often no longer the case, as Moral suggested over three decades ago: "It is 'plaçage honnête'—that is, monogamy—that best characterizes matrimonial status in today's rural society."[21] The reason for this shift toward monogamy, he believed, was the same one that leads many rural people to avoid marriage in the first place: formal unions are costly. "If the considerable growth of *plaçage* is to be explained in part by economic factors," continued Moral, "the form that *plaçage* now takes is greatly influenced by the poverty spreading throughout the countryside."

Allman's review suggests that contemporary sexual unions are considerably more complex than the bipolar model just described. In a survey in which women who had sexual relations with the same partner for a minimum of three months were considered to be "in union," interviews revealed an emic typology with five major categories: three of these—*rinmin, fiyanse,* and *viv avèk*—did not usually involve cohabitation and engendered only slight economic support; two others—*plase* and *marye*—were deemed much stronger unions, generally involving cohabitation as well as economic support.[22]

In addition, a number of other sexual practices have often been loosely termed "prostitution," in Haiti a largely urban phenomenon and much understudied.[23] It is clear, however, that unemployed women from rural areas may become involved in occasional and often clandestine sex work (variously described by terms such as *ti degaje, woulman*) when other options are exhausted. There are few avenues of escape for those caught in the web of urban migration, greater than 60 percent unemployment, and extreme poverty.[24]

How are these forms of sexual union related to the dynamics of HIV transmission? To those working in rural clinics, *plasaj* is often implicated in the spread or persistence of sexually transmitted diseases such as gonorrhea and chlamydial disease. Treatment of one or two members of a network is of course inadequate, as even women who have but one sexual partner are indirectly in regular sexual contact with any other *plase* partners of their mate. Regarding HIV, polygamous *plasaj* may be considered a preexisting sociocultural institution that serves to speed the spread of HIV and that constitutes a risk in and of itself, particularly for monogamous women. Women throughout the world bear similar risks—which are compounded wherever gender inequality erodes women's power over condom use.

The unremitting immiseration of Haiti has clearly undermined stable patterns of union such as marriage and *plasaj* by creating economic pressures to which women with dependents are particularly vulnerable. In the wake of these pressures, new patterns have emerged: "serial monogamy" might describe the monogamous but weak unions that lead to one child but last little longer than a year or two. After such unions have dissolved, the woman finds herself with a new dependent and even more in need of a reliable partner.

Equally dangerous, as we have seen, is the quest for a union with a financially "secure" partner. In rural Haiti, men of this description once included a substantial fraction of all peasant landholders. In recent decades, however, financial security has become elusive for all but a handful of truck drivers, representatives of the state (such as soldiers and petty officials), and landholders (*grandòn*). As noted, truck drivers and soldiers are clearly groups with above average rates of HIV infection.

Gender Inequality

"The ability of young women to protect themselves from [HIV] infection becomes a direct function of power relations between men and women."[25] Gender inequality has weakened women's ability to negotiate safe sexual encounters, and this sapping of agency is especially amplified by poverty. The Haitian economy counts a higher proportion of economically active women—most of them traders—than any other developing society, with the exception of Lesotho.[26] It is not surprising, then, that the *machismo* that has so marked other Latin American societies is less pronounced in Haiti.[27] (Even the head of the Duvaliers' dreaded paramilitary force was a woman.) But gender inequality is certainly a force in political, economic, and domestic life. It would be difficult to argue with Neptune-Anglade when she states that, in all regards, rural women "endure a discrimination and a pauperization that is worse than that affecting [rural] men."[28]

Preliminary ethnographic research in the Do Kay area suggests that many rural women do not wield sufficient authority to demand that *plase* partners (or husbands) use condoms. A growing literature documents similar patterns throughout the developing world and in the inner cities of the United States.[29] These considerations lead us to agree with those calling for preventive efforts that are "women-centered." "In societies where the female has a weaker hand," Desvarieux and Pape argue, "effective methods of prevention have a better chance of working if the woman does not have to rely on either the consent or the willingness of her partner."[30]

Other "Cultural" Considerations

Practices such as the widespread and unregulated use of syringes by "folk" practitioners unschooled in aseptic techniques received a fair amount of attention as possible sources of HIV transmission. But far more frequently invoked were "voodoo practices," which played a peculiarly central role in early speculations about the nature of the AIDS epidemic. These speculations, which sparked waves of anti-Haitian sentiment, had the added disadvantage of being incorrect; none of these leads, when investigated, panned out. In urban Haiti, GHESKIO did not even consider these hypotheses worthy of serious investigation.

In our small-scale but in-depth study of AIDS in the Central Plateau, we did not find any strong implication of nonsexual transmission of HIV.[31] Similarly, the Collaborative Study Group of AIDS in Haitian-Americans initiated the first and (so far) only controlled study of risk factors for AIDS among Haitians living in the United States. Compiling data from several North American research centers, the investigators reached the following conclusion: "Folklore rituals have been suggested as potential risk factors for [HIV] transmission in Haiti. Our data do not support this hypothesis."[32] Such hypotheses reflect less an accurate reading of existing data and more a series of North American folk theories about Haitians.[33]

There have been few ethnographic studies of Haitian understandings of AIDS, and most of these have been conducted in Montreal, New York, or Miami. To my knowledge, the only such study conducted in rural Haiti demonstrated that such understandings were in fact changing, at first quite rapidly. Over time, however, a stable illness representation of *sida*—as AIDS is termed—seemed to evolve.[34]

In the Do Kay region, serial interviews with the same group of villagers permitted us to delineate a complex model of illness causation, one linked fairly closely to understandings of tuberculosis. Villagers often, but not always, cited sorcery in discussions about *sida*, which nonetheless came to be seen as a fatal illness that could be transmitted by sexual contact. Local understandings of *sida* did not seem to affect disease distribution, but certainly they may hamper preventive efforts if not taken into account when designing interventions. Far more disabling, however, has been the nation's political situation.

Political Disruption

It is unfortunate indeed that HIV arrived in Haiti shortly before a period of massive and prolonged social upheaval. Political unrest has clearly undermined preventive efforts and may have helped, through other mechanisms, to spread HIV. Although many commentators observed that political struggles served to divert the public's interest away from AIDS, this was not the case in the Do Kay region. In fact, periods of increased strife were associated with increased public discourse about the new sickness.

But the same political disruptions that may have stimulated commentary about AIDS also served to paralyze coordinated efforts to prevent HIV transmission. For example, although the Haitian Ministry of Health has identified AIDS prevention as one of its top priorities, the office charged with coordinating preventive efforts has been hamstrung by six coups d'état, which have led, inevitably, to personnel changes—and to more significant disruptions. At the time GESCAP was founded, in 1991, *there had been no comprehensive effort to prevent HIV transmission in rural Haiti.* Even in Port-au-Prince, what has been accomplished thus far has often been marred by messages that are either culturally inappropriate or designed for a small fraction of the population (for example, Haitians who are francophone, literate, and television-owning). These messages are especially unsuccessful in rural areas, where even well-funded "social marketing" schemes have had little cultural currency.

A sense of hopefulness, rare in Haiti, returned to the public health community in 1991, when the country's first democratic elections brought to office a social-justice government headed by a progressive priest. A new Ministry of Health promised to make AIDS, tuberculosis, and other infectious pathogens its top priority. But in September of that year, a violent military coup brought a swift end to Haiti's democratic experiment. The impact on the population's health was incalculable.[35]

Political upheaval did not simply hobble coordinated responses to the AIDS epidemic. It has had far more direct effects. One of the most epidemiologically significant events of recent years may prove to be the coup d'état of September 1991. As noted earlier, surveys of asymptomatic adults living in Cité Soleil revealed seroprevalence rates of approximately 10 percent, whereas surveys of asymptomatic rural people were likely to find rates an order of magnitude lower. Following the coup, the army targeted urban slums for brutal repression. A number of journalists and health care professionals estimated that fully half of the adult residents of Cité Soleil fled to rural areas following the army's lethal incursions. It takes little imagination to see that such flux substantially changes the equations describing the dynamics of HIV transmission in rural areas sheltering the refugees.[36] Similar patterns have been noted elsewhere, particularly in sub-Saharan Africa:

Women living in areas plagued by civil unrest or war may be in a situation of higher risk. In many countries, relatively high percentages of male military and police personnel are infected and their unprotected (voluntary or forced) sexual encounters with local women provide an avenue for transmission. Patterns of female infection have been correlated with the movements of members of the military in parts of Central and Eastern Africa.[37]

Concurrent Disease

The progression of HIV disease depends on host variables such as age, sex, and nutritional status; viral load, CD_4-cell number and function; and concurrent disease. Concurrent illness can alter this progression in at least three ways: first, any serious illness, including opportunistic infections (most notably, tuberculosis), may hasten the progression of HIV disease; second, various diseases can heighten an individual's "net state of immunosuppression," rendering him or her increasingly vulnerable to infection; and, third, certain infections seem to increase the risk of *acquiring* HIV—the point considered here.

Sexually transmitted diseases have been cited as AIDS co-factors in a number of studies, especially those conducted in tropical and subtropical regions.[38] Researchers view STDs as particularly important in the hetero-sexual spread of HIV, as the virus is less efficiently transmitted from women to men than vice versa. Thus vaginal and cervical diseases—even those as ostensibly minor as trichomoniasis—may increase the risk of HIV transmission through "microwounds" and even through mere inflammation (as certain lymphocytes are, after all, the target cells of HIV).[39]

Although researchers are now collecting important data about STDs in Port-au-Prince,[40] few studies have focused on rural areas.[41] But there is no evidence to suggest that villagers are more sexually active than their urban counterparts; there is even less evidence to suggest that rural Haitians are more sexually active than age-matched controls from North America. What is evident is that a majority of STDs go untreated—which certainly implies that sores, other lesions, and inflammation will persist far longer in rural Haiti than in most areas of the world.

Other diseases—including leprosy, yaws, endemic syphilis, and various viruses—have been suggested as possible co-factors in "tropical" AIDS, but their roles have not been clarified. It seems safe to add, however, that serious co-infections do enhance the net state of immunosuppression. Similarly, malnutrition clearly hastens the advent of advanced, symptomatic disease among the HIV-infected, although this dynamic may lessen the risk of transmission: the Haitian variant of "slim disease" is now popularly associated with AIDS, and visible cachexia is likely to drive away potential sexual partners.[42]

Access to Medical Services

Finally, in seeking to understand the Haitian AIDS epidemic, it is necessary to underline the contribution, or lack thereof, of a nonfunctioning public health system. Medical care in Haiti is something of an obstacle course, one that places innumerable barriers before poor people seeking care. Failure to have an STD treated leads to persistence of important co-factors for HIV infection; failure to treat active tuberculosis causes rapid progression of HIV disease and death—to say nothing of its impact on HIV-negative individuals, for HIV-infected patients with tuberculosis have been shown to be efficient transmitters of tuberculosis.[43] Contaminated blood transfusions alternate with no transfusions at all. Condoms are often not available even to those who want them. The cost of pharmaceuticals, always prohibitive, has skyrocketed in recent years. Antivirals are in essence unavailable to most Haitians: in February 1990, "local radio stations announced . . . that for the first time, the drug AZT is available in Haiti. It might as well have been on Mars. A bottle of 100 capsules costs $343—more than most Haitians make in a year."[44] Since that time, it has become possible to find newer, highly active antiretroviral agents in Haiti—but for a prince's ransom.

▶AIDS, Analysis, Accountability

Identifying and weighting the various social forces that shape the HIV epidemic is a perennial problem, but one too rarely addressed by medical anthropology, which is often asked to elucidate the "cultural component" of particular subepidemics. By combining social analysis with ethnographically informed epidemiology, however, we can identify the most significant of these forces. The factors listed here are differentially weighted, of course, but each demonstrably plays a role in determining HIV transmission in rural Haiti:

1. Deepening poverty
2. Gender inequality
3. Political upheaval
4. Traditional patterns of sexual union
5. Emerging patterns of sexual union
6. Prevalence of and lack of access to treatment for STDs
7. Lack of timely response by public health authorities
8. Lack of culturally appropriate prevention tools

Many of these factors are a far cry from the ones that anthropologists were exhorted to explore—for example, ritual scarification, animal sacrifice, sexual behavior in "exotic subcultures"—during the first decade of AIDS. But the forces underpinning the spread of HIV to rural Haiti are as economic and political as they are cultural, and poverty and inequality seem to underlie all of them. Although many working elsewhere would agree that poverty and social inequalities are the strongest enhancers of risk for exposure to HIV, international conferences on AIDS have repeatedly neglected this subject. Of the hundreds of epidemiology-track posters presented in 1992 in Amsterdam, for example, only three used "poverty" as a keyword; two of these were socioculturally naïve and did not seem to involve the collaboration of anthropologists.

What were anthropologists doing in the early years of AIDS? The mid-to late 1980s saw the formation of task forces and research groups as well as an increasing number of AIDS-related sessions at our professional meetings. The central themes of many of the early sessions focused on the "special understanding of sexuality" that was, suggested certain speakers, the province of anthropologists. The scenario most commonly evoked was one in which ethnographers, steeped in local lore after years of participant-observation, afforded epidemiologists and public health authorities detailed information about sexual behavior, childbearing, and beliefs about blood and blood contact. This knowledge transfer was deemed indispensable to determining which "behaviors" put individuals and communities at risk for HIV infection.

Fifteen years into the AIDS pandemic, after at least a decade of social science studies of AIDS, we must ask, How substantial were these claims? How many secret, AIDS-related "behaviors" have we unearthed in the course of our ethnography? Anthropologists deeply involved in AIDS prevention now know that many such claims were immodest. Everywhere, it seems,

HIV spreads from host to host through a relatively restricted set of mechanisms. We've also learned that preventive efforts, even the most culturally appropriate ones, are least effective in precisely those settings in which they are most urgently needed. Africa, long a favored proving ground for anthropology, offers the most obvious and humbling example. Haiti offers another.

In the interest of enhancing the efficacy of interventions, it's important to pause and take stock of the situation. How might anthropology best contribute to efforts to prevent HIV transmission or to alleviate AIDS-related suffering? One major contribution would be to help show where the pandemic is going, which leads us back to analytic challenges such as these:

> Identifying and differentially weighting the major factors promoting or retarding HIV transmission

> Linking the sexual choices made by individual actors to the various shifting conditions that restrict choice, especially among the poor

> Understanding the contribution of the culturally specific—not only local sexualities but also kinship structures and shifting representations of disease—without losing sight of the large-scale economic forces shaping the AIDS pandemic

> Investigating the precise mechanisms by which such forces as racism, gender inequality, poverty, war, migration, colonial heritage, coups d'état, and even structural-adjustment programs become embodied as increased risk

Anthropology, the most radically contextualizing of the social sciences, is well suited to meeting these analytic challenges, but we will not succeed by merely "filling in the cultural blanks" left by epidemiologists, physicians, scientists, and policy makers. Nor will we succeed without a new vigilance toward the analytic traps that have hobbled our understanding of the AIDS pandemic.[45]

First, we often find widespread, if sectarian, ascription to behaviorist, cognitivist, or culturalist reductionism. Just as many physicians regard social considerations as outside the realm of the central, so too have psychologists tended to reify individual psychology, while economists have reified the economic. Anthropologists writing of AIDS have of course tended to reify culture. We must avoid confusing our own desire for personal efficacy with sound analytic purchase on an ever-growing pandemic: HIV cares little for our theoretical stances or our disciplinary training. AIDS demands broad biosocial approaches. Jean Benoist and Alice Desclaux put it well:

> The conditions limiting or promoting transmission, illness representations, therapeutic itineraries, and health care practices—none of these subjects are captured by disciplinary approaches. They evade even the distinction between biology and social sciences, so tightly are biological realities tied to behaviors and representations, revealing links that have not yet been fully explored.[46]

Second, much anthropologic analysis focuses overmuch (or exclusively) on local factors and local actors, which risks exaggerating the agency of the poor and marginalized. Constraints on the agency of individual actors should be brought into stark relief so that prevention efforts do not come to grief, as they have to date. To explore the relation between personal agency and supraindividual structures—once the central problematic of social theory—we need to link our ethnography to systemic analyses that are informed by history, political economy, and a critical epidemiology. It is not possible to explain the strikingly patterned distribution of HIV by referring exclusively to attitude, cognition, or affect. Fine-grained psychological portraits and rich ethnography are never more than part of the AIDS story.

Third, the myths and mystifications that surround AIDS and slow AIDS research often serve powerful interests. If, in Haiti and in parts of Africa, economic policies (for example, structural-adjustment programs) and political upheaval are somehow related to HIV transmission, who benefits when attention is focused largely or solely on "unruly sexuality" or alleged "promiscuity"? The lasting influence of myths and immodest claims has helped to mask the effects of social inequalities on the distribution of HIV and on AIDS outcomes.

The recent advent of more effective antiviral therapy could have an enormous impact on what it means to have AIDS at the close of the twentieth century—if you don't happen to live in Africa or Haiti or Harlem. Protease inhibitors and other drugs raise the possibility of transforming AIDS into a chronic condition to be managed over decades, but they also remind us that there are two emerging syndromes: an AIDS of the North, and an AIDS of the South.

Perhaps this does not sound much like an anthropologist speaking. Why talk of latitude (North/South) and class (rich/poor) before speaking of culture? One answer to this question is that, for many of us, the view that AIDS is a culturally constructed phenomenon is not open to debate. AIDS, like sexuality, is inevitably embedded in local social context; representations and responses must necessarily vary along cultural lines. The contribution of cultural factors to the lived experience of AIDS is and will remain enormous. Indeed, the true and vast variation of HIV lies not, as we had been led to believe, in its modes of spread, nor is it found in the mechanisms by which the virus saps the host. The variation of HIV lies, rather, in its highly patterned distribution, in its variable clinical course among the infected, and in the ways in which we respond, socially, to a deadly pathogen.

Chapter
15

Special Topics

At Risk and Neglected: Four Key Populations

UNAIDS

This chapter focuses on four populations: sex workers; men who have sex with men; injecting drug users; and prisoners. In most countries, these populations tend to have a higher prevalence of HIV infection than that of the general population because (i) they engage in behaviours that put them at higher risk of becoming infected and (ii) they are among the most marginalized and discriminated against populations in society. At the same time, the resources devoted to HIV prevention, treatment and care for these populations are not proportional to the HIV prevalence—a serious mismanagement of resources and a failure to respect fundamental human rights.

In countries with low-level and concentrated epidemics, well-designed and adequately funded HIV prevention programmes among these populations have proven decisive in slowing or even stopping the epidemic in its tracks. For example, in the late 1980s, Thailand moved decisively to implement its brothel-based "100% condom use" programme, which provided concentrated HIV prevention services to sex workers and their clients. Had it not done so, adult HIV prevalence today would be an estimated 15%—10 times the current level of about 1.5% (MAP, 2005). Countries with generalized epidemics that place a high priority on HIV programming for these populations, guided by epidemiological surveillance, will ensure the most effective use of resources.

Sex workers, men who have sex with men, injecting drug users and prisoners are largely under-represented and voiceless in the decision-making processes that affect their lives, including those related to HIV. Yet where they have been engaged in responses to the epidemic, they have often been among the most effective actors in those responses. Civil society's involvement in responding to AIDS began with associations of men who have sex with men in industrialized countries, followed by organized groups of sex workers and injecting drug users in various parts of the world.

> ## HIV RISK AND VULNERABILITY
>
> HIV risk can be defined as the probability of an individual becoming infected by HIV either through his or her own actions, knowingly or not, or via another person's actions. For example, injecting drugs using contaminated needles or having unprotected sex with multiple partners increases a person's risk of HIV infection. Vulnerability to HIV reflects an individual's or community's inability to control their risk of HIV infection. Poverty, gender inequality and displacement as a result of conflict or natural disasters are all examples of social and economic factors that can enhance people's vulnerability to HIV infection. Both risk and vulnerability need to be addressed in planning comprehensive responses to the epidemic (UNAIDS, 1998).

Many other populations are also vulnerable to HIV (e.g. women and girls, young people, people living in poverty, migrant labourers, people in conflict and post-conflict situations, refugees and internally displaced people) and their HIV prevention needs should also be addressed.

▶ Sex Workers

While it is not possible to accurately count the number of people selling sex, it is estimated that sex workers may number in the tens of millions worldwide—and their clients in the hundreds of millions. While sex workers can be of all ages, most are young and the great majority are female; their clients (for both male and female sex workers) are mostly male. In many countries, a high percentage of sex workers are migrants.

Although countries may criminalize sex work and thereby subject the act of buying or selling sex for money to criminal sanction, sex workers have the same human rights as everyone else, particularly rights to education, information, the highest attainable standard of health and freedom from discrimination and violence, including sexual violence.

Governments have a responsibility to protect these rights and, in the context of the HIV epidemic, to reach sex workers and their clients with the full panoply of HIV information, commodities and services. Furthermore, ways must be found to empower sex workers to use these HIV services and to actively participate in the design and provision of the health services they need.

High Rates of HIV Infection

In Asia, a high proportion of new HIV infections are contracted during paid sex, and a relatively high HIV prevalence has been found among sex workers in many countries. In Viet Nam, HIV prevalence among female sex workers increased rapidly throughout the 1990s, from 0.06% in 1994 to 6% in 2002. In Indonesia, the rate of HIV infection among female sex workers is 3.1% nationally but varies significantly from region to region. In Jakarta, it reached 6.4% in 2003 (MAP, 2005). In China, it is estimated that sex workers and their clients account for just less than 20% of the total number of people living with HIV (Ministry of Health, People's Republic of China/UNAIDS, 2005a).

High HIV prevalence is also found in the Caribbean and Latin America (Pan Caribbean Partnership on HIV/AIDS, 2002). In Suriname, HIV prevalence among female sex workers was found to be 21% in a 2005 study, while in Guyana, levels of almost 27% were recorded in 2004. Jamaica reported an HIV prevalence of 20% among female sex workers in 2002 (Ministry of Health of Jamaica 2002), while in El Salvador, 16% of street-based sex workers in San Salvador and Puerto de Acajutla tested HIV-positive in the same year (Ministerio de Salud Pública y Asistencia Social de El Salvador, 2003).

While little is known about sex work in the Middle East and North African countries, one exception is Tamanrasset, where HIV prevalence rose from 1.7% in 2000 to 9% in 2004 among sex workers (World Bank, 2005). More is known about Eastern Europe and Central Asia. For example, a study in St Petersburg, Russian Federation, found that 33% of sex workers under 19 years of age tested HIV-positive (Central and Eastern European Harm Reduction Network/OSI, 2005).

In major urban areas of sub-Saharan Africa, various studies over the past eight years have recorded HIV infection among female sex workers at levels as high as 73% in Ethiopia, 68% in Zambia, 50% in Ghana and South Africa, 40% in Benin, 31% in Côte d'Ivoire, 27% in Djibouti and Kenya, and 23% in Mali (UNAIDS, 2003). These data underscore the need for HIV prevention efforts to be scaled up among sex workers, even in countries with generalized epidemics.

Sex Work and Drug Use

In many parts of the world, sex work and injecting drug use are intricately linked: drug users resort to sex work to fund their habit, while sex workers turn to injecting drugs to escape the pressures of their work. Sex workers who also inject drugs are at further risk, not least because the combination of their work and drug taking puts them beyond the protection of the law and so opens them to exploitation and abuse, including sexual violence and harm, and incapacity to negotiate condom use.

High rates of HIV and sexually transmitted infections have been found among sex workers in countries with large populations of injecting drug users. In China, Indonesia, Kazakhstan, Ukraine, Uzbekistan and Viet Nam, the large overlap between injecting drug use and sex work is linked to growing HIV epidemics (UNAIDS, 2005a). In Manipur, India, which has a well-established HIV epidemic driven by injecting drug use, 20% of female sex workers said they injected drugs, according to behavioural surveillance (MAP, 2005). In Ho Chi Minh City, in 2002, 49% of sex workers who reported injecting drugs were found to be HIV-positive, compared to 19% of sex workers who used drugs without injecting them and 8% of those who did not use drugs at all. Research also showed that drug-using sex workers in Viet Nam were about half as likely to use condoms compared with those who did not use drugs (Tran et al., 2004).

Young and Ill-Informed

Most women and men enter sex work in their teens or early 20s. It is estimated that 80% of sex workers in eastern European and central Asian regions are under 25 years of age, and that sex workers who inject drugs may be even younger than those who do not.

Many sex workers lack information about HIV and about services that might help protect them. A 2003 study carried out along major transport routes in Africa found that the average age of sex workers was 22.8 years and the average education level was grade six (upper primary school). Only 33% knew that they were at risk if they had unprotected sex. None reported seeking HIV counselling and testing services (Omondi et al., 2003). Sex workers are frequently less likely than the general population to access public health services, and may

---

MALE AND TRANSGENDER SEX WORKERS

While not as numerous as female sex workers, male and transgender sex workers also sell sex, predominantly to men. Among these populations, HIV prevalence is frequently high. A recent study in Spain found HIV infection rates of over 12% in male sex workers who visited HIV testing clinics in 19 Spanish cities (Belza, 2005). In Indonesia, a study found HIV prevalence of 22% among transgender sex workers and 3.6% among male sex workers. Approximately 60% of the transgender sex workers and 65% of the male sex workers reported recent unprotected anal intercourse with clients. Almost 55% of the male sex workers reported having had sex with female partners in the preceding year (Pisani et al., 2004). A recent survey by municipal health authorities found that 5% of male sex workers in Shenzhen, a city in southern China, were HIV-positive (South China Morning Post, 2005).

---

not know about or be able to afford treatment for sexually transmitted infections, which can increase physiological vulnerability to HIV. In Dili, one-quarter of sex workers surveyed in 2003 were diagnosed with gonorrhoea or chlamydial infections, and 60% were infected with herpes simplex virus 2 (Pisani and Dili STI survey team, 2004). Among incarcerated sex workers in a juvenile detention facility in the Russian Federation, 58% had at least one bacterial sexually transmitted infection and 4% were HIV-positive (Shakarishvili et al., 2005).

Impact of the Sex Work Environment

Sex workers operate in a variety of different environments, ranging from highly organized brothels and massage parlours to the street, markets and vehicles or cinemas, bars, hotels and homes. Each location carries with it its own degree of risk and vulnerability in terms of stigma, discrimination or the potential for violence, as well as the obvious danger of HIV infection. Moreover, the sex trade is not fixed but is evolving in reaction to social and economic conditions. This means HIV prevention programmes must adapt to address these changes. In Thailand, for example, there has been a large increase in the number of non-brothelbased sex service establishments, such as massage parlours. The sex workers in these establishments are largely unaffected by "100% condom use" programming, which concentrates on brothel-based sex work, and must therefore be reached in other ways. Similarly, many cities in India have reported an increase in non-brothelbased sex workers (UNAIDS, 2005a).

Clients of Sex Workers

The majority of HIV interventions that address sex work are aimed at the sex workers themselves, with insufficient attention paid to their clients or the contexts in which they work. In many countries, the fact that there is consistent demand for sex work is often ignored by government policies, which focus solely on repressing or regulating supply. The prevalence of purchasing sex varies greatly. For example, a general population study in 24 Peruvian cities found that 44% of men aged 18–29 years said they paid for sex in 2002. Of these, 45% said they did not consistently use condoms with sex workers (Guanira et al., 2004). In some Asian countries, levels as high as 15% of men in the general population and 44% of men in mobile, high-risk populations (e.g. long-distance truckers and men who work in mines or forests far from home) reported buying sex during 2004 (MAP, 2005).

SEX WORK, HUMAN TRAFFICKING AND HIV

Every year, an estimated 600 000 to 800 000 people are trafficked across international borders (US Department of State, 2004). When those trafficked within their own countries are added, the annual toll of people trafficked may come to 4 million, including 1.2 million children under 18 years (ILO, 2002). All regions of the world are affected, although there are some well-established routes along which large numbers of people are trafficked. Within the South Asia region, for example, India and Pakistan are the main destinations for trafficked girls aged under 16 years, especially from Bangladesh and Nepal (UNAIDS, 2005b).

There are few data on HIV prevalence among trafficked women and girls. However, even in countries where HIV rates are low, trafficked women and girls are highly vulnerable to infection because they are often placed in situations where they cannot negotiate condom use, are forced to endure multiple sex partners and are subjected to violent sex (Burkhalter, 2003).

Trafficked women and girls come mostly from sectors of society and settings where there is poverty, indebtedness, high unemployment and gender discrimination (ILO, 2004). Efforts to overcome these factors with the objective of preventing human trafficking should be supported. However, until such efforts can show decisive success, interventions which address immediate needs—including HIV prevention and care services for potential and actual victims of human trafficking—are required.

▶ HIV Programming

There is substantial evidence that HIV prevention programmes for sex workers are effective and that sex workers can be strong participants in HIV prevention programmes. The Thai "100% condom use" policy has been replicated with success in countries from South-East Asia to the Caribbean, while the lessons learnt from organized sex workers in India (Kolkata), have been a touchstone for sex worker projects around the world (UNAIDS, 2000).

In Santo Domingo, low HIV infection levels of 3–4% among sex workers are thought to partly reflect consistent condom use and other safer behaviours promoted in the city's "100% condom use" programme. A recent survey found that 87% of sex workers reported using a condom the last time they had sold sex and 76% said they always used a condom during paid sex (Secretaria de Estado de Salud Póblica y Asistencia Social de Republica Dominica, 2005).

Many projects seek to provide sex workers with alternative ways of earning income. In Ethiopia, for example, the Sister Self-Help Association was formed by a small group of sex workers to try to provide themselves with a regular income and better health provision. The income-generating activities include a restaurant, a convenience store (a shop with extended opening hours, stocking a limited range of household goods and groceries) and a catering service for local hotels.

Successful HIV programmes use a mix of strategies, taking into account factors such as whether sex workers are brothel-based, if they work in one area or are mobile and the legal status of sex work. Effective strategies include (UNAIDS, 2002):

- promotion of safer sexual behaviour among sex workers, their partners and clients (e.g. promotion of condom use and negotiation skills) and of sex worker solidarity and local organization (in particular, so that clients cannot search for sex workers who are willing to have sex without a condom); provision of sexually transmitted infection prevention and care services, and access to commodities such as male and female condoms and lubricants; peer education and outreach work, including health, social and legal services;

- care for sex workers living with HIV; and
- policy and law reform, along with efforts to ensure that those in authority, such as police and public health staff, respect and protect sex workers' human rights.

These strategies should be accompanied by programmes to prevent entry into sex work, assistance to help women get out of it and anti-trafficking measures, including protection and assistance to women and girls who have been trafficked into the sex trade. Overall, programming works best if it has the active involvement of sex workers themselves in all phases of projects, from development to evaluation, and aims to decrease their vulnerability by addressing the conditions and context (e.g. economic and gender issues) surrounding sex work.

▶ Men Who Have Sex with Men

The term "men who have sex with men" describes a social and behavioural phenomenon rather than a specific group of people. It includes not only self-identified gay and bisexual men, but also men who engage in male–male sex and self-identify as heterosexual or who do not self-identify at all, as well as transgendered males. Men who have sex with men are found in all countries, yet are largely invisible in many places.

Current indicators suggest that globally fewer than one in twenty men who have sex with men have access to the HIV prevention and care services they need (see 'Overview' chapter). Many factors contribute to this situation including denial by society and communities, stigma and discrimination, and human rights abuse.

Complex gender issues, social and legal marginalization and lack of access to HIV information affect how many of these men perceive, or do not perceive, their HIV-related risks. Traditional gender norms of masculinity and femininity contribute strongly to homophobia and the related stigma and discrimination against men who have sex with men, transgendered and 'third-gender' people. (An example of the latter is the *hijaras* who live in various regions of South Asia and who may define themselves as neither men nor women, but as a third gender.) Homophobia has been identified as one of the primary obstacles to effective HIV responses in the move towards universal access to treatment.

Not Enough Data?

In some regions of the world, epidemiological information about male-to-male HIV transmission is relatively scarce. This is partly because of the fact that many of the men involved are married to women and are thus regarded as part of the general population, rather than a distinct subpopulation. Crucially, in many parts of the world, men who have sex with men have no separate social identity (unlike self-identified "gay" men) and sex between men is not commonly talked about or acknowledged, even by the men concerned.

Nevertheless, much useful research has been carried out over the years in many low- and middle-income countries, and the burden of HIV infection in men who have sex with men is becoming increasingly clear. Sex between men is central to the HIV epidemic in nearly all Latin American countries (UNAIDS, 2006). In Bogotá, for example, an HIV prevalence of 20% has been registered among men who have sex with men (Montano et al., 2005). But sex between men also has important implications in many other regions. In Bangkok, and Mumbai, for example, HIV infection levels of 17% have been found in men who have sex with men (UNAIDS, 2005a). Unfortunately, even in the many countries where data indicate that men who have sex with men are severely affected by HIV, their prevention needs have been largely ignored or underfunded (see 'National responses' chapter).

Lack of HIV Information and Awareness of Risk

Many men who have sex with men do not regard themselves as homosexual and therefore rule themselves out of being exposed to HIV. Even among men who readily identify themselves as gay, bisexual or transgender, there is still considerable lack of awareness of HIV and what constitutes sexual risk behaviour. A peer-to-peer study among men who have sex with men in south-eastern Europe discovered misconceptions about modes of HIV transmission, with some men reporting sexual risk behaviours (Longfield et al., 2004). In Beijing, only 15% of a sample of 482 men who have sex with men understood that they were at risk of HIV infection, and many had misconceptions about HIV transmission routes and limited knowledge about condoms. Some 49% of the participants reported unprotected anal intercourse with men during the previous six months. Less than one-quarter obtained free condoms and condom lubricants in the previous two years (Gibson et al., 2004).

Sex with Both Men and Women

Many men who have sex with men also have sex with women. In the study in Beijing just described, 28% of the men surveyed reported having sex with both men and women during the previous six months and 11% had unprotected intercourse with both men and women (Gibson et al., 2004). A large study, conducted in Andhra Pradesh, found that 42% of men in the sample who have sex with men are married, that 50% had had sexual relations with a woman within the past three months and that just under half had not used a condom (Dandona et al., 2005).

Criminalized and Marginalized

Vulnerability to HIV infection is dramatically increased where sex between men is criminalized. In Jamaica, men having sex with men can be convicted of a crime and sentenced to jail. Same-sex relations between men in Malawi attract a 14-year penal sentence (Goyer, 2003). Criminalization and homophobia severely limit the ability of many men who have sex with men to access HIV prevention information, commodities and treatment and care (USAID, 2004). Faced with legal or social sanctions, men having sex with men are either excluded from, or exclude themselves from, sexual health and welfare agencies because they fear being identified as homosexual.

Prevention Efforts Losing Ground?

In some countries, self-identified homosexual men have taken their places within mainstream society through a process of activism, legal reform and changes in social attitudes. They have been at the forefront of HIV prevention since the early years of the epidemic, and continue to be so. A five-city survey of men who have sex with men in India recently found that use of peers to distribute and promote condoms resulted in significant increases in condom use, especially in Mumbai, where peer educators distributed more than two-thirds of the condoms used by the survey population (MAP, 2005).

Yet some of the success against HIV achieved by men who have sex with men is apparently being eroded. For example, sexual risk-taking among men who have sex with men is increasing in many countries, some of it closely linked with alcohol or drug use. For example, the United States has witnessed a rapid growth in recent years in the use of the stimulant crystal methamphetamine. Research indicates that in Los Angeles, men who use this drug and have sex with men have an HIV infection rate more than three times higher than non-methamphetamine-using men who have sex with men (Peck et al., 2005). In San Francisco, approximately one in five men who have sex with men have recently reported that they use the drug, while in New York City, the figure was one in seven, and in Chicago and Los Angeles it was one in ten (Chicago Department of Public Health, 2005; de Herrera et al., 2005).

The resurgence of sexual risk behaviours has a number of possible explanations. One may be the erroneous belief that with widespread access to antiretroviral therapy, AIDS is more or less curable and protected sex is therefore optional. At the same time, public health authorities in most countries are devoting fewer resources to men who have sex with men than epidemiological evidence suggests is necessary. Rising HIV prevalence among this population in many countries confirms this is a short-sighted and irresponsible public policy.

A Range of Responses

A range of responses aimed at reducing the risk behaviours and vulnerability to HIV of men who have sex with men has proved successful in a variety of settings (UNAIDS, 2000b). These include:

- general and targeted promotion of high-quality condoms and water-based lubricants, and ensuring their continuing availability;
- safer-sex campaigns and skills training, focusing mainly on reducing the number of partners, increasing condom use and alternatives to penetrative sex;
- peer education among men who have sex with men, along with outreach programmes by volunteers or professional social or health workers;
- provision of education and outreach to female partners of men who have sex with men; and
- programmes tailored to particular subpopulations such as the police and military personnel, prisoners and male sex workers.

In addition to these prevention measures, a number of activities must be encouraged among managers of health systems and governments. First, it is important to support organizations of self-identified gay men, enabling them to promote HIV prevention and care programmes. Alliances should be built between epidemiologists, social scientists, politicians, human rights groups, lawyers, clinicians, journalists, organized groups of men who have sex with men and other civil society organizations. Laws that criminalize same-sex acts between consenting adults in private need to be reviewed, and antidiscrimination or protective laws enacted to reduce human rights violations based on sexual orientation. Finally, but crucially, public commitment is needed from governments, national AIDS commissions, community organizations and donors to include men who have sex with men in their HIV programming and funding priorities. National AIDS action frameworks should have specific prevention, treatment and care plans for men who have sex with men.

SEXUAL PARTNERS (MALE AND FEMALE) OF MEN WHO HAVE SEX WITH MEN

Ignoring the risks of unprotected anal sex not only makes men who have sex with men vulnerable to HIV infection, but also puts their female sexual partners at risk. In high-income countries, a relatively high incidence of HIV continues among men who have sex with men. Recent research indicates that many either do not disclose their HIV serostatus to their sexual partners or may be becoming complacent about sexual risk behaviour. HIV-positive men who have sex with men surveyed recently in Los Angeles and Seattle in the United States were found to be unlikely to disclose their HIV serostatus to sexual partners because they consider it "nobody's business" or because they are in denial, have a low viral load or fear rejection (Gorbach et al., 2004).

▶ Injecting Drug Users

Injecting drug use is estimated to account for just less than one-third of new infections outside sub-Saharan Africa. Once HIV enters a community of injecting drug users, progress of the infection into the rest of the population can be very rapid if appropriate measures are not taken early. Yet in spite of the importance of injecting drug users in the response to HIV, coverage of HIV prevention for this population is at best 5% across the globe (USAID et al., 2004).

There are approximately 13 million injecting drug users worldwide, of whom 8.8 million live in eastern Europe and Central, South and South-East Asia. There are around 1.4 million injecting drug users in North America and 1 million in Latin America (UNODC, 2004). Use of contaminated injection equipment during drug use is the major route of HIV transmission in eastern Europe and Central Asia, where it accounts for more than 80% of all HIV cases. It is also the entry point for HIV epidemics in a wide range of countries in the Middle East, North Africa, South and South-East Asia and Latin America. Alarmingly, new epidemics of injecting drug use are being witnessed in countries of sub-Saharan Africa (UNAIDS, 2005c).

Risk and Vulnerability

Certain drug-use practices contribute significantly to HIV infection among drug users, with the biggest risk being use of contaminated needles and syringes; sexual risk practices also contribute, but to a lesser extent. For instance, sex workers in Ho Chi Minh City who inject drugs were about half as likely to use condoms as those who did not use drugs (MAP, 2004). A high prevalence of sexually transmitted infections among drug users reflects their unsafe sexual practices.

Beyond the physical risks associated with drug injection, drug users are vulnerable to HIV because of their social and legal status. Ironically, in many countries this means that HIV interventions are not available to drug users, or that drug users are unable or unwilling to access them for fear of recrimination. For example, about 80% of Russians living with HIV became infected through using contaminated needles and syringes, and it is estimated that between 1.5% and 8% of all Russian men younger than 30 years have injected drugs at some time in their lives (Molotilov et al., 2003). Despite the proven efficacy of HIV prevention measures for injecting drug users such as needle and syringe exchanges and drug substitution treatment, the Russian Federation has been slow to take advantage of such measures. A recent survey found that funding for needle and syringe exchange programmes had actually fallen by 29% between 2002 and 2004. Although some regional legislators have contributed funds to needle and syringe exchange projects and to AIDS centres offering HIV treatment, this support was neither universal nor sufficiently widespread to approach the levels of coverage needed to contain HIV epidemics driven by injecting drug use. However, new funding may help to begin to redress the balance. The first grant to the Russian Federation from the Global Fund to Fight AIDS, Tuberculosis and Malaria supported 23 exchange projects in 10 regions, and its funding of treatment for people living with HIV explicitly included injecting drug users among those targeted (Wolfe, 2005).

Harm Reduction: A High Priority

Some 20 years of research and experience confirm that HIV epidemics among injecting drug users can be prevented, stabilized and even reversed using a comprehensive package of HIV prevention and care activities. This package was recently summarized in a UNAIDS position paper on HIV prevention as "a comprehensive, integrated and effective system of measures that consists of the full range of treatment options, (notably drug substitution treatment) and the implementation of harm reduction measures (through, among others, peer outreach to injecting drug users, and sterile needle and syringe programmes), voluntary confidential HIV counselling and testing, prevention of sexual transmission of HIV among drug users (including condoms and prevention and treatment for sexually transmitted infections), access to primary health care and access to antiretroviral therapy. Such an approach must be based on promoting, protecting and respecting the human rights of drug users" (UNAIDS, 2005d).

Numerous studies in diverse epidemiological settings have demonstrated that harm reduction strategies are cost effective in preventing the spread of HIV (Sullivan et al., 2005). Since the 1990s, maintenance programmes using methadone have reported success in helping to contain HIV epidemics in areas as diverse as Australia, China, Hong Kong Special Administrative Region, Sweden, Thailand and the United States (Mattick et al., 2003). Such maintenance programmes provide an opportunity for stabilizing the health and social situations of drug users and enhancing antiretroviral treatment compliance. Despite the evidence, however, certain aspects of harm reduction remain controversial in some parts of the world (Beckley Foundation, 2005). For example, counterproductive laws and policies in some countries prohibit substitution therapy using methadone or buprenorphine.

WHO added methadone and buprenorphine to the *WHO Model List of Essential Medicines* in 2005, and has been advocating for their introduction into drug programmes in countries where use of opioids (e.g. opium and heroin) is prevalent, as an essential component of both HIV prevention and treatment. This has included supporting the development of national guidelines for methadone substitution therapy and the scaling up of harm reduction programmes in countries such as China, Myanmar and Ukraine.

The lessons of comprehensive HIV prevention are being applied in an increasing number of countries. Despite a strong commitment to compulsory treatment for drug dependence and abstinence-based programmes, Malaysia has recently decided to introduce harm reduction programmes. In 2004, the country had an estimated 117 000 to 240 000 injecting drug users, and approximately 52 000 people who were living with HIV, the vast majority of them young men aged 20–29 years (Ministry of Health Malaysia and WHO, 2004; Huang and Hussein, 2004). After sustained advocacy by nongovernmental organizations and the health community, pilot methadone maintenance programmes have been established, and pilot needle and syringe exchange programmes are planned to start in 2006. In addition, antiretroviral therapy

EVIDENCE FOR HARM REDUCTION

HIV transmission and HIV/AIDS impact associated with injecting drug use can best be contained by implementing a core package of interventions . . . There is strong and consistent evidence that this package of harm reduction interventions significantly reduces injecting drug use and associated risk behaviours and hence prevents, halts and reverses HIV epidemics associated with injecting drug use. Conversely, there is no convincing evidence of major negative consequences of such interventions, such as initiation of injecting drug use among people who have previously not injected or an increase in the duration of frequency of illicit drug use or drug injection (UNAIDS, 2005c).

is now being provided to injecting drug users resident in drug-dependence treatment facilities. In 2005, a judicial order in the Islamic Republic of Iran stipulated that individuals who use illegal drugs would no longer be targets of criminal repression but would instead be treated as patients by the public health system (Asian Harm Reduction Network, 2005).

In Central Asia, the Kyrgyz Government supports needle and syringe exchange programmes in three cities and in prisons in the country, and was the first member of the Commonwealth of Independent States to offer methadone maintenance therapy. Although such programmes have yet to be implemented on a wide scale, early evidence suggests that the country has benefited from its active search for technical assistance and its strong engagement of nongovernmental organizations in formulating and implementing national HIV prevention efforts (Wolfe, 2005).

China has also embraced comprehensive HIV prevention among injecting drug users, having established 91 needle and syringe exchange programmes in various parts of the country (Ministry of Health, People's Republic of China/UNAIDS, 2005). It is currently in the process of establishing 1500 methadone maintenance programmes to cover 300 000 opioid users over a period of three years, and linking these services to sites delivering antiretroviral drugs.

HIV Treatment for Injecting Drug Users

The International Treatment Preparedness Coalition recommends that global and national treatment goals specify targets for key at-risk populations. This is in response to evidence that in many countries injecting drug users, prisoners, men who have sex with men, sex workers and certain mobile populations face acute barriers to proper HIV care and treatment (International Treatment Preparedness Coalition, 2005).

This is especially true in the case of injecting drug users. The reasons for this are complex. Because of the illegality of drug use and the stigma associated with it, injecting drug users are often estranged from the health-care system and perceive little reason to seek medical services. In the Russian Federation, for example, a drug user will be officially registered with government authorities if he or she seeks treatment for addiction or otherwise accesses various health or social services.

While injecting drug users on antiretroviral drugs can achieve clinical outcomes comparable to those of patients on antiretroviral therapy who do not inject drugs, they require experienced clinicians with the ability to address the many serious and potentially life-threatening conditions that must be managed in tandem with HIV infection. Injecting drug users who are infected with HIV are especially prone to severe bacterial infections, such as infective endocarditis and pulmonary tuberculosis (Gordon and Lowy, 2005).

In hospital settings, providing care and treatment to injecting drug users frequently presents special challenges. Those who have had chaotic lifestyles frequently try to continue injecting drugs when in hospital, find it difficult to adjust to hospital rules and sometimes feel stigmatized by hospital staff. Some innovative approaches have been developed to deal with these challenges. Clinicians in Vancouver have long been concerned with the fact that injecting drug-using patients frequently leave hospital before treatment for bacterial infections has been completed, leading to long-term health problems and repeated hospital stays. In response, the public health authority has recently piloted a transitional care unit designed to accommodate the complex needs of drug-using patients. The apartment-style unit provides care 24 hours a day, not only for immediate medical problems—including the AIDS-related illnesses frequently found in this population—but also access to drug treatment programmes and social services such as housing when they leave. Since the project began in early 2005, monitoring has found improved health outcomes among patients, higher levels of satisfaction in both patients and staff, and significantly lower costs in comparison with hospital care (Vancouver Coastal Health Authority, 2005).

Accommodating Drug Control Objectives and Public Health Policy

The tension between law enforcement objectives and public health concerns may never be fully resolved with regard to injecting drug use. However, as a matter of both basic ethical principle and proven public health practice, drug control policies should reduce, not increase, the HIV risk faced by injecting drug users (for example, they should not deprive them of access to medical care or reduce their access to sterile injection equipment). At the same time, HIV prevention activities should not inadvertently promote illegal drug use. In practice, there needs to be clear government policies and legislation that authorize the implementation of all elements of the comprehensive package of HIV prevention and care activities, as well as sufficient funding so they can be carried out on a sufficiently large scale. As with all HIV programmes aimed at vulnerable populations, policies and programmes that deal with injecting drug users and their families should also conform to international human rights standards.

▶ Prisoners

> "It was Dostoevsky, of course, who said that the degree of civilization in society can be judged by entering its prisons. He was a wise man. . . . . We cannot allow discrimination and stigma to stand between us and a solution. Injecting drug users in prison must have access to the same care offered to people on the outside."
>
> Speech by Antonio Maria Costa, Executive Director, UNODC, 1 April 2005

It is estimated that at any given time there are over nine million people in prisons, with an annual turnover of 30 million moving from prison to the community and back again (Walmsley, 2005). Conditions reigning in most prisons make them extremely high-risk environments for HIV transmission, leading them to be called 'incubators' of HIV infection, as well as of hepatitis C and tuberculosis (OSI, 2004). Prisons are sites for illicit drug use, unsafe injecting practices, tattooing with contaminated equipment, violence, rape and unprotected sex. They are often overcrowded and offer poor nutrition, limited access to health care and high rates of airborne and bloodborne diseases.

Although data from low- and middle-income countries are relatively scarce, the evidence available confirms that the prevalence of HIV infection in prisons is almost invariably higher than that in the general population. In South Africa, estimates put the figure as high as 41% in the general prison system and higher yet in individual prisons. In Cameroon, HIV prevalence at the New Bell prison in the city of Douala was 12.1% in 2005. A recent report from Zambia's prison headquarters stated that, in 2004 alone, some 449 inmates had died of AIDS-related illnesses (Simooya and Sanjobo, 2006). HIV prevalence in prisons in the Russian Federation has been estimated to be at least four times higher than that in the wider population (Russian Ministry of Justice, 2004). Nor is HIV confined to male prisoners: in the United States it is estimated that women prisoners are 15 times more likely to be HIV-positive than women in the general population (De Groot, 2005).

The risk factors explaining these prevalence levels are clear. To begin with, both male and female prisoners often come from marginalized populations, such as injecting drug users or sex workers, who are already at an elevated risk of HIV infection. Use of contaminated or non-sterile injecting equipment is almost invariably higher inside prisons than among injecting drug users outside of prison, while the prevalence of male–male sexual activity is often higher in prison than in the general population (WHO, 2005; Dolan et al., 2004). Tattooing represents another risk factor for the transmission of bloodborne viruses as contaminated instruments are often used. There is generally no access to sterile injecting equipment and condoms—the basic tools against HIV transmission.

HIV Prevention and Care

If countries are reluctant to introduce harm reduction programmes to the general population, or to recognize and condone sex between men, they are even more unlikely to do so in their prisons. There is considerable anecdotal evidence that some public officials feel that prisoners who inject drugs or participate in male–male sex "get what they deserve." More pragmatically, many worry that harm reduction measures and condom provision in prison might lead to an increase in sex between men or injecting drug use.

In fact, there is no empirical evidence for these fears. In European prison systems there has been no increase in sexual risk behaviours as a result of harm reduction programmes for inmates (WHO, 2005). Rather, provision of HIV prevention services in prisons has been a considerable success story in many countries (Stoöver and Nelles, 2003). Following successful pilot programmes beginning in the late 1990s, Spain has expanded its provision of needle and syringe exchanges to more than 30 prisons. Other countries are only beginning to see the benefits of such programmes. In Ukraine, a 2005 study found that most prisoners' knowledge of HIV was generally poor, with only 39% having basic knowledge of how to prevent the sexual transmission of HIV. However, among prisoners who had been reached by prevention programmes in prison, two-thirds knew how to protect themselves against HIV (Ministry of Health of Ukraine, 2005). Following implementation of a peer-based health education programme in a prison setting in the Siberia region of the Russian Federation, HIV-related knowledge and condom use among prisoners increased, while the prevalence of tattooing declined (Dolan et al., 2004).

Prisons are not closed off from the world. Prisoners are eventually released and infection acquired inside prison can be readily transmitted outside it. HIV prevention and treatment for prisoners is also therefore a strategy with high potential benefits for the rest of society. To be truly effective, national AIDS programmes must significantly expand their provision of comprehensive HIV prevention, treatment, care and support services in prison.

In October 2004, WHO convened an international meeting on prisons and health in De Leeuwenhorst. The resulting *Status Paper on Prisons, Drugs and Harm Reduction* recommended that all prison systems adopt an approach based on public health and human rights "even if this means acknowledging the limitations in depending on an official enforcement of total abstinence [from drug use and sex]" (WHO, 2005). Recommended HIV-related measures for prisons include:

- providing what is required so that prison staff can ensure that all prisoners are given basic information relating to HIV and other bloodborne diseases and how they spread;
- providing clinical management of drug-dependent prisoners at a standard equivalent to that in the local community;
- ensuring that adequate information and guidance are provided before prisoners are released; and
- providing follow-up care with links to community services, which is important for all prisoners with health problems, but is essential for those dependent on drugs.

All prison systems are urged to move as quickly as resources allow to introduce important additional harm reduction action:

- developing a planned and comprehensive clinical treatment programme for drug-dependent prisoners, including the use of opiate substitution maintenance therapy;
- developing a needle and syringe exchange programme equivalent to that available in the community, especially if the local prevalence of HIV or hepatitis C is high or if injecting drug use is known to occur in the prison; and
- providing an effective method for disinfecting needles and syringes and tattooing instruments along with appropriate information and training should needle and syringe exchange programmes be considered not necessary or feasible.

A Matter of Human Rights

HIV prevention and treatment efforts in prisons should be important components of national AIDS strategies not only because of the undoubted benefits in public health terms but also as

---

HIV PREVENTION: AS NECESSARY OUTSIDE OF PRISON AS INSIDE

The United Nations Office on Drugs and Crime (UNODC) emphasizes that the presence of drugs and HIV in prisons presents two distinct dilemmas. First, drugs in prison represent a failure of security and a breach in the rule of law. Second, injecting drug use among prison populations results in high rates of HIV transmission between prisoners and to uninfected sexual partners once the prisoner is released. Two population streams—new inmates who may be uninfected and inmates who are already HIV-positive—flow in and out of prisons on a regular basis.

Experience in various countries has shown that evidence-based HIV prevention programming is effective in prisons. But UNODC, along with WHO and other UNAIDS Cosponsors, emphasize that prison authorities alone cannot fix the problem. Coordinated efforts with other government entities, particularly health and justice agencies, are necessary to break the chain of HIV transmission that accompanies incarceration and release, and to care for prisoners living with HIV—whether they are in prison or have served their sentence and are outside.

a matter of fundamental human rights. People retain the majority of their human rights when they enter prison, losing only those that are necessarily and explicitly limited because of their imprisonment. They retain such rights as freedom from cruel and inhuman punishment, and the right to the highest attainable standard of health and security of the person. Courts in many parts of the world have ruled that governments actually have greater obligations to prisoners than to the general public because governments are the sole source of essential services provided to prisoners, including health care.

In a presentation to the United Nations Commission on Human Rights in April 1996, UNAIDS stated (UNAIDS 1996):

> "[By] entering prisons, prisoners are condemned to imprisonment for their crimes; they should not be condemned to HIV and AIDS. There is no doubt that governments have a moral and legal responsibility to prevent the spread of HIV among prisoners and prison staff and to care for those infected."

Some 10 years later, this position has not changed.

Towards a Definition of Orphaned and Vulnerable Children

*Donald Skinner, N. Tsheko, S. Mtero-Munyati,
M. Segwabe, P. Chibatamoto, S. Mfecane,
B. Chandiwana, N. Nkomo, S. Tlou, G. Chitiyo*

The HIV epidemic presents challenges including orphans and a large mass of children rendered vulnerable by the epidemic and other societal forces. Focus on orphaned and vulnerable children (OVC) is important, but needs accurate definition. Twelve focus group interviews of service providers, leaders in these communities, OVC and their caretakers were conducted at six project sites across Botswana, South Africa and Zimbabwe to extend this definition. The loss of a parent through death or desertion is an important aspect of vulnerability. Additional factors leading to vulnerability included severe chronic illness of a parent or caregiver, poverty, hunger, lack of access to services, inadequate clothing or shelter, overcrowding, deficient caretakers, and factors specific to the child, including disability, direct experience of physical or sexual violence, or severe chronic illness. Important questions raised in this research include the long-term implications for the child and community, and the contribution of culture systems.

▶ Introduction

The importance of considering the situation of children orphaned by AIDS has been made clear both by projections of the number of orphans expected, and the lack of adequate caring mechanisms and service structures to support them. However, looking at the situation of these orphans does not address the full scale of the problem, since the epidemic and surrounding poverty are generating a context in which large numbers of children are becoming vulnerable. The term orphaned and vulnerable children (OVC) was introduced due to the limited usefulness of the tight definition of the construct of "orphanhood" in the scenario of HIV/AIDS. The term OVC in turn has its own difficulties as a construct, since it has no implicit definition or clear statement of inclusion and exclusion. It therefore works as a theoretical construct, but requires explanation and definition at ground level.

Orphans are the focus of much academic and popular writing. Such work includes counts or projections of numbers of orphans, examination of interventions required to provide adequate assistance, descriptions of the context and caring of orphans, and descriptions of the impact of HIV on children. Some of the material, particularly that in the popular literature, has sensationalized the issue. Examples of the "worst-case" studies of orphans are identified and these situations are extrapolated to all orphans in the region. Some projects have more recently extended their scope and worked more with the concept of vulnerability and services to assist these children.

An orphan is defined by UNAIDS as a child under 15 years of age who has lost their mother (maternal orphan) or both parents (double orphan) to AIDS. Many researchers and intervention groups usually increase the age range to 18 years, but a number appear to use the UNAIDS definition. It is also being more generally accepted that the loss of the father would also classify the child as an orphan. The UNAIDS definition has come under criticism for its lack of breadth and sensitivity to the situation on the ground for many children. The criticism acknowledges that increasing the age covered by the definition to 18 does have policy implications, since this definition increases the number of children affected, but the context demands this acknowledgement.

Within the orphan grouping, layers of vulnerability are addressed as one system for adding descriptive understanding to the context of the OVC. There appear to be some implicit classification systems for orphans, such as the nature of their caregivers i.e., extended families, foster parents, community caregivers, child-headed households and those under institutional care, the level of additional assistance that is required, and between maternal, paternal and double orphans.

"Vulnerability" is much more difficult to define. The complexity increases when it is considered that this definition needs to guide work with children in multiple contexts around the world, and needs to avoid being construed as stigmatizing. World Vision listed some identifiers, such as children who live in a household in which one person or more is ill, dying or deceased; children who live in households who receive orphans; children whose caregivers are too ill to continue to look after them; and children living with very old and frail caregivers. A consultative meeting in Kenya defined children as vulnerable if they lived in households with a chronically ill parent or caregiver, and in terms of access to key resources such as food, shelter, education, psychosocial and emotional support and love. These categories focus on factors related to HIV. There is an entire set of variables that needs to be considered that relate to more general aspects of the child's context, such as poverty, access to shelter, education and other basic services, disability, impact of drought, stigma and political repression—all factors that could influence vulnerability.

A range of definitions has been used for describing vulnerability in children across a number of African countries. In Botswana, children seen as vulnerable were street children, child laborers, children who are sexually exploited, who are neglected, those with handicaps and children in remote areas who are part of indigenous minorities. By contrast, in Rwanda, vulnerable children include those in child-headed households, in foster care, in institutions, in conflict with the law, street children, disabled children, children affected by armed conflict, children who are sexually exploited or abused, working children, children with parents in prison, children in very poor households, refugee or displaced children and children who get married before the age of majority. The definition of vulnerable children from South Africa included those children who are neglected, destitute or abandoned, living with terminally ill parents, those born to single mothers, with unemployed caretakers, who are abused or ill-treated by caretakers or are disabled. Finally, in Zambia, a state of vulnerability was assigned to children who were not at school, children from female/aged/disabled-headed households, children whose parents are ill, children from families where there is insufficient food, and children who live in poor housing.

With the creation of terms to name or define a group, especially a group seen to be having as many problems as OVC, they become objectified or automatically become targets for stigma. Care must therefore be taken with how the term is used, in both the academic and popular literature, as well as in care programs.

Community definitions of the orphan and the vulnerable child are also often different from the definitions used by government and external agencies. For instance, assistance to children by the government is directed by particular age limits—any child that falls outside those limits may be excluded. There was general consensus during the focus groups that the government should adopt a "bottom-up" approach, taking guidance from community level when setting parameters for assistance. To get a real sense of where to introduce interventions or support, a clear understanding of the community's perspective is required. Time has to be spent in the community listening to people who are doing work there already, particularly the caretakers and the vulnerable children themselves. Work in this project, to obtain a common definition of OVC across the three countries of Botswana, South Africa and Zimbabwe, is one contribution to establishing a basic definition that can be used as a basis for planning around OVC at a general level, while acknowledging the specifics of each intervention site.

▶ Methods

This research forms part of a much larger study aimed at developing interventions with OVC across seventeen research sites in Botswana, South Africa and Zimbabwe. The full study has multiple objectives, with the key aim being the development, implementation and evaluation of best practice interventions for OVC as well as their households and communities, to act as models for other sites in Africa and further afield. The aim of these interviews was to obtain a definition of OVC drawn from and having meaning for the communities in which the research project is being done. Ethical approval for this work was obtained as part of the ethical approval of the entire study from the ethics board of the University of the Witwatersrand in Johannesburg.

Research Design and Sample

The essential method of obtaining a definition was via focus group discussions with people in the communities, including service providers and orphans and caretakers, as well as broader members of the community. Group members were recruited on a purposive basis to try to ensure that there was an adequate representation of different sectors of the community who have

TABLE 15.1   Site of interviews with nature of the respondents and number in each group

Site of Interviews	Nature of the Respondents	Number
Botswana		
Letlhakeng	Primary caregivers in households of OVC	8
Letlhakeng	Community leaders including a chief and teachers and NGO staff including nurses and family welfare officers	10
Palapye	Members of the dominant NGO providing services, primary caregivers in households of OVC and OVC	10
Zimbabwe		
Bulilimamangwe	Traditional Chiefs and Headmen, Rural district council officers, social welfare representatives, local government representatives, staff of NGOs working with OVC	14
Bulilimamangwe	Primary caregivers in households of OVC including parents, volunteers who assist in the care of OVC and Church members who also provide assistance	30
Chimanimani	Traditional Chiefs, Rural district council officers, social welfare representatives, local government representatives, staff of NGOs working with OVC	15
Chimanimani	Primary caregivers in households of OVC including parents, volunteers who assist in the care of OVC and Church members who also provide assistance	20
South Africa		
Mathjabeng	Department of Health (DoH) home based caregivers for people with HIV/AIDS, DoH official and representatives from faith based organisations (FBO)	15
Mathjabeng	Representatives from a day care centre, an FBO and an NGO providing support to OVC and interested members of the community	9
Mathjabeng	Members of a the local task team set up to address issues of OVC, including representatives from the DoH, Dept. of Social Development and NGOs	8
Klerksdorp	Representatives from NGOs, a traditional healer and a volunteer from a local clinic	12

contact with and work with OVC. These interviews were done as a first phase of research during the initial period of meeting with communities and requesting access, so would have been the first contact with people in the communities. The full list of interviews undertaken is provided in Table 15.1. All interviews were conducted in the language of the persons being interviewed.

Research Question

Rather than using a fixed question or discussion schedule, the following statement was read to the group as a basis for discussion:

> With the HIV epidemic, poverty and other social problems, many children have been put at risk by the loss of parents or the increasing pressure that the epidemic and poverty have put on their community. The vulnerability can be seen in terms of illness, unemployment, violence, HIV, crime, desertion, etc. We are looking for a definition of such a vulnerable child. The definition will be used to guide a community-wide intervention directed at

orphaned and vulnerable children, and will act a basis for the research. To repeat, we would like to get a definition of those children the community considers to be vulnerable.

A checklist of the major potential areas of vulnerability also guided the interviewers. These included principally the age limitations to childhood, definitions of orphanhood and vulnerability, indicators of vulnerability and orphanhood. Within the definition of vulnerability interviewers were asked to check specifically for issues around hunger, loss of schooling, illness, emotional issues, loss of resources, loss of caretakers, and also to probe for any new ideas from the group members. Finally for the identification of and provision of services for OVC, interviewers were also asked to identify differences between a vulnerable child and a secure child, places and situations where these children would be found, and to specify the rights of the OVC to services, inherited property, security, a home, food, etc.

Analysis

A thematic content analysis method was used in analyzing the data. The analysis went through a number of stages. Transcriptions of audiotapes of the groups were used for the analysis. The researchers in each country developed a report based on the interviews done there using a content analysis method. The content analysis was done by hand, without the use of computer programs. There was no fixed process to the analysis nor were there preset critical themes, other than what was provided in the research question. However the researcher had met previously and discussed the research question and approach, so there was a common understanding as to the nature of the task and the analysis required. The authors of the study were responsible for the analysis, all of which have considerable experience in qualitative analysis. Again there had been discussion on methods of analysis at a previous inter-country meeting to agree on an overall approach. The process was not overly pre-structured to limit the potential for bias and to allow for new ideas to emerge from each country. The reports were then drawn together into this document. All the research staff that worked on establishing definition reports for their own countries and sites agreed on the final analysis and definition as outlined in this document.

Within this document the construct for the OVC requires consideration of a number of components of the broad term, i.e. definition of a child and of an orphan, and of what constitutes vulnerability. These sub-definitions were outlined first, before the full definition was drawn together. There was considerable agreement on many of the constructs across all the groups and sites in the three countries. Some important variations in and nuances to the explanations according to context have to be addressed.

▶ Results

Definition of a Child

A child is primarily defined by age, with most common agreement being 18 years, which is the legal age of majority in many of the sub-Saharan countries. Ultimately, age definitions were felt to depend on the period of dependence of the child on the parents or caretakers of the household. The period of dependence could be extended considerably by many situations, including unemployment, extended studies, physical or mental handicap, or severe illness. Such individuals would not be considered as children, but would remain dependent and remain part of the load on the household.

Definition of an Orphan

The most accepted definition of an orphan is a child who has lost one or both parents through death. This definition was immediately extended in most of the groups to include loss of parents through desertion or if the parents are unable or unwilling to provide care. In most cases the absent parent is the father. The feeling among some respondents was that fathers seldom return, even after the death or absence of the mother.

An initial question often raised was whether the loss of one parent constituted orphan status, and whether there was a difference according to which parent died or left. For most the loss of one parent was sufficient to classify the child as an orphan, especially if the primary caregiver was lost. A distinction was made here between a wage earner, usually the father, and a carer at home, usually the mother. Both were considered vital to the survival of the household and for the healthy development of the child.

A second concern was whether the child who still had a caregiver should be considered an orphan, since they still have extended family or caregivers from their community. This was raised particularly in view of the African context, where many stated that "orphan" is not a recognized term. Group participants pointed out that their community is not aware of the difference between orphan and a vulnerable child: ". . . a child remains a child right through, that is the African culture." However, others in the same group felt that some distinctions are made between orphaned and other vulnerable children, which impact on the provision of assistance to the children concerned.

The claim that African culture did not define orphan status was contradicted by statements made in one of the groups from Botswana. According to them, in Setswana there are two terms that describe an orphan: "lesiela" (lost one parent), and "khutsana" (lost both parents). "Lesiela" is widely used because it is user-friendly and less derogatory; with "khutsana," there is the implication that the child has absolutely nobody to care for him or her, which is contrary to extended family norms. The absence of guardians certainly increased the potential vulnerability of the orphan. In Zimbabwe orphans were divided into two groups, those with and those without guardians. This emphasized the point made in many of the groups that being an orphan did not always mean that the child became vulnerable—it would depend on the quality of caretaking from there on.

It was often stated in the groups that in African culture as soon as a child was in need they would be cared for. While the sentiment is generous, there are many children who have had to suffer in communities without adequate care, and in fact have experienced abuse. The problem is even more pronounced now with communities overwhelmed by the burden of AIDS that is leaving behind considerable numbers of orphans and vulnerable children. The extended family also contributes to vulnerability on occasions, by taking from the child their inheritance and family land, and even sometimes abusing their social support grants. These are monthly grants provided by government departments to assist in the ongoing maintenance of orphaned and other children who live in very poor circumstances. This contradiction has to be addressed, since romantic notions about care in Africa could be detrimental to planning and leave children without care.

Definition of a Vulnerable Child

A vulnerable child was seen as someone who has little or no access to basic needs or rights. They may have both parents, but the child might be compromised in other ways. The definition of vulnerability was felt to reflect certain aspects of the context of the child. Participants drew on personal experience, knowledge of context, and documents such as national constitutions. Vulnerability was contextualized for many as the child not having certain of their basic rights fulfilled, and identification of problems in the environment of the child or problems that the child faces.

The basic rights of children identified across the groups were to a name and nationality including recognition via birth registration; a safe home and community environment; education; love; family care and support; sufficient food and basic nutrition, protection from maltreatment, neglect, abuse both in and outside the home; security from abuse and violence from both the community and the government; health care and good hygiene; recreational facilities; adequate clothing; and the right to make choices concerning their way of living, e.g., not being forced into early marriage.

A set of inherent and contextual factors indicating vulnerability was also developed. This arose out of identified problems or gaps in the provision of needs, or specific threats that existed in the communities, and includes the individual, family and community contexts that make the child vulnerable.

Some specific indicators for vulnerability in children, any physical or mental handicap or any other long-term difficulty that would make it difficult for the child to function independently; illness, either HIV or other major illness; and emotional or psychological problems. Particularly in the case of the latter indicators that need to be checked include apathy or helplessness that might show in the child being unhappy, dull, not performing well in class, being miserable or demotivated; or neglect of schoolwork, not attending school regularly, not performing well at school. Also at the physical level indicators could include signs that the child does not receive sufficient healthy food and constantly shows signs of hunger; constantly showing signs of not sleeping well; has poor hygiene or cannot engage in personal care; and does not have clothing or clothing is dirty or damaged. The final set of core indicators included abuse at emotional, physical or sexual level; use of drugs, e.g., glue, alcohol, cigarettes, marijuana or crack; and not receiving care, particularly love, guidance and support.

The family situations that make the child vulnerable include caregivers who are not able or willing to care for the children under their care, including alcoholic, poor and emotionally disturbed parents; handicapped (physically and mentally) or chronically very sick parents, e.g., confined to bed; or parents or caregivers not equipped to provide the care giving role. With the increasing pressure of the number of children being orphaned the danger of households being overcrowded or the ratio of children to caregivers is too high was raised. Of particular concern were abusive family members or caregivers, including those who commit sexual and/or physical abuse. The latter should also cover the use of excessive discipline and corporal punishment. Children of divorced parents were felt to be at risk. Finally there were concerns that the caregivers may lack financial resources to adequately care for the child; or lack skills in parental guidance and direction.

The community context in which the child lives also influences vulnerability. The group members identified the following areas of concern in terms of risk of being exposed to dangerous situations. Unsafe environments such as informal settlements without adequate housing, lack of toilets leading to the presence of raw sewage, or high levels of crime and exposure to and/or participation in crime, gangs and drug use were particular external threats. A lack of facilities for children to allow for safe entertainment and play, and for extramural activities; was felt to possibly deny children opportunities for enjoyment of the space of being a child and put limits on development. High levels of poverty were acknowledged as a general threat as this meant the child having to go without many crucial resources. Finally, there were concerns about any community situations that prevent children from having a normal life, e.g. obtaining schooling, having time and space to play, being safe from physical or emotional threats etc.

Vulnerability is not an absolute state. There are degrees of vulnerability, depending on the situation of the child. As shown above, a number of factors contribute to a child's vulnerability. Each of these could add to the cumulative load that the child carries. The extent of the crisis and additional problems associated with it will also affect the impact on the child. Other factors that influence the impact of a stressor include—the age at which the loss of parents and assets took place, the state of development of internal resources within the child, and any coping strategies or support structures put in place. The most vulnerable are those children who have no caretakers, with street children being the most vulnerable among them. Street children are found at shops and malls, on streets, in market areas and abandoned buildings, and at road junctions and refuse disposal sites.

It is important to note that a balance of aspects in the child's context determines vulnerability, so even if one component goes wrong the child could suffer considerably. One example provided is that a child may be provided with all their basic needs, but be abused by the caretaker. One group expressed concern that although parents may show love and care, and provide well for a child, they may also practice excessive discipline or abuse the child. Ultimately, each child has to be examined individually to determine their own vulnerability, but it remains important to establish some central constructs for this definition. There was a particular fear of children being abused behind closed doors, and a sense of a lack of power to do anything about the risk.

> Families cannot be relied upon; a case of an uncle who took children under his protection. It later turned out that he was abusing them. We tried to call the police after we visited him and found out but he has since disappeared. He used to buy books, clothes, etc.; now these children are at my home and my mother is also unemployed.

Definition of a Caretaker

A caretaker is the person who plays the key caring role for the OVC. The person should be able to provide all aspects of care and be responsible for the child under their care. The roles for caretakers are seen as being to protect the rights of the children in their care as far as they are able; provision of basic requirements of life and development such as shelter, food, education, clothing and health care; provision of environment for psychosocial development and to support, moral, cultural and religious instruction, as well as basic hygiene; being responsible if anything happens to a child and being there to attend to the child; and ensuring that the conditions exist for adequate emotional development.

In many debates there is talk of a primary caretaker, but this needs further definition. In the focus groups there was division as to whether the primary caretaker is the person who provides emotional care, or the person who brings in the financial support. While they were seen as separate with strong gender overtones as to who could effectively provide is each role, both were considered as being of key importance to the ongoing survival of the child.

Overall Definition

An overall definition is required for intervention and research, which raises considerable complications—especially if an absolute answer is sought. The definition needs rather to incorporate a range of factors that may be important.

There appeared to be agreement that the age limit for definition of a child should be 18 years. An orphan is a child who has lost either one or both parents. The remainder of the definition needs to centre around three core areas. The relative importance of each will be defined by context: *Material problems,* including access to money, food, clothing, shelter, health care and education; *Emotional problems,* including experience of caring, love, support, space to grieve and containment of emotions; *Social problems,* including lack of a supportive peer group, of role models to follow, stigma or of guidance in difficult situations, and risks in the immediate environment; Vulnerability may be defined according to what is immediately seen in a situation and what is more easily measurable.

An initial attempt to operationalize and measure from the definition is provided below. One danger of this approach is that it is biased against hidden problems such as emotional issues and abuse, and can put excessive emphasis on income and financial security. The discussions within the groups and critical examination of the definition raised a number of questions, which need to be addressed.

The community factors that form part of the vulnerability of a child affect all children in a community. This raises the question of whether all children living in certain contexts should be considered OVC. One method of addressing this would be to look at likely exposure to the negative influences, or whether the impact of these community factors is variable across the community.

A clearer discussion of what is meant by vulnerability is also required. As a starting-point it implies real risk of long-term damage. This would include vulnerability to infection with HIV, dropping out of school and losing out on an education, experiencing development problems through lack of food, or having social problems due to not being cared for or being denied a role model. These points can start the discussion, but the complexity of the definition requires more thorough debate and more inputs.

In order to be able to measure vulnerability using a survey or general data source, easily measurable criteria are required. For this exercise two aspects of measurement have to be considered, namely the ease or even possibility of measurement, and the likely accuracy of the results. Constructs that are more easily measurable include death or desertion of parents; severe chronic illness of parents; illness of child; disability of child; poverty/income levels, including difficulty in accessing to grants; poor housing; difficulties in accessing services, e.g., schooling, health and social services; and inadequate clothing. However, even here considerable problems must be recognized and it may be difficult in any situation to get full and accurate measures of these variables.

Some of the more difficult variables to measure are emotional problems; occurrence of abuse, including excessive discipline; and substance abuse by caregivers or the child.

These are often hidden or are less tangible, and so less open to measurement. However, their implications for the child can be as great as or greater than those more easily calculated, so they also have to be considered. There are options for the use of psychometric scales or observational research methods to collect this information.

▶ Conclusions

This discussion provides a starting point for the construction of a definition of OVC that can be used for the development of interventions, and for the development of further research to adequately understand the position of OVC. The variation across contexts requires specific consideration, as stated under "Methodology." However, there was strong agreement across all the sites and as to the content of this report. The results are also similar to those obtained from research in many other countries. It is useful to note that similar debates and decisions around definition and support were generated in Rwanda in discussions about assisting vulnerable children after the genocide.

There are a number of immediate confusions around the levels of need of OVC, the relative readiness of governments to step in and assist the people in the country, and the role of culture in responding to the situation of HIV. The influence of these and other contextual variables on vulnerability and on the nature of the vulnerability that the child would experience have to be considered in the ongoing development of a construct of vulnerability. For example, if a rural community is experiencing a drought, then access to food and water becomes core to the care of the children living there. However, even given these needs for flexibility, it is possible to develop an overarching set of constructs that can be used to understand the vulnerability that children face in certain communities.

At the basis of all of this work is the desire to address the needs of OVC. A definition of such vulnerable children provides a basis for understanding the range and nature of needs that vulnerable children face. In each context, greater specificity about needs will have to be obtained, but this is part of the development of interventions that seek to roll back the impact of HIV and other challenges to childhood development.

▶ Acknowledgements

We would like to acknowledge the W. K. Kellogg Foundation for their funding of the study and interventions, and for their continued support of this program.

The direct contribution of the Masiela Trust in Botswana, the Family AIDS Caring Trust in Zimbabwe and the Nelson Mandela Children's Fund in South Africa also need to be acknowledged for assisting in facilitating access and for their collaboration on the overall project.

Finally, those who participated directly in the project are, particularly the OVC, caregivers, NGO members, and service providers.

▶ References

1. Appleton, J. (2000). At my age I should be sitting under that tree: The impact of AIDS on Tanzanian lakeshore communities. *Gender and Development, 8*(2), 19–27.

2. Bhargava, A., and Bigombe, B. (2003). 21 June. Public policies and the orphans of AIDS in Africa. *British Medical Journal, 326,* 1387–1389.

3. Baylies, C. (2000). The impact of HIV on family size preference in Zambia. *Reproductive Health Matters, 8*(15), 77–86.

4. Bicego, G., Rutstein, S., and Johnson, K. (2003). Dimensions of the emerging orphan crisis in sub-Saharan Africa. *Social Science and Medicine, 56,* 1235–1247.

5. Evans, R. (2003). Voices of the stigmatised: Listening to the street children of Tanzania. Lawyers for Human Rights. Available at: http://www.lhr.org.za/child/page0.php. Accessed March 17, 2004.

6. Hunter, S. (1991). The impact of AIDS on children in sub-Saharan African urban centers. *African Urban Quarterly, 6*(1&2), 108–128.

7. ICAD HIV/AIDS and Policies Affecting Children. (2001). Interagency coalition on AIDS and development. Available at: www.icad-cisd.com. Accessed March 17, 2004.

8. Krift, T., and Phiri, S. (2004). Developing a strategy to strengthen community capacity to assist HIV/AIDS-affected children and families: The COPE Program of Save the Children Federation in Malawi. Available at: http://www.cindi.org.za/papers/papers7.htm. Accessed March 17, 2004.

9. Masland, T., Nordland, R., Kaheru, S., Santoro, L., Haller, V., and Bagely, S. (2000). 10 million orphans. *Newsweek,* 17 January, 42–45.

10. NACC Taskforce on OVC, Nairobi. (2002). Proceedings of a consultative meeting of OVC. 16–19 December, 2002. Available at: http://www.fhi.org/en/HIVAIDS/Publications/Archive/confrpts/Orphans_HIV_Research.htm. Accessed March 17, 2004.

11. Nyambedha, E., Wandibba, S., and Aagaard-Hansen, J. (2003). Changing patterns of orphan care to the HIV epidemic in western Kenya. *Social Science and Medicine, 57,* 301–311.

12. Peterson, A. (2004). Situation update. Paper presented at the XV International AIDS Conference 2004, 11–16 June, Bangkok: Thailand.

13. RAISA. (2002). Regional AIDS Initiative of Southern Africa: Orphans and vulnerable children and HIV/AIDS national workshop report. Bronte Hotel, Harare, Zimbabwe, 28–29 November 2002.

14. Robinson, S. (1999). Orphans of AIDS. *Time,* 13 December, 60–61.

15. Smart, R. A. (2003). Policies for orphans and vulnerable children: A framework for moving ahead. Washington: Policy project, USAID.

16. UNICEF/UNAIDS. (1999). Children orphaned by AIDS. Frontline responses from eastern and southern Africa. New York: UNICEF Division of Communication.

17. UNICEF. (2004). Factsheet: Children without primary caregivers and in institutions. Geneva: UNICEF.

18. Whiteside, A. (2000). The real challenges: The orphan generation and employment creation. *AIDS Analysis Africa, 10*(4), 14–15.

19. Women's Commission for Refugee Women & Children. (2004). Rwanda's Women and children: The long road to reconciliation, 1997. Available at: http://www.womenscommission.org/report/rw/rwanda.html Accessed March 17, 2004.

20. World Bank. (2004). Operational guidelines for supporting early child development (ECD) in multi-sectoral HIV/AIDS programs in Africa, 2004. Available at: http://www.worldbank.org/children/ECDAIDSRevised.htm. Accessed March 17, 2004.

21. World Vision. (2002). *Summary of OVC programming approaches.* Geneva: World Vision International/HIV/AIDS Hope Initiative, 2002.

▶ Suggested Readings and Resources for Part 4

UNAIDS: 2006 Report on the global epidemic
Chapter 4: The Impact of AIDS on People and Societies
http://www.unaids.org/en/HIV_data/2006GlobalReport/default.asp

UNAIDS: 2006 Report on the global epidemic
Chapter 9: The Essential Role of Civil Society
http://www.unaids.org/en/HIV_data/2006GlobalReport/default.asp

Women, HIV and AIDS
http://www.avert.org/wwhiv.htm

Women's Health Information Center, December 2006
http://www.womenshealth.gov/hiv/gender/

Women's Health Information Center, December 2006
http://www.womenshealth.gov/hiv/worldwide/

Kawachi & Wamala (2007). Case Study: The Zambia PRSP. Poverty and HIV: Chapter 14
Excerpt: The Globalization of Health. 236–240.

Working with Religious Leaders to Prevent the Spread of HIV/AIDS in Senegal
FHI/UNAIDS Best Practices in HIV/AIDS Prevention
http://www.fhi.org/en/HIVAIDS/pub/guide/bestpractices.htm

Working with the Church in Kenya to Prevent the Spread of HIV/AIDS FHI/UNAIDS
Best Practices in HIV/AIDS Prevention
http://www.fhi.org/en/HIVAIDS/pub/guide/bestpractices.htm

UNAIDS: 2006 Report on the global epidemic
Chapter 3: Progress in Countries
http://www.unaids.org/en/HIV_data/2006GlobalReport/default.asp

AIDS Around the World
http://www.avert.org/aids-countries.htm

HIV Prevention Around the World
http://www.avert.org/hivprevention.htm

UNAIDS: 2006 Report on the global epidemic
Chapter 8: Reducing the Impact of AIDS
http://www.unaids.org/en/HIV_data/2006GlobalReport/default.asp

AIDS Epidemic Update: WHO 2006
http://www.who.int/hiv/mediacentre/news62/en/index.html

Okie (2006): Fighting HIV: Lessons from Brazil. The New England Journal of Medicine; 354:19:1977–1981.

Merson, Black & Mills (2006). Chapter 2 Excerpt: Case Study: The Slim Disease: HIV/AIDS in Sub-Saharan Africa. International Public Health 2nd Edition.

FHI/UNAIDS Best Practices in HIV/AIDS Prevention
http://www.fhi.org/en/HIVAIDS/pub/guide/bestpractices.htm

HIV Prevention, Harm Reduction and Injecting Drug Use
http://www.avert.org/wwhiv.htm

HIV Prevention and Sex Workers
http://www.avert.org/wwhiv.htm

Older People and HIV and AIDS
http://www.avert.org/wwhiv.htm

HIV/AIDS Prevention and Education for Refugees: Implementing Effective Emergency Projects, FHI/UNAIDS Best Practices in HIV/AIDS Prevention
http://www.fhi.org/en/HIVAIDS/pub/guide/bestpractices.htm

Children, HIV and AIDS
http://www.avert.org/wwhiv.htm

AIDS Orphans
http://www.avert.org/wwhiv.htm

Child-Headed Households: International Perspectives on children left behind by HIV/AIDS
http://www.ovcsupport.net/graphics/OVC/documents/0000015e02.pdf

Child-Headed Households, 2005 Office of the UN High Commissioner for Human Rights
http://www.crin.org/docs/resources/treaties/crc.40/GDD_2005_Plan_Finland.pdf

Critical Thinking

1. Select a social condition discussed and research information on what is being done to address this particular issue with HIV.
2. What would you say to someone who says that a person deserves to get HIV/AIDS if they behave inappropriately?
3. What does poverty have to do with the spread of sexually transmitted infections?
4. What are the challenges to prevention in rural areas?

Discussion Questions

1. How are women affected by HIV?
2. List and describe the four at risk populations for HIV.
3. How is stigma involved with HIV?
4. How are children affected by HIV?
5. How are culture and poverty associated with HIV?

Appendix
A

Male and Female Reproductive System

Janet Stein Carter

▶ Male Reproductive System

The male reproductive system is illustrated to the right. **Sperm** are produced in the **testes** located in the **scrotum**. Normal body temperature is too hot thus is lethal to sperm so the testes are outside of the abdominal cavity where the temperature is about 2° C (3.6° F) lower. Note also that a woman's body temperature is lowest around the time of ovulation to help insure sperm live longer to reach the egg. If a man takes too many long, very hot baths, this can

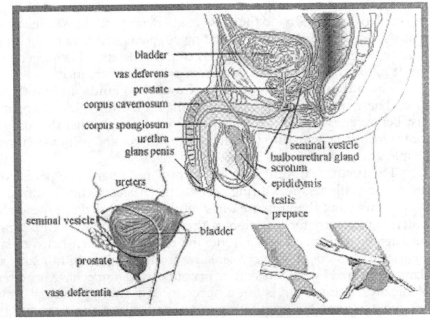

reduce his sperm count. Undescended testes (testes are supposed to descend before birth) will cause sterility because their environment is too warm for sperm viability unless the problem can be surgically corrected.

From there, sperm are transferred to the **epididymis,** coiled tubules also found within the scrotum, that store sperm and are the site of their final maturation.

In **ejaculation,** sperm are forced up into the **vas deferens** (plural = vasa deferentia). From the epididymis, the vas deferens goes up, around the front of, over the top of, and behind the bladder. A **vasectomy** is a fairly simple, outpatient operation that involves making a small slit in each scrotum, cutting the vasa deferentia near where they begin, and tying off the cut ends to prevent sperm from leaving the scrotum. Because this is a relatively non-invasive procedure (as compared to doing the same to a woman's oviducts), this is a popular method of permanent birth control once a couple has had all the children they desire. Couples should carefully weigh their options, because this (and the corresponding female procedure) is not designed to be a reversible operation.

The ends of the vasa deferentia, behind and slightly under the bladder, are called the **ejaculatory ducts**. The **seminal vesicles** are also located behind the bladder. Their secretions are about 60% of the total volume of the **semen** (= sperm and associated fluid) and contain mucus, amino acids, fructose as the main energy source for the sperm, and prostaglandins to stimulate female uterine contractions to move the semen up into the uterus. The seminal vesicles empty into the ejaculatory ducts. The ejaculatory ducts then empty into the **urethra** (which, in males, also empties the urinary bladder).

The initial segment of the urethra is surrounded by the **prostate gland** (note spelling!). The prostate is the largest of the accessory glands and puts its secretions directly into the urethra. These secretions are alkaline to buffer any residual urine, which tends to be acidic, and the acidity of the woman's vagina. The prostate needs a lot of **zinc** to function properly, and insufficient dietary zinc (as well as other causes) can lead to enlargement which potentially can constrict the urethra to the point of interfering with urination. Mild cases of prostate **hypertrophy** can often be treated by adding supplemental zinc to the man's diet, but severe cases require surgical removal of portions of the prostate. This surgery, if not done very carefully can lead to problems with urination or sexual performance.

The **bulbourethral glands** or **Cowper's glands** are the third of the accessory structures. These are a small pair of glands along the urethra below the prostate. Their fluid is secreted just before emission of the semen, thus it is thought that this fluid may serve as a lubricant for inserting the penis into the vagina, but because the volume of these secretions is very small, people are not totally sure of this function.

The urethra goes through the **penis**. In humans, the penis contains three cylinders of spongy, **erectile tissue**. During arousal, these become filled with blood from the arteries that supply them and the pressure seals off the veins that drain these areas causing an **erection,** which is necessary for insertion of the penis into the woman's vagina. In a number of other animals, the penis also has a bone, the **baculum,** which helps to stiffen it. The head of the penis, the **glans penis,** is very sensitive to stimulation. In humans, as in other mammals, the glans is covered by the foreskin or **prepuce,** which may have been removed by **circumcision**. Medically, circumcision is not a necessity, but rather a cultural "tradition." Males who have not been circumcised need to keep the area between the glans and the prepuce clean so bacteria and/or yeasts don't start to grow on accumulated secretions, etc. there. There is some evidence that uncircumcised males who do not keep the glans/prepuce area clean are slightly more prone to penile cancer.

▶ Female Reproductive System

The female reproductive system is illustrated on the next page. "**Eggs**" are produced in the **ovaries,** but remember from our discussion of meiosis, that these are not true eggs, yet, and will never complete meiosis and become such unless/until first fertilized by a sperm. Within the ovary, a **follicle** consists of one precursor egg cell surrounded by special cells to nourish and protect it. A human female typically has about 400,000 follicles/potential eggs, all formed before birth. Only several hundred of these "eggs" will actually ever be released during her reproductive years. Normally, in humans, after the onset of puberty, due to the

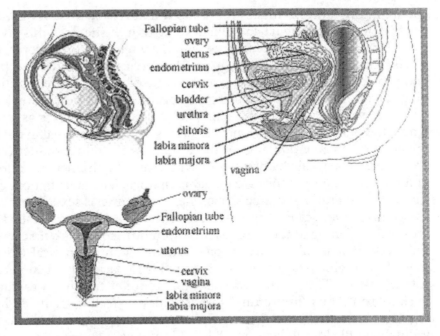

stimulation of **follicle-stimulating hormone (FSH)** one "egg" per cycle matures and is released from its ovary. **Ovulation** is the release of a mature "egg" due to the stimulation of **leutenizing hormone (LH),** which then stimulates the remaining follicle cells to turn into a **corpus luteum** which then secretes **progesterone** to prepare the uterus for possible implantation. If an egg is not fertilized and does not implant, the corpus luteum disintegrates and when it stops producing progesterone, the lining of the uterus breaks down and is shed.

Each "egg" is released into the abdominal cavity near the opening of one of the **oviducts** or **Fallopian tubes**. Cilia in the oviduct set up currents that draw the egg in. If sperm are present in the oviduct (if the couple has recently had intercourse), the egg will be fertilized near the far end of the Fallopian tube, will quickly finish meiosis, and the embryo will start to divide and grow as it travels to the uterus. The trip down the Fallopian tube takes about a week as the cilia in the tube propel the unfertilized "egg" or the embryo down to the **uterus**. At this point, if she had intercourse near the time of ovulation, the woman has no idea whether an unfertilized "egg" or a new baby is travelling down that tube. During this time, progesterone secreted by the corpus luteum has been stimulating the **endometrium,** the lining of the uterus, to thicken in preparation for possible implantation, and when a growing embryo finally reaches the uterus, it will implant in this nutritious environment and begin to secrete its own hormones to maintain the endometrium. If the "egg" was not fertilized, it dies and disintegrates, and as the corpus luteum also disintegrates, its progesterone production falls, and the unneeded, built-up endometrium is shed.

The **uterus** has thick, muscular walls and is very small. In a **nulliparous** woman, the uterus is only about 7 cm long by 4 to 5 cm wide, but it can expand to hold a 4 kg baby. The lining of the uterus is called the **endometrium,** and has a rich capillary supply to bring food to any embryo that might implant there.

The bottom end of the uterus is called the **cervix.** The cervix secretes mucus, the consistency of which varies with the stages in her menstrual cycle. At ovulation, this **cervical mucus** is clear, runny, and conducive to sperm. Post-ovulation, the mucus gets thick and pasty to block sperm. Enough of this mucus is produced that it is possible for a woman to touch a finger to the opening of her vagina and obtain some of it. If she does this on a daily basis, she can use the information thus gained, along with daily temperature records, to tell where in her cycle she is. If a woman becomes pregnant, the cervical mucus forms a plug to seal off the uterus and protect the developing baby, and any medical procedure which involves removal of that plug carries the risk of introducing pathogens into the nearly-sterile uterine environment.

The **vagina** is a relatively-thin-walled chamber. It serves as a repository for sperm (it is where the penis is inserted), and also serves as the birth canal. Note that, unlike the male, the female has separate opening for the urinary tract and reproductive system. These openings are covered externally by two sets of skin folds. The thinner, inner folds are the **labia minora** and the thicker, outer ones are the **labia majora.** The labia minora contain erectile tissue like that in the penis, thus change shape when the woman is sexually aroused. The opening around the genital area is called the **vestibule.** There is a membrane called the **hymen** that partially covers the opening of the vagina. This is torn by the woman's first sexual intercourse (or sometimes other causes like injury or some kinds of vigorous physical activity). In women, the openings of the vagina and urethra are susceptible to bacterial infections if fecal bacteria are wiped towards them. Thus, while parents who are toilet-training a toddler usually wipe her from back to front, thus "imprinting" that sensation as feeling "right" to her, it is important, rather, that that little girls be taught to wipe themselves from the front to the back to help prevent vaginal and bladder infections. Older girls and women who were taught the wrong way need to make a conscious effort to change their habits.

At the anterior end of the labia, under the pubic bone, is the clitoris, the female equivalent of the penis. This small structure contains **erectile tissue** and many nerve endings in a sensitive **glans** within a **prepuce** which totally encloses the glans. This is the most sensitive point for female sexual stimulation, so sensitive that vigorous, direct stimulation does not feel good. It is better for the man to gently stimulate near the clitoris rather than right on it. Some cultures do a procedure, similar to circumcision, as a puberty rite in teenage girls in which the prepuce is cut, exposing the extremely-sensitive clitoris. There are some interesting speculations on the cultural significance of this because the sensitivity of the exposed clitoris would probably make having sexual intercourse a much less pleasant experience for these women.

Appendix
B

HIV/AIDS Epidemiology, Pathogenesis, Prevention and Treatment

Viviana Simon, David D. Ho,
Quarraisha Abdool Karim

The HIV-1 pandemic is a complex mix of diverse epidemics within and between countries and regions of the world, and is undoubtedly the defining public-health crisis of our time. Research has deepened our understanding of how the virus replicates, manipulates, and hides in an infected person. Although our understanding of pathogenesis and transmission dynamics has become more nuanced and prevention options have expanded, a cure or protective vaccine remains elusive. Antiretroviral treatment has transformed AIDS from an inevitably fatal condition to a chronic, manageable disease in some settings. This transformation has yet to be realised in those parts of the world that continue to bear a disproportionate burden of new HIV-1 infections and are most affected by increasing morbidity and mortality. This Seminar provides an update on epidemiology, pathogenesis, treatment, and prevention interventions pertinent to HIV-1.

▶ HIV Pandemic

An estimated 38 · 6 (33 · 4 – 46 · 0) million people live with HIV-1 worldwide, while about 25 million have died already.[1] In 2005 alone, there were 4 · 1 million new HIV-1 infections and 2 · 8 million AIDS deaths.[1] These estimates mask the dynamic nature of this evolving epidemic in relation to temporal changes, geographic distribution, magnitude, viral diversity, and mode of transmission. Today, there is no region of the world untouched by this pandemic (Figure B-1).[2]

503

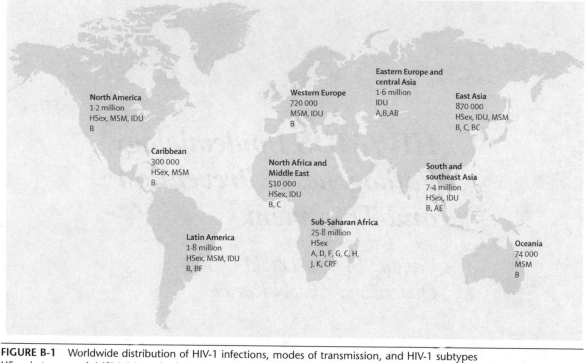

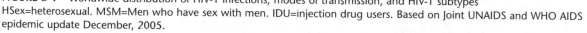

FIGURE B-1   Worldwide distribution of HIV-1 infections, modes of transmission, and HIV-1 subtypes HSex=heterosexual. MSM=Men who have sex with men. IDU=injection drug users. Based on Joint UNAIDS and WHO AIDS epidemic update December, 2005.

Heterosexual transmission remains the dominant mode of transmission and accounts for about 85% of all HIV-1 infections. Southern Africa remains the epicentre of the pandemic and continues to have high rates of new HIV-1 infections.[3] Although overall HIV-1 prevalence remains low in the emerging epidemics in China and India, the absolute numbers, which are fast approaching those seen in southern Africa, are of concern.[1] Outside of sub-Saharan Africa, a third of all HIV-1 infections are acquired through injecting drug use, most (an estimated 8 · 8 million) of which are in eastern Europe and central and southeast Asia.[1] The rapid spread of HIV-1 in these regions through injecting drug use is of importance, since it is a bridge for rapid establishment of more generalised epidemics.

A defining feature of the pandemic in the current decade is the increasing burden of HIV-1 infections in women,[4] which has additional implications for mother-to-child transmission. Women now make up about 42% of those infected worldwide; over 70% of whom live in sub-Saharan Africa.[1] Overall, a quarter of all new HIV-1 infections are in adults aged younger than 25 years.[1] HIV-1 infection rates are three to six times higher in female adolescents than in their male counterparts,[1,5–7] and this difference is attributed to sexual coupling patterns of young women with older men. Population prevalence of HIV-1 infection, concurrent sexual relationships, partner change, sexual practices, the presence of other sexually transmitted diseases,[8–11] and population mobility patterns[12–14] for economic and other reasons (eg, natural disasters and wars) further increase the probability of HIV-1 acquisition.[3,15] Emerging data accord with strong links between risk of sexual HIV-1 acquisition and episodic recreational drug or alcohol use.[16]

SEARCH STRATEGY AND SELECTION CRITERIA

A comprehensive literature review was undertaken by searching the PubMed database online, for English language publications between January 2000, and June 2006. The database search terms included keywords such as "HIV/AIDS", "epidemiology", "prevention", "pathogenesis", "HSV-2", "male circumcision", "PMTCT", "scaling up treatment", "resource constrained settings", "antiretroviral pre-exposure prophylaxis", "HAART", "restriction", "host factor", "HIV pathogenesis", "resistance", "latency". Various combinations of these words were entered. All duplicate articles were removed. A subset of relevant articles was chosen and full-text manuscripts were summarised.

Although sub-Saharan Africa continues to bear a disproportionate burden of HIV-1 infections, there is now an increasing number of countries reporting stabilisation or declines in prevalence (eg, Zambia, Tanzania, Kenya, Ghana, Rwanda, Burkina Faso, and Zimbabwe).[1] There is some evidence to attribute these reductions to effective changes in sexual behaviour, such as postponement of sexual debut, reduction in casual relationships, and more consistent condom use in casual relationships.[17,18] However, increasing morbidity and mortality rates associated with a maturing HIV-1 epidemic need to be considered when interpreting these data.[19] For example, the death of a few high-risk individuals who are key to transmission chains could exert a major effect on sexual networks and result in major reductions in infection rates.[20] Additionally, since most HIV-1 estimates are based on surveys in antenatal populations, increasing morbidity and mortality could cause the numbers of women in this group to decrease, and thus lead to underestimates of the true prevalence in these countries.[19]

Although the relative contribution of cell-free virus compared with cell-associated virus in HIV-1 transmission remains unclear, there is growing evidence that viral load is predictive of transmission risk.[21,22] The highest levels of viraemia are seen during acute infection and advanced HIV-1 disease.[22] Further, co-infections with other sexually transmitted diseases in asymptomatic HIV-1 infected people can increase viral shedding to levels similar to those seen during acute infection.[23] Thus, sexually transmitted diseases could enhance HIV-1 transmission to rates similar to those seen during primary infection.[24] This observation could help to explain why the efficiency of HIV-1 transmission exceeds, in some settings, the earlier mathematical projections.[25] Thus, identification and treatment of recently infected people is an important means to reduce transmission. However, most people are unaware of their HIV-1 status during these crucial first months of infection. Several screening strategies based on laboratory testing and clinical algorithms are being developed and tested[26] for efficient identification of early infection before antibody development.[27] Additionally, a more aggressive management of sexually transmitted infections in settings with generalised epidemics has the potential to affect current epidemic trajectories.[24]

Based on their genetic make-up, HIV-1 viruses are divided into three groups (eg, M [main], N, and O group, Figure B-2). These HIV-1 groups and HIV-2 probably result from distinct cross-species transmission events.[28] Pandemic HIV-1 has diversified into at least nine subtypes (figures B-1 and B-2) and many circulating recombinant forms,[29,30] which encode genetic structures from two or more subtypes (eg, A/E=CRF01; A/G=CRF02). The continuously evolving HIV-1 viral diversity poses an immense challenge to the development of any preventive or therapeutic intervention.[29]

In terms of viral diversity, subtype C viruses continue to dominate and account for 55–60% of all HIV-1 infections worldwide (Figure B-1).[30] Non-subtype B isolates might differ in their

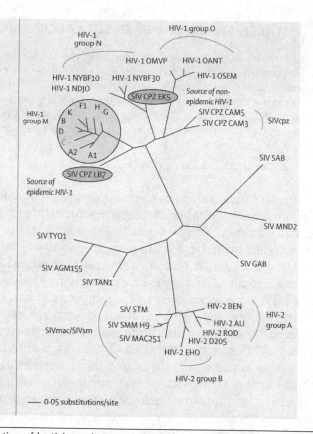

FIGURE B-2 Phylogenetic relation of lentiviruses in man and non-human primates

The HIV-1 pandemic is largely due to viral isolates belonging to the HIV-1 M-group, with HIV-1 subtype C being the most prevalent (red). Recombinant circulating forms cluster with the M-group but have been omitted for clarity. HIV-1 M group and the contemporary SIV strains identified in wild chimpanzees in Cameroon (SIVcpzLB7/EK5[28]) are highlighted. HIV-1 sequences cluster closely with SIV from chimpanzees (SIVcpz), whereas HIV-2 resembles SIV from macaques and sooty mangabeys (SIVmac/SIVsm).

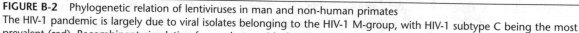

virological characteristics from the subtype B isolates (eg, viral load, chemokine co-receptor usage, transcriptional activation in specific biological compartments).[31–33] However, the clinical consequences of subtype variations remain unclear.

Infection with two or more genetically distinct viruses could lead to new recombinant viruses. Recombination takes place at a higher rate than initially predicted,[30] and circulating recombinant forms account for as much as 20% of infections in some regions (eg, southeast Asia).[31] These findings are in agreement with the occurrence of co-infections with multiple distinct isolates in a close temporal context.[34–36] Further, superinfections in which time points of virus acquisition are months to years apart have been described, although at a much lower frequency than co-infections.[34,37–39] Collectively, these observations challenge the assumption that HIV-1 acquisition happens only once with a singular viral strain and that, thereafter, the infected individual is protected from subsequent infections.[40] This lack of immunisation has substantial implications for vaccine development. Emerging evidence suggests that clinical progression to AIDS might be more rapid in individuals with dual infections,[35] and encouraging safer sex practices in viraemic HIV-1-infected people might be appropriate to keep recurrent exposure to new viral strains to a minimum.

▶ Pathogenesis of HIV-1

The worldwide spread of HIV-1 indicates that the virus effectively counteracts innate, adapted, and intrinsic immunity.[41,42] Despite its modest genome size (less than 10 kb) and its few genes (Figure B-3), HIV-1 excels in taking advantage of cellular pathways while neutralising and hiding from the different components of the immune system.[43–45] Notably, our understanding of pathogenesis is often derived from studies of subtype B viruses and non-human primate studies.

The HIV-1 life cycle is complex (Figure B-3) and its duration and outcome is dependent on target cell type and cell activation.[46] In the early steps, HIV-1 gains access to cells without causing immediate lethal damages but the entry process can stimulate intracellular signal cascades, which in turn might facilitate viral replication.[47,48] The two molecules on the HIV-1 envelope, the external glycoprotein (gp120) and the transmembrane protein (gp41), form the spikes on the virion's surface.[49] During the entry process, gp120 attaches to the cell membrane by first binding to the CD4+ receptor. Subsequent interactions between virus and chemokine co-receptors (eg, CCR5, CXCR4) trigger irreversible conformational changes.[49,50] The actual fusion event takes place within minutes by pore formation,[50,51] and releases the viral core into the cell cytoplasm. After the core disassembles, the viral genome is reverse transcribed into DNA by the virus' own reverse transcriptase enzyme.[46] Related yet distinct viral variants can be generated during this process since reverse transcriptase is error prone and has no proof-reading activity.[46] At the midpoint of infection, the viral protein integrase in conjunction with host DNA repair enzymes inserts the viral genome into gene-rich, transcriptionally active domains of the host's chromosomal DNA.[52–54] An integrase binding host factor, LEDGF/p75 (lens epithelium-derived growth factor), facilitates integration,[55,56] which marks the turning point by irreversibly transforming the cell into a potential virus producer. In the late steps, production of viral particles needs host driven as well as virus driven transcription.[46] Viral proteins are transported to and assemble in proximity to the cell membrane. Virus egress from the cell is not lytic and takes advantage of the vesicular sorting pathway (ESCRT-I, II, III), which normally mediates the budding of endosomes into multivesicular bodies.[57,58] HIV-1 accesses this protein-sorting pathway by binding TSG101 via its late domain, a short sequence motif in p6 of Gag.[59,60] Cleavage of the Gag-Pol polyprotein by the viral protease produces mature infectious virions.[46,61]

Since cytoplasmic molecules of the producer cell and components from its cell surface lipid bilayer are incorporated into the new viral particle, virions bear characteristics of the cells in which they were produced.[62] Incorporated host molecules can determine the virus' phenotype in diverse ways (eg, shape the replicative features in the next cycle of infection or mediate immune activation of bystander cells[62]).

Studies of the early events that happen after HIV-1 breaches the mucosal barrier suggest the existence of a window period in which viral propagation is not yet established and host defences could potentially control viral expansion.[63] The important co-receptors for HIV-1 infection are two chemokine receptors—CCR5 and CXCR4. Independently of the transmission route, most new infections are established by viral variants that rely on CCR5 usage.[64] CXCR4-tropic viruses generally appear in late stages of infection and have been associated with increased pathogenicity and disease progression.[65]

Compelling evidence from non-human primate models (eg, simian immunodeficiency virus [SIV] infection of rhesus macaques) suggest that vaginal transmission results in infection of a small number of CD4+ T lymphocytes, macrophages, and dendritic cells located in the lamina propria.[63] Potential pathways for virus transmission involve endocytosis,

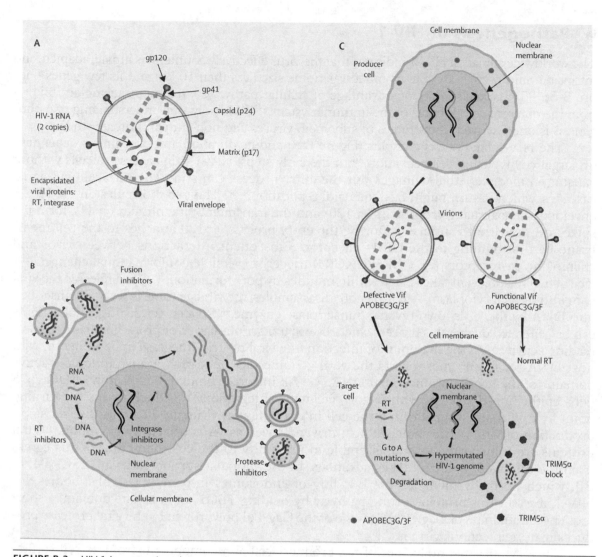

FIGURE B-3   HIV-1 is a retrovirus that encodes three structural genes (Gag, Pol, and Env)
(A) Envelope glycoproteins gp120/41 form the spikes on the virion's surface. During maturation the gag protein is cleaved and Gag p24 forms the core. The viral genome, viral reverse transcriptase (RT), integrase as well as a number of host proteins are encapsidated. (B) Different steps of the viral life cycle on a cellular level and the potential targets for treatment interventions. (C) HIV-1 has evolved strategies to counteract the restriction factors TRIM5α and APOBEC3G/3F. If left unchecked by HIV-1 Vif, APOBEC3G/3F is encapsidated into the egressing virion, and on infection of a target cell leads to G-to-A hypermutations in the viral genome. Rhesus TRIM5α inhibits HIV-1 replication early after infection of the target cell before the step of reverse transcription.

transcytosis, and virus attachment to mannose C-type lectin receptors (eg, DC-SIGN) located on dendritic cells and macrophages.[66] The initial replication takes place in the regional lymph organs (eg, draining lymph nodes) and is composed of few viral variants, and leads to modest primary amplification. With migration of infected T lymphocytes or virions into the bloodstream, secondary amplification in the gastrointestinal tract, spleen, and bone marrow results in massive infection of susceptible cells. In close temporal relation with the resulting peak of viraemia (eg, 10^6 to 10^7 copies per mL plasma), clinical symptoms can be manifested during primary HIV-1 infection (Figure B-4). The level of viraemia characteristic for the chronic phase of infection in an individual (viral set point) differs from the peak viraemia by one or two orders of magnitude. This reduction is largely attributed to HIV-1 specific CD8+ responses but target cell limitation could also play a part. The viral population is most homogeneous early after transmission, but as viral quasi-species diversify in distinct biological compartments, mutant viruses that are resistant to antibody neutralisation, cytotoxic T cells, or antiretroviral drugs are generated and archived in long-lived cells (ie, viral reservoirs).

A pronounced depletion of activated as well as memory CD4+ T cells located in the gut-associated lymphoid tissues has been seen in individuals identified early after infection.[67] The preferential depletion of the CD4+ cells in the mucosal lymphoid tissues remains despite years of antiretroviral treatment, a striking observation that contrasts with the fact that the number of CD4+ T lymphocytes in the peripheral blood can return to normal under antiretroviral treatment.

A gradual destruction of the naive and memory CD4+ T-lymphocyte populations is the hallmark of HIV-1 infection, with AIDS being the last disease stage (Figure B-4).[68] Despite

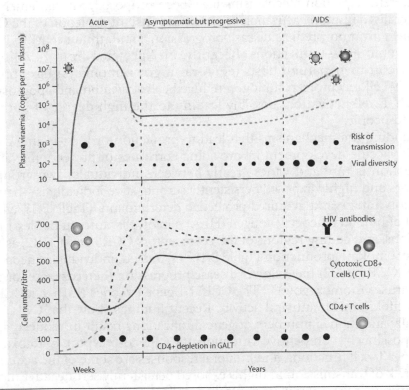

FIGURE B-4   The course of HIV-1 infection defined by the level of viral replication
Plasma viraemia (top), and dynamic changes of the CD4+ T-lymphocyte compartments (bottom). Primary infection characterised by high plasma viraemia (red line, top), low CD4 cells (green line, bottom), and absence of HIV-1 specific antibodies (orange line, bottom). Viraemia drops as cytotoxic CD8+ T-lymphocytes (CTL) develop (blue line, bottom) and an individual viral-load set point is reached during chronic infection. Viral set points differ greatly among individuals (eg, red dotted line, top) and predict disease progression. Viral diversity increases through out the disease (closed circles, top). The risk of transmission is highest in the first weeks when viraemia peaks (closed circles, top). GALT=gut-associated lymphoid tissues.

TABLE B.1 Some of the host factors affecting susceptibility to HIV-1 infection

Innate	Genetic	Acquired	Intrinsic
Autoantibodies	HLA haplotype	Cytotoxic T-cell activity	APOBEC3G/3F
Chemokines	CCR5 gene/promoter	Helper T-cell function	TRIM5α
Cytokines	CCR2 gene/promoter	Neutralising antibodies	
	CCL3L1 gene copy number		

HLA=human leucocyte antigen. CCR5=chemokine receptor 5. CCR2=chemokine receptor 2. CCL3L1=CC chemokine ligand like-1, APOBEC3G/3F=apolipoprotein B mRNA editing complex 3.

the frequent absence of symptoms during early and chronic phase, HIV-1 replication is dynamic throughout the disease. The half-life of a single virion is so short that half the entire plasma virus population is replaced in less than 30 minutes,[69] and the total number of virions produced in a chronically infected person can reach more than 10^{10} particles per day.[69,70] The turnover rates of lymphocyte populations are upregulated many fold during HIV-1 infection, whereas cell proliferation decreases once viral replication is reduced by antiretroviral treatment.[71,72] Different depletion mechanisms have been proposed, with an emerging consensus favouring generalised immune activation as cause for constant depletion of the CD4+ cell reservoir.[73] Immune activation predicts disease progression[74] and, thus, seems to be a central feature of pathogenic HIV-1 infections. Recently, Nef proteins from SIV lineages that are non-pathogenic in their natural hosts (eg, African green monkeys) have proved to downregulate CD3-T-cell receptors, resulting in reduced cell activation and apoptosis.[75] HIV-1 Nef fails to quench T-cell activation, possibly leading to the high degree of immune activation seen in infected people.

Understanding the mechanisms that lead to protection or long-lasting control of infection will guide vaccine development by providing correlates of protection. Natural resistance to HIV-1 infection is rare and varies greatly between individuals. Two groups—long-term non-progressors and highly exposed persistently seronegative individuals—have been studied widely to identify innate and acquired protective determinants (Table B.1).[76] Host resistance factors consist of human leucocyte antigen (HLA) haplotypes, autoantibodies, mutations in the promoter regions, and coding regions of the co-receptors CCR5 and CCR2, as well as the up-regulation of chemokine production (Table B.1).[76,77] Indeed, individuals encoding a truncated CCR5 version (CCR5ΔG32) have slower disease progression (heterozygote) or are resistant to CCR5-using viruses (homozygote).[78] The CCL3L1 gene encodes MIP1α, a CCR5 co-receptor ligand and chemokine with antiviral activity. Recent findings show that CCL3L1 gene copies vary individually and higher numbers of gene duplications result in reduced susceptibility to infection,[77,79] possibly by competitive saturation of CCR5 co-receptor. Cytotoxic T-lymphocyte responses, helper T-cell functions, and humoral responses are some of the acquired factors that modulate the risk of transmission in highly exposed persistently seronegative individuals,[76] and could also contribute to spontaneous control of replication in long-term non-progressors. The putative protective role of cytotoxic T-lymphocyte activity has been suggested in seronegative sex workers and in some long-term nonprogressors.[76,80]

Mammalian cells are not welcoming micro-environments, but rather deploy a defensive web to curb endogenous and exogenous viruses. HIV-1's ability to circumvent these defences is as impressive as its efficiency to exploit the cellular machinery. APOBEC3G/3F and TRIM5α are recently described intrinsic restriction factors that are constitutively expressed in many cells.[81,82] Both gene loci have been under strong selective pressure throughout primate evolution,[83] indicating an ancient need to neutralise foreign DNA and maintain genome stability that precedes the current HIV-1 pandemic.

APOBEC3 enzymes (A3) belong to the superfamily of cytidine deaminases,[84] a group of intracellular proteins with DNA/RNA editing activity.[84, 85] Most representatives of the APOBEC3 group have some mutagenic potential and restrict endogenous retroviruses and mobile genetic elements. The deaminases A3G, A3F, and A3B have potent antiviral activity, with the first two being expressed in cells that are susceptible to HIV-1 infection (T-lymphocytes, macrophages). HIV-1 evades APOBEC3 mutagenesis by expressing Vif, which leads to APOBEC3G/3F but not A3B degradation.[42,86–90]

We still need to establish how the mechanisms of DNA editing and antiviral activity are interwoven, since some antiviral activity can be maintained despite defective DNA editing.[91] The early replication block in non-stimulated CD4+ T cells has been attributed to low molecular mass complexes of APOBEC3G.[92] Hypermutated genomes in HIV-1 infected patients[93] and mutations in Vif resulting in abrogated or differential APOBEC3 neutralisation capacity have been described.[94, 95] The degree to which APOBEC3G/3F mRNA expression predicts clinical progression remains an area of intensive investigation.[96,97]

Several representatives of the heterogeneous family of tripartite motif proteins (TRIM) inhibit retroviruses in a species-specific manner.[81,98] TRIM5α from rhesus macaques and African green monkeys inhibit HIV-1 replication, whereas the human homologue is inactive against SIV and HIV-1, leading to the recorded susceptibility of human cells to both viruses.[81] Rhesus TRIM5α recognises the capsid domain of HIV-1 Gag and manipulates the kinetics of HIV-1 core disassembly within minutes after cell entry.[99,100] Thus, experimental approaches to render HIV-1 resistant to rhesus TRIM5α could lead to immunodeficiency viruses capable of replicating in rhesus macaques. Such a non-primate model would allow testing of antiviral treatment and vaccine interventions with HIV-1 viruses instead of SIV or SIV/HIV chimeric viruses.

▶ Clinical Management

Diagnosis

The diagnosis of HIV-1 infection is based on the detection of specific antibodies, antigens, or both, and many commercial kits are available. Serological tests are generally used for screening. A major advance has been the availability of rapid HIV-1 antibody tests. These assays are easy to do and provide results in as little as 20 minutes,[101] enabling specimen collection and proper diagnosis at the same visit. Rapid tests are important tools for surveillance, screening, and diagnosis, and can be reliably done on plasma, serum, whole blood, or saliva by healthcare providers with little laboratory expertise. The two limitations of these serological tests are detection of infection during primary infection when antibodies are absent, and in infants younger than 18 months who might bear maternal HIV-1 antibodies. In these instances direct virus detection is the only option (eg, quantification of viral RNA [standard] or p24 antigen in heat denatured serum [less expensive]).

For staging purposes, measurement of CD4+ cells and viraemia is required. Plasma viral load is widely used to monitor therapeutic success on antiretroviral treatment. Several commercially available tests provide sensitive quantification of plasma HIV-1 RNA copies. The newer versions of the Amplicor and Quantiplex (Roche, Indianapolis, IN, USA, and Bayer Diagnostics, Walpole, MA, USA, respectively) assays have overcome initial suboptimum performance for non-B subtypes.[102] While the viral load determines the rate of destruction of the immune system, the number of CD4+ cells reveals the degree of immunodeficiency and is, therefore, used to assess the stage of infection. CD4+ cell counts together with clinical manifestations (eg, occurrence of opportunistic infections) are key criteria for HIV-1 disease classification. Flow cytometry analysis is the standard method for CD4+ cells quantification.

Standard methods for quantifying viral load and CD4+ cell counts need advanced laboratory infrastructures, and assays require a specimen to be tested within a short time of collection. These requirements pose challenges for resource-constrained settings. The use of dried blood spot specimen has resolved some of the difficulties associated with transportation of samples needed for virological assessments.[103] Measurement of reverse transcriptase activity in plasma samples, simplification of gene amplification methods (eg, Taqman technology), and paper-strip quantification (dipstick assays) might provide cost-effective alternatives for the future.[104–106] Similarly microcapilliary flow-based systems, CD4+ chips, or total white counts (panleucocyte gating) provide alternatives for establishment of the level of immunodeficiency in resource-limited settings.[107–110]

▶ Drug Treatment

Antiretroviral Compounds

Antiretroviral treatment is the best option for longlasting viral suppression and, subsequently, for reduction of morbidity and mortality. However, current drugs do not eradicate HIV-1 infection and lifelong treatment might be needed.

20 of the 21 antiretroviral drugs currently approved by the US Food and Drug Administration target the viral reverse transcriptase or protease (Table B.2). Eight nucleoside/nucleotide analogues and three non-nucleoside reverse transcriptase inhibitors inhibit viral replication after cell entry but before integration. Fixed-dose combination tablets simplify treatment regimens by reducing the daily pill burden, and drugs with long half-lives allow once or twice daily dosing. Eight protease inhibitors prevent the maturation of virions resulting in production of non-infectious particles. The recently approved darunavir (June, 2006) is the first of its class that retains activity against viruses with reduced susceptibility to protease inhibitors. Enfuvirtide targets a gp41 region of the viral envelope and stops the fusion process before the cell is infected. This drug needs to be injected twice daily and its use is reserved for treatment of heavily drug-experienced patients since it can help overcome existing drug resistance.[111,112] Development of new antiretrovirals focuses on molecules that target entry, reverse transcription, integration, or maturation. Compounds that have been designed to inhibit resistant viruses are urgently needed since many patients treated during the past decades harbour viral strains with reduced susceptibilities to many if not all available drugs (Table B.3).

The goal of antiretroviral treatment is to decrease the morbidity and mortality that is generally associated with HIV-1 infection. A combination of three or more active drugs is needed to achieve this aim in most patients. Effective treatment returns to near normal the turnover rates of both CD4+ and CD8+ T-cell populations.[72] Potent but well tolerated drugs with long half-lives and simplified regimens improve the options for first-line and second-line chemotherapeutic interventions.

TABLE B.2   Antiretroviral drugs currently approved by US Food and Drug Administration

	Entry	Reverse Transcriptase			Protease
		Nucleoside	Nucleotide	Non-nucleoside	
Single compound tablets	Enfuvirtide	Abacavir Didanosine Emtricitabine Lamivudine Stavudine Zalcitabine Zidovudine	Tenofovir	Delaviridine Efavirenz Nevirapine	(Fos)-Amprenavir Atazanavir Darunavir Indinavir Nelfinavir Ritonavir Saquinavir Tripanavir Lopinavir/ritonavir
Fixed-dose combination tablets		Abacavir/lamivudine (Epzicom) Zidovudine/lamivudine (Combivir) Tenofovir/emtricitabine (Truvada) Abacavir/lamivudine/zidovudine (Trizavir) Tenofovir/emtricitabine/efavirenz (Atripla)			

Drugs belong to five drug classes and target three different viral steps (entry, reverse transcription, or protease). Availability of these drugs In resource-limited countries is subject to country specific licensing agreements.

Combination Antiretroviral Treatment

High rate of viral replication, low fidelity of reverse transcription, and the ability to recombine are the viral characteristics that lead to the diversity of HIV-1 species (quasi-species) in chronically infected individuals. This high genetic variability provided the rationale for highly active antiretroviral treatments (HAART). By combination of several potent antiretroviral agents, viral replication is suppressed to such low levels that emergence of drug resistant HIV-1 variants was, if not prevented, at least delayed. By doing so, CD4+ T-lymphocyte numbers increase, leading to a degree of immune reconstitution that is sufficient to reverse clinically apparent immunodeficiency. Widespread introduction of HAART in industrialised countries resulted in a striking decrease in morbidity and mortality, putting forward the hope that HIV-1 infection can be transformed into a treatable chronic disease.[113–115]

A set of criteria composed of plasma viraemia concentration, absolute or relative CD4+ cell counts, and clinical manifestations, is used to recommend initiation of HAART. The benefits of treatment clearly outweigh the potential side-effects in patients with clinical signs of immunodeficiency (eg, AIDS defining illnesses) or with CD4+ numbers less than 200 per μL (recommendation of US Department of Health and Human Services, October, 2005). However, the best time point to begin treatment remains controversial in asymptomatic patients with modest depletion of CD4+ T cells (eg, more than 350 per μL) and modest levels of viraemia (eg, less than 100 000 copies per mL).[116] Studies with clinical endpoints supporting the validity of early versus late interventions in asymptomatic patients are difficult to do and insufficient clinical data are currently available. Early depletion of gut CD4+ T lymphocytes,[117] increasing viral diversity, and the poor regenerative abilities of key populations of the immune system provide arguments for beginning treatment as early as possible. The wide application of this principle is restricted by long-term drug toxicities that lead to reduction of quality of life, and by treatment costs. Toxicities (eg, renal, hepato, mitochondrial), metabolic changes

TABLE B.3 Antiretrovirals currently in phase II/III of clinical development

	Drug	Mechanism	Activity Against PI and RT Resistant Strains
Maraviroc	MVC	CCR5 inhibitor	Yes, but not X4 variants
Vicriviroc	SCH D		Yes, but not X4 variants
Etravirine	TMC-125	Non-nucleoside reverse transcriptase inhibitor	Yes, also NNRTI-resistant strains
	TMC-278		Yes, also NNRTI-resistant strains
n/a	MK-0518	Integrase strand transfer inhibitor	Yes
n/a	GS-9137		Yes

(eg, lipodystrophy, diabetes mellitus), and immune reconstitution disease are some of the long-term problems that complicate decade-long HAART.[118–121]

One strategy addressing life-long daily compliance to HAART has been structured treatment interruptions. The rationale for this approach was based on the premise that the body's own immune system could keep the virus in check if exposed to a very modest level of viral replication. If successful, this strategy could limit drug toxicity and reduce treatment costs.[122] Although preliminary findings for this strategy were mixed in terms of benefits,[123–125] the recent early closure of the SMART trial was based on increased morbidity and mortality in the treatment interruption arm.[126] Thus, in the absence of clinical benefits, most investigators strongly discourage treatment interruptions except as needed to address treatment intolerance.

HAART in Resource-Constrained Settings

The transformation of AIDS into a chronic disease in industrialised countries has yet to be realised in resource-constrained settings. Access to HAART is an absolute humanitarian necessity to avert mortality in people who are central to the future survival of their countries.[127] Despite restricted health infrastructures and diverse co-morbidities in these regions, remarkable therapeutic success rates have been shown, with adherence rates at least comparable with those reported in industrialised countries.[128–131] WHO and UNAIDS treatment guidelines focusing on resource-limited settings suggest use of standard first-line regimen followed by a set of more expensive second-line options[132] and proposes the use of standardised decision-making steps (eg, when to start, to substitute for side-effects, to switch for virological failure).[132,133] In many countries, treatment options are limited not only by the costs of HAART but also by restrictive licensing policies, and current estimates suggest that 80% of people infected with HIV-1 with a clinical need for treatment do not yet have access to antiretroviral drugs.[1] Thus, efforts and strategies to further scale up treatment access are crucial,[134–137] since antiretroviral treatment is also an effective intervention for prevention.[138]

Drug Resistance

Emergence of drug resistance is the most common reason for treatment failure. Insufficient compliance, drug side-effects, or drug-drug interactions can lead to suboptimum drug concentrations, resulting in viral rebound. Viral resistance has been described to every antiretroviral drug and therefore poses a serious clinical as well as public-health problem.[139] HIV-1 subtypes differ in the sequence of mutations leading to drug resistance, and some naturally occurring polymorphisms might actually modulate resistance.[140,141] Drug-resistant HIV-1 is transmissible and can be detected in up to 20% of newly infected individuals in countries with broad access to antiretrovirals.[34] The prevalence of drug resistance in the untreated population remains low in regions with poor access to treatment.[142]

Short-term antiretroviral-based interventions are effective in prevention of mother-to-child transmission. However, these interventions could result in drug resistant viral variants in the mother, baby, or both.[143] Around half the women who received one dose of nevirapine to prevent mother-to-child transmission harbour viruses resistant to non-nucleoside reverse transcriptase inhibitors (NNRTI).[144,145] These resistant viruses replicate efficiently and can be transmitted by breast milk,[146] and minor resistant populations present long after the intervention can possibly decrease the effectiveness of subsequent NNRTI-based treatment regimens.[147] The combination of short-course zidovudine, lamivudine, and nevirapine prevents peripartum transmission while reducing the risk of nevirapine resistant viruses.[148]

Viral Reservoirs

Viral reservoirs consist of anatomical sanctuaries and a small pool of infected long-lived memory T lymphocytes. HIV-1 latency in long-lived cell populations (eg, memory T lymphocytes, macrophages) poses an obstacle to eradication because current antiviral combination treatments fail to eliminate integrated proviruses from resting cells. Different strategies, including immune-modulatory molecules (interleukin 2, anti-CD3 mAb, interleukin 7), have been used to reactivate resting cells in the setting of HAART. Histone deacetylase-1 inhibitors, like valproic acid, release an inherent transcriptional block and by doing so facilitate viral long terminal repeat-driven expression.[149] Augmenting standard antiretroviral treatment with enfuviridine and valproic acid reduced the number of latently infected CD4+ T cells (29–84%), but to establish the relative contribution of each drug with respect to the final outcome is difficult.[150]

▶ Prevention

Mother-to-Child Transmission

Prevention of mother-to-child transmission has seen advances in both industrialised and resource-constrained settings.[151–153] Intrapartum transmission has been reduced by increasing access to interventions such as one dose of nevirapine to mother and newborn baby.[154] Concerns about drug-resistant viral strains have led to several trials with combination treatments to reduce transmission during the intrapartum period.[148,152,155] In some settings, elective delivery by caesarean section can further reduce HIV-1 transmission during the intrapartum period, but the benefits of the intervention could be countered by post-partum sepsis and increasing maternal mortality.[156]

Because HIV-1 can be transmitted by breastfeeding, replacement feeding is recommended in many settings. Poor access to clean running water precludes, however, the use of formula feeding under these circumstances,[157] and exclusive breastfeeding with abrupt weaning is one option for reducing transmission.[158] A potential novel intervention still being tested is the daily use of antiretrovirals during breastfeeding. More attention is starting to focus on the pregnant mother, especially initiation of antiretroviral therapy in mothers with low CD4+ counts during pregnancy and thereafter.[159,160] Only limited data are available regarding the health of uninfected children born to HIV-1-positive mothers.[161] In a European cohort of exposed-uninfected children, no serious clinical manifestations were apparent, at least in the short term to medium term (median follow-up 2 years).[162]

Sexual Transmission

Reduction of heterosexual transmission is crucial for control of the epidemic in many parts of the world.[1,163] Prevention is achieved through reduction in the number of discordant sexual acts or reduction of the probability of HIV-1 transmission in discordant sexual acts. The first can be achieved through abstinence and sex between concordantly seronegative individuals. Abstinence and lifelong monogamous relationships might not be adequate solutions for many people and therefore several interventions aimed at lowering the risk of transmission per discordant sexual act are in the process of clinical testing. Male and female condoms provide a proven and affordable prevention option.[164,165] In combination, these options are also more commonly referred to as the ABC (abstinence, be faithful, condom use) approach.

Other biomedical prevention interventions include male circumcision, antiretrovirals for prevention (eg, pre-exposure or post-exposure), chemoprophylactic treatment of herpes simplex virus-2 (HSV-2), microbicides, and vaccines. Results from one of three independent phase III male circumcision trials underway in South Africa, Kenya, and Uganda has helped to allay some of the ambivalence around the protective effect of male circumcision.[8,166] The findings from the South African trial show a 60% protective effect of male circumcision.[167] The possible mechanism relates to the fact that the foreskin has apocrine glands that secrete lysozymes but also Langerhans cells expressing CD4 and other receptors.[168,169] These skin-specific dendritic cells can uptake virus and are believed to play a part in transport of the virus to susceptible T cells. Immunofluorescence studies of foreskin mucosa suggest that these tissues might be more susceptible to HIV-1 infection than cervical mucosa.[170] Findings from this proof-of-concept trial need to be compared with evidence from the two trials still underway in Kenya and Uganda, and to acceptability data, behaviour change after circumcision, surgical complication rates, and logistics of undertaking the procedures before policy formulation and wide-scale access as a prevention strategy.[171-173]

Since high plasma viraemia increases the risk of transmission by as much as an order of magnitude,[21] does reducing viral load in the infected partner through, for example, antiretroviral treatment reduce the risk of HIV-1 transmission in the uninfected sexual partner? A trial to explore this question is currently being run jointly by the HIV Prevention Trials Network (www.hptn.org) and the Adult Clinical Trials Group. Mathematical projections estimate up to 80% HIV-1 reduction,[174,175] but scarce observational data currently exist.[176] Post-exposure prophylaxis is recommended after occupational (eg, needle stick)[177] and non-occupational (eg, rape, sexual abuse)[178] exposure, although data for efficacy and optimum drug combinations are few.[179] Some clinical trials assessing the benefits of once daily pre-exposure chemoprophylaxis with antiretroviral compounds with long biological half-life (eg, tenofovir) have been put on hold or stopped.[175,180] Neither the overall idea of pre-exposure prophylaxis nor the drug itself, which is well tolerated, was at the root of the protests. Concerns were centred on clinical trials in resource-poor settings and the perceived scarcity of adequate interventions protecting these vulnerable populations.

HSV-2 might increase both the risk of transmitting and acquiring HIV-1.[181,182] Antivirals (eg, aciclovir, valaciclovir) are effective in reducing viral shedding[183–185] and HSV-2 transmission in discordant heterosexual couples.[182] The future of HSV-2 prevention might reside in the vaccine that is currently under development.[186] Whether prophylactic use of aciclovir in populations with high HSV-2 prevalence and incidence rates results in reduced HIV-1 incidence rates remains unresolved but several trials addressing this issue are underway, including HPTN039.

Gender disparities lie at the centre of women's vulnerability. Prevention options need to be provided that can be used by women independently of their male sexual partner's knowledge or consent.[187] Notwithstanding that redressing these disparities is a long-term challenge, several preventive interventions can be implemented in the interim on the basis of our incomplete understanding at a biological level of HIV-1 risk for women. For example, there seems to be a correlation between levels of sexual hormones (eg, progesterone) and transmission risk.[188] Observational studies also highlight the relation between abnormal vaginal flora and increased risk of HIV-1 infection.[189,190] The high prevalence of vaginal infections such as bacterial vaginosis (30–50%), vulvovaginal candidosis (10–13%), and trichomonas vaginalis (7–23%) in African women is associated with a substantial risk of HIV-1 acquisition.[189] In addition to increasing access to female condoms and treatment of other sexually transmitted infections, trials are underway to assess the use of other barrier methods such as cervical caps, invisible condoms, diaphragms, and diaphragms combined with micro bicides.[190] The control of vaginal infections is a potentially important method for decreasing HIV-1 acquisition that has yet to be tested. Periodic presumptive treatment for vaginal infections is being explored as an HIV-1 prevention strategy.[191]

Microbicides

Microbicides are an additional important biomedical intervention technology that is covert and under women's control.[192] These topical products potentially could be used to prevent rectal and vaginal transmission of HIV-1, but proof of concept has been elusive. Although the three phase III trial results of the first microbicidal product (nonoxynol-9) done in the mid-1980s and 1990s did not show protective effects,[193,194] they have informed the medical knowledge in terms of product selection, clinical testing, and safety assessments. The past 5 years have seen major advances in investment and product development.[66,195,197] Early clinical testing of multiple products including the launch of advanced clinical trials for five different products is continuing (Table B.4). The development of antiretroviral gels increased the specificity of these third generation microbicides in relation to surfactants, vaginal enhancers, or entry inhibitors that have dominated the product pipeline so far (Figure B-5). The first antiretroviral gel to undergo early testing is tenofovir gel, and the findings in terms of safety profile, tolerance, low systemic absorption, and slight adverse events are promising.[192] As with vaccines, a major obstacle is the absence of a surrogate marker of protection. Additional challenges are adherence to product use and the high rates of pregnancy in trial participants.

Vaccines

A safe, protective, and inexpensive vaccine would be the most efficient and possibly the only way to curb the HIV pandemic.[198] Despite intensive research, development of such a candidate vaccine remains elusive. Safety concerns prohibit the use of live-attenuated virus as

TABLE B.4   Summary of microbicides currently undergoing advanced clinical testing

	Phase	Mode of Action	Effective Against
Carraguard	III	Seaweed polymer, entry inhibitor	HIV-1/HIV-2, human papilloma virus, herpes simplex virus
Cellulose sulphate	III	Entry inhibitor	Broad range of sexually transmitted diseases; also active as contraceptive
PRO2000	III	Entry inhibitor	HIV-1/HIV-2, human papillomavirus, chlamydia
Savvy (C31G)	III	Surfactant	Broad range of sexually transmitted diseases; also active as contraceptive
Tenofovir gel	IIb	Nucleotide reverse transcriptase inhibitor	HIV-1/HIV-2
Buffer gel+PRO2000	IIb/III	Natural vaginal defence/ entry inhibitor	HIV-1/HIV-2, chlamydia, gonorrhoea, human papillomavirus, bacterial vaginosis
Tenofovir gel+oral	II	Nucleotide reverse transcriptase inhibitor	HIV-1/HIV-2

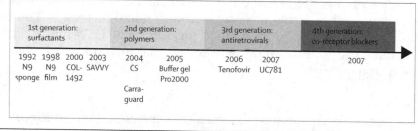

FIGURE B-5   Timeline of microbicide development of different product generation with trial initiation dates as reference N9=nonoxonol-9. CS=cellulose sulphate.

immunogen.[199] Many different approaches with recombinant technologies have been pursued over the past two decades. Initially, efforts were focused on generating neutralising antibodies with recombinant monomeric envelope gp120 (AIDSVAX) as immunogen.[200,201] This vaccine did not induce neutralising antibodies and, not unexpectedly, the phase III trials failed to show protection.[202,203] Antibody mediated HIV-1 neutralisation is complicated by the high genetic diversity of the variable Env regions, epitopes masked by a carbohydrate shield (glycosylation), and conformational or energetic constraints.[204] Since CD8 T-cell responses control to some extent viral replication in vivo, recent vaccine development has focused on eliciting cellular immune responses. Overcoming pre-existing immunity against replication incompetent immunogenic vectors (eg, recombinant adenovirus type 5) is one of the challenges.[205] Safety and immunogenicity studies using replication defective vaccine vectors are continuing after preliminary studies in non-human primates showed some protection.[204] The immune system generally fails to spontaneously clear HIV-1 and the true correlates of protection continue to be ill defined.[198,206] However, the general belief is that approaches aimed at eliciting both humoral and cell mediated immunity are most promising to prevent or at least control retroviral infection.[198]

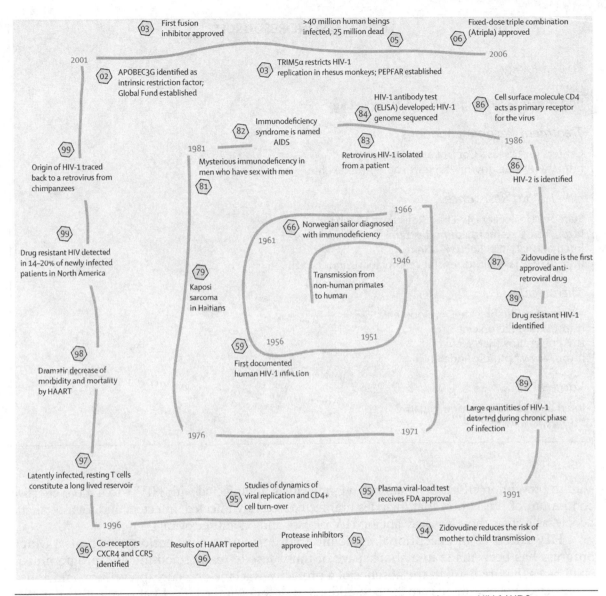

FIGURE B-6 Selected observations, scientific developments, and treatment options pertinent to HIV-1/AIDS Estimates place the cross species transmission events leading to the worldwide spread of HIV-1 to the early decades of the 20th century. Numbers circled by a hexagon identify the specific year of an event.

▶ Conclusions

An important gateway to both prevention and care is knowledge of HIV-1 status.[207] Fear of knowledge of status, including stigma and discrimination, has discouraged many from seeking voluntary counselling and testing services.[208] As access to antiretroviral interventions (prevention of mother-to-child transmission, antiretroviral treatment) increases, the opportunities for HIV-1 testing will grow and create opportunities for a prevention-care continuum, with the voluntary counselling and testing services as a point of entry. These changes will result in a

---

PANEL: ONLINE RESOURCES

Epidemiology

UNAIDS
http://www.unaids.org/en/HIV_data/default.asp

Treatment Recommendations

Centers for Disease Control and Prevention
http://www.cdc.gov/hiv/topics/treatment/index.htm

HIV-1 Drug Resistance

Stanford University HIV Drug Resistance Database
http://hivdb.stanford.edu/index.html
International AIDS Society–USA
http://www.iasusa.org/resistance_mutations/index.html

Microbicide

Alliance for Microbicide Development
http://www.microbicide.org
HIV Prevention Trials Network
http://www.hptn.org/index.htm

Vaccine

International AIDS Vaccine Initiative
http://www.iavi.org

---

shift in prevention efforts from a focus on individuals not infected with HIV-1 to a more effective continuum of prevention that includes uninfected, recently infected, infected, and asymptomatic people, as well as those with advancing HIV disease and on antiretroviral therapy.

HIV/AIDS is an exceptional epidemic that demands an exceptional response. Much progress has been made in a short space of time, despite many scientific and programmatic challenges (Figure B-6). In the absence of a protective vaccine or a cure, prevention and access to antiretroviral treatments are the best options to slow down the HIV-1 pandemic. Broad implementation of these principles needs improved infrastructures in resource-constrained regions, which have been and will continue to be most affected. The fact that HIV-1 is predominantly sexually transmitted and disproportionately affects populations that are already socially or challenges.

In view of the immediacy of the problem, and the fact that both research and programmes are mainly funded by the public sector, there is a greater demand from civil society for co-ownership of research and accountability for use of public funds. On the one hand, this co-ownership defines a changing role and responsibility of science in society, and on the other hand, shows a necessary synergy between activism and science. This partnership has been invaluable for antiretroviral drug development, treatment access in resource-constrained settings, and the scale-up of interventions to reduce mother-to-child transmission.

The increasing number of infected women and the disproportionate burden of infection in resource-constrained settings creates a scientific imperative to ensure research is done for people and in settings who stand to benefit most. The most affected countries face many other economic, political, and development challenges, which have raised issues in undertaking multicentre and multicountry research. Research addressing women-specific topics (such as effect of sexual hormones on transmission and disease progression, viral diversity, and antiretroviral potency) and women-specific prevention interventions including microbicides is crucial. We are probably at one of the most hopeful and optimistic points in our response to the pandemic. There is definitely more attention being directed to HIV-1, more resources (panel), more civil society mobilisation, more governments speaking up, more possibilities for treatment, and more evidence about what prevention and treatment strategies will work than in previous years. The unrelenting growth of the pandemic tells us that current strategies are not enough. Clearly, we need to do some things differently, while also increasing the scale and magnitude of current strategies in keeping with the pandemic.

▶ Acknowledgments

We thank P D Bieniasz, W Cates, L Chakrabarti, C Cheng-Mayer, J Coovadia, H Gayle, P A Fryd, R Gray, S Abdool Karim, L Kuhn, K Mayer, P Mane, L C F Mulder, L Myer, and M Wawer for helpful discussions. M Boettiger and C Baxter assisted with literature searches. This work was supported by NIH grant RO1AI064001 (VS), by grant 1 U19AI51794 (QAK) from CAPRISA that forms part of the Comprehensive International Program of Research on AIDS (CIPRA) funded by the National Institute of Allergy and infectious Disease (NIAID), National Institutes of Health (NIH) and the US Department of Health and Human Services (DHHS) and grant D43 TW00231 (QAK) from the Columbia University-Southern African Fogarty AIDS International Training and Research Program.

▶ Conflict of Interest Statement

D D Ho sits on the scientific advisory boards for Monogram, Osel, Achillion, Valiant, Oyagen, Lavipharm, and XTL. Products or work from these companies are not discussed in the review. He holds patents on vaccine candidates. The other authors declare no conflict of interest.

▶ References

1. UNAIDS. 2006 report on the global AIDS epidemic: a UNAIDS 10th anniversary special edition. http://www.unaids.org/en/HIV_data/2006GlobalReport/default.asp (accessed July 20, 2006).

2. Inciardi JA, Williams ML. Editor's introduction: the global epidemiology of HIV and AIDS. *AIDS Care* 2005; **17**(suppl 1): S1–8.

3. Hayes R, Weiss H. Epidemiology. Understanding HIV epidemic trends in Africa. *Science* 2006; **311**: 620–21.

4. Quinn TC, Overbaugh J. HIV/AIDS in women: an expanding epidemic. *Science* 2005; **308**: 1582–83.

5. Abdool-Karim Q, Abdool-Karim SS. The evolving HIV epidemic in South Africa. *Int J Epidemiol* 2002; **31:** 37–40.

6. Pettifor AE, Rees HV, Kleinschmidt I, et al. Young people's sexual health in South Africa: HIV prevalence and sexual behaviors from a nationally representative household survey. *AIDS* 2005; **19:** 1525–34.

7. Shisana O, Davids A. Correcting gender inequalities is central to controlling HIV/AIDS. *Bull World Health Organ* 2004; **82:** 812.

8. Siegfried N, Muller M, Volmink J, et al. Male circumcision for prevention of heterosexual acquisition of HIV in men. *Cochrane Database Syst Rev* 2003; **3:** CD003362.

9. Aral SO, Padian NS, Holmes KK. Advances in multilevel approaches to understanding the epidemiology and prevention of sexually transmitted infections and HIV: an overview. *J Infect Dis* 2005; **191** (suppl 1): S1–6.

10. Rottingen JA, Cameron DW, Garnett GP. A systematic review of the epidemiologic interactions between classic sexually transmitted diseases and HIV: how much really is known? *Sex Transm Dis* 2001; **28:** 579–97.

11. Korenromp EL, White RG, Orroth KK, et al. Determinants of the impact of sexually transmitted infection treatment on prevention of HIV infection: a synthesis of evidence from the Mwanza, Rakai, and Masaka intervention trials. *J Infect Dis* 2005; **191**(suppl 1): S168–78.

12. Bloom SS, Urassa M, Isingo R, Ng'weshemi J, Boerma JT. Community effects on the risk of HIV infection in rural Tanzania. *Sex Transm Infect* 2002; **78:** 261–66.

13. Nunn AJ, Wagner HU, Kamali A, Kengeya-Kayondo JF, Mulder DW. Migration and HIV-1 seroprevalence in a rural Ugandan population. *AIDS* 1995; **9:** 503–06.

14. Lurie MN, Williams BG, Zuma K, et al. The impact of migration on HIV-1 transmission in South Africa: a study of migrant and nonmigrant men and their partners. *Sex Transm Dis* 2003; **30:** 149–56.

15. Abdool Karim Q, Abdool Karim SS, Singh B, Short R, Ngxongo S. Seroprevalence of HIV infection in rural South Africa. *AIDS* 1992; **6:** 1535–39.

16. Buchbinder SP, Vittinghof E, Heagerty PJ, et al. Sexual risk, nitrite inhalant use, and lack of circumcision associated with HIV seroconversion in men who have sex with men in the United States. *J Acquir Immune Defic Syndr* 2005; **39:** 82–89.

17. Halperin DT, Epstein H. Concurrent sexual partnerships help to explain Africa's high HIV prevalence: implications for prevention. *Lancet* 2004; **364:** 4–6.

18. Cates W Jr. Review of non-hormonal contraception (condoms, intrauterine devices, nonoxynol-9 and combos) on HIV acquisition. *J Acquir Immune Defic Syndr* 2005; **38**(suppl 1): S8–10.

19. Gray RH, Wawer MJ, Serwadda D, et al. Population-based study of fertility in women with HIV-1 infection in Uganda. *Lancet* 1998; **351:** 98–103.

20. Gregson S, Garnett GP, Nyamukapa CA, et al. HIV decline associated with behavior change in eastern Zimbabwe. *Science* 2006; **311:** 664–66.

21. Quinn TC, Wawer MJ, Sewankambo N, et al. Viral load and heterosexual transmission of human immunodeficiency virus type 1. Rakai Project Study Group. *N Engl J Med* 2000; **342:** 921–29.

22. Wawer MJ, Gray RH, Sewankambo NK, et al. Rates of HIV-1 transmission per coital act, by stage of HIV-1 infection, in Rakai, Uganda. *J Infect Dis* 2005; **191:** 1403–09.

23. Galvin SR, Cohen MS. The role of sexually transmitted diseases in HIV transmission. *Nat Rev Microbiol* 2004; **2**: 33–42.

24. Cohen MS, Pilcher CD. Amplified HIV transmission and new approaches to HIV prevention. *J Infect Dis* 2005; **191**: 1391–93.

25. Aral SO, Peterman TA. Measuring outcomes of behavioural interventions for STD/HIV prevention. *Int J STD AIDS* 1996; **7**(suppl 2): 30–38.

26. Price MA, Miller WC, Kaydos-Daniels SC, et al. Trichomoniasis in men and HIV infection: data from 2 outpatient clinics at Lilongwe Central Hospital, Malawi. *J Infect Dis* 2004; **190**: 1448–55.

27. Sharghi N, Bosch RJ, Mayer K, Essex M, Seage GR 3rd. The development and utility of a clinical algorithm to predict early HIV-1 infection. *J Acquir Immune Defic Syndr* 2005; **40**: 472–78.

28. Keele BF, Van Heuverswyn F, Li Y, et al. Chimpanzee reservoirs of pandemic and nonpandemic HIV-1. Science 2006; published online May 25, 2006.

29. Korber B, Gaschen B, Yusim K, Thakallapally R, Kesmir C, Detours V. Evolutionary and immunological implications of contemporary HIV-1 variation. *Br Med Bull* 2001; **58**: 19–42.

30. Thomson MM, Najera R. Molecular epidemiology of HIV-1 variants in the global AIDS pandemic: an update. *AIDS Rev* 2005; **7**: 210–24.

31. Blackard JT, Cohen DE, Mayer KH. Human immunodeficiency virus superinfection and recombination: current state of knowledge and potential clinical consequences. *Clin Infect Dis* 2002; **34**: 1108–14.

32. Laeyendecker O, Li X, Arroyo M, et al. The effect of HIV subtype on rapid disease progression in Rakai, Uganda. 13th Conference on Retroviruses and Opportunitic Infections, Denver, CO, USA; Feb 6–9, 2006.

33. Centlivre M, Sommer P, Michel M, et al. The HIV-1 clade C promoter is particularly well adapted to replication in the gut in primary infection. *AIDS* 2006; **20**: 657–66.

34. Steain MC, Wang B, Dwyer DE, Saksena NK. HIV-1 co-infection, superinfection and recombination. *Sex Health* 2004; **1**: 239–50.

35. Gottlieb GS, Nickle DC, Jensen MA, et al. Dual HIV-1 infection associated with rapid disease progression. *Lancet* 2004; **363**: 619–22.

36. Yerly S, Jost S, Monnat M, et al. HIV-1 co/super-infection in intravenous drug users. *AIDS* 2004; **18**: 1413–21.

37. Chohan B, Lavreys L, Rainwater SM, Overbaugh J. Evidence for frequent reinfection with human immunodeficiency virus type 1 of a different subtype. *J Virol* 2005; **79**: 10701–08.

38. van der Kuyl AC, Kozaczynska K, van den Burg R, et al. Triple HIV-1 infection. *N Engl J Med* 2005; **352**: 2557–59.

39. Smith DM, Richman DD, Little SJ. HIV superinfection. *J Infect Dis* 2005; **192**: 438–44.

40. McCutchan FE, Hoelscher M, Tovanabutra S, et al. In-depth analysis of a heterosexually acquired human immunodeficiency virus type 1 superinfection: evolution, temporal fluctuation, and intercompartment dynamics from the seronegative window period through 30 months postinfection. *J Virol* 2005; **79**: 11693–704.

41. Mahalingam S, Meanger J, Foster PS, Lidbury BA. The viral manipulation of the host cellular and immune environments to enhance propagation and survival: a focus on RNA viruses. *J Leukoc Biol* 2002; **72**: 429–39.

42. Bieniasz PD. Intrinsic immunity: a front-line defense against viral attack. *Nat Immunol* 2004; **5:** 1109–15.

43. Coffin JM. Retroviridae: the viruses and their replication. In: Knipe DM, Howley PM, Griffin DE, et al, eds. Fields virology 3rd edn. Philadelphia, New York: Lippencott-Raven, 1996: 1767–847.

44. Barre-Sinoussi F. HIV as the cause of AIDS. *Lancet* 1996; **348:** 31–35.

45. Emerman M, Malim MH. HIV-1 regulatory/accessory genes: keys to unraveling viral and host cell biology. *Science* 1998; **280:** 1880–84.

46. Coffin JM, Hughes SH, Varmus HE, eds. Retroviruses. Plainview, NY, USA: Cold Spring Harbor Laboratory Press, 1997.

47. Balabanian K, Harriague J, Decrion C, et al. CXCR4-tropic HIV-1 envelope glycoprotein functions as a viral chemokine in unstimulated primary CD4+ T lymphocytes. *J Immunol* 2004; **173:** 7150–60.

48. Cicala C, Arthos J, Selig SM, et al. HIV envelope induces a cascade of cell signals in non-proliferating target cells that favor virus replication. *Proc Natl Acad Sci USA* 2002; **99:** 9380–85.

49. Ray N, Doms RW. HIV-1 coreceptors and their inhibitors. *Curr Top Microbiol Immunol* 2006; **303:** 97–120.

50. Eckert DM, Kim PS. Mechanisms of viral membrane fusion and its inhibition. *Annu Rev Biochem* 2001; **70:** 777–810.

51. Platt EJ, Durnin JP, Kabat D. Kinetic factors control efficiencies of cell entry, efficacies of entry inhibitors, and mechanisms of adaptation of human immunodeficiency virus. *J Virol* 2005; **79:** 4347–56.

52. Schroder A. HIV-1 integration in the human genome favors active genes and local hotspots. *Cell* 2002; **110:** 521–29.

53. Mitchell RS, Beitzel BF, Schroder AR, et al. Retroviral DNA integration: ASLV, HIV, and MLV show distinct target site preferences. *PLoS Biol* 2004; **2:** E234.

54. Scherdin U, Rhodes K, Breindl M. Transcriptionally active genome regions are preferred targets for retrovirus integration. *J Virol* 1990; **64:** 907.

55. Ciuffi A, Llano M, Poeschla E, et al. A role for LEDGF/p75 in targeting HIV DNA integration. *Nat Med* 2005; **11:** 1287–89.

56. Turlure F, Maertens G, Rahman S, Cherepanov P, Engelman A. A tripartite DNA-binding element, comprised of the nuclear localization signal and two AT-hook motifs, mediates the association of LEDGF/p75 with chromatin in vivo. *Nucleic Acids Res* 2006; **34:** 1663–75.

57. Martin-Serrano J, Zang T, Bieniasz PD. Role of ESCRT-I in retroviral budding. *J Virol* 2003; **77:** 4794–804.

58. Bieniasz PD. Late budding domains and host proteins in enveloped virus release. *Virology* 2006; **344:** 55–63.

59. Martin-Serrano J, Zang T, Bieniasz PD. HIV-1 and Ebola virus encode small peptide motifs that recruit Tsg101 to sites of particle assembly to facilitate egress. *Nat Med* 2001; **7:** 1313–19.

60. Garrus JE, von Schwedler UK, Pornillos OW, et al. Tsg101 and the vacuolar protein sorting pathway are essential for HIV-1 budding. *Cell* 2001; **107:** 55–65.

61. Zhu T, Mo H, Wang N, et al. Genotypic and phenotypic characterization of HIV-1 patients with primary infection. *Science* 1993; **261:** 1179–81.

62. Cantin R, Methot S, Tremblay MJ. Plunder and stowaways: incorporation of cellular proteins by enveloped viruses. *J Virol* 2005; **79:** 6577–87.

63. Haase AT. Perils at mucosal front lines for HIV and SIV and their hosts. *Nat Rev Immunol* 2005; **5:** 783–92.

64. Briggs JA, Grunewald K, Glass B, Forster F, Krausslich HG, Fuller SD. The mechanism of HIV-1 core assembly: insights from three-dimensional reconstructions of authentic virions. *Structure* 2006; **14:** 15–20.

65. Connor RI, Sheridan KE, Ceradini D, Choe S, Landau NR. Change in coreceptor use correlates with disease progression in HIV-1-infected individuals. *J Exp Med* 1997; **185:** 621–28.

66. Shattock RJ, Moore JP. Inhibiting sexual transmission of HIV-1 infection. *Nature Rev Microbiol* 2003; **1:** 25–34.

67. Mehandru S, Poles MA, Tenner-Racz K, et al. Primary HIV-1 infection is associated with preferential depletion of CD4+ T lymphocytes from effector sites in the gastrointestinal tract. *J Exp Med* 2004; **200:** 761–70.

68. Douek DC, Picker LJ, Koup RA. T cell dynamics in HIV-1 infection. *Annu Rev Immunol* 2003; **21:** 265–304.

69. Ramratnam B, Bonhoeffer S, Binley J, et al. Rapid production and clearance of HIV-1 and hepatitis C virus assessed by large volume plasma apheresis. *Lancet* 1999; **354:** 1782–85.

70. Simon V, Ho DD. HIV-1 dynamics in vivo: implications for therapy. *Nat Rev Microbiol* 2003; **1:** 181–90.

71. Kovacs JA, Lempicki RA, Sidorov IA, et al. Identification of dynamically distinct subpopulations of T lymphocytes that are differentially affected by HIV. *J Exp Med* 2001; **194:** 1731–41.

72. Mohri H, Perelson AS, Tung K, et al. Increased turnover of T lymphocytes in HIV-1 infection and its reduction by antiretroviral therapy. *J Exp Med* 2001; **194:** 1277–87.

73. De Boer RJ, Mohri H, Ho DD, Perelson AS. Turnover rates of B cells, T cells, and NK cells in simian immunodeficiency virus-infected and uninfected rhesus macaques. *J Immunol* 2003; **170:** 2479–87.

74. Giorgi JV, Hultin LE, McKeating JA, et al. Shorter survival in advanced human immunodeficiency virus type 1 infection is more closely associated with T lymphocyte activation than with plasma virus burden or virus chemokine coreceptor usage. *J Infect Dis* 1999; **179:** 859–70.

75. Schindler M, Muench J, Kutsch O, et al. Nef mediated suppression of T cell activation was lost in a lentiviral lineage that gave rise to HIV-1. *Cell* 2006; **125:** 1055–67.

76. Kulkarni PS, Butera ST, Duerr AC. Resistance to HIV-1 infection: lessons learned from studies of highly exposed persistently seronegative (HEPS) individuals. *AIDS Rev* 2003; **5:** 87–103.

77. Telenti A, Bleiber G. Host genetics of HIV-1 suceptibility. *Future Virology* 2006; **1:** 55–70.

78. Carrington M, Dean M, Martin MP, O'Brien S. Genetics of HIV-1 infection: chemokine receptor CCR5 polymorphism and its consequences. *Hum Mol Genet* 1999; **8:** 1939–45.

79. Gonzalez E, Kulkarni H, Bolivar H, et al. The influence of CCL3L1 gene-containing segmental duplications on HIV-1/AIDS susceptibility. *Science* 2005; **307:** 1434–40.

80. Valdez H, Carlson NL, Post AB, et al. HIV long-term non-progressors maintain brisk CD8 T cell responses to other viral antigens. *AIDS* 2002; **16:** 1113–18.

81. Stremlau M, Owens CM, Perron MJ, Kiessling M, Autissier P, Sodroski J. The cytoplasmic body component TRIM5alpha restricts HIV-1 infection in Old World monkeys. *Nature* 2004; **427:** 848–53.

82. Sheehy AM, Gaddis NC, Choi JD, Malim MH. Isolation of a human gene that inhibits HIV-1 infection and is suppressed by the viral Vif protein. *Nature* 2002; **418:** 646–50.

83. Sawyer SL, Emerman M, Malik HS. Ancient adaptive evolution of the primate antiviral DNA-editing enzyme APOBEC3G. *PLoS Biol* 2004; **2:** E275.

84. Jarmuz A, Chester A, Bayliss J, et al. An anthropoid-specific locus of orphan C to U RNA-editing enzymes on chromosome 22. *Genomics* 2002; **79:** 285–96.

85. Petersen-Mahrt SK, Neuberger MS. In vitro deamination of cytosine to uracil in single-stranded DNA by apolipoprotein B editing complex catalytic subunit 1 (APOBEC1). *J Biol Chem* 2003; **278:** 19583–86.

86. Mangeat B, Trono D. Lentiviral vectors and antiretroviral intrinsic immunity. *Hum Gene Ther* 2005; **16:** 913–20.

87. Cullen BR. Role and mechanism of action of the APOBEC3 family of antiretroviral resistance factors. *J Virol* 2006; **80:** 1067–76.

88. Huthoff H, Malim MH. Cytidine deamination and resistance to retroviral infection: towards a structural understanding of the APOBEC proteins. *Virology* 2005; **334:** 147–53.

89. Harris RS, Liddament MT. Retroviral restriction by APOBEC proteins. *Nat Rev Immunol* 2004; **4:** 868–77.

90. Schrofelbauer B, Yu Q, Landau NR. New insights into the role of Vif in HIV-1 replication. *AIDS Rev* 2004; **6:** 34–39.

91. Navarro F, Bollman B, Chen H, et al. Complementary function of the two catalytic domains of APOBEC3G. *Virology* 2005; **333:** 374–86.

92. Chiu YL, Soros VB, Kreisberg JF, Stopak K, Yonemoto W, Greene WC. Cellular APOBEC3G restricts HIV-1 infection in resting CD4+ T cells. *Nature.* 2005; **435:** 108–14.

93. Kieffer TL, Kulon P, Nettles RE, Han Y, Ray SC, Siliciano RF. G→A hypermutation in protease and reverse transcriptase regions of human immunodeficiency virus type 1 residing in resting CD4+ T cells in vivo. *J Virol* 2005; **79:** 1973–80.

94. Tian C, Yu X, Zhang W, Wang T, Xu R, Yu XF. Differential requirement for conserved tryptophans in human immunodeficiency virus type 1 Vif for the selective suppression of APOBEC3G and APOBEC3F. *J Virol* 2006; **80:** 3112–15.

95. Simon V, Zennou V, Murray D, Huang Y, Ho DD, Bieniasz PD. Natural variation in Vif: differential impact on APOBEC3G/3F and a potential role in HIV-1 diversification. *PLoS Pathog* 2005; **1:** e6.

96. Jin X, Brooks A, Chen H, Bennett R, Reichman R, Smith H. APOBEC3G/CEM15 (hA3G) mRNA levels associate inversely with human immunodeficiency virus viremia. *J Virol* 2005; **79:** 11513–16.

97. Cho SJ, Drechsler H, Burke RC, Arens MQ, Powderly W, Davidson NO. APOBEC3F and APOBEC3G mRNA levels do not correlate with human immunodeficiency virus type 1 plasma viremia or CD4+ T-cell count. *J Virol* 2006; **80:** 2069–72.

98. Nisole S, Stoye JP, Saib A. Trim family proteins: retroviral restriction and antiviral defence. *Nat Rev Microbiol* 2005; **3:** 799–808.

99. Perez-Caballero D, Hatziioannou T, Zhang F, Cowan S, Bieniasz PD. Restriction of human immunodeficiency virus type 1 by TRIM-CypA occurs with rapid kinetics and independently of cytoplasmic bodies, ubiquitin, and proteasome activity. *J Virol* 2005; **79:** 15567–72.

100. Stremlau M, Perron M, Lee M, et al. Specific recognition and accelerated uncoating of retroviral capsids by the TRIM5{alpha} restriction factor. *Proc Natl Acad Sci USA* 2006; **103:** 5514–19.

101. Greenwald JL, Burstein GR, Pincus J, Branson B. A rapid review of rapid HIV antibody tests. *Curr Infect Dis Rep* 2006; **8:** 125–31.

102. Berger A, Scherzed L, Sturmer M, Preiser W, Doerr HW, Rabenau HF. Comparative evaluation of the Cobas Amplicor HIV-1 Monitor Ultrasensitive test, the new Cobas AmpliPrep/Cobas Amplicor HIV-1 Monitor Ultrasensitive test and the Versant HIV RNA 3.0 assays for quantitation of HIV-1 RNA in plasma samples. *J Clin Virol* 2005; **33:** 43–51.

103. Uttayamakul S, Likanonsakul S, Sunthornkachit R, et al. Usage of dried blood spots for molecular diagnosis and monitoring HIV-1 infection. *J Virol Methods* 2005; **128:** 128–34.

104. Jennings C, Fiscus SA, Crowe SM, et al. Comparison of two human immunodeficiency virus (HIV) RNA surrogate assays to the standard HIV RNA assay. *J Clin Microbiol* 2005; **43:** 5950–56.

105. Lombart JP, Vray M, Kafando A, et al. Plasma virion reverse transcriptase activity and heat dissociation-boosted p24 assay for HIV load in Burkina Faso, West Africa. *AIDS* 2005; **19:** 1273–77.

106. Tuaillon E, Gueudin M, Lemee V, et al. Phenotypic susceptibility to nonnucleoside inhibitors of virion-associated reverse transcriptase from different HIV types and groups. *J Acquir Immune Defic Syndr* 2004; **37:** 1543–49.

107. Rodriguez WR, Christodoulides N, Floriano PN, et al. A microchip CD4 counting method for HIV monitoring in resource-poor settings. *PLoS Med* 2005; **2:** e182.

108. Spacek LA, Shihab HM, Lutwama F, et al. Evaluation of a low-cost method, the Guava EasyCD4 assay, to enumerate CD4-positive lymphocyte counts in HIV-infected patients in the United States and Uganda. *J Acquir Immune Defic Syndr* 2006; **41:** 607–10.

109. Mofenson LM, Harris DR, Moye J, et al. Alternatives to HIV-1 RNA concentration and CD4 count to predict mortality in HIV-1-infected children in resource-poor settings. *Lancet* 2003; **362:** 1625–27.

110. Ceffa S, Erba F, Assane M, Coelho E, Calgaro M, Brando B. Panleucogating as an accurate and affordable flow cytometric protocol to analyse lymphocyte subsets among HIV-positive patients on HAART treatment in Mozambique. *J Biol Regul Homeost Agents* 2005; **19:** 169–75.

111. Lazzarin A, Clotet B, Cooper D, et al. Efficacy of enfuvirtide in patients infected with drug-resistant HIV-1 in Europe and Australia. *N Engl J Med* 2003; **348:** 2186–95.

112. Lalezari JP, Henry K, O'Hearn M, et al. Enfuvirtide, an HIV-1 fusion inhibitor, for drug-resistant HIV infection in North and South America. *N Engl J Med* 2003; **348:** 2175–85.

113. Mocroft A, Vella S, Benfield TL, et al. Changing patterns of mortality across Europe in patients infected with HIV-1. EuroSIDA Study Group. *Lancet* 1998; **352:** 1725–30.

114. Hogg RS, Heath KV, Yip B, et al. Improved survival among HIV-infected individuals following initiation of antiretroviral therapy. *JAMA* 1998; **279:** 450–54.

115. Palella FJ Jr, Delaney KM, Moorman AC, et al. Declining morbidity and mortality among patients with advanced human immunodeficiency virus infection. HIV Outpatient Study Investigators. *N Engl J Med* 1998; **338:** 853–60.

116. Mocroft A, Lundgren JD. Starting highly active antiretroviral therapy: why, when and response to HAART. *J Antimicrob Chemother* 2004; **54:** 10–03.

117. Mehandru S, Tenner-Racz K, Racz P, Markowitz M. The gastrointestinal tract is critical to the pathogenesis of acute HIV-1 infection. *J Allergy Clin Immunol* 2005; **116:** 419–22.

118. Nolan D, Mallal S. Antiretroviral-therapy-associated lipoatrophy: current status and future directions. *Sex Health* 2005; **2:** 153–63.

119. French MA, Price P, Stone SF. Immune restoration disease after antiretroviral therapy. *AIDS* 2004; **18:** 1615–27.

120. Wyatt CM, Klotman PE. Antiretroviral therapy and the kidney: balancing benefit and risk in patients with HIV infection. *Expert Opin Drug Saf* 2006; **5:** 275–87.

121. Calza L, Manfredi R, Chiodo F. Dyslipidaemia associated with antiretroviral therapy in HIV-infected patients. *J Antimicrob Chemother* 2004; **53:** 10–14.

122. Hirschel B. Planned interruptions of anti-HIV treatment. *Lancet Infect Dis* 2001; **1:** 53–59.

123. Powers AE, Marden SF, McConnell R, et al. Effect of long-cycle structured intermittent versus continuous HAART on quality of life in patients with chronic HIV infection. *Aids* 2006; **20:** 837–45.

124. Dybul M, Nies-Kraske E, Daucher M, et al. Long-cycle structured intermittent versus continuous highly active antiretroviral therapy for the treatment of chronic infection with human immunodeficiency virus: effects on drug toxicity and on immunologic and virologic parameters. *J Infect Dis* 2003; **188:** 388–96.

125. Abbas UL, Mellors JW. Interruption of antiretroviral therapy to augment immune control of chronic HIV-1 infection: risk without reward. *Proc Natl Acad Sci* USA 2002; **99:** 13377–78.

126. El-Sadr W, Neaton J. Episodic CD4-guided use of ART is inferior to continuous therapy: results of the SMART study. 13th Conference on Retroviruses and Opportunitic Infections; Denver, CO, USA: Feb 6–9, 2006.

127. Kim JY, Gilks C. Scaling up treatment—why we can't wait. *N Engl J Med* 2005; **353:** 2392–94.

128. Orrell C. Antiretroviral adherence in a resource-poor setting. *Curr HIV/AIDS Rep* 2005; **2:** 171–76.

129. Ferradini L, Jeannin A, Pinoges L, et al. Scaling up of highly active antiretroviral therapy in a rural district of Malawi: an effectiveness assessment. *Lancet* 2006; **367:** 1335–42.

130. Coetzee D, Hildebrand K, Boulle A, et al. Outcomes after two years of providing antiretroviral treatment in Khayelitsha, South Africa. *AIDS* 2004; **18:** 887–95.

131. Levy NC, Miksad RA, Fein OT. From treatment to prevention: the interplay between HIV/AIDS treatment availability and HIV/AIDS prevention programming in Khayelitsha, South Africa. *J Urban Health* 2005; **82:** 498–509.

132. WHO. Scaling up antiretroviral therapy in resource-limited settings: treatment guidelines for a public health approach: 2003 revision. Geneva, Switzerland: WHO, 2004.

133. Badri M, Bekker LG, Orrell C, Pitt J, Cilliers F, Wood R. Initiating highly active antiretroviral therapy in sub-Saharan Africa: an assessment of the revised World Health Organization scaling-up guidelines. *AIDS* 2004; **18:** 1159–68.

134. Calmy A, Klement E, Teck R, Berman D, Pecoul B, Ferradini L. Simplifying and adapting antiretroviral treatment in resource-poor settings: a necessary step to scaling-up. *AIDS* 2004; **18:** 2353–60.

135. Kober K, Van Damme W. Scaling up access to antiretroviral treatment in southern Africa: who will do the job? *Lancet* 2004; **364:** 103–07.

136. Libamba E, Makombe S, Harries AD, et al. Scaling up antiretroviral therapy in Africa: learning from tuberculosis control programmes—the case of Malawi. *Int J Tuberc Lung Dis* 2005; **9:** 1062–71.

137. Gupta R, Irwin A, Raviglione MC, Kim JY. Scaling-up treatment for HIV/AIDS: lessons learned from multidrug-resistant tuberculosis. *Lancet* 2004; **363:** 320–24.

138. Bachmann MO. Effectiveness and cost effectiveness of early and late prevention of HIV/AIDS progression with antiretrovirals or antibiotics in Southern African adults. *AIDS Care* 2006; **18:** 109–20.

139. Deeks SG. Treatment of antiretroviral-drug-resistant HIV-1 infection. *Lancet* 2003; **362:** 2002–11.

140. Kantor R, Katzenstein DA, Efron B, et al. Impact of HIV-1 subtype and antiretroviral therapy on protease and reverse transcriptase genotype: results of a global collaboration. *PLoS Med* 2005; **2:** e112.

141. Parkin NT, Schapiro JM. Antiretroviral drug resistance in non-subtype B HIV-1, HIV-2 and SIV. *Antivir Ther* 2004; **9:** 3–12.

142. Wensing AM, Boucher CA. Worldwide transmission of drug-resistant HIV. *AIDS Rev* 2003; **5:** 140–55.

143. Toni TD, Masquelier B, Lazaro E, et al. Characterization of nevirapine (NVP) resistance mutations and HIV type 1 subtype in women from Abidjan (Cote d'Ivoire) after NVP single-dose prophylaxis of HIV type 1 mother-to-child transmission. *AIDS Res Hum Retroviruses* 2005; **21:** 1031–34.

144. Eshleman SH, Jackson JB. Nevirapine resistance after single dose prophylaxis. *AIDS Rev* 2002; **4:** 59–63.

145. Flys TS, Chen S, Jones DC, et al. Quantitative analysis of HIV-1 variants with the K103N resistance mutation after single-dose nevirapine in women with HIV-1 subtypes A, C, and D. *J Acquir Immune Defic Syndr* 2006; published online June 12, 2006. DOI: 10.1097/01.qai .0000221686.67810.20.

146. Lee EJ, Kantor R, Zijenah L, et al. Breast-milk shedding of drug-resistant HIV-1 subtype C in women exposed to single-dose nevirapine. *J Infect Dis* 2005; **192:** 1260–64.

147. Palmer S, Boltz V, Martinson N, et al. Persistence of nevirapine-resistant HIV-1 in women after single-dose nevirapine therapy for prevention of maternal-to-fetal HIV-1 transmission. *Proc Natl Acad Sci USA* 2006; **103:** 7094–99.

148. Chaix ML, Ekouevi DK, Rouet F, et al. Low risk of nevirapine resistance mutations in the prevention of mother-to-child transmission of HIV-1: Agence Nationale de Recherches sur le SIDA Ditrame Plus, Abidjan, Cote d'Ivoire. *J Infect Dis* 2006; **193:** 482–87.

149. Ylisastigui L, Archin NM, Lehrman G, Bosch RJ, Margolis DM. Coaxing HIV-1 from resting CD4 T cells: histone deacetylase inhibition allows latent viral expression. *AIDS* 2004; **18:** 1101–08.

150. Lehrman G, Hogue IB, Palmer S, et al. Depletion of latent HIV-1 infection in vivo: a proof-of-concept study. *Lancet* 2005; **366:** 549–55.

151. Luzuriaga K, Sullivan JL. Prevention of mother-to-child transmission of HIV infection. *Clin Infect Dis* 2005; **40:** 466–67.

152. McIntyre J. Strategies to prevent mother-to-child transmission of HIV. *Curr Opin Infect Dis* 2006; **19:** 33–38.

153. Newell ML. Current issues in the prevention of mother-to-child transmission of HIV-1 infection. *Trans R Soc Trop Med Hyg* 2006; **100:** 1–5.

154. Ekouevi DK, Tonwe-Gold B, Dabis F. Advances in the prevention of mother-to-child transmission of HIV-1 infection in resource-limited settings. *AIDS Read* 2005; **15:** 479–80.

155. Cressey TR, Jourdain G, Lallemant MJ, et al. Persistence of nevirapine exposure during the postpartum period after intrapartum single-dose nevirapine in addition to zidovudine prophylaxis for the prevention of mother-to-child transmission of HIV-1. *J Acquir Immune Defic Syndr* 2005; **38:** 283–88.

156. Read JS, Newell MK. Efficacy and safety of cesarean delivery for prevention of mother-to-child transmission of HIV-1. *Cochrane Database Syst Rev* 2005; **4:** CD005479.

157. Magoni M, Bassani L, Okong P, et al. Mode of infant feeding and HIV infection in children in a program for prevention of mother-to-child transmission in Uganda. *AIDS* 2005; **19:** 433–37.

158. Rollins N, Meda N, Becquet R, et al. Preventing postnatal transmission of HIV-1 through breast-feeding: modifying infant feeding practices. *J Acquir Immune Defic Syndr* 2004; **35:** 188–95.

159. Duerr A, Hurst S, Kourtis AP, Rutenberg N, Jamieson DJ. Integrating family planning and prevention of mother-to-child HIV transmission in resource-limited settings. *Lancet* 2005; **366:** 261–63.

160. Welty TK, Bulterys M, Welty ER, et al. Integrating prevention of mother-to-child HIV transmission into routine antenatal care: the key to program expansion in Cameroon. *J Acquir Immune Defic Syndr* 2005; **40:** 486–93.

161. Tuomala RE, Shapiro DE, Mofenson LM, et al. Antiretroviral therapy during pregnancy and the risk of an adverse outcome. *N Engl J Med* 2002; **346:** 1863–70.

162. Exposure to antiretroviral therapy in utero or early life: the health of uninfected children born to HIV-infected women. *J Acquir Immune Defic Syndr* 2003; **32:** 380–87.

163. Chan DJ. Factors affecting sexual transmission of HIV-1: current evidence and implications for prevention. *Curr HIV Res* 2005; **3:** 223–41.

164. de Vincenzi I. A longitudinal study of human immunodeficiency virus transmission by heterosexual partners. European Study Group on Heterosexual Transmission of HIV. *N Engl J Med* 1994; **331:** 341–46.

165. Weller S, Davis K. Condom effectiveness in reducing heterosexual HIV transmission. *Cochrane Database Syst Rev* 2002; **1:** CD003255.

166. Siegfried N, Muller M, Deeks J, et al. HIV and male circumcision—a systematic review with assessment of the quality of studies. *Lancet Infect Dis* 2005; **5**: 165–73.

167. Auvert B, Taljaard D, Lagarde E, Sobngwi-Tambekou J, Sitta R, Puren A. Randomized, controlled intervention trial of male circumcision for reduction of HIV infection risk: the ANRS 1265 Trial. *PLoS Med* 2005; **2**: e298.

168. Szabo R, Short RV. How does male circumcision protect against HIV infection? *BMJ* 2000; **320**: 1592–94.

169. Soto-Ramirez LE, Renjifo B, McLane MF, et al. HIV-1 Langerhans' cell tropism associated with heterosexual transmission of HIV. *Science* 1996; **271**: 1291–93.

170. Patterson BK, Landay A, Siegel JN, et al. Susceptibility to human immunodeficiency virus-1 infection of human foreskin and cervical tissue grown in explant culture. *Am J Pathol* 2002; **161**: 867–73.

171. Halperin DT, Fritz K, McFarland W, Woelk G. Acceptability of adult male circumcision for sexually transmitted disease and HIV prevention in Zimbabwe. *Sex Transm Dis* 2005; **32**: 238–39.

172. Garenne M. Male circumcision and HIV control in Africa. *PLoS Med* 2006; **3**: e78.

173. Bailey RC. Editorial comment: male circumcision to reduce HIV acquisition—not quite yet. *AIDS Read* 2005; **15**: 136–37.

174. Blower SM, Gershengorn HB, Grant RM. A tale of two futures: HIV and antiretroviral therapy in San Francisco. *Science* 2000; **287**: 650–54.

175. Gray RH, Wawer MJ, Brookmeyer R, et al. Probability of HIV-1 transmission per coital act in monogamous, heterosexual, HIV-1-discordant couples in Rakai, Uganda. *Lancet* 2001; **357**: 1149–53.

176. Nicolosi A, Correa Leite ML, Musicco M, Arici C, Gavazzeni G, Lazzarin A. The efficiency of male-to-female and female-to-male sexual transmission of the human immunodeficiency virus: a study of 730 stable couples. Italian Study Group on HIV Heterosexual Transmission. *Epidemiology* 1994; **5**: 570–75.

177. Puro V, Cicalini S, De Carli G, et al. Post-exposure prophylaxis of HIV infection in healthcare workers: recommendations for the European setting. *Eur J Epidemiol* 2004; **19**: 577–84.

178. Winston A, McAllister J, Amin J, Cooper DA, Carr A. The use of a riple nucleoside-nucleotide regimen for nonoccupational HIV post-exposure prophylaxis. *HIV Med* 2005; **6**: 191–97.

179. Bassett IV, Freedberg KA, Walensky RP. Two drugs or three? Balancing efficacy, toxicity, and resistance in postexposure prophylaxis for occupational exposure to HIV. *Clin Infect Dis* 2004; **39**: 395–401.

180. Blower SM, Gershengorn HB, Grant RM. A tale of two futures: HIV and antiretroviral therapy in San Francisco. *Science* 2000; **287**: 650–54.

181. Grosskurth H, Gray R, Hayes R, Mabey D, Wawer M. Control of sexually transmitted diseases for HIV-1 prevention: understanding the implications of the Mwanza and Rakai trials. *Lancet* 2000; **355**: 1981–87.

182. Corey L, Wald A, Celum CL, Quinn TC. The effects of herpes simplex virus-2 on HIV-1 acquisition and transmission: a review of two overlapping epidemics. *J Acquir Immune Defic Syndr* 2004; **35**: 435–45.

183. Nagot N, Foulongne V, Becquart P, et al. Longitudinal assessment of HIV-1 and HSV-2 shedding in the genital tract of West African women. *J Acquir Immune Defic Syndr* 2005; **39:** 632–34.

184. Gupta R, Wald A, Krantz E, et al. Valacyclovir and acyclovir for suppression of shedding of herpes simplex virus in the genital tract. *J Infect Dis* 2004; **190:** 1374–81.

185. Corey L, Wald A, Patel R, et al. Once-daily valacyclovir to reduce the risk of transmission of genital herpes. *N Engl J Med* 2004; **350:** 11–20.

186. Hosken NA. Development of a therapeutic vaccine for HSV-2. *Vaccine* 2005; **23:** 2395–98.

187. Duffy L. Culture and context of HIV prevention in rural Zimbabwe: the influence of gender inequality. *J Transcult Nurs* 2005; **16:** 23–31.

188. Gray RH, Li X, Kigozi G, et al. Increased risk of incident HIV during pregnancy in Rakai, Uganda: a prospective study. *Lancet* 2005; **366:** 1182–88.

189. Schwebke JR. Abnormal vaginal flora as a biological risk factor for acquisition of HIV infection and sexually transmitted diseases. *J Infect Dis* 2005; **192:** 1315–17.

190. van der Straten A, Kang MS, Posner SF, Kamba M, Chipato T, Padian NS. Predictors of diaphragm use as a potential sexually transmitted disease/HIV prevention method in Zimbabwe. *Sex Transm Dis* 2005; **32:** 64–71.

191. Myer L, Denny L, Telerant R, Souza M, Wright TC Jr, Kuhn L. Bacterial vaginosis and susceptibility to HIV infection in South African women: a nested case-control study. *J Infect Dis* 2005; **192:** 1372–80.

192. Stein ZA. Vaginal microbicides and prevention of HIV infection. *Lancet* 1994; **343:** 362–63.

193. Van Damme L, Ramjee G, Alary M, et al. Effectiveness of COL-1492, a nonoxynol-9 vaginal gel, on HIV-1 transmission in female sex workers: a randomised controlled trial. *Lancet* 2002; **360:** 971–77.

194. Hillier SL, Moench T, Shattock R, Black R, Reichelderfer P, Veronese F. In vitro and in vivo: the story of nonoxynol 9. *J Acquir Immune Defic Syndr* 2005; **39:** 1–8.

195. Weber J, Desai K, Darbyshire J. The development of vaginal microbicides for the prevention of HIV transmission. *PLoS Med* 2005; **2:** e142.

196. Dhawan D, Mayer KH. Microbicides to prevent HIV transmission: overcoming obstacles to chemical barrier protection. *J Infect Dis* 2006; **193:** 36–44.

197. Malcolm RK, Woolfson AD, Toner CF, Morrow RJ, McCullagh SD. Long-term, controlled release of the HIV microbicide TMC120 from silicone elastomer vaginal rings. *J Antimicrob Chemother* 2005; **56:** 954–56.

198. Ho DD, Huang Y. The HIV-1 vaccine race. *Cell* 2002; **110:** 135–38.

199. Sheppard HW. Inactivated- or killed-virus HIV/AIDS vaccines. *Curr Drug Targets Infect Disord* 2005; **5:** 131–41.

200. Wyatt R, Sodroski J. The HIV-1 envelope glycoproteins: fusogens, antigens, and immunogens. *Science* 1998; **280:** 1884–88.

201. Pantophlet R, Burton DR. GP120: target for neutralizing HIV-1 antibodies. *Annu Rev Immunol* 2006; **24:** 739–69.

202. Cohen J. Public health. AIDS vaccine trial produces disappointment and confusion. *Science* 2003; **299:** 1290–91.

203. Francis DP, Heyward WL, Popovic V, et al. Candidate HIV/AIDS vaccines: lessons learned from the world's first phase III efficacy trials. *AIDS* 2003; **17**: 147–56.

204. Garber DA, Silvestri G, Feinberg MB. Prospects for an AIDS vaccine: three big questions, no easy answers. *Lancet Infect Dis* 2004; **4**: 397–413.

205. Roberts DM, Nanda A, Havenga MJ, et al. Hexon-chimaeric adenovirus serotype 5 vectors circumvent pre-existing anti-vector immunity. *Nature* 2006; **441**: 239–43.

206. Jamieson BD, Ibarrondo FJ, Wong JT, et al. Transience of vaccine-induced HIV-1-specific CTL and definition of vaccine "response". *Vaccine* 2006; **24**: 3426–31.

207. Rennie S, Behets F. Desperately seeking targets: the ethics of routine testing in low income countries. *Bull World Health Organ* 2006; **84**: 52–57.

208. Manzi M, Zachariah R, Teck R, et al. High acceptability of voluntary counselling and HIV-testing but unacceptable loss to follow up in a prevention of mother-to-child HIV transmission programme in rural Malawi: scaling-up requires a different way of acting. *Trop Med Int Health* 2005; **10**: 1242–50.

▶ Further Readings and Resources

Funding the Fight Against AIDS
http://www.avert.org/wwhiv.htm

Funding AIDS Grassroots Organizations
http://www.avert.org/wwhiv.htm

What is PEPFAR
http://www.avert.org/wwhiv.htm

What is PEPFAR doing in its focus countries
http://www.avert.org/wwhiv.htm

PEPFAR's Partners
http://www.avert.org/wwhiv.htm

PEPFAR Description
http://www.cgdev.org/section/initiatives/_active/hivmonitor/funding/pepfar_overview

Bill and Melinda Gates Foundation
http://www.gatesfoundation.org/GlobalHealth/RelatedInfo/GlobalHealthFactSheet-021201.htm
http://www.gatesfoundation.org/AboutUs/QuickFacts/Timeline/default.htm

amFar
http://www.amfar.org/cgi-bin/iowa/amfar/history/record.html?record=6

FHI/UNAIDS Best Practices in HIV/AIDS Prevention
htt://www.fhi.org/en/HIVAIDS/pub/guide/bestpractices.htm

Glossary

Acronyms

ACTG AIDS clinical trial group

AIDS acquired immunodeficiency syndrome

ARV AIDS-related virus

AZT azathioprine (this is not zidovudine or azidothymidine)

CD4 reception site on a T4 cell to which HIV most often binds

CDC Centers for Disease Control and Prevention (part of PHS)

3TC Lamivudine; nucleoside analog

CTS Counseling and Testing Services

DHHS Department of Health and Human Services

DNA deoxyribonucleic acid

d4T stavudine; nucleoside analog

ddC dideoxycytosine; nucleoside analog

ddI dideoxyinosine; nucleoside analog

FDA Food and Drug Administration (part of PHS)

HTLV-I human T cell lymphotropic virus, type I

HTLV-II human T cell lymphotropic virus, type II

HTLV-III human T cell lymphotropic virus, type III

IDAV immune deficiency associated virus

IDU injection Drug User

LAV lymphadenopathy-associated virus

NCI National Cancer Institute (part of NIH)

NEI National Eye Institute (part of NIH)

NHLBI National Heart, Lung and Blood Institute (part of NIH)

NIAID National Institute of Allergy and Infectious Diseases (part of NIH)

NIDA National Institute on Drug Abuse (part of PHS)

NIDR National Institute of Dental Research (part of NIH)

NIH National Institutes of Health (part of PHS)

NIMH National Institute of Mental Health (part of PHS)

NINCDS National Institute of Neurological and Communicative Disorders and Stroke (part of NIH)

OTA Office of Technology Assessment (part of U.S. Congress)

PHS Public Health Service (part of DHHS)

RNA ribonucleic acid

ZDV Zidovudine major drug in treating HIV/AIDS persons; nucleoside analog

Terms

Acquired immunodeficiency syndrome (AIDS): A life-threatening disease caused by a virus and characterized by the breakdown of the body's immune defenses. (See AIDS.)

Active immunity: Protection against a disease resulting from the production of antibodies in a host that has been exposed to a disease causing antigen.

Acute: Sudden onset, short-term with severe symptoms.

Acyclovir (Zovirax): Antiviral drug for herpes I and 2 and herpes zoster.

AIDS (acquired immunodeficiency syndrome): A disease believed to be caused by a retrovirus called HIV and characterized by a deficiency of the immune system. The primary defect in AIDS is an acquired, persistent, quantitative functional depression within the T4 subset of lymphocytes. This depression often leads to infections caused by opportunistic microorganisms in HIV-infected individuals. A rare type of cancer (Kaposi's sarcoma) usually seen in elderly men or in individuals who are severely immunocompromised may also occur. Other associated diseases are currently under investigation and will probably be included in the final definition of AIDS.

AIDS dementia: Neurological complications affecting thinking and behavior; intellectual impairment.

Allergic reaction: A reaction that results from extreme sensitivity to a drug or agent and is not dependent on the amount of drug given. These may be classified into two types, immediate and delayed, based on the time it takes for the reaction to occur.

Anemia: Low number of red blood cells.

Anorexia: Prolonged loss of appetite that leads to significant weight loss.

Antibiotic: A chemical substance capable of destroying bacteria and other microorganisms.

Antibody: A blood protein produced by mammals in response to a specific antigen.

Antigen: A large molecule, usually a protein or carbohydrate, which when introduced into the body stimulates the production of an antibody that will react specifically with that antigen.

Antigen-presenting cells: B cells, cells of the monocyte lineage (including macrophages and dentritic cells) and various other body cells that 'present' antigen in a form that T cells can recognize.

Antiserum: Serum portion of the blood that carries the antibodies.

Antiviral: Means against virus; drugs that destroy or weaken virus.

ARC: AIDS-related complex.

Arthritis: Inflammation of the joints and the surrounding tissues.

Arthropod: An insect-like animal.

Aspiration: The removal of fluids by suction.

Asymptomatic carrier: A host which is infected by an organism but does not demonstrate clinical signs or symptoms of the disease.

Asymptomatic seropositive: HIV-positive without signs or symptoms of HIV disease.

Ataxia: Inability to coordinate movement of muscles.

Atrophy: The wasting away or decrease in size and function of a body part.

Attenuated: Weakened.

Atypical: Irregular; not of typical character.

Autoimmunity: Antibodies made against self tissues.

Autoinoculation: A secondary infection originating from an infection site already present in the body.

B lymphocytes or B cells: Lymphocytes that produce antibodies. B lymphocytes proliferate under stimulation from factors released by T lymphocytes.

Bacterium: A microscopic organism composed of a single cell. Many but not all bacteria cause disease.

Blood count: A count of the number of red and white blood cells and platelets.

Bone marrow: Soft tissue located in the cavities of the bones. The bone marrow is the source of all blood cells.

Cancer: A large group of diseases characterized by uncontrolled growth and spread of abnormal cells.

Candida albicans: A fungus; the causative agent of vulvovaginal candidiasis or yeast infection.

Candidiasis: A fungal infection of the mucous membranes (commonly occurring in the mouth, where it is known as Thrush) characterized by whitish spots and/or a burning or painful sensation. It may also occur in the esophagus. It can also cause a red and itchy rash in moist areas, e.g., the vagina.

Capsid: The protein coat of a virus particle.

Carcinogen: Any substance that causes cancer.

Carcinoma: A form of skin cancer that occurs in tissues that cover or line body organs, e.g., intestines, lungs, breasts, uterus, etc.

Cardiovascular: Pertaining to the heart and blood vessels.

CC-CKR-5 (CKR-5): Receptor for human chemokines and a necessary receptor for HIV entrance into macrophage.

CD: Cluster differentiating type antigens found on T lymphocytes. Each CD is assigned a number: CD1, CD2, etc.

CD4(T4): White blood cell with type 4 protein embedded in the cell surface-target cell for HIV infection.

CD8: Suppressor white blood cell with type 8 protein embedded in the cell surface.

Cell-mediated immunity: The reaction to antigenic material by specific defensive cells (macrophages) rather than antibodies.

Cellular immunity: A collection of cell types that provide protection against various antigens.

Central nervous system (CNS): The brain and spinal cord.

Cerebral spinal fluid (CSF): The fluid which surrounds the brain and spinal cord.

Chain of infection: A series of infections that are directly or immediately connected to a particular source.

Chemokines: Chemicals released by T cell lymphocytes and other cells of the immune system to attract a variety of cell types to sites of inflammation.

Chemotherapy: The use of chemicals that have a specific and toxic effect upon a disease-causing pathogen.

Chlamydia: A species of bacterium, the causative organism of *Lymphogranuloma venereum,* chlamydial urethritis and most cases of newborn conjunctivitis.

Chromosomes: Physical structures in the cell's nucleus that house the genes. Each human cell has 22 pairs of autosomes and two sex chromosomes.

Chronic: Having a long and relatively mild course.

Clade: Related HIV variants classified by degree of genetic similarity; nine are known for HIV.

Clinical latency: Infectious agent developing in a host without producing clinical symptoms.

Clinical manifestations: The signs of a disease as they pertain to or are observed in patients.

Cofactor: Factors or agents which are necessary or which increase the probability of the development of disease in the presence of the basic etiologic agent of that disease.

Cohort: A group of individuals with some characteristics in common.

Communicable: Able to spread from one diseased person or animal to another, either directly or indirectly.

Condylomata acuminatum (venereal warts): Viral warts of the genital and anogenital area.

Congenital: Acquired by the newborn before or at the time of birth.

Core proteins: Proteins that make up the internal structure or core of a virus.

Cryptococcal meningitis: A fungal infection that affects the three membranes (meninges) surrounding the brain and spinal cord. Symptoms include severe headache, vertigo, nausea, anorexia, sight disorders and mental deterioration.

Cryptococcosis: A fungal infectious disease often found in the lungs of AIDS patients. It characteristically spreads to the meninges and may also spread to the kidneys and skin. It is due to the fungus *Oyptococcus neoformans.*

Cryptosporidiosis: An infection caused by a protozoan parasite found in the intestines of animals. Acquired in some people by direct contact with the infected animal, it lodges in the intestines and causes severe diarrhea. It may be transmitted from person to person. This infection seems to be occurring more frequently in immunosuppressed people and can lead to prolonged symptoms which do not respond to medication.

Cutaneous: Having to do with the skin.

Cytokines: Powerful chemical substances secreted by cells. Cytokines include lymphokines produced by lymphocytes and monokines produced by monocytes and macrophages.

Cytomegalovirus (CMV): One of a group of highly host specific herpes viruses that affect humans and other animals. Generally produces mild flu-like symptoms but can be more severe. In the immunosuppressed, it may cause pneumonia.

Cytopathic: Pertaining to or characterized by abnormal changes in cells.

Cytotoxic: Poisonous to cells.

Cytotoxic T cells: A subset of T lymphocytes that carry the T8 marker and can kill body cells infected by viruses or transformed by cancer.

Dementia: Chronic mental deterioration sufficient to significantly impair social and/or occupational function. Usually patients have memory and abstract thinking loss. They may have impairment of more specific higher cortical functions. Frequently progressive and irreversible.

Dendritic cells: White blood cells found in the spleen and other lymphoid organs. Dendritic cells typically use threadlike tentacles to "hold" the antigen, which they present to T cells.

Dermatitis: Inflammation of the skin.

Diagnosis: The identification of a disease by its signs, symptoms and laboratory findings.

Didanosine: Also known as videx; see ddI—inhibits HIV replication.

Direct transmission: A manner of transmitting disease organisms in which the agent moves immediately from the infected person to the susceptible person, as in person-to-person contact and in droplet contact.

Disease intervention specialist (DIS): A person who performs STD patient interviewing/counseling and field investigation.

Dissemination: Spread of disease throughout the body.

DNA (deoxyribonucleic acid): A linear polymer, made up of deoxyribonucleotide repeating units. It is the carrier of genetic information in living organisms and some viruses.

DNA viruses: Contain DNA as their genetic material.

Dysentery: Inflammation of the intestines, especially the colon, producing pain in the abdomen and diarrhea containing blood and mucus.

Efficacy: Effectiveness.

ELISA test: A blood test *which* indicates the presence of antibodies to a given antigen. Various ELISA tests are used to detect a variety of infections. The HIV ELISA test does not detect AIDS but only indicates if viral infection has occurred.

Endemic: Prevalent in or peculiar to community or group of people.

Enteric infections: Infections of the intestine.

ENV: HIV gene that codes for protein gp160

Envelope proteins: Proteins that comprise the envelope or surface of a virus, gp120 and gp41.

Enzyme: A catalytic protein that is produced by living cells and promotes the chemical processes of life without itself being altered or destroyed.

Epidemic: When the incidence of a disease surpasses the expected rate in any well-defined geographical area.

Epidemiologic studies: Studies concerned with the relationships of various factors determining the frequency and distribution of certain diseases.

Epidemiology: The study of the factors that impact on the spread of disease in an area.

Epitopes: Characteristic shapes of antigens found on an organism or virus.

Epivir: See 3TC.

Epstein-Barr virus (EBV): A virus that causes infectious mononucleosis. It is spread by saliva. EBV lies dormant in the lymph glands and has been associated with Burkitt's lymphoma, a cancer of the lymph tissue.

Etiologic agent: The organism which causes a disease.

Etiology: The study of the cause of disease.

Extracellular: Found outside the cell wall.

Exudate: To produce liquid in response to disease.

Factor VIII: A naturally occurring protein in plasma that aids in the coagulation of blood. A congenital deficiency of Factor VIII results in the bleeding disorder known as hemophilia A.

Factor VIII concentrate: A concentrated preparation of Factor VIII that is used in the treatment of individuals with hemophilia A.

Fallopian tube: A slender 4-inch-long tube extending from the ovary to the uterus. Eggs released during ovulation pass through this tube to reach the uterus.

False negative: Failure of a test to demonstrate the disease or condition when present.

False positive: A positive test result caused by a disease or condition other than the disease for which the test is designed.

Fellatio: Oral sex involving the penis.

Follicular dendritic cells: Found in germinal centers of lymphoid organs.

Fomite: An inanimate object that can hold infectious agents and transfers them from one individual to another.

Fulminant: Rapid onset, severe.

Fungus: Member of a class of relatively primitive organisms. Fungi include mushrooms, yeasts, rusts, molds and smuts.

Gammaglobulin: The antibody component of the serum.

Ganciclovir (DHPG): An experimental antiviral drug used in the treatment of CMV retinitis.

Gene: The basic unit of heredity; an ordered sequence of nucleotides. A gene contains the information for the synthesis of one polypeptide chain (protein).

Gene expression: The production of RNA and cellular proteins.

Genitourinary: Pertaining to the urinary and reproductive structures; sometimes called the GU tract or system.

Genome: The genetic endowment of an organism.

GP41: Glycoprotein found in envelope of HIV.

GP120: Glycoprotein found in outer level of HIV envelope.

GP160: Precusor glycoprotein to forming gp41 and gp120.

Giardiasis: Infection of the intestinal tract with *Giardia lamblia* (a protozoan) which may cause intermittent diarrhea of lengthy duration.

Globulin: That portion of serum which contains the antibodies.

Glycoproteins: Proteins with carbohydrate groups attached at specific locations.

Glycosylation: The attachment of a carbohydrate molecule to another molecule such as a protein.

Gonococcus: The specific etiologic agent of gonorrhea discovered by Neisser and named *Neisseria gonorrhoeae*.

Granulocytes: Phagocytic white blood cells filled with granules containing potent chemicals that allow the cells to digest microorganisms. Neutrophils, eosinophils, basophils and mast cells are examples of granulocytes.

Hemoglobin: The oxygen-carrying portion of red blood cells which gives them a red color.

Hemophilia: A hereditary bleeding disorder caused by a deficiency in the ability to synthesize one or more of the blood coagulation proteins, e.g., FactorVIII (hemophilia A) or Factor IX (hemophilia B).

Hepatitis: Inflammation of the liver; due to many causes including viruses, several of which are transmissible through blood transfusions and sexual activities.

Hepatosplenomegaly: Enlargement of the liver and spleen.

Herpes simplex virus 1 (HSV-I): A virus that results in cold sores or fever blisters, most often on the mouth or around the eyes. Like all herpes viruses, it may lie dormant for months or years in nerve tissues and flare up in times of stress, trauma, infection or immunosuppression. There is no cure for any of the herpes viruses.

Herpes simplex virus II (HSV-II): Causes painful sores on the genitals or anus. It is one of the most common sexually transmitted diseases in the United States.

Herpes varicella zoster virus (HVZ): The varicella virus causes chicken pox in children and may reappear in adulthood as herpes zoster. Herpes zoster, also called shingles, is characterized by small, painful blisters on the skin along nerve pathways.

High-risk behavior: A term used to describe certain activities that increase the risk of disease exposure.

High-risk groups: Those groups of people that show a behavioral risk for exposure to a disease or condition.

Histoplasmosis: A disease caused by a fungal infection that can affect all the organs of the body. Symptoms usually include fever, shortness of breath, cough, weight loss and physical exhaustion.

HIV (human immunodeficiency virus): A newly discovered retrovirus that is said to cause AIDS. The target organ of HIV is the T4 subset of T lymphocytes, which regulate the immune system.

HIV-positive: Presence of the human immunodeficiency virus in the body.

Homophobia: Negative bias towards or fear of individuals who are homosexual.

Human leukocyte antigens (HLA): Protein markers of self used in histocompatibility testing. Some HLA types also correlate with certain autoimmune diseases.

Humoral immunity: The production of antibodies for defense against infection or disease.

Hybridoma: A hybrid cell created by fusing a B lymphocyte with a long-lived neoplastic plasma cell, or a T lymphocyte with a lymphoma cell. A B-cell hybridoma secretes a single specific antibody.

Idiotypes: The unique and characteristic parts of an antibody's variable region, which can themselves serve as antigens.

Immunity: Resistance to a disease because of a functioning immune system.

Immune complex: A cluster of interlocking antigens and antibodies.

Immune response: The reaction of the immune system to foreign substances.

Immune status: The state of the body's natural defense to diseases. It is influenced by heredity, age, past illness history, diet and physical and mental health. It includes production of circulating and local antibodies and their mechanism of action.

Immunoassay: The use of antibodies to identify and quantify substances. Often the antibody is linked to a marker such as a fluorescent molecule, a radioactive molecule or an enzyme.

Immunocompetent: Capable of developing an immune response

Immunoglobulins: A family of large protein molecules, also known as antibodies.

Immunostimulant: Any agent that will trigger a body's defenses.

Immunosuppression: When the immune system is not working normally. This can be the result of illness or certain drugs (commonly those used to fight cancer).

Incidence: The total number of new cases of a disease in a given area within a specified time, usually 1 year.

Incubation period: The time between the actual entry of an infectious agent into the body and the onset of disease symptoms.

Indinavir: Crixivan, a protease inhibitor drug.

Indirect transmission: The transmission of a disease to a susceptible person by means of vectors or by airborne route.

Infection: Invasion of the body by viruses or other organisms.

Infectious disease: A disease which is caused by microorganisms or viruses living in or on the body as parasites.

Inflammatory response: Redness, warmth and swelling in response to infection; the result of increased blood flow and a gathering of immune cells and secretions.

Injection drug use: Use of drugs injected by needle into a vein or muscle tissue.

Innate immunity: Inborn or hereditary immunity.

Inoculation: The entry of an infectious organism or virus into the body.

Integrase: HIV enzyme used to insert HIV DNA into host cell DNA.

Interferon: A class of glycoproteins important in immune function and thought to inhibit viral infection.

Interleukins: Chemical messengers that travel from leukocytes to other white blood cells. Some promote cell development, others promote rapid cell division.

Intracellular: Found within the cell wall.

In utero: In the uterus

In vitro: 'In glass' pertains to a biological reaction in an artificial medium.

In vivo: 'In the living' pertains to a biological reaction in a living organism.

IV: Intravenous.

Kaposi's sarcoma: A multifocal, spreading cancer of connective tissue, principally involving the skin; it usually begins on the toes or the feet as reddish blue or brownish soft nodules and tumors.

Keratin: A waterproofing protein in the skin.

Lamivudine: Nucleoside analog inhibits HIV replication.

Langerhans cells: Dendritic cells in the skin that pickup antigen and transport it to lymph nodes.

Latency: A period when a virus or other organism is still in the body but in an inactive state.

Latent viral infection: The virion becomes part of the host cell's DNA.

Lentiviruses: Viruses that cause disease very slowly. HIV is believed to be this type of virus.

Lesion: Any abnormal change in tissue due to disease or injury.

Leukocyte: A white blood cell.

Leukopenia: A decrease in the white blood cell count.

Log: 10-fold difference.

Lymph: A transparent, slightly yellow fluid that carries lymphocytes, bathes the body tissues and drains into the lymphatic vessels.

Lymph nodes: Gland-like structures in the lymphatic system which help to prevent spread of infection.

Lymphadenopathy: Enlargement of the lymph nodes.

Lymphadenopathy syndrome (LAS): A condition characterized by persistent, generalized, enlarged lymph nodes, sometimes with signs of minor illness such as fever and weight loss, which apparently represents a milder reaction to HIV infection. LAS is also known as generalized lymphadenopathy syndrome.

Lymphatic system: A fluid system of vessels and glands which is important in controlling infections and limiting their spread.

Lymphocytes: Specialized white blood cells involved in the immune response.

Lymphoid organs: The organs of the immune system where lymphocytes develop and congregate. They include the bone marrow, thymus, lymph nodes, spleen and other clusters of lymphoid tissue.

Lymphokines: Chemical messengers produced by T and B lymphocytes. They have a variety of protective functions.

Lymphoma: Malignant growth of lymph nodes.

Lymphosarcoma: A general term applied to malignant neoplastic disorders of lymphoid tissue, not including Hodgkin's disease.

Lytic infection: When a virus infects the cell, the cell produces new viruses and breaks open (lyse) releasing the viruses.

Macrophage: A large and versatile immune cell that acts as a microbe-devouring phagocyte, an antigen-presenting cell and an important source of immune secretions.

Macule: A discolored spot or patch on the skin which is not raised or thickened.

Major histocompatibility complex (MHC): A group of genes that controls several aspects of the immune response. MHC genes code for self markers on all body cells.

Malaise: A general feeling of discomfort or fatigue.

Malignant tumor: A tumor made up of cancerous cells. The tumors grow and invade surrounding tissue, then the cells break away and grow elsewhere.

Messenger RNA (mRNA): RNA that serves as the template for protein synthesis; it carries the information from the DNA to the protein synthesizing complex to direct protein synthesis.

Microbes: Minute living organisms including bacteria, viruses, fungi and protozoa.

Microorganisms: Microscopic plants or animals.

Molecule: The smallest amount of a specific chemical substance that can exist alone. To break a molecule down into its constituent atoms is to change its character. A molecule of water, for instance, reverts to oxygen and hydrogen.

Monocyte: A large phagocytic white blood cell which, when it enters tissue, develops into a macrophage.

Monokines: Powerful chemical substances secreted by monocytes and macrophages. They help direct and regulate the immune response.

Morbidity: The proportion of people with a disease in a community.

Morphology: The study of the form and structure of organisms.

Mortality: The number of people who die as a result of a specific cause.

Mucosal immunity: Resistance to infection across, mucous membranes.

Mucous membrane: The lining of the canals and cavities of the body which communicate with external air, such as the intestinal tract, respiratory tract and the genitourinary tract.

Mucous patches: White, patchy growths, usually found in the mouth, that are symptoms of secondary syphilis and are highly infectious.

Mucus: A fluid secreted by membranes

Neisseria gonorrhoeae: The bacterium that causes gonorrhea.

Neonatal: Pertaining to the first 4 weeks of life.

Neuropathy: Group of nerve disorders, symptoms range from tingling sensation, numbness to paralysis.

Nevirapine: Non-nucleostide analog inhibits HIV replication.

Nodule: A small node which is solid and can be detected by touch.

Notifiable disease: A notifiable disease is one that, when diagnosed, health providers are required, usually by law, to report to state or local public health officials. Notifiable diseases are those of public interest by reason of their contagiousness, severity, or frequency.

Nucleic acids: Large, naturally occurring molecules composed of chemical building blocks known as nucleotides. There are two kinds of nucleic acid, DNA and RNA.

Nucleoside analog: Synthetic compounds generally similar to one of the bases of DNA.

Nucleotide of DNA: Made up of one of four nitrogen-containing bases (adenine, cytosine, guanine or thymine), a sugar and a phosphate molecule.

Oncogenic: Anything that may give rise to tumors, especially malignant ones.

Opportunistic disease: Disease caused by normally benign microorganisms or viruses that become pathogenic when the immune system is impaired.

p24 antigen: A protein fragment of HIV. The p24 antigen test measures this fragment. A positive test result suggests active HIV replication and may mean the individual has a chance of developing AIDS in the near future.

Parenteral: Not taken in through the digestive system.

Parasite: A plant or animal that lives, grows and feeds on another living organism.

Pathogen: Any disease-producing microorganism or substance.

Pathogenic: Giving rise to disease or causing symptoms.

Pathology: The science of the essential nature of diseases, especially of the structural and functional changes in tissues and organs caused by disease.

Perianal glands: Glands located around the anus.

Perinatal: Occurring in the period during or just after birth.

Phagocytes: Large white blood cells that contribute to the immune defense by ingesting microbes or other cells and foreign particles.

PID (pelvic inflammatory disease): Inflammation of the female pelvic organs; often the result of gonococcal or chlamydial infection.

Plasma: The fluid portion of the blood which contains all the chemical constituents of whole blood except the cells.

Plasma cells: Derived from B cells, they produce antibodies.

Platelets: Small oval discs in blood that are necessary for blood to clot.

PLWA: Persons Living With AIDS.

Polymerase chain reaction: Method to detect and amplify very small amounts of DNA in a sample.

Poppers: Slang term for the inhalant drug amyl nitrate.

Positive HIV test: A sample of blood that is reactive on an initial ELISA test, reactive on a second ELISA run of the same specimen and reactive on Western blot, if available.

Pneumocystis carinii pneumonia (PCP): A rare type of pneumonia primarily found in infants and now common in patients with AIDS.

Prenatal: During pregnancy.

Prevalence: The total number of cases of a disease existing at any time in a given area.

Primary immune response: Production of antibodies about 7 to 10 days after an infection.

Prophylactic treatment: Medical treatment of patients exposed to a disease before the appearance of disease symptoms.

Protease: Enzyme that cuts proteins into peptides.

Protense inhibitors: Compounds that inhibit the action of protease.

Proteins: Organic compounds made up of amino acids. Proteins are one of the major constituents of plant and animal cells.

Protocol: Standardization of procedures so that results of treatment or experiments can be compared.

Protozoa: A group of one-celled animals, some of which cause human disease including malaria, sleeping sickness and diarrhea.

Provirus: The genome of an animal virus integrated into the chromosome of the host cell, and thereby replicated in all of the host's daughter cells.

Pruritis: Itching.

Rate: A rate is a measure of some event, disease, or condition in relation to a unit of population, along with some specification of time.

Receptors: Special molecules located on the surface membranes of cells that attract other molecules to attach to them. (For example CD4, CD8, and CC-CKR-5)

Recombinant DNA techniques: Techniques that allow specific segments of DNA to be isolated and inserted into a bacterium or other host (e.g., yeast, mammalian cells) in a form that will allow the DNA segment to be replicated and expressed as the cellular host multiplies.

Rectum: The end part of the large intestine through which feces are excreted from the body.

Remission: The lessening of the severity of disease or the absence of symptoms over a period of time.

Retroviruses: Viruses that contain RNA and produce a DNA analog of their RNA using an enzyme known as reverse transcriptase.

Reverse transcriptase: An enzyme produced by retroviruses that allows them to produce a DNA analog of their RNA, which may then incorporate into the host cell.

Ritonavir: Novir, a protease inhibitor drug.

RNA (ribonucleic acid): Any of various nucleic acids that contain ribose and uracil as structural components and are associated with the control of cellular chemical activities.

RNA viruses: Contain RNA as their genetic material.

Salmonella: A bacterium that may cause diarrhea with cramps and sometimes fever.

Sarcoma: A form of cancer that occurs in connective tissue, muscle, bone and cartilage.

Saquinavir: Invirase, a protease inhibitor drug.

Secondary immune response: On repeat exposure to an antigen, there is an accelerated production of antibodies.

Sensitivity: The probability that a test will be positive when the infection is present.

Septicemia: A disease condition in which the infectious agent has spread throughout the lymphatic and blood systems causing a general body infection.

Seroconversion: The point at which an individual exposed to the AIDS virus becomes serologically positive.

Serologic test: Laboratory test made on serum.

Serum: The clear portion of any animal liquid separated from its more solid elements, especially the clear liquid which separates in the clotting of blood (blood serum).

Shigella: A bacterium that can cause dysentery.

Specificity: The probability that a test will be negative when the infection is not present.

Spirochete: A corkscrew-shaped bacterium; e.g., *Treponema pallidum.*

Spleen: A lymphoid organ in the abdominal cavity that is an important center for immune system activities.

Squamous: Scaly or plate-like; a type of cell.

Stavudine: Also known as Zerit; See d4T—inhibits HIV replication.

Sterilizing immunity: Immune response that completely prevents an infection.

STD (sexually transmitted disease): Any disease which is transmitted primarily through sexual practices.

Subclinical infections: Infections with minimal or no apparent symptoms.

Subunit vaccine: A vaccine that uses only one component of an infectious agent rather than the whole to stimulate an immune response.

Suppressor T cells: A subset of T cells that carry the T8 marker and turn off antibody production and other immune responses.

Surrogate marker: A substitute; a person or agent that replaces another, an alternate.

Surveillance: The process of accumulating information about the incidence and prevalence of disease in an area.

Susceptible: Inability to resist an infection or disease.

Symptomatology: The combined symptoms of a disease.

Syndrome: A set of symptoms which occur together.

Systemic: Affecting the body as a whole.

T cell growth factor (TCGF, also known as interleukin-2): A glycoprotein that is released by T lymphocytes on stimulation by antigens and which functions as a T cell growth factor by inducing proliferation of activated T cells.

T Helper cells (also called T4 cells): A subset of T cells that carry the T4 marker and are essential for turning on antibody production, activating cytotoxic T cells and initiating many other immune responses.

T lymphocytes or T cells: Lymphocytes that mature in the thymus and which mediate cellular immune reactions. T lymphocytes also release factors that induce proliferation of T lymphocytes and B lymphocytes.

T8 cells: A subset of T cells that may kill virus-infected cells and suppress immune function when the infection is over.

Thrush: A disease characterized by the formation of whitish spots in the mouth. It is caused by the fungus *Candida albicans* during times of immunosuppression.

Thymus: A primary lymphoid organ high in the chest where T lymphocytes proliferate and mature.

Titer: Level or amount.

Tolerance: A state of nonresponsiveness to a particular antigen or group of antigens.

Toxic reaction: A harmful side effect from a drug; it is dose dependent, i.e., becomes more frequent and severe as the drug dose is increased. All drugs have toxic effects if given in a sufficiently large dose.

Toxoplasmosis: An infection with the protozoan *Taxoplasma gondii,* frequently causing focal encephalitis (inflammation of the brain). It may also involve the heart, lungs, adrenal glands, pancreas and testes.

Transcription: The synthesis of messenger RNA on a DNA template; the resulting RNA sequence is complementary to the DNA sequence. This is the first step in gene expression.

Translation: The process by which the genetic code contained in a nucleotide sequence of messenger RNA directs the synthesis of a specific order of amino acids to produce a protein.

Treponema pallidum: The bacterial spirochete that causes syphilis.

Tropism: Involuntary turning, curving, or attraction to a source of stimulation.

Tumor: A swelling or enlargement; an abnormal mass that can be malignant or benign. It has no useful body function.

Urethra: The tube conveying urine from the bladder out of the body.

Urethritis: Inflammation of the urethra.

Uterus: The womb; a pear-shaped, muscular organ which holds the fetus during pregnancy.

V3 loop: Section of the gp120 protein on the surface of HIV; appears to be important in stimulating neutralizing antibodies.

Vaccine: A preparation of dead organisms, attenuated live organisms, live virulent organisms, or parts of microorganisms that is administered to artificially increase immunity to a particular disease.

Vagina: The canal which leads from the external female genitalia to the cervix.

Vector: The means by which a disease is carried from one human to another.

Venereal warts: Viral *Condylomata acuminata* on or near the anus or genitals.

Vesicle: A small blister on the skin.

Viremia: The presence of virus in the blood.

Virulence: The ability on the part of an infectious agent to induce, incite or produce pathogenic changes in the host.

Virus: Any of a large group of submicroscopic agents capable of infecting plants, animals and bacteria; characterized by a total dependence on living cells for reproduction and by a lack of independent metabolism.

Vulva: The external parts of the female genitalia including the labia majora, labia minora, mons pubis, clitoris, perineum and vestibulum vagina.

Western Blot: A blood test used to detect antibodies to a given antigen. Compared to the ELISA test, the Western Blot is more specific and more expensive. It can be used to confirm the results of the ELISA test.

X-ray: Radiant energy of extremely short wavelength used to diagnose and treat cancer.

Zalcitabine: Also known as HIVID; see ddC—inhibits HIV replication.

Zidovudine: Also known as Retrovir; see ZDV—inhibits HIV replication.